Hypertension Society of India

Manual of
Hypertension

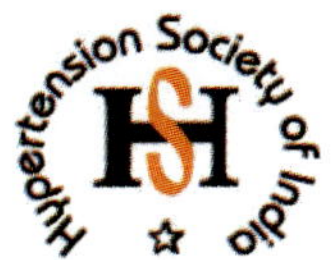

Hypertension Society of India

Manual of Hypertension

Second Edition

Editor-in-Chief

BA Muruganathan

MD FICP FRCP (Glasgow, London and Ireland) FACP (USA) FPCP (Philippines)

Emeritus Professor, The Tamil Nadu Dr MGR Medical University
Chairman, AG Hospital
Tirupur, Tamil Nadu, India

Editors

YP Munjal MD FRCP FACP FICP FIAMS

Senior Consultant
Department of Endocrinology
Artemis Hospital and Research
Institute
Gurugram, Haryana, India

M Maiya MD

Former Professor
Department of Medicine
Government Medical
Colleges
Bengaluru, Karnataka,
India

Gurpreet S Wander MD DM

Professor and Head
Department of Cardiology
Hero DMC Heart Institute
Dayanand Medical College and
Hospital
Ludhiana, Punjab, India

Assistant Editor

Bhivaji R Bansode MD FICP FCCP

Physician and Cardiologist
Department of Medicine and Cardiology
Dr BAM Hospital
Mumbai, Maharashtra, India

Foreword

Siddharth N Shah

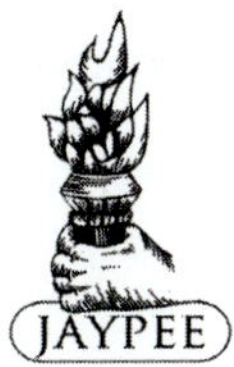

JAYPEE BROTHERS MEDICAL PUBLISHERS
The Health Sciences Publisher
New Delhi | London

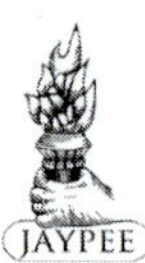

Jaypee Brothers Medical Publishers (P) Ltd

Headquarters

Jaypee Brothers Medical Publishers (P) Ltd
4838/24, Ansari Road, Daryaganj
New Delhi 110 002, India
Phone: +91-11-43574357
Fax: +91-11-43574314
Email: jaypee@jaypeebrothers.com

Overseas Offices

J.P. Medical Ltd
83 Victoria Street, London
SW1H 0HW (UK)
Phone: +44 20 3170 8910
Fax: +44 (0)20 3008 6180
Email: info@jpmedpub.com

Website: www.jaypeebrothers.com
Website: www.jaypeedigital.com

HSI Manual of Hypertension

First Edition: **2016**
Second Edition: **2020**

ISBN: 978-93-5270-708-9

Printed at: Sterling Graphics Pvt. Ltd. India.

Contributors

EDITOR-IN-CHIEF

BA Muruganathan MD FICP FRCP (Glasgow, London and Ireland) FACP (USA) FPCP (Philippines)
Emeritus Professor
The Tamil Nadu Dr MGR Medical University
Chairman, AG Hospital
Tirupur, Tamil Nadu, India

EDITORS

YP Munjal MD FRCP FACP FICP FIAMS
Senior Consultant
Department of Endocrinology
Artemis Hospital and Research
Institute
Gurugram, Haryana, India

M Maiya MD
Former Professor
Department of Medicine
Government Medical
Colleges
Bengaluru, Karnataka, India

Gurpreet S Wander MD DM
Professor and Head
Department of Cardiology
Hero DMC Heart Institute
Dayanand Medical College and
Hospital
Ludhiana, Punjab, India

ASSISTANT EDITOR

Bhivaji R Bansode MD FICP FCCP
Physician and Cardiologist
Department of Medicine and Cardiology, Dr BAM Hospital
Mumbai, Maharashtra, India

CONTRIBUTING AUTHORS

Akash Singh MBBS
Postgraduate Student
Department of General Medicine
SAMC and PGI
Indore, Madhya Pradesh, India

Alladi Mohan MD FAMS FRCP
(Edinburgh) FCCP (USA) FICP PG Dip
in Epidemiology (PHFI-IIPH)
Professor and Head, Department
of Medicine, Sri Venkateswara
Institute of Medical Sciences
Tirupati, Andhra Pradesh, India

Alpa Hemant Bharati MD
Chief Cardiac Imaging
Consultant
Holy Family Hospital
BJ Wadia Hospital for Children
Mumbai, Maharashtra, India

Amit A Saraf MD FRCP (London)
FACP (USA) FCPS
Consultant Physician
Department of Medicine
Jupiter Hospital
Mumbai, Maharashtra, India

AN Rai MD MRCP (UK) FRCP
(Glasgow) FICP FICC FICN
Former Professor and Head
Department of Medicine
Principal
Anugrah Narayan Magadh
Medical College and Hospital
Chairman
Abhay Institute of Medical
Sciences
Gaya, Bihar, India

Anandakumar Amutha MSc RD PGDDE PhD
Scientist
Department of Epidemiology
Dr Mohan's Diabetes Specialities
Centre and Madras Diabetes
Research Foundation
Chennai, Tamil Nadu, India

Ananthi Mathiyalagan MD
Medical Officer
Department of General Medicine
NLC IL General Hospital
Neyveli, Tamil Nadu, India

Anish K Gupta M Pharm
Research Associate
Department of Internal Medicine
Max Super Speciality Hospital
Ghaziabad, Uttar Pradesh, India

Anita Jaiswal Ektate MD
Additional Chief Health Director
Department of General Medicine
Dr Babasaheb Ambedkar
Memorial Hospital
Mumbai, Maharashtra, India

Anjan Lal Dutta MD DM
Senior Consultant and Head
Department of Cardiology
Peerless Hospital and
BK Roy Research Centre
Kolkata, West Bengal, India

Anusha Singh MBBS DNB FNIC
Senior Resident
Department of Clinical and
Preventive Cardiology
Medanta Heart Institute
Medanta – The Medicity
Gurugram, Haryana, India

Arathi N MD
Assistant Professor
Department of Medicine
Government Medical College
Alappuzha, Kerala, India

Ashish Mishra MBBS
Postgraduate Student
Department of General Medicine
SAMC and PGI
Indore, Madhya Pradesh, India

Ashraya Nayaka TE MS FLVPEI-FVRS
Consultant Vitreoretinal Surgeon
Retina and Uvea Services
The Eye Foundation
Coimbatore, Tamil Nadu, India

Ashutosh Chaturvedi MD
Consultant Physician and
Diabetologist
Department of Internal Medicine
Maxwell Hospital and
Jain Chest Care Centre
Jaipur, Rajasthan, India

Avathvadi Venkatesan Srinivasan MD DM PhD DSc (Hon) FRCP (London) FAAN FIAN
Emeritus Professor
The Tamil Nadu Dr MGR Medical
University
Former Head
Institute of Neurology
Madras Medical College
Chennai, Tamil Nadu, India

B Khandelwal MD
Associate Dean, Research and
Development
Professor and Head
Department of General Medicine
Sikkim Manipal Institute of
Medical Sciences
Sikkim Manipal University
Gangtok, Sikkim, India

BA Muruganathan MD FICP FRCP (Glasgow, London and Ireland) FACP (USA) FPCP (Philippines)
Emeritus Professor, The Tamil
Nadu Dr MGR Medical University
Chairman, AG Hospital
Tirupur, Tamil Nadu, India

Barjinderjit K Dhillon MSc PhD
Senior Biotechnologist
Department of Biochemistry
Dayanand Medical College and
Hospital
Ludhiana, Punjab, India

BC Kalmath MD DM DNB MNAMS FACC
Associate Honorary Cardiologist
Associate Professor
Department of Cardiology
Bombay Hospital Institute of
Medical Sciences
Consultant Cardiologist
Jupiter Hospital and Thane Clinic
Mumbai, Maharashtra, India

Bhanu Kesavamurthy DNB DM
Director
Department of Neurology and
Neurosurgery, Mehtas Hospitals
Former Head and Director
Institute of Neurology
Madras Medical College
Chennai, Tamil Nadu, India

Bhivaji R Bansode MD FICP FCCP
Physician and Cardiologist
Department of Medicine and
Cardiology, Dr BAM Hospital
Mumbai, Maharashtra, India

Chamma Gupta Integrated MSc (Medical Biotechnology)
Senior Research Fellow
Department of Biochemistry
Sikkim Manipal Institute of
Medical Sciences
Sikkim Manipal University
Gangtok, Sikkim, India

Chandni Radhakrishnan MD PhD PGDMLE FICP FRCP (Edinburgh)
Professor and Head
Department of Emergency
Medicine
Government Medical College
Kozhikode, Kerala, India

Chandrasekhar Valupadas MD
Professor and Head
Department of General
Medicine
Kakatiya Medical College/
Mahatma Gandhi Memorial
Hospital
Warangal, Telangana, India

Chirag Uppal
Junior Biotechnologist
Department of Biochemistry
Dayanand Medical College and
Hospital
Ludhiana, Punjab, India

Dev B Pahlajani MD FACC FSCAI
Chief
Department of Interventional
Cardiology
Breach Candy Hospital
Mumbai, Maharashtra, India

Dilip A Kirpalani MD DM
Consultant and Assistant
Professor
Department of Nephrology
Bombay Hospital Institute of
Medical Sciences
Mumbai, Maharashtra, India

Divya Saxena Dip Diab (USA UK)
MD FICP FIEC FICCM FIAMS
Director and Head
Department of Diabetes
Tulip Multispeciality Hospital
Sonipat, Haryana, India

Divyansh Mathur MBBS
NKP Salve Institute of
Medical Sciences
Nagpur, Maharashtra, India

Donald J DiPette MD FACP
FAHA
Health Sciences Distinguished
Professor
University of South Carolina
University of South Carolina
School of Medicine Columbia,
South Carolina, USA

E Dhandapani MD FCIP FIMSA
FACP
Professor and Head
Department of General
Medicine
Sree Balaji Medical College and
Hospital
Chennai, Tamil Nadu, India

Fraz A Mir MA MBBS FRCP
Consultant
Addenbrooke's Hospital
Cambridge University Hospitals
NHS Foundation Trust
Cambridge, England, United
Kingdom

Gayathri Ranie AP MBBS
Postgraduate Student
Department of Medicine
Maulana Azad Medical College
New Delhi, India

Ghan Shyam Pangtey MD
Senior Consultant Physician
Department of Medicine
LHMC and Associated
Hospital
New Delhi, India

Girish Mathur MD FRCP
(Glasgow) FICP FACP (USA) FIACM
Senior Consultant
Department of Internal
Medicine
Alka Diagnostic Centre
Kota, Rajasthan, India

Gurleen Kaur MD
Chief Research Fellow
Department of Nephrology
Emory University
Atlanta, Georgia, USA

Gurpreet S Wander MD DM
Professor and Head
Department of Cardiology
Hero DMC Heart Institute
Dayanand Medical College and
Hospital
Ludhiana, Punjab, India

Harish Jayakumar MD
MRCP (UK) DM
Junior Neurologist
Department of Neurology
JK Institute of Neurology
Madurai, Tamil Nadu, India

Jagdish C Mohan MD DM
Chairman
Institute of Heart and Vascular
Diseases, Jaipur Golden Hospital
Delhi, India

Jatinder Singh MS
Consultant Vitreoretinal Surgeon
Retina and Uvea Services
The Eye Foundation
Coimbatore, Tamil Nadu, India

Jinu Johnson MD
Senior Resident
Department of Medicine
Government Medical College
Kozhikode, Kerala, India

JPS Sawhney DM FESC FACC
Chairperson
Department of Cardiology
Dharma Vira Heart Center
Sir Ganga Ram Hospital
New Delhi, India

Jyotirmoy Pal MD
Professor, RG Kar Medical
College and Hospital
Kolkata, West Bengal, India

K Mugundhan MD DM
FRCP (Glasgow)
Professor and Head
Department of Neurology
Government Kilpauk Medical
College
Chennai, Tamil Nadu, India

Kalyani Sridharan MD DM
Senior Resident
Department of Endocrinology,
Diabetes and Metabolism
Christian Medical College
Vellore, Tamil Nadu, India

Kamlesh Patidar MBBS
Postgraduate Student
Department of General Medicine
SAMC and PGI
Indore, Madhya Pradesh, India

KK Pareek MD FACP (USA) FICP
FFIACM FGSI FRCP (Glasgow)
Director
SN Pareek Memorial Hospital
and Research Center
Kota, Rajasthan, India

Kushal Madan PhD FAHA
Cardiac Rehabilitation Consultant
Department of Cardiology
Sir Ganga Ram Hospital
New Delhi, India

M Chenniappan MD DM FRCP
Emeritus Professor
The Tamil Nadu, Dr MGR Medical
University, Chennai
Senior Consultant Cardiologist
Ramakrishna Medical Centre and
Apollo Speciality Hospitals
Trichy, Tamil Nadu, India

M Gowri Sankar MD
Assistant Professor
Department of General Medicine
Government Medical College
and ESI Hospital
Coimbatore, Tamil Nadu, India

Mangesh Tiwaskar MD FRCP
(London, Ireland and Glasgow) FACP
FICP FGSI FDI Diploma in Advanced
Diabetology, Denmark
Consultant Physician and
Diabetologist, Karuna Hospital
Shilpa Medical Research Centre
Mumbai, Maharashtra, India

Marc G Jaffe MD
Resolve to Save Lives, Vital
Strategies
New York, USA
Kaiser Permanente South San
Francisco Medical Center South
San Francisco, California, USA

Michaela M Watts RGN
Clinical Nurse Lead
Department of Ambulatory
Care/Acute Medicine
Addenbrooke's Hospital
Cambridge University Hospitals
NHS Foundation Trust
Cambridge, England, United
Kingdom

Milind Y Nadkar MD FICP FACP
Additional Dean (Academics)
Professor and Head
Department of Medicine
Seth GS Medical College and
KEM Hospital
Mumbai, Maharashtra, India

Minal Mohit MBBS MD FDE FPAE
FRCP FACP FICN FIACM FDI FRSSDI
Consultant, Department of
Endocrinology, Manipal Hospital
Jaipur, Rajasthan, India

Mrinal Kanti Das MD DM FICP
FICC FCSI
Consultant and Interventional
Cardiologist
CK Birla Group of Hospitals
Kolkata, West Bengal, India

Mritunjay Kumar Singh MD
Consultant, Department of
Nephrology, Abhay Institute of
Medical Sciences
Gaya, Bihar, India

Narinder P Singh MD MBA FAMS
FRCP (Edinburgh) FACP FISN FICP
Medical Advisor and Senior
Director
Department of Internal Medicine
Max Super Specialty Hospital
Ghaziabad, Uttar Pradesh, India

Navjot Bajwa
Professor and Head
Department of Biochemistry
Dayanand Medical College and
Hospital
Ludhiana, Punjab, India

Neeta Rajram Narang DNB CPS
(HIV) Fellowship in Critical Care
Consultant
Sai Charities
Karnal, Haryana, India

Nihal Thomas MBBS MD MNAMS
DNB (Endo) FRACP (Endo) FRCP
(Edinburgh) FRCP (Glasgow) FRCP
(London) PhD (Copenhagen)
Professor and Head
Unit-I, Department of
Endocrinology, Diabetes and
Metabolism
Christian Medical College
Vellore, Tamil Nadu, India

Nihar Mehta MD DNB (Medicine)
DNB (Cardiology)
Consultant Cardiologist
Department of Cardiology
Jaslok Hospital and Research
Centre
Mumbai, Maharashtra, India

Niharika Aggarwal MD
Associate Professor
Department of Medicine
LHMC and Associated Hospital
New Delhi, India

NN Anand MD FRCP
Professor
Department of General Medicine
Sree Balaji Medical College and
Hospital
Chennai, Tamil Nadu, India

Norm RC Campbell MD
O'Brien Institute for Public
Health
Libin Cardiovascular Institute of
Alberta
University of Calgary
Calgary, Alberta, USA

NR Rau MD FICP
Former Professor and Head
Department of Medicine
Kasturba Medical College
Manipal, Karnataka, India

Packiamary Jerome MD
Deputy General Superintendent
Department of General
Medicine
NLC IL General Hospital
Neyveli, Tamil Nadu, India

Pedro Ordunez MD PhD
Pan American Health
Organization (PAHO)/WHO
Regional Advisor
Additional Specialties-NCDs
Washington DC, USA

Pradip Sarkar MD
Senior Registrar
Department of Cardiology
Vivekananda Institute of Medical
Sciences
Kolkata, West Bengal, India

Prashant Wankhade DNB
Senior Resident
Department of Cardiology
Dharma Vira Heart Center
Sir Ganga Ram Hospital
New Delhi, India

Pritam Gupta MD ICP FACP FRCP
FIAMS
Senior Consultant and Head
Department of Medicine
Sunder Lal Jain Hospital
Senior Consultant
Department of Medicine
Fortis Hospital
New Delhi, India

Purbasha Biswas MBBS
Junior Resident
Department of General Medicine
RG Kar Medical College and
Hospital
Kolkata, West Bengal, India

R Rajasekar MD FICP FACP (USA)
FRCP (Glasgow) FRCP (Ireland)
Senior Consultant Physician and
Diabetologist, Department of
Heart and Diabetes, Heart and
Diabetes Therapy Centre
Kumbakonam, Tamil Nadu, India

Rajeev Gupta MD PhD FACC FESC
Chairman
Department of Preventive
Cardiology and Internal Medicine
Eternal Heart Care Centre and
Research Institute
Academic and Research
Development Unit, Rajasthan
University of Health Sciences
Jaipur, Rajasthan, India

Rajendra Pradeepa MSc PhD
Senior Scientist and Head
Department of Research
Operations, Dr Mohan's Diabetes
Specialities Centre and Madras
Diabetes Research Foundation
Chennai, Tamil Nadu, India

Rajib Ratna Chaudhary MD
Professor and Head
Department of Medicine
Rohilkhand Medical College and
Hospital
Bareilly, Uttar Pradesh, India

Ramamurthy D MD DNB
Chairman, Retina and Uvea
Services, The Eye Foundation
Coimbatore, Tamil Nadu, India

Raman Puri MD
Senior Consultant
Department of Cardiology
Indraprastha Apollo Hospital
New Delhi, India

Ramanpreet Kaur
Associate Biotechnologist
Department of Biochemistry
Dayanand Medical College and
Hospital
Ludhiana, Punjab, India

Ravi R Kasliwal MD DM FIMSA
MNAMS FASE
Adjunct Professor
Department of Cardiology
Chairman, Division of Clinical
and Preventive Cardiology
Medanta – The Medicity
Gurugram, Haryana, India

Renu Moti Pandita
Biotechnologist
Department of Biochemistry
Dayanand Medical College and
Hospital
Ludhiana, Punjab, India

Riddhi Das Gupta MD DM
Associate Professor
Department of Endocrinology,
Diabetes and Metabolism
Christian Medical College
Vellore, Tamil Nadu, India

RK Jha MD
Professor and MS
Department of General Medicine
SAMC and PGI
Indore, Madhya Pradesh, India

Rohit Kapoor MD FCSI FISC FICP
FACC FRCP (Edinburgh) FACP FDI
FRSSDI
Medical Director
Care Well Heart and Super
Speciality Hospital
Amritsar, Punjab, India

Sadanand R Shetty MD DM
FACC FESC
Interventional Cardiologist
Department of Cardiology
KJ Somaiya Superspeciality
Hospital
Mumbai, Maharashtra, India

Saket Goyal MD DM FACC FSCAI
Chief Interventional Cardiologist
Kota Heart Institute
Kota, Rajasthan, India

Sankar D Navaneethan MD
MS MPH FASN
Associate Professor
Department of Medicine
Director of Clinical Research,
Section of Nephrology
Associate Director
Institute of Clinical and
Translational Research
Baylor College of Medicine
Houston, Texas, USA

Santanu Guha MD DM FCSI FICC FESC FACC
Professor and Head
Department of Cardiology
Medical College
Kolkata, West Bengal, India

Sasidharan PK MD FICP
Former Professor and Head
Department of Medicine
Government Medical College
Kozhikode, Kerala, India

Saurabh Dhariya DNB
Senior Resident
Department of Cardiology
Jaslok Hospital and Research
Centre
Mumbai, Maharashtra, India

SC Manchanda DM
Professor and
Senior Consultant
Department of Cardiology
Dharma Vira Heart Center
Sir Ganga Ram Hospital
New Delhi, India

Sekhar Chakraborty MD MRCP
FRCP (Ireland) FRCP (Glasgow) FACP
(USA) FICP (India)
Consultant Physician and
Diabetologist
Medical Director
Kins Care Research Foundation
and Kins Hospital
Siliguri, West Bengal, India

Shivashankara MD
Professor
Department of Medicine
Kasturba Medical College
Manipal, Karnataka, India

Shraddha More MD
Assistant Professor
Department of Medicine
Seth GS Medical College and
KEM Hospital
Mumbai, Maharashtra, India

Shreya Gupta MBBS
Junior Resident
Department of Medicine
Mahatma Gandhi Medical College
Jaipur, Rajasthan, India

Siddharth N Shah MD
Professor, Consultant Physician
and Diabetologist
Saifee Hospital, SL Raheja
Hospital, Bhatia Hospital
Global Hospital
Mumbai, Maharashtra, India

Sidhartha Mani MD DM
Consultant Interventional
Cardiologist, Department of
Cardiology, Medical College
Kolkata, West Bengal, India

Simran Sawhney MBBS
Postgraduate Student
Department of Medicine
St. Stephen's Hospital
New Delhi, India

Sonia Y Angell MD MPH DTM&H
Chief of the Noncommunicable
Disease Unit and Senior Advisor
for Global Noncommunicable
Diseases, Division of Global
Health Protection in the Center
for Global Health
Centers for Disease Control and
Prevention (CDC)
New York, USA

Soumik Chaudhuri MD DM
Consultant Cardiologist
Peerless Hospital and BK Roy
Research Centre
Kolkata, West Bengal, India

Soumitra Kumar MD DM FCSI
FICP FACC FESC FSCAI FICC FIAE
Professor and Head
Department of Cardiology
Vivekananda Institute of
Medical Sciences
Kolkata, West Bengal, India

SS Iyengar MD DM FRCP
(Edinburgh)
Consultant, Department of
Cardiology, Manipal Hospital
Bengaluru, Karnataka, India

Sujatha Sudarsan MASLP
Audiologist and Speech
Therapist, Vidya Sagar
Chennai, Tamil Nadu, India

Sunita Aggarwal MD FICP
FIMSA FIACM
Professor
Department of Medicine
Maulana Azad Medical College
New Delhi, India

Suresh T Yavagal MD DM
Former Professor and Head
Department of Cardiology
Sri Jayadeva Institute of
Cardiovascular Sciences and
Research
Bengaluru, Karnataka, India

T Ravikumar MD
Professor and Head
Department of General Medicine
Government Medical College
and ESI Hospital
Coimbatore, Tamil Nadu, India

Tanuka Mandal MBBS
Postgraduate Trainee
Department of Medicine
RG Kar Medical College
Kolkata, West Bengal, India

Tarun Kumar Paria MBBS
Postgraduate Trainee
Department of Medicine
RG Kar Medical College
Kolkata, West Bengal, India

Tiny Nair MD DM FACC FRCP
Head, Department of Cardiology
PRS Hospital
Thiruvananthapuram,
Kerala, India

Uddalak Chakraborty MBBS
Postgraduate Trainee
Department of Medicine
RG Kar Medical College
Kolkata, West Bengal, India

V Mohan MD FRCP (London,
Edinburgh, Glasgow, Ireland) PhD
DSc DSc (Hon Causa) FNASc FASc
FNA FAC FACE FTWAs MACP
Chairman and
Chief Diabetologist
Madras Diabetes Research
Foundation and Dr Mohan's
Diabetes Specialities Centre
Chennai, Tamil Nadu, India

V Padma MD FRCP (Glasgow)
Professor,
Department of Medicine
Sree Balaji Medical College
Chennai, Tamil Nadu, India

Vasili Pradeep MBBS
Postgraduate Junior Resident
Department of Medicine
Sri Venkateswara Institute of
Medical Sciences
Tirupati, Andhra Pradesh, India

Viplav Deogaonkar DNB
Resident, Department of
Medicine, Jupiter Hospital
Mumbai, Maharashtra, India

Virendra KR Chauhan DNB
Resident, Department of
General Medicine, Dr Babasaheb
Ambedkar Memorial Hospital
Mumbai, Maharashtra, India

VT Shah MD FCSI FSCAI (USA)
Interventional Cardiologist
Surana Sethia Hospitals
Raheja Fortis Hospital
Breach Candy Hospital
Prince Aly Khan Hospital
Wockhardt Hospital
Saifee Hospital, Jupiter Hospital
Mumbai, Maharashtra, India

YP Munjal MD FRCP FACP FICP
FIAMS
Senior Consultant
Department of Endocrinology
Artemis Hospital and Research
Institute
Gurugram, Haryana, India

Foreword

Dr BA Muruganathan, a dynamic leader in the field of medicine has compiled the *Second Edition* of *"Manual of Hypertension"* keeping in mind the basic and also the modern approach to the management of hypertension and its complications.

Everyone concerned with the care of hypertensive patient is aware of the immense burden of misery that can be inflicted by long-term complication of the disease, e.g. stroke, cardiovascular complications, renal failure, blindness and many more. The person afflicted with hypertension also has comorbid conditions such as diabetes, dyslipidemia, renal failure and obesity. This monogram makes an attempt to understand all this in a comprehensive manner.

The newer version of monogram has been divided into 14 sections covering the entire field of hypertension. The content of each chapter has been carefully selected to be useful to the primary care physicians, postgraduates and medical community at large. The approach taken by the authors in the monograph is both clinical and scientific. Each chapter deals with the pathophysiological background which leads on to a practically orientated review of clinical features and management. Dr BA Muruganathan has added Genetics in Hypertension and Interventional Interventions in Hypertension covering recent aspects. Guidelines and meta-analysis, economical and organizational issues have been covered. Miscellaneous section covers all the important aspects faced by physicians in day-to-day practice for efficient management of hypertension.

There are three principal approaches to learning medicine and keeping abreast of latest developments—*lectures, journals, and textbooks*. Each approach has its place in the educational armamentarium and each leads itself to imparting certain facts, ideas and best concepts. Dr BA Muruganathan has taken a combination of this approach by revising the *Manual of Hypertension*.

The book also deals with chapters on therapy beyond medicine and comorbidities in hypertension along with nonpharmacological and pharmacological therapy of hypertension. I recommend this book for internists, intensivists, nephrologists, cardiologists, medical practitioners and postgraduate students as a referral book which covers all aspects of hypertension.

Dr BA Muruganathan has done an excellent job in compiling this monogram and I trust it will be useful to broad array of physicians who wish to remain active in the field of hypertension and will have most updated information with references at their fingertips.

Siddharth N Shah MD
Executive Chairman
Hypertension Society of India

Preface to the Second Edition

Books are Tools, Doctors are Craftsmen

Osler

I take this opportunity to thank all the members of Hypertension Society of India, particularly Dr Siddharth N Shah (Executive Chairman), for having faith in me and encouraging me to bring out the *Second Edition* of the *"Manual of Hypertension"*. I also thank Editors Dr YP Munjal, Dr M Maiya, Dr Gurpreet S Wander and Dr Bhivaji R Bansode (General Secretary) for their contributions.

Hypertension is a hemodynamic malignancy and an important risk factor for many diseases such as cardiovascular diseases and kidney diseases; however, control of hypertension rates remains dismal. In India, there are nearly 200 million patients with high blood pressure. Indeed proper control of hypertension could prevent more than 30% of the estimated 1.5 million deaths attributed to hypertension in India. We would like to emphasize the importance of home blood pressure monitoring, combination therapy and simplified protocols for effective management of hypertension.

Every physician needs to know the updates and changes so that they can confidently approach the patient with hypertension. In this edition, we have included the following topics which would be useful for the physicians to improve their knowledge and skill in the field of hypertension:

- Epidemiology: Recent statistics and the importance of social determinants of hypertension, treatment and control in India
- Pathophysiology: Overview of various pathogenic mechanisms in essential hypertension and the renin-angiotensin-aldosterone system
- Molecular basis of hypertension: Role of cell membrane (red blood cells and platelets) in essential hypertension, role of cytokines and inflammation in hypertension and multiple roles of eicosanoids in blood pressure regulation
- Guidelines: Every guideline stresses the significance of correct methodology of blood pressure and importance of out-of-office blood pressure monitoring
- Evaluation of hypertension: Clinical examination is the forgotten art and the author has described clearly step-by-step as to how to arrive at the diagnosis and how ECG is helpful in decision making. A separate chapter is given on Imaging Studies in Hypertension.

Target organ damage—evaluation and clinical importance:

- Special conditions and situations: Hypertension in pregnancy, metabolic syndrome and hypertension, perioperative hypertension and blood pressure variability and target organ damage

- Secondary hypertension: Management of hypertension in chronic kidney disease, primary hyperaldosteronism other mineralocorticoid hypertension, pheochromocytoma, genomic insights and coarctation of the aorta
- Therapeutic aspects—pharmacologic and nonpharmacologic interventions: Nonpharmacological intervention in hypertension and their impact, role of yoga in hypertension, combination therapy in hypertension (fixed or variable) as per the recommendation of various guidelines, simplified protocols.

Genetics and Hypertension:

- Interventions in hypertension: Rhoa/rho–kinase signaling pathway in vascular smooth muscle contraction biochemistry, physiology and pharmacology
- Guideline and meta-analysis: Comparison of various guidelines in hypertension–which is best for India? Meta-analysis in hypertension: What we have learnt? and what we have to learn
- Miscellaneous: How to organize and run a hypertension clinic, dilemmas in hypertension management, hypertensive crisis, lipid and hypertension.

Every contributor has given considerable amount of newer information in this book and we are sure this would be useful for the practitioners in their clinical practice to handle various problems of hypertension. I hope this book would serve as an important reference guide for postgraduate students, junior doctors, clinicians and hypertension specialists.

Our special thanks to Shri Jitender P Vij (Group Chairman), Mr MS Mani (Group President), Dr Richa Saxena (Chief Editor), Dr Ekta (Senior Development Editor) and the team of Jaypee Brothers Medical Publishers (P) Ltd, New Delhi. My personal thanks to my personal assistant Mr K Venkatesan for his contribution to bring out this book.

Editor-in-Chief
BA Muruganathan
MD FICP FRCP (Glasgow, London and Ireland) FACP (USA) FPCP (Philippines)
Emeritus Professor, The Tamil Nadu Dr MGR Medical University
Chairman, AG Hospital, Tirupur, Tamil Nadu, India

Preface to the First Edition

I take this opportunity to thank all the members of Hypertension Society of India, particularly Dr Siddharth N Shah (Executive Chairman) and Dr Bhivaji R Bansode (General Secretary) for having faith in me and encouraging me to bring out this Manual of Hypertension for the first time. Hypertension is a very common problem faced by physicians in day-to-day practice. The hypertension epidemic is sweeping across the country like a deluge probably because of television watching, sedentary life, rapid urbanization, and wrong food culture of the people. In India, there are nearly 100 million patients with high blood pressure. The asymptomatic nature of the initial stage of the disease leads to a high number of undiagnosed cases. Among the Indian population, only about half (55%) of the hypertensive patients were aware of their disease state, only a third (36%) of these known hypertensive subjects were under treatment, and furthermore, only a quarter (28.2%) of this treatment group patients had their blood pressure under control. According to the Chennai Urban Rural Epidemiology Study (CURES), 15.4% of the total hypertensive group only had blood pressure under control.

Various clinical trials, international guidelines, Association of Physicians of India guidelines, recommendations, new updates, and new information regarding hypertension are pouring everyday into the literature. With all the available information, we have better understanding about the diagnosis, management of hypertension, and its complications. Every practitioner needs to know the updates and changes so that they can confidently approach the patient with hypertension.

In this book, I have tried to cover:

- Epidemiology, socioeconomic factors and hypertension awareness, treatment, and control in India
- Pathophysiology in hypertension: gut microbiota—diet, genetic basis of blood pressure, blood pressure variability, the renin-angiotensin-aldosterone system
- Secondary hypertension: various forms of hypertension
- Examinations and investigations: ambulatory blood pressure monitoring and central aortic pressure and pulse wave velocity. My trust is on home blood pressure monitoring. I want every physician to popularize home blood pressure monitoring just like home blood sugar monitoring
- Pharmacology therapy: new directions in management of hypertension, combination therapy for hypertension in Asia Pacific region, parental antihypertensive drugs, emerging anti-hypertensive drugs, and pharmacogenomics in management of hypertension
- Therapy beyond medicine: interventions in hypertension management
- Comorbidities in hypertension: hypertension and diabetes, hypertension and coronary artery disease

- Special situation in hypertension: hypertension in pregnancy, resistant hypertension, blood pressure response to acute physical and mental stress, hypertension in elderly, and Indian scenario of hypertension in young
- Guidelines/trials in hypertension: overview of the guidelines and interventional trials—the lesson learned and compliance to treatment in hypertension.

I welcome the hypertension specialists to do hypertension registry and more research suitable for our Indian context. We have given considerable amount of newer information in this book and I am sure this would be useful for the practitioners in their clinical practice to handle various problems of hypertension. I hope this book would serve as an important reference guide for postgraduate students, junior doctors, clinicians, and hypertension specialists.

My special thanks to Shri Jitender P Vij (Group Chairman), Dr Neeraj Choudhary (Senior Acquisition Editor-Corporate), Ms Neha Bhatia (Development Editor), Ms Shweta Tiwari (Editorial Coordinator), and his team of Jaypee Brothers Medical Publishers (P) Ltd, New Delhi. My personal thanks to my personal assistant Mr K Venkatesan for his contribution to bring out this book.

Editor-in-Chief
BA Muruganathan
MD FICP FRCP (Glasgow, London and Ireland) FACP (USA) FPCP (Philippines)

Emeritus Professor, The Tamil Nadu Dr MGR Medical University
Chairman, AG Hospital, Tirupur, Tamil Nadu, India

Email: a.muruganathan@gmail.com
Website: www.muruganathan.com

Contents

Section 10: Therapeutic Aspects: Pharmacologic and Nonpharmacologic Interventions

PLATE 1

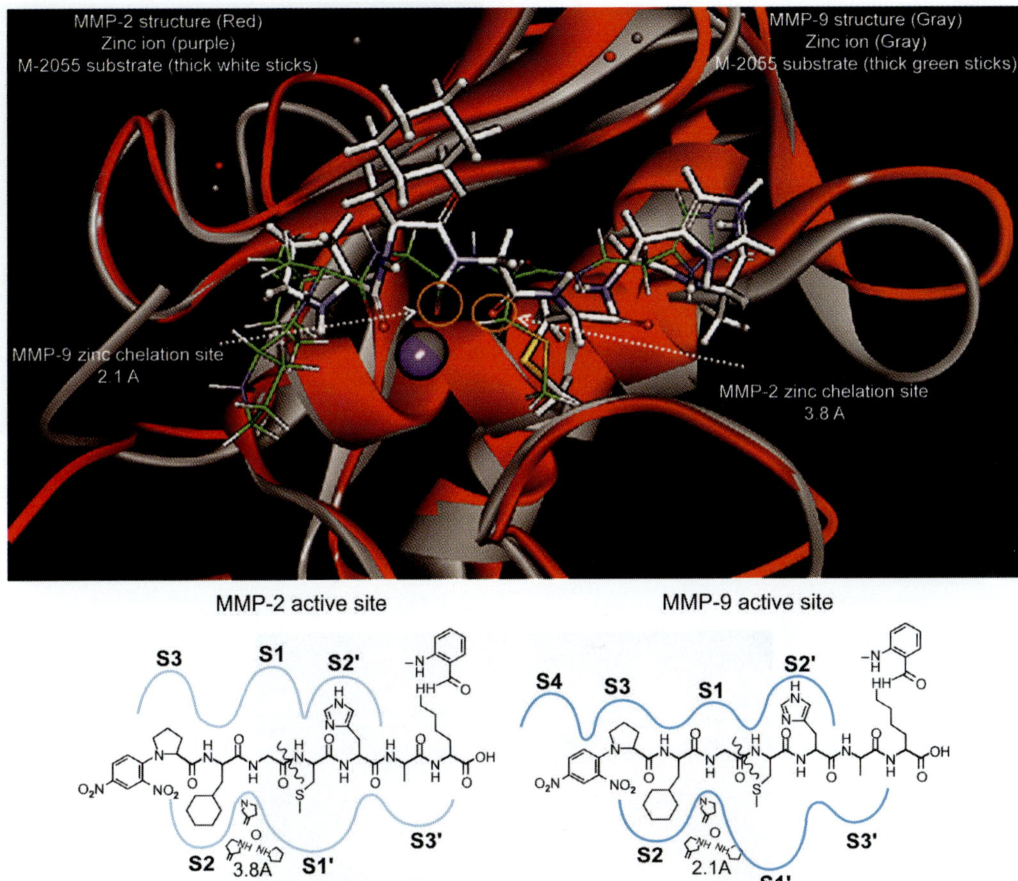

Fig. 1: Docked complexes of 1 substrate and the catalytic domain of human MMP-2 (PDB code 1QIB) and MMP-9 (PDB code 1GKC). The MMP-substrate docked complexes are merged with zinc as the same point of view. MMP-2 structure is shown in red, zinc as purple and 1 substrate (white sticks) docked within MMP-2 active site. MMP-9 is shown in gray, zinc as green and 1 substrate (thin green sticks) docked within its active site. (Bottom) Schematic representation of 1: active site binding interaction in human MMP-2 and MMP-9. MMP-2 and MMP-9 enzyme binding pockets are shown in red and green, respectively. Substrate chemical structure and its scissile bond are shown in black. The zinc ion is indicated in blue. *(Chapter 7)*

PLATE 2

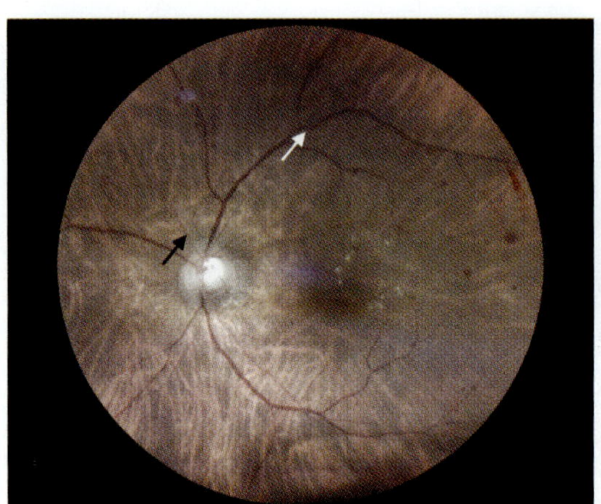

Fig. 1: Mild hypertensive retinopathy: generalized arteriolar attenuation (black arrow) with arteriovenous nicking (white arrow). *(Chapter 19)*

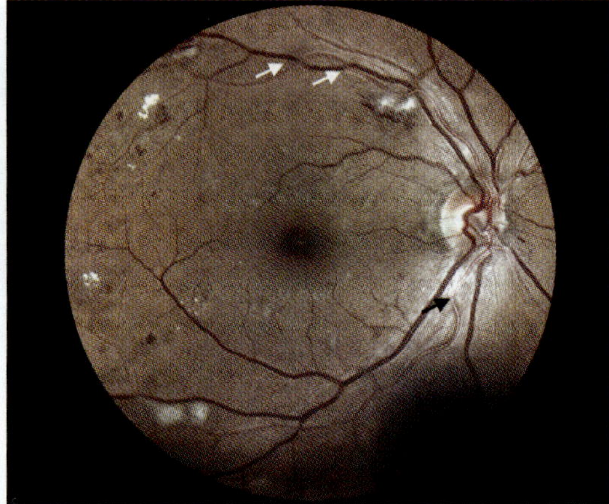

Fig. 2: Moderate hypertensive retinopathy: Arteriolar narrowing (white arrow) with arteriovenous nicking (black arrow). *(Chapter 19)*

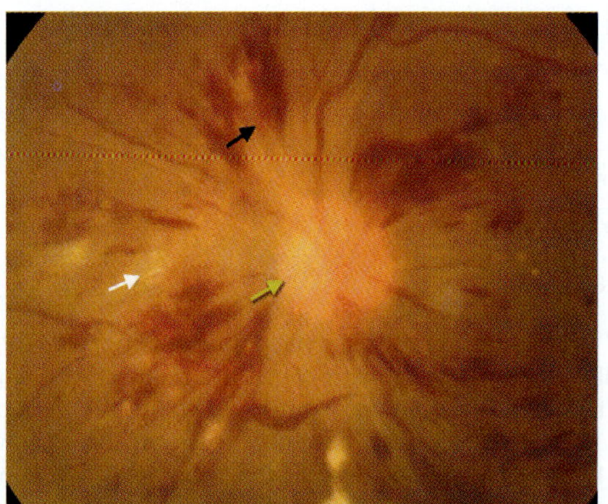

Fig. 3: Malignant retinopathy: Disc edema (yellow arrow) with cotton wool spots (white arrow) and flame shaped hemorrhage (black arrow). *(Chapter 19)*

SECTION 1

History and Epidemiology

Historical Aspects of Hypertension

M Gowri Sankar

"Study the past if you would define the future"

—Confucius (Chinese Philosopher)

INTRODUCTION

History is a blend of huge sacrifices, sufferings, trials and failures. Also, it tells the tale for the younger generations to explore the science and its roots. Hypertension is an ancient disease, which has come a long way and has challenged even the most famous physicians for centuries. Moreover, there is a long list of physicians and scientific researchers who have spent their whole life in advancing the Blood pressure (BP) measuring techniques. As of now, the management of hypertension has become the greatest medical success story of the 20th century. Nowadays the BP instruments are available everywhere in the world but this instrument was actually invented in late 19th century and moreover it has taken around 200 years to get an accurate measurement of BP.

HISTORICAL PERSPECTIVES ON HYPERTENSION[1]

The historical aspects of hypertension go back a long way from Sushruta, who was the foundation figure of Indian medicine and considered as the "Father of Indian Medicine". In fact, he authored a book called "Sushruta Samhita". This was one of the ancient treatises and the source of knowledge about medicine in ancient India. He has explained about medicine in general and also showcased his extraordinary surgical skills and methods. He further developed many special and practical techniques in dissections and also studied the anatomy of human body including the structure of the heart and its role in circulation. Moreover, he mentioned and described about hritshoola (meaning heart pain), circulation of body fluids (blood-rakta dhatu, lymph-rasa dhatu), madhumeha (diabetes), obesity (medoroga) and hypertension as sira-kunchan and rakta-poornata and its symptom as vatarakta. It is remarkable that Sushruta had described these conditions before Hippocrates.

HARD PULSE DISEASE[1,2]

Today, what we now call as hypertension could have been identified only by the quality of the pulse in the ancient period. The traditional Tamil system of Siddha medicine is also called as Siddha Vaidya which was originated in between 10,000 BCE and 4,000 BCE. In fact, the Siddhars who had attained eight supernatural powers had laid the foundation for this traditional medicine. Subsequently, a wrist pulse reading called Naadi method was developed by the Siddha practitioners of the past which became the window for cardiovascular system.

Furthermore, the early history related to hypertension was portrayed in "Classics in Arterial Hypertension" by Dr Ruskin. He described that in the Yellow Emperor's Classic of Internal Medicine dated as early as 2600 BC that "The usage of too much salt in food will harden the pulse". Then he had indicated the relationship between hypertension and congestive heart failure by stating, "When the pulse is abundant but tense and hard like a cord there are dropsical swellings".

Subsequently, the Roman patrician "Cornelius Celsus" was much concerned with the pulse in his days and he has explained about the increased heart rate and tense pulse with exercise, emotion, and even physician's arrival; which we call as "White-Coat" effect today. Later, the ancient Egyptian physicians in the Ebers Papyrus (1550 BCE) had described the relationship between the palpated pulse and the development of heart and brain disease.

In addition, Hippocrates had revealed that the sudden death occurred more commonly in fat people than in the lean.

In ancient times the "hard pulse disease" was treated by doing venesection, bleeding by leeches and acupuncture methods. These methods were advocated by the Yellow Emperor of China, Celsus, Galen and Hippocrates.

However, the modern history of hypertension began with the work of William Harvey (1578–1657), who described the fundamentals of circulation that blood circulates in the body in one direction. In 1628, he penned and published a book titled "On the Motion of the Heart and Blood in Animals", which explained the above stated fundamental through his scientific and experimental methods which became a gigantic milestone in medicine.

■ EVOLUTION OF BLOOD PRESSURE MEASUREMENTS[3,4]

Stephen Hales (1677–1761) was an English clergyman, who gave the first description of measurement of the force of the blood (BP) in modern era. In 1733, he carried out catheterization of a live horse by inserting fine tubes into carotid artery and measured the BP by assessing the rise in column of blood in a glass tube of 9 feet 6 inches in height initially and which gradually fell. The animals died when the blood in the tube fell to approximately 2 feet bound into an artery. Thus, he demonstrated that amount of pressure generated by heart could be measured through the displacement of blood.

Jean Louis Poiseuille (1797–1869) was a French physiologist, dedicated himself to research in the early 17th century for the invention of U-tube mercury manometer. He called the mercury instrument as hydrodynamometer. By using this, he greatly reduced the height of the column needed for measuring the BP. Thereupon, he measured the pressures in arteries of horses and dogs by inserting a hollow tube into artery and attached to a manometer on another end. He then identified the BP by measuring the amount of mercury displacement. Moreover, he was the first who introduced the "mm Hg" units. In 1846, he explained the physics of blood flow in small vessels by his Poiseuille's equation which states that the blood flow (Q) is related to the viscosity (n) of the blood, the difference in BP in two ends (P), length (L) and diameter (r) of the vessel.

Karl von-Vierordt (1818–1884) was a German physiologist. He discovered the instrument sphygmograph in 1854. Furthermore, he was the first to develop the noninvasive technique to estimate BP by using his newly invented sphygmograph. His instrument made up of weights and levers through which he postulated that to measure the BP accurately, it is necessary to stop the pulse. Therefore, he did by applying weight (counter pressure) on an artery and obliterated the radial arterial pulse. Furthermore, he published his investigations titled as "A Treatise on the Arterial Pulse".

Etienne Jules Marey (1830–1904) was a French physiologist. He upgraded the von-Vierordt cumbersome sphygmograph to a wearable sphygmograph to measure BP. He refined the technique to measure the BP by enclosing the arm in a water filled glass chamber and increasing the water pressure until no circulation occurred.

Karl Samuel Ritter von Basch (1837–1905) was an Austrian physiologist, who created the new device called sphygmomanometer and further introduced the aneroid manometer for the measurement of BP. Subsequently, he inaugurated the first noninvasive clinical measurements of BP. Here, he placed a rubber bag around a manometer bulb and inflated it with water. As the water pressure increased, the mercury in the manometer was displaced enabling the measurement of the pressure. The bag was placed over the distal pulse and inflated until the pulse stopped being felt; the pressure at that point was noted as the systolic pressure.

Pierre Potain (1825–1901) was a French cardiologist, who contributed enormously to the field of cardiology. He was also credited for his significant modifications done in sphygmomanometer by using air rather than water in the compressed bag.

Scipione Riva-Rocci (1863–1937), an Italian physician, is best known for his invention and initiation of an easy-to-use upper arm cuff-based mercury sphygmomanometer for measuring of brachial BP in the year 1896. He developed the apparatus by using copper pipes, bicycle tubes and mercury barometer and also he designed an inflatable rubber cuff to encircle the arm. He further did a palpation of radial artery and measured the peak systolic BP by observing the cuff pressure at which there was disappearance of the radial pulse on palpation. During 1896 and 1897, he published a series of four articles regarding his new method of BP measurement. Dr Harvey Cushing, an American neurosurgeon, was an early adopter of Riva-Rocci mercury sphygmomanometer. He successfully used his apparatus to monitor his patients during anesthesia and surgery in Johns Hopkins Hospital.

Heinrich von Recklinghausen (1867–1942) was a German physician. Subsequent to the work of Dr Riva-Rocci, he increased the width of the cuff from 5 to 14 cm to obtain better accuracy on the adult arm and he was recognized for the same.

Nikolai Korotkov (1874–1920), a Russian surgeon, further proceeded to improvize the Riva-Rocci–von Recklinghausen inflatable cuff by attaching with a stethoscope. In the year 1905, he invented the auscultatory technique for BP measurement. By applying cuff on upper arm and slowly deflating, he described both the appearance and disappearance of sounds over brachial artery, measured as systolic and diastolic BP. Since this method was found to be easy and accurate, it was considered as a "gold standard" for BP measurement.

■ GROWTH OF KNOWLEDGE IN HYPERTENSION[3,4]

18th and 19th Century

Thomas Young (1773-1829) was a British polymath and physician. He was considered as a man of universal interest, who had contributed in various fields of medicine. In physiology, he made a significant contribution to hemodynamics by measuring the percent fall in BP in dogs from aorta to mesenteric arteries. Subsequently, he derived a formula for the wave speed of the pulse and stated that the quality of the arterial pulsation depended on the force of the heart. He further presented his experimental research as the "Functions of the Heart and Arteries" in the Croonian lecture during 1808.

Richard Bright (1789-1858) was an English physician and early pioneer in the research of kidney disease. He was considered as the Father of Nephrology. He brought his various observations such as albuminuria, hardening of the pulse and dropsy with inflammation, or hardening of the kidneys together named as Bright's disease. In 1836, he further observed and disclosed that hypertrophy of left ventricle could be noticed in advanced kidney disease.

Additionally, **Samuel Wilks** described about the hardening of arteries in Bright's disease in 1853. During the year 1872, **Gull and Sutton** proposed that Bright's disease occurred due to the generalized hyaline fibrinoid deposits in arterioles and capillaries which in turn led to left ventricular hypertrophy and contracted kidneys.

Afterward, the first report to disclose that the elevated BP could even occur without primary renal disease was by **Frederick Akbar Mahomed** (1849-1884) an Indian origin-Irish physician who had an extensive contribution in the field of medicine. Moreover, he modified the device sphygmograph while he was a medical student. By using his quantitative sphygmogram, he measured the arterial tension in Troy ounces and published his modified instrument in 1872. Subsequently, he was the first to report the elevation of BP in a patient without the evidence of kidney disease, which he assessed by measuring proteins in urine. Furthermore, he was one of the first who correlated the pathological effects of elevated BP and its postmortem changes such as cardiac hypertrophy, thickening and fibrosis of the arterial wall, aneurysm formation, and arteriocapillary fibrosis. He then described it as "High pressure diathesis". Additionally, he explained the characteristics of pulse in patients with high BP and in persons with arteriosclerosis consequent on aging. He further stated that hypertension could occur without arteriosclerosis and vice versa.

William Gowers (1845-1915) was a British neurologist. The greatest clinical neurologist of all times, he was an early adopter of the ophthalmoscope for systemic diseases. He gave the clear description about the constricted retinal vessels in relation to hypertension in 1876.

Sir Thomas Clifford Allbutt (1836-1925) was an English physician who was well-known for his invention of the clinical thermometer. He also disclosed the concept of hypertensive disease as a generalized circulatory disease in 1896 and he called the disease as "hyperpiesia" a term continued to use in England until 1930. In his textbook "Diseases of the Arteries, Including Angina Pectoris" (1915), he exhibited the role of excessive salt, stress and anxiety in elevated BP.

Early 20th Century[3,4]

The term called Essential Hypertension (Essentielle Hypertonie) was coined by German physician **Eberhard Frank** in

1911. He was the first to describe that the hypertension occurs without any other obvious cause.

Theodore Caldwell Janeway (1872–1917), an American physician, was the first fulltime professor of medicine in United States. He collaborated with Sir Harvey Cushing, who was one of the supporters of sphygmomanometer. Both together researched on hypertension and mainly focused on determining the accurate apparatus and a range of normal values for BP. In 1913, they described the varied course of hypertension and called the disorder as "Hypertensive Cardiovascular Disease".

Even in early 20th century, physicians could not recognize the need for aggressive management of hypertension which has been proved by the following quotes.

Paul Dudley White, one of the leading cardiologists and a prominent advocate of preventive medicine who suggested that "Hypertension may be an important compensatory mechanism that should not be tampered with, even where it is certain that we could control it..."

In 1928, another term called malignant hypertension was coined by Mayo Clinic physicians, who had described that a high BP with organ damage causes retinopathy and impaired renal function and which possibly leads to death within a year from stroke, heart failure or kidney failure.

However, the impact of untreated hypertension came to public attention only after the ill effect on American President Franklin D Roosevelt. The President's physician gave a clean chit of health with documented BP of 200/100 mm Hg. While at Yalta conference in February 1945, Winston Churchill's personal physician had recorded President Roosevelt's BP of 260/150 mm Hg and further noted his signs and symptoms of cardiac failure. Unfortunately, on April 12, 1945, the President Roosevelt had severe occipital headache followed by loss of consciousness with BP of 300/190 mm Hg and ultimately had a fatal hemorrhagic stroke. Finally, his death brought hypertension as a deadly malady to the limelight.[5]

Three years later from Roosevelt's death, the President Truman had signed the National Heart Act which created the new path for several cardiac studies including Framingham Heart Study. Prior to Framingham studies, in fact nothing was known about the epidemiology of hypertension or atherosclerotic cardiovascular disease. Consequently, this study introduced the term "risk factor" which clearly showed that hypertension and hyperlipidemia are risk factors associated with cardiovascular morbidities and leading to premature deaths.

Low-salt Diets

Thereafter, the nonpharmacological methods to treat hypertension came to light through Ambard and Beaujard, who were the medical students from France. They discovered the direct relationship between sodium chloride retention and hypertension in 1904. Later in 1922, Allen and Sherrill confirmed their investigations. But the use of low-salt diet in the treatment of hypertensive patients became popular only during 1940.

Surgical Sympathectomy

The first surgical sympathectomy for hypertension was done by the surgeon Fritz Bruening in 1923, based on the hypothesis that reduction of sympathetic outflow will lead to reduction in BP. The experience with surgical sympathectomy had paved the way for the development of drugs causing chemical sympathectomy by the ganglion-blocking agents like tetraethylammonium chloride, hexamethonium pentaquine, bretylium and others.

■ THE BEGINNING OF DRUG ERA[3,4]

Before the Second World War, there were no effective antihypertensive drugs. Only sodium thiocyanate was the first chemical used by Treupel and Edinger in 1900. But the drug was poorly tolerated due to its toxicity. After the Second World War, the drugs like hexamethonium, hydralazine and reserpine were put on trial. Subsequently, the first effective drug treatment of malignant hypertension was introduced in the year 1947 with the use of the antimalarial agent, pentaquine. In fact, James A Shannon, the head of the Squibb Institute for Medical Research, had found that large oral doses of pentaquine led to a marked reduction of BP with severe orthostatic hypotension. Also, pentaquine use demonstrated the reversal of pathological manifestations of malignant hypertension by effectively reducing BP. But, its role was overtaken by the development of newer antihypertensive drugs with less side effects.

A major breakthrough in the treatment of hypertension had occurred only after the introduction of chlorothiazide in 1958, which was achieved by the scientist Novello and Sprague of Merck & Co. In 1964, a landmark randomized controlled trial by the Veterans Administration study compared hydrochlorothiazide plus reserpine and hydralazine versus placebo. First time in the history of drug treatment, the antihypertensive drugs were found more beneficial in lowering moderate-to-severe hypertension with remarkable decrease in the incidence of mortality and cardiovascular events. In order to honor their remarkable work, the Lasker Special Public Health Award was presented to the team in 1975.

At the same time, the Scottish physician Dr James Black had shown interest in finding the effects of adrenaline on the heart developed beta-blockers. His drug named propranolol was initially used for angina then turned out to lower BP. Eventually, his ground breaking work was honored with Lasker Award in 1976 and with most prestigious Nobel Prize in Physiology or Medicine in 1988. In addition, Prichard and Gillam were the first to demonstrate the effectiveness of the beta-blocking drugs in hypertension.

Dr Albrecht Fleckenstein, a German pharmacologist, had contributed himself to the discovery of calcium channel blockers. He described that his drug verapamil as a calcium antagonist in 1964. He further coined the term calcium antagonist and its inhibitory actions of excitation-contraction coupling. He subsequently identified nifedipine, a dihydropyridine to lower BP.

Development of Angiotensin-converting Enzyme Inhibitors[6]

At the beginning, the development of angiotensin-converting enzyme (ACE) inhibitors was the serendipitous discovery of ACE in plasma by an American Biochemist Leonard T Skeggs in 1956. Later in 1965, Brazilian scientist Sergio Henrique Ferreira had reported that a Bradykinin-Potentiating factor is present in the venom of Bothrops Jararaca, a South American pit viper, a world's deadliest snake. In 1967, Kevin KF Ng and John Vane (Nobel Prize winner) showed plasma ACE is too slow to account for the conversion of angiotensin I to angiotensin II in vivo. Subsequently, his investigation had showed that rapid conversion occurs during its passage through the pulmonary circulation. In 1968, studies carried out by John Vane, had proved that peptides from the Brazilian viper's venom inhibited the activity of ACE. Then Vane suggested ACE as a target for research at The Squibb Institute. Furthermore, the American chemist Dr David Cushman, Dr Miguel Ondetti and colleagues at the same institute had advanced their studies on peptide analogs to observe the structure of ACE and created the first ACE inhibitor captopril in 1975, which was approved by the United States Food and Drug Administration in 1981 and entered into the antihypertensive armamentarium.

World Hypertension League

The World Hypertension League, an umbrella to organizations of 85 National Hypertension Societies and Leagues, was launched in 2005 to create a global awareness campaign. It has dedicated May 17th of each year as the World Hypertension Day.

■ CONCLUSION

Diagnose the disease, detect its root cause, Discern its cure and then act aptly.

- (Tamil saint Thiruvalluvar)

"Hypertension" is an ancient disease with a long journey. Now it is the most prevalent chronic noncommunicable disease in the world. Hypertension has been challenging physicians for centuries and with an exhaustive list of scientific researches and efforts of physicians who have advanced the BP measuring techniques by investing their whole life. Measuring BP is essential and needs no excuse.

■ REFERENCES

1. Bansal A. (2012). India's contribution to medical science. [online] Available from: Indiamedicalscience.blogspot.com [Last accessed January 2019].
2. Harold JG. Harold on Hypertension/historical perspectives on hypertension, Cardiology magazine (2017). Available from: www.acc.org
3. Freis ED. Historical development of antihypertensive treatment. In: Laragh JH, Brenner BM (Eds). Hypertension: Pathophysiology, Diagnosis, and Management, 2nd edition. New York: Raven Press Ltd; 1995. Pp. 2741-51.
4. Wikipedia. [online] Available from: www.wikipedia.com [Last accessed January 2019].
5. Saklayen MG, Deshpande NV. Timeline of history of hypertension treatment. Front Cardiovasc Med. 2016;3:3.
6. Bryan J. From snake venom to ACE inhibitor—The discovery and rise of captopril. Pharm J. 2009.

Hypertension Epidemiology in 21st Century India: High Prevalence and Low Control Paradigm

Rajeev Gupta

■ INTRODUCTION

Hypertension is a major public health problem in India. Recent nationwide studies have reported a high prevalence of hypertension.[1-3] Mathematical extrapolations show that using current definitions (systolic BP ≥140 mm Hg and/or diastolic BP ≥90 mm Hg or individuals on treatment), there are more than 200 million patients with hypertension in the country.[3] Reports from the World Health Organization (WHO),[4] Global Burden of Diseases (GBDs) Study,[5] and UK-based Noncommunicable Disease Risk Factor Collaboration (NCD-RisC)[6] have highlighted that hypertension is the most important cause of mortality and morbidity in India. This is also an important risk factor target that is amenable to control. Indeed, proper control of hypertension could prevent more than 30% of the estimated 1.5 million deaths attributed to hypertension in India.[7] Although recent studies and reports have assessed the burden of hypertension in India, none has comprehensively studied unique features of hypertension in the country that include regional differences, socioeconomic differences, younger age of onset, and low treatment and control rates. In this review, we highlight some of these issues.

■ REVIEWS OF EPIDEMIOLOGICAL STUDIES

Reviews of hypertension in epidemiological studies in India have reported significant and increasing burden of hypertension.[1,2] This increase has been reported from urban as well as rural populations. In mid-1950s, epidemiological studies from urban populations in India used older WHO criteria for diagnosis of hypertension (known hypertension or BP ≥160 mm Hg systolic and/or ≥95 mm Hg diastolic) and reported it in 1.2–4.0% adults.[8] Subsequent studies using similar criteria have reported that prevalence in urban populations has increased from 3.0–4.5% in 1960s to 11.0–15.5% in mid-1990s.[8] Although rural populations have lower prevalence, there has been an increase in hypertension in them also from >1% in 1960s to 5–7% in 1990s.[8]

Systolic BP of ≥140 mm Hg and/or diastolic BP of ≥90 mm Hg is the currently accepted threshold for diagnosis of hypertension. Many epidemiological studies of hypertension prevalence that have defined it by the standard criteria have been performed. These studies are mostly regional and show increasing trend in hypertension prevalence from mid-1990s to the present in urban as well as rural populations.[9] There are only a few multicentric studies in India that have determined prevalence of hypertension using similar tools. All these studies have reported that hypertension is more in urban populations versus rural populations.[3,8] A recent review reported that in 21st century, hypertension has increased more rapidly in rural populations as compared to the urban populations and there is an urban-rural convergence in its prevalence.[2] These studies also show that one in four adults in India have hypertension, which is similar to other developing countries.[5] Limitations of these studies include representation of small geographical region and wide variability in methodology. Other limitations include variability in age-groups studied (>20 years, 20–75 years, 35–64 years, 35–70 years, etc.), different types of BP instruments (mercury, aneroid, or electronic), number of readings (1 vs. 3), days of measurement (usually single but more than a day in some), and method of averaging (all three, last two readings, or the lowest reading).[3] Systematic reviews of these local and regional hypertension epidemiological studies in India have reported that hypertension is present in 25–30% urban and 10–20% rural adults.

■ NATIONAL FAMILY HEALTH SURVEY-4

The Fourth National Family Health Survey (NFHS-4) has obtained multiple adult socio-economic, demographic, and lifestyle factors using a nationally representative sample.[10] This survey also determined prevalence of hypertension among young and middle-aged men and women in India using a representative national sampling.[11] A uniform sampling method was adopted in all districts of the country. Details have been reported.[11,12]

Hypertension prevalence in various states of India among men and women is shown in Figure 1. The sample sizes were population proportionate and data shows that there are significant differences in prevalence of hypertension in different states of the country. Of the 33 states that are represented in these data, hypertension prevalence of >15% was observed in 8 (24.2%). The NFHS-4 has reported that the overall country-level prevalence of hypertension among the younger age individuals (men 15–49 years, women 15–54 years) was 13.6% in men, 8.8% in women, and 11.3% overall (Fig. 1). In this study, the prevalence of hypertension was highest in Northern and Northeastern states that include Punjab, Himachal Pradesh, Assam and Northeastern states while the lowest prevalence is observed in central Indian states extending from Rajasthan in the West to Bihar in the East. The NFHS-4 data also shows that prevalence of hypertension is significantly greater in urban as compared to rural locations—men 15.1% versus 12.6%, women 9.6% versus 8.5% (p <0.01).[3] However, the urban-rural difference is not large. This urban-rural convergence in hypertension in India is a new phenomenon.[2] Rapidly changing social and economic structures of rural India could be implicated.[13]

A major shortcoming of the overall NFHS program (NFHS-1 to NFHS-4 studies) has been exclusion of older age adults.[12] It is well-known that hypertension prevalence increases with age, and if this high-risk group is excluded, the prevalence of hypertension would be lower as compared to previous studies. On the other hand, the Prospective Studies Collaboration (Oxford) has reported that intervention and control of hypertension at a younger age is associated with greater benefit in terms of vascular protection and reduction of cardiovascular (CV) mortality and morbidity.[14] The NCD-RisC Collaboration has reported that highest rates of hypertension in the young men and women (<30 years age) are from South Asia and therefore, these data are important.[6] High burden of hypertension in

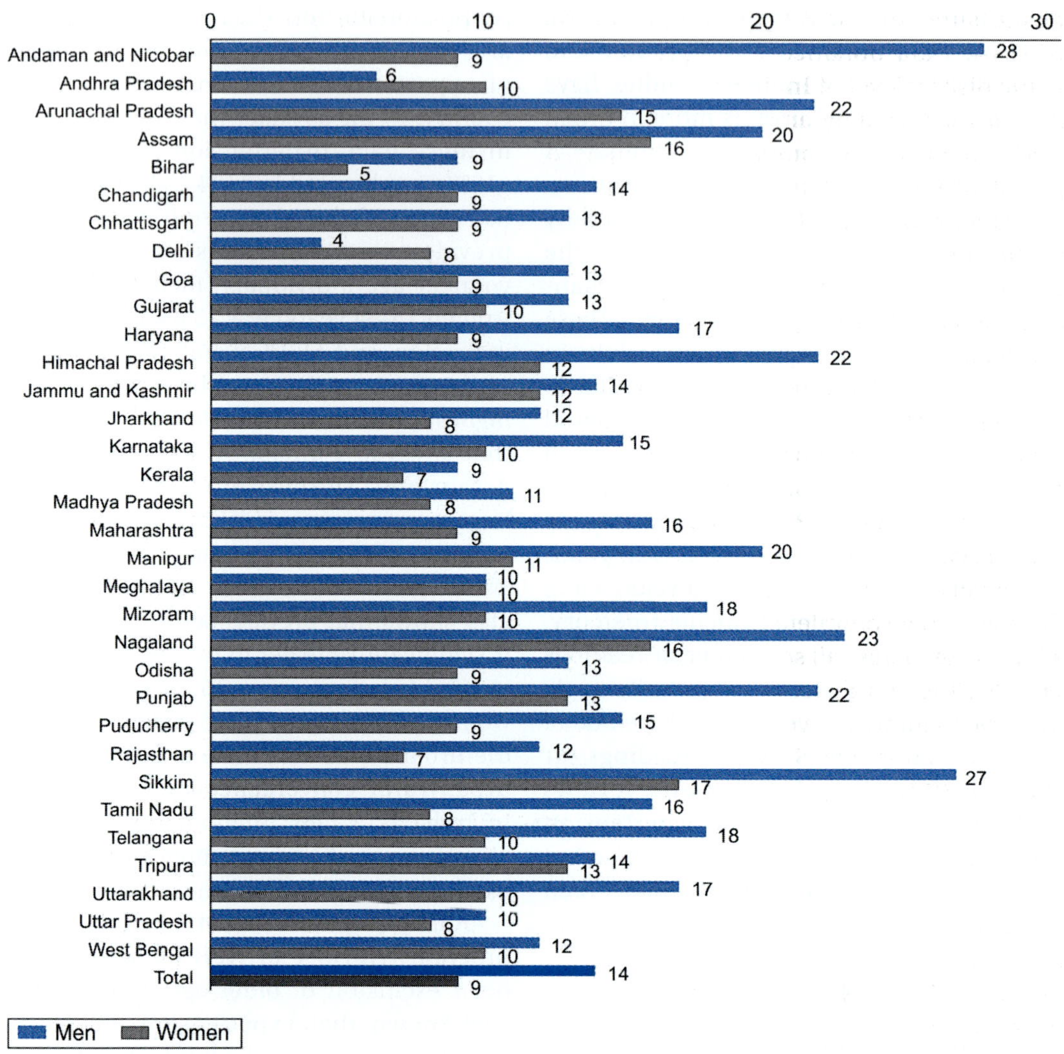

Fig. 1: Hypertension prevalence (%) in young and middle-aged men (15–54 years) and women (15–49 years) in different states of India in the National Family Health Survey-4 (Manhattan plot).

the young also conveys an important message to healthcare providers and policy-makers for prevention efforts.

■ DISTRICT LEVEL HOUSEHOLD SURVEY-4 AND ANNUAL HEALTH SURVEY

A more robust survey employing district level health data has been performed by the Government of India to estimate important CV risk factors (overweight, obesity, hypertension and diabetes) in all states of the country.[15] In this program, a standardized measurement of BP, similar to NFHS-4, and data on hypertension prevalence were obtained. Geldsetzer et al. pooled data from the District Level Household Survey-4 (DLHS-4) and Annual Health Survey (AHS).[16] These large surveys were undertaken between the years 2012–2014 and methodology of measurement of BP was similar to the NFHS-4. Data obtained are representative at the district level of India and jointly cover 29 states. In this study, among 1,320,555 adults (46.9% men, 53.1% women), the unadjusted prevalence of hypertension was 25.3% [95% confidence intervals (CIs) 25.0–25.6%] with greater prevalence in men (27.4%, CI 27.0–27.7%) as compared to women (23.6%, CI 23.3–23.8%) (p <0.001).[16] Age-standardized prevalence was also significantly greater in men (24.5%, CI 24.2–24.9%) as compared to women (20.0%, CI 19.7–20.3%). Hypertension prevalence in different states is shown in Figure 2. The prevalence in different states ranged from a low of 13.5% among women in Chhattisgarh to a high of 43.5% among men in Daman and Diu. This study concluded that there was a high prevalence of hypertension in all the states across all socioeconomic groups in India. The prevalence of hypertension was high even among the young age individuals. This is similar to NFHS-4 and other regional studies in India.

Regional variation of hypertension as reported in the abovementioned Indian studies is similar to reports from many countries and in large continents such as North America and Europe. Within country variations in hypertension, prevalence has been reported from large countries such as USA,[17] UK,[18] China,[19] Russia,[20] Brazil,[21] Indonesia,[22] Pakistan,[23] Bangladesh,[24] etc. The European Society of Cardiology has reported large intercountry differences in hypertension within Europe.[25] Most of the studies reported a greater prevalence of hypertension in rural populations in developed countries and vice versa for developing countries.[26] Greater prevalence of hypertension has also been reported in counties and countries with lower human and social development in most developed countries.[4-6,26,27] In contrast to these countries, a unique feature of hypertension in India is lower prevalence in rural populations (reported in both NFHS-4 and DLHS-4). Prevalence of hypertension in India is also lower in states with lower human development index (Fig. 3).

■ HYPERTENSION DETERMINANTS

There are multiple determinants of hypertension that range from macrolevel socioeconomic determinants and individual risk factors to genetic factors and their interactions.[28] There are no large prospective studies that have identified determinants of hypertension in Indian populations. Almost all the studies that have evaluated determinants of hypertension are cross-sectional in nature. Multiple determinants have been identified including macrolevel and microlevel factors.[29-34] Some of these factors as shown in Table 1.

Social Factors

Apart from the well-known social determinants of health,[30] macrolevel factors also include political and cultural determinants of health.[35,36] The WHO has identified 10 social determinants as important—(1) the social gradient, (2) stress, (3) early life, (4) social exclusion, (5) work, (6) unemployment, (7) social support, (8) addiction, (9) food, and (10) transport.[30] The strongest predictor for hypertension and other chronic diseases is position on the social gradient measured by income, education, place of residence, or occupation. Traditionally, in India, hypertension and other noncommunicable diseases are considered diseases of the affluent.[33] Some regional studies in the last 2 decades have reported that prevalence of hypertension is now greater in men and women with low educational status.[37-39] On the other hand, DLHS-4/AHS study reported that, at the national level, better socioeconomic status is associated with greater hypertension prevalence.[16] The

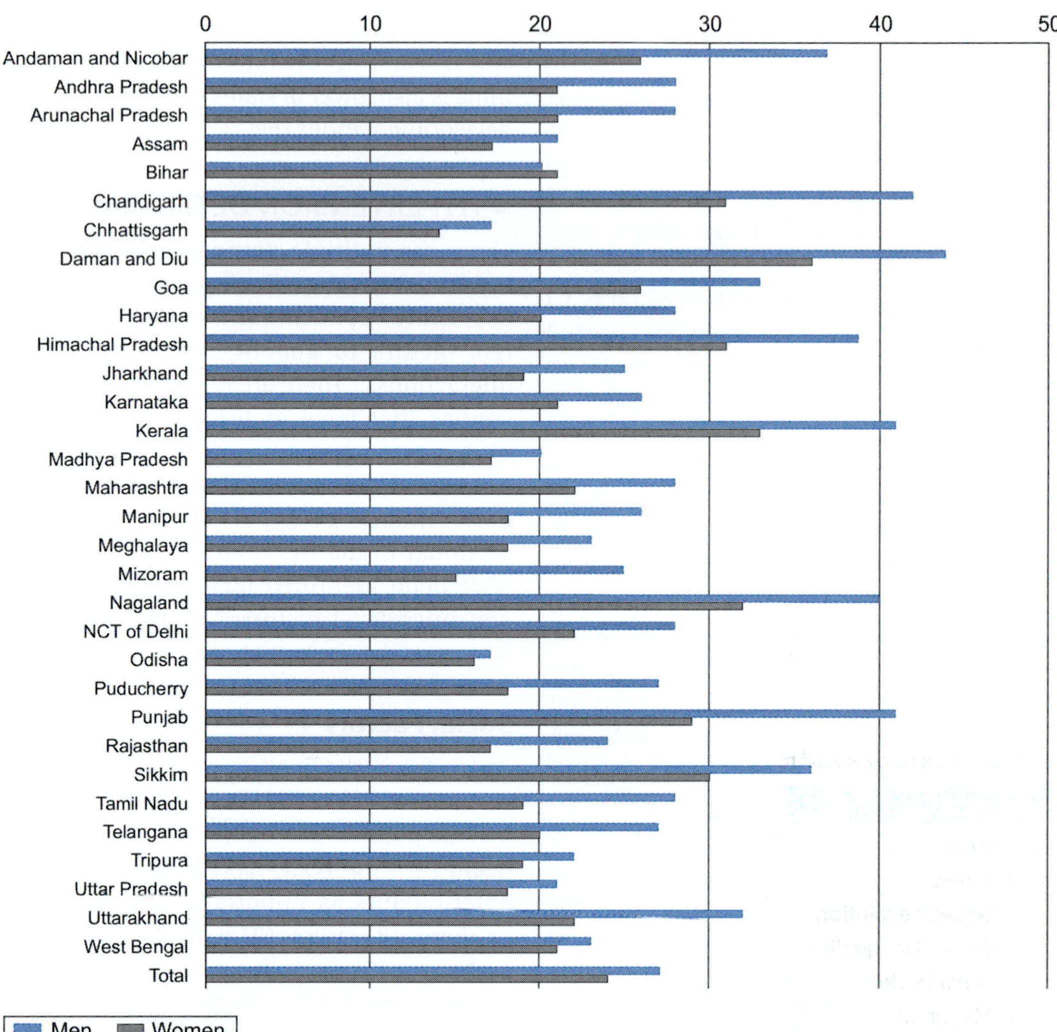

Fig. 2: Age-adjusted hypertension prevalence (%) in men and women in different states of India in the District Level Household Survey-4 and Annual Health Survey.

difference between the richest versus the poorest household was small (Δrural 4.15%, Δurban 3.47%) and this suggests convergence of urban-rural and a poor-rich difference in hypertension prevalence in India.

Healthcare delivery systems are important for noncommunicable disease management.[4] In India, very little focus has been placed on social determinants of health and, unlike Western countries, there is no focus on political and cultural factors.[40] At a macrolevel, we determined association of healthcare availability and healthcare quality with hypertension prevalence in various states of India.[3] No correlation was observed showing that healthcare delivery system in India is still focused on communicable, maternal and childhood issues. There is a need for changing the system to focus more on chronic diseases. In absence of focus on these macrolevel factors (Table 1), hypertension control in India shall always remain suboptimal and poor. Recently

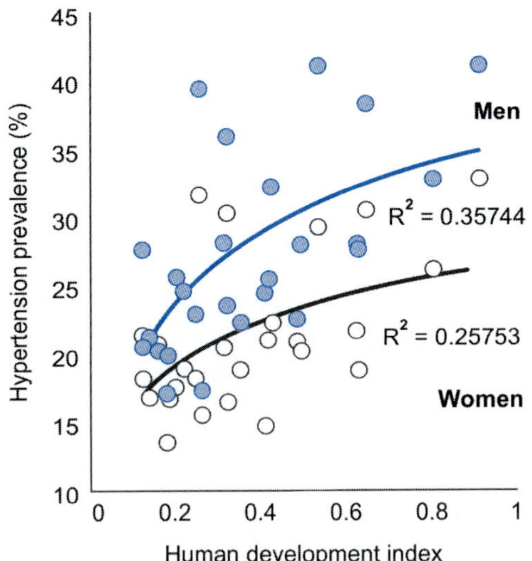

Fig. 3: Association of state level human development index with hypertension prevalence in men and women in India (logarithmic correlation R², men = 0.36, women = 0.26).

launched national universal healthcare programs are important in this regard.[41]

Biological Factors

Multiple individual level factors are important as hypertension risk factors. These include unhealthy lifestyles including sedentary habits, unhealthy diet (high calorie, high unrefined carbohydrate, high fat, high salt and high alcohol intake), combined with low fruits and vegetables intake, stress, overweight, obesity, abdominal obesity and insulin resistance. Complex interplay of these factors is involved in pathogenesis of hypertension.[28] All these factors are widely prevalent in India.[4]

Age is the strongest determinant of hypertension worldwide. All the studies have reported that hypertension prevalence increases with age in India.[8,9] However,

TABLE 1: Macrolevel and microlevel social and clinical determinants of hypertension.

Macrolevel and social determinants of health	Individual and clinical factors

• Macrolevel social factors:
  ○ Human and social development
  ○ Societal evolution
  ○ Societal inequality
  ○ Urbanization
  ○ Migration
  ○ Area-based measures
• Macroeconomic factors:
  ○ Measures of income
  ○ Gini coefficient
  ○ Education
  ○ Food availability
  ○ Transport
• Political determinants
• Cultural determinants
• Healthcare service delivery:
  ○ Universal health coverage
  ○ High quality primary care
  ○ Availability of medicines
  ○ Medicine costs
	• Individual-level socioeconomic factors:
	  ○ Lifetime social class
	  ○ Education
	  ○ Income
	  ○ Occupation
	  ○ Employment status
	  ○ Exclusion
	  ○ Stress
	  ○ Addiction
	• Anthropometric factors:
	  ○ Age
	  ○ Gender
	  ○ Body mass index
	  ○ Waist circumference, waist-hip ratio
	• Adherence to healthy lifestyles:
	  ○ Smoking/tobacco use
	  ○ Healthy/unhealthy diet
	  ○ Alcohol abuse
	• Primary prevention (risk factor management)
	• Secondary prevention (disease management)

the Global Burden of Hypertension Study by NCD-RisC[6] and DLHS-4/AHS[16] studies have highlighted an important difference. It was reported that, as compared to various global populations, at age-group 20–39 years, the mean BP levels and the prevalence of hypertension were the highest in South-Asian populations (Fig. 4).[6,16] Reasons for greater hypertension among the young in India may be due to multiple factors including adverse socioeconomic circumstances.

Other factors that are unique in South-Asian Indians include high prevalence of sedentary lifestyles, overweight and obesity especially abdominal adiposity, and diabetes as hypertension risk factors and comorbidities. The Prospective Urban Rural Epidemiology (PURE) study evaluated physical activity in multiple regions of the world using validated physical activity questionnaires.[42] Physical activity levels (leisure time, work related, or household activity) were the lowest in low-income countries including India. Prevalence of hypertension was also high in Indian participants in this study.[26] In a large study, mobile phone-app measured physical activity was also found to be low in Indian population.[43]

Obesity and abdominal obesity are important and rapidly increasing problems in India.[44,45] Multiple studies have reported significant association of obesity and abdominal obesity with hypertension in India.[1,9] Studies from India have also reported a linear association of systolic as well as diastolic BP with body mass index.[46,47] Babu et al. performed a meta-analysis of multiple observational studies (n = 18) in India and reported that the pooled odds ratio of obesity with hypertension was 3.82 (95%

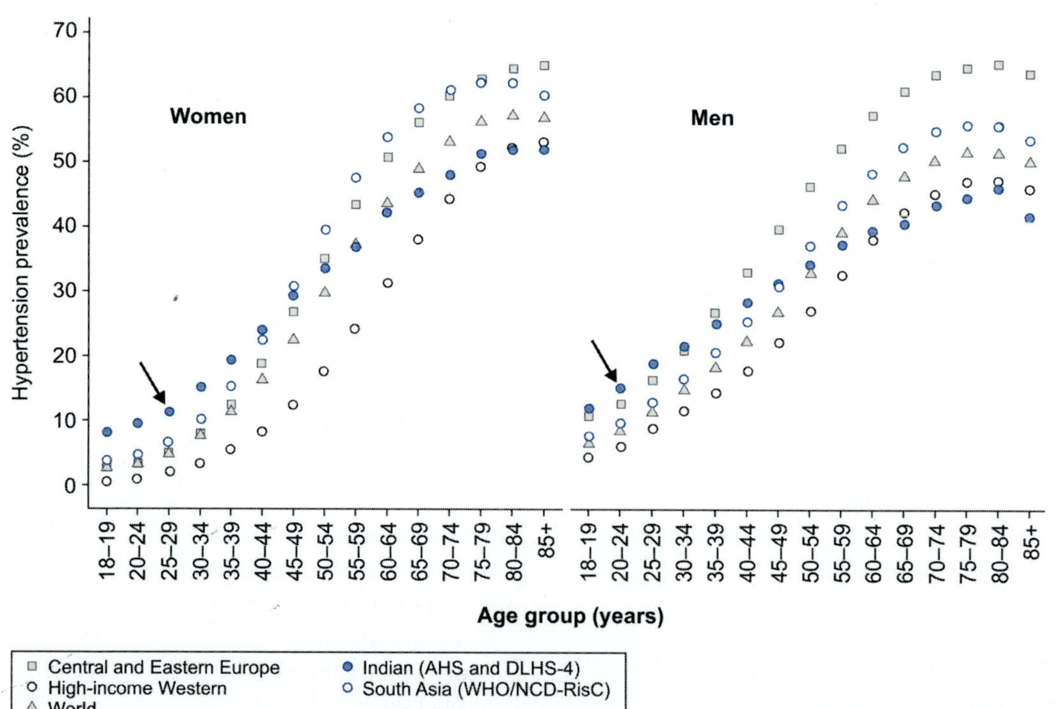

Fig. 4: Greater hypertension prevalence at younger age groups in India (dark circles, marked by arrows) as compared to other countries in South Asia, Eastern and Central Europe, high-income Western countries.

CI 3.39–4.25).[48] Obesity was also reported a stronger risk factor for hypertension as compared to abdominal obesity.[49] Similar associations have been reported in various international studies and NCD-RisC reports.[50]

High prevalence of diabetes is a unique Indian phenotype.[51] Population-based studies in India have reported diabetes in 30–40% of patients of hypertension which is more than double the population prevalence rates.[52] Similarly, more than 60% of patients with type 2 diabetes mellitus in India have hypertension.[53] Indian patients are more insulin resistant than their Caucasian counterparts, which may predispose them to hypertension.[51] Studies have reported high prevalence of insulin resistance in patients with hypertension in India.[51] This syndemic of diabetes and hypertension is attributed to a common soil hypothesis wherein both conditions have common genetic, epigenetic and proteomic abnormalities leading to cardiovascular diseases (CVDs).[54]

■ HYPERTENSION TREATMENT AND CONTROL

Although hypertension is highly prevalent in India, there is low awareness, treatment and control in urban as well as rural populations.[1] Awareness status has increased in the last 30 years, but it remains low especially in rural populations. Awareness increased from <30% in 1980s among urban populations to about 60% presently and from <10% in rural areas in 1980s to 35–40% presently.[3]

Anchala et al. reviewed hypertension awareness, treatment and control status including all the recent studies in India.[1] This meta-analysis reported that aware-ness of hypertension in India was 42% (CI 35–49%) for urban and 25% (CI 21–29%) for rural populations. The awareness levels for hypertension were consistently above 35% in almost all the studies from urban areas. In urban populations, the treatment and control status of those with known hypertension was 38% (95% CI 24–51%) and control in 20% (CI 12–29%). While in rural populations, the treatment status for those with known hypertension was 25% (CI 17–33%) and control status was in 11% (CI 6–15%). Treatment status varied by location and in urban parts of India, the percentage treated for hypertension varied from a low of 19% to high of 80%. The treated percentage among hypertensive patients showed greater variation in rural parts of India, ranging from 1% to 47%. Overall, only 38% of urban Indians suffering from hypertension are being treated. The BP control among both urban and rural parts of India was poor ranging from 12% to 29% in urban and 6–15% in rural populations. South-Asian cohorts in the PURE study reported similar low rate of hypertension awareness, treatment and control, respectively, in urban (46%, 38% and 15%) as well as rural (33%, 24% and 9%) locations.[55] No data on hypertension awareness, treatment and control are available from the NFHS-4 and DLHS-4/AHS studies.

Only a few studies in India have reported on trends of hypertension prevalence using serial studies.[56-59] We prospectively performed multiple cross-sectional studies (Jaipur Heart Watch studies, JHW-1 to JHW-6) among urban population in Jaipur over the past 25 years to assess prevalence of various CV risk factors.[60] The age-adjusted hypertension prevalence among adults in successive JHW studies increased from 29.5% to 36.1% (R^2 = 0.41). Increasing trends were also observed for hypertension awareness (R^2 = 0.63); treatment in all (R^2 = 0.68) and aware participants with hypertension (R^2 = 0.46); and control in all (R^2 = 0.82), aware (R^2 = 0.54), and treated (R^2 = 0.80) participants with hypertension.[60] Projections to year 2030 show increase in prevalence to 44% (95% CI 43–45%), awareness to 82% (95% CI 81–83%), treatment to 62% (95% CI 61–63%), and control to 36%

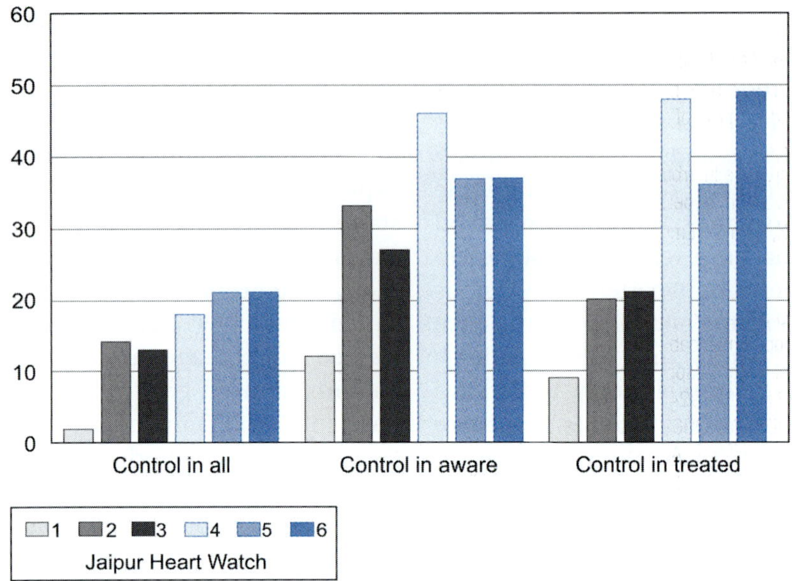

Fig. 5: 25-year secular trends in hypertension control in Jaipur Heart Watch (JHW) studies among participants with all, aware and treated hypertension.

(95% CI 35–37%). The rates of hypertension treatment and control among urban populations in India are lower than the targets set by the WHO Global Monitoring Framework and UN Sustainable Development Goals.[61,62] Rural patients with hypertension in India have much lower rates of treatment and it is likely that these projections are an overestimate.[63] Many middle-income countries are, however, on track to achieve the WHO Global Framework Goals in contrast to India.[64] Slow increase in BP control rates in India, even among those with treated hypertension, is a concern (Fig. 5). This highlights need for clinicians in India to focus on BP control in every patient with hypertension rather than focusing on pharmacological treatment with no control.[65]

CONCLUSION

This review shows that hypertension is endemic in the 21st century India. Burden of hypertension is increasing and there are large regional variations. Nationwide NFHS-4 study among the young (Fig. 1) and DLHS-4/AHS studies (Fig. 2) among general population have highlighted large regional variations. States with lower human development have less burden of hypertension (Fig. 3). However, this shall change with development as it has happened in high-income and middle-income countries,[34] and in not too distant future, the poorer states in the country shall have greater hypertension burden. Hypertension among the younger population in India is an important concern. The WHO Global Monitoring Framework has provided an ambitious 25 × 25 target for noncommunicable diseases control.[61] However, hypertension treatment and control rates have to be substantially increased in India to achieve this target.[60,65] A war-like response is required involving policy-makers, health bureaucrats, and medical and paramedical personnel at all levels of healthcare to achieve levels of hypertension control that can prevent CVDs.

■ REFERENCES

1. Anchala R, Kannuri NK, Pant H, et al. Hypertension in India: a systematic review and meta-analysis of prevalence, awareness, and control of hypertension. J Hypertens. 2014;32:1170-7.
2. Gupta R. Convergence in urban-rural prevalence of hypertension in India. J Hum Hypertens. 2016;30:79-82.
3. Gupta R, Gaur K, Ram CV. Emerging trends in hypertension epidemiology in India. J Hum Hypertens. 2018. [Epub ahead of print].
4. World Health Organization (WHO). (2014). Global Status Report on Noncommunicable Diseases 2014. [online] Available from https://apps.who.int/iris/bitstream/handle/10665/148114/9789241564854_eng.pdf;jsessionid=D0F919E0BD5E3D30B093A4C4CA4ED16C?sequence=1. [Last accessed from April, 2019].
5. Forouzanfar MH, Liu P, Roth GA, et al. Global Burden of Hypertension and Systolic Blood Pressure of at Least 110 to 115 mm Hg, 1990-2015. JAMA. 2017;317:165-82.
6. NCD Risk Factor Collaboration (NCD-RisC). Worldwide trends in blood pressure from 1975 to 2015: a pooled analysis of 1479 population-based measurement studies with 19.1 million participants. Lancet. 2017;389:37-55.
7. Gupta R, Xavier D. Hypertension: the most important non-communicable disease risk factor in India. Indian Heart J. 2018;70:565-72.
8. Gupta R, al-Odat NA, Gupta VP. Hypertension epidemiology in India: meta-analysis of 50 year prevalence rates and blood pressure trends. J Hum Hypertens. 1996;10:465-72.
9. Gupta R. Trends in hypertension epidemiology in India. J Hum Hypertens. 2004;18:73-8.
10. National Family Health Survey (NFHS-4). (2017). Introduction. [online] Available from http://rchiips.org/nfhs/NFHS-4Reports/India.pdf. [Last accessed from April, 2019].
11. Ram F, Paswan B, Singh SK, et al. National Family Health Survey-4 (2015-16). Econ Pol Weekly. 2017;52:66-70.
12. Gupta R, Gaur K, Mohan I, et al. Urbanization, human development and literacy and syndemics of obesity, hypertension and hyperglycemia in Rajasthan: National Family Health Survey-4. J Assoc Physicians India. 2018;66:17-24.
13. Joshi V. India at the cusp. In: Lane A (Ed). India's Long Road: The Search for Prosperity. Haryana: Penguin Random House India; 2016. pp. 3-33.
14. Lewington S, Clarke R, Qizilbash N, et al. Age-specific relevance of usual blood pressure to vascular mortality: a meta-analysis of individual data for one million adults in 61 prospective studies. Lancet. 2002;360:1903-13.
15. District Level Household and Facility Survey (DLHS-4). (2018). Hypertension (age 18 years and above) (%)—DLHS IV. [online] Available from https://data.gov.in/resources/hypertension-age-18-years-and-above-dlhs-iv. [Last accessed from April, 2019].
16. Geldsetzer P, Manne-Goehler J, Theilmann M, et al. Diabetes and Hypertension in India: A Nationally Representative Study of 1.3 Million Adults. JAMA Intern Med. 2018;178:363-72.
17. Roth GA, Johnson CO, Abate KH, et al. The Burden of Cardiovascular Diseases Among US States, 1990-2016. JAMA Cardiol. 2018;3:375-89.
18. Steel N, Ford JA, Newton JN, et al. Changes in health in the counties of the UK and 150 English Local Authority areas 1990-2016: a systematic analysis for the Global Burden of Disease Study 2016. Lancet. 2018;392:1647-61.
19. Zhang G, Yu C, Zhou M, et al. Burden of Ischaemic heart disease and attributable risk factors in China from 1990 to 2015: findings from the global burden of disease 2015 study. BMC Cardiovasc Disord. 2018;18:18.
20. GBD 2016 Russia Collaborators. The burden of disease in Russia from 1980 to 2016: a systematic analysis for the Global Burden of Disease Study 2016. Lancet. 2018;392:1138-46.
21. Malta DC, Santos NB, Perillo RD, et al. Prevalence of high blood pressure measured in the Brazilian population, National Health Survey 2013. Sao Paulo Med J. 2016;134:163-70.
22. Hussain MA, Mamun AA, Reid C, et al. Prevalence, Awareness, Treatment and Control of Hypertension in Indonesian Adults Aged ≥40 Years: Findings from the Indonesia Family Life Survey ((IFLS). PLoS One. 2016;11:e0160922.
23. Jafar TH, Haaland BA, Rahman A, et al. Non-communicable diseases and injuries in Pakistan: strategic priorities. Lancet. 2013;381:2281-90.
24. Rahman M, Zaman MM, Islam JY, et al. Prevalence, treatment patterns, and risk factors of hypertension and pre-hypertension among Bangladeshi adults. J Hum Hypertens. 2018;32:334-48.
25. Williams B, Spiering W, Rosei EA, et al. 2018 ESC/ESH guidelines for the management of arterial hypertension. Eur Heart J. 2018;39:3021-104.
26. Chow CK, Teo KK, Rangarajan S, et al. Prevalence, awareness, treatment and control of hypertension in rural and urban communities in high-, middle-, and low-income countries. JAMA. 2013;310:959-68.
27. Whelton PK, Carey RM, Aronow WS, et al. 2017 ACC/AHA/AAPA/ABS/ACPM/AGS/APhA/ASH/ASPC/NMA/PCNA guideline for the prevention, detection, evaluation and management of high blood pressure in adults: executive summary. J Am Coll Cardiol. 2018;71:2199-269.
28. Poulter N, Prabhakaran D, Caulfield M. Hypertension. Lancet. 2015;386:801-12.
29. Kaplan GA, Keil JE. Socioeconomic factors and cardiovascular disease: a review of the literature. Circulation. 1993;88:1973-98.

30. Wilkinson RG, Marmot M. Social Determinants of Health: The Solid Facts. Copenhagen: WHO Regional Office for Europe; 1998.

31. Berkman LF, Kawachi I. Social Epidemiology. New York: Oxford University Press; 2000. pp. 13-94.

32. Marmot M. The Status Syndrome: How Social Standing Affects Our Health and Longevity. New York: Henry Holt Co; 2004. pp. 139-7.

33. Gupta R, Gupta KD. Coronary heart disease in low socioeconomic status subjects in India: an evolving epidemic. Indian Heart J. 2009;61:358-67.

34. Marmot M. Social determinants of health inequalities. Lancet. 2005;365:1099-104.

35. Napier AD, Ancarno C, Butler B, et al. Culture and health. Lancet. 2014;384:1607-39.

36. Barnish M, Tørnes M, Nelson-Home B. How much evidence is there that political factors are related to population health outcomes? An internationally comparative systematic review. BMJ Open. 2018;8:020866.

37. Gupta R, Gupta VP, Ahluwalia NS. Educational status, coronary heart disease and coronary risk factor prevalence in a rural population of India. BMJ. 1994;309:1332-6.

38. Reddy KS, Prabhakaran D, Jeemon P, et al. Educational status and cardiovascular risk profile in Indians. PNAS. 2007;104:16263-8.

39. Gupta R, Kaul V, Agrawal A, et al. Cardiovascular risk according to educational status in India. Prev Med. 2010;51:408-11.

40. Horton R. Offline: India's health crisis: will democracy deliver? Lancet. 2019;393:390.

41. Gupta R. Universal healthcare ahoy! RUHS J Health Sci. 2018;3:179-81.

42. Lear S, Hu W, Rangarajan S, et al. The effect of physical activity on mortality and cardiovascular disease in 130,000 people from 17 high-income, middle-income and low-income countries: The PURE Study. Lancet. 2017;390:2643-54.

43. Althoff T, Sosic R, Hicks JL, et al. Large scale physical activity data reveal worldwide activity inequality. Nature. 2017;547:336-9.

44. Misra A, Soares MJ, Mohan V, et al. Body fat, metabolic syndrome and hyperglycemia in South Asians. J Diabetes Complications. 2018;32:1068-75.

45. Misra A, Jayawardena R, Anoop S. Obesity in South Asia: Phenotype, Morbidities, and Mitigation. Curr Obes Rep. 2019;8:43-52.

46. Gupta R, Keswani P, Al-Odat NA, et al. Correlation of body-mass index with hypertension in urban and rural Indian populations. South Asian J Prev Cardiol. 1998;2:93-100.

47. Gupta PC, Gupta R, Pednekar M. Hypertension prevalence and blood pressure trends in 88,653 subjects in Mumbai, India. J Hum Hypertens. 2004;18:907-10.

48. Babu GR, Murthy GV, Ana Y, et al. Association of obesity with hypertension and type 2 diabetes mellitus in India: A meta-analysis of observational studies. World J Diabetes. 2018;9:40-52.

49. Gupta R, Gupta VP, Bhagat N, et al. Obesity is a major determinant of coronary risk factors in India: Jaipur Heart Watch Studies. Indian Heart J. 2008;60:26-33.

50. NCD Risk Factor Collaboration (NCD-RisC). Worldwide trends in body-mass index, underweight, and obesity from 1975 to 2016: a pooled analysis of 2416 population-based measurement studies in 128.9 million children, adolescents, and adults. Lancet. 2017;390:2627-42.

51. Unnikrishnan R, Anjana RM, Mohan V. Diabetes mellitus and its complications in India. Nat Rev Endocrinol. 2016;12:357-70.

52. Gupta R, Deedwania PC, Achari V, et al. Normotension, prehypertension and hypertension in Asian Indians: prevalence, determinants, awareness, treatment and control. Am J Hypertens. 2013;26:83-94.

53. Gupta A, Gupta R, Sharma KK, et al. Prevalence of diabetes and cardiovascular risk factors in middle-class urban populations in India. BMJ Open Diabetes Res Care. 2014;2:e000048.

54. Stern MP. Diabetes and cardiovascular disease: The common soil hypothesis. Diabetes. 1995;44:369-74.

55. Gupta R, Kaur M, Islam S, et al. Association of household wealth, educational status and social capital with hypertension awareness, treatment and control in South Asia. Am J Hypertens. 2017;30:373-81.

56. Ahlawat SK, Singh MM, Kumar R, et al. Time trends in the prevalence of hypertension and associated risk factors in Chandigarh. J Indian Med Assoc. 2002;100:547-55.

57. Oommen AM, Abraham VJ, George K, et al. Rising trend of cardiovascular risk factors between 1991-1994 and 2010-2012: a repeat cross-sectional survey in urban and rural Vellore. Indian Heart J. 2016;68:263-9.

58. Goyal A, Kahlon P, Jain D, et al. Trend in prevalence of coronary artery disease and risk factors over two decades in rural Punjab. BMJ Heart Asia. 2017;9:e010938.

59. Roy A, Praveen PA, Amarchand R, et al. Changes in hypertension prevalence, awareness, treatment and control rates over twenty years in National Capital Region of India. BMJ Open. 2017;7:e015639.

60. Gupta R, Gupta VP, Agrawal A, et al. 25-year trends in hypertension prevalence, awareness, treatment and control in an urban population in India. Indian Heart J. 2018;64:802-7.

61. World Health Organization (WHO). (2013). Draft comprehensive global monitoring framework and targets for the prevention and control of noncommunicable diseases. [online] Available from https://apps.who.int/iris/bitstream/handle/10665/105633/A66_8-en.

pdf?sequence=1&isAllowed=y. [Last accessed from April, 2019].

62. United Nations. (2019). Sustainable Development Goals. [online] Available from http://www.un.org/pga/wp-content/uploads/sites/3/2015/08/120815_outcome-document-of-Summit-for-adoption-of-the-post-2015-development-agenda.pdf. [Last accessed from April, 2019].

63. Lloyd-Sherlock P, Beard J, Minicucci N, et al. Hypertension among older adults in low- and middle-income countries: prevalence, awareness and control. Int J Epidemiol. 2015;43:116-28.

64. Niessen LW, Mohan D, Akuoku JK, et al. Tackling socio-economic inequalities and non-communicable diseases in low-income and middle income countries under the Sustainable Development agenda. Lancet. 2018;391: 2036-46.

65. Gupta R, Yusuf S. Towards better hypertension control in India. Ind J Med Res. 2014;139:657-60.

SECTION **2**

Overview of
Risk Factors in Hypertension:
Old and New

Social Determinants of Hypertension Treatment and Control in India

Rajeev Gupta, Shreya Gupta

■ INTRODUCTION

High blood pressure (BP) and hypertension is now the most important risk factor for global disease burden. The latest iteration of Global Burden of Diseases (GBD) study has reported that in 2017, high systolic BP was the leading risk factor accounting for 10.2 million [95% uncertainty intervals (UI) 9.2–11.3 million] deaths and 208 million (UI 188–227 million) disability-adjusted life years (DALYs). Overall, 8.6% (UI 7.7–9.6) of total DALYs were attributable to high systolic BP. Most of the burden attributable to high systolic BP was due to ischemic heart disease and stroke and high systolic BP accounted for 55% (UI 48–63%) and 56% (UI 49–63%) of DALYs due to ischemic heart disease and stroke, respectively.[1] In India also, it has emerged as the most important risk factor for deaths and disability.[2] According to hypertension-focused reports from the World Health Organization (WHO),[3] GBD study,[4] and Non-Communicable Disease Risk Factor Collaboration (NCDRiSC)[5] the prevalence of hypertension is increasing globally and currently more than 1 billion people have NCDRiSC study reported that number of adults with high BP increased from 594 million in 1975 to 1·13 billion in 2015 and the increase was mostly in low-income and middle-income countries.[5]

■ BURDEN OF HYPERTENSION IN INDIA

Gupta R et al. reviewed 50-year trends in the prevalence of hypertension in India and reported escalating burden of this condition from the 1950s to 1990s in both the urban and rural areas.[6] Population-based epidemiological studies, conducted during mid-1950s and early 1960s, among the urban subjects used the older WHO criteria for making diagnosis (known hypertension or systolic BP more than or equal to 160 mm Hg and/or diastolic BP 95 mm Hg). Prevalence of hypertension was reported to be 1–4%. Since then, in many Indian locations, the prevalence of hypertension has been evaluated. It has been documented that steady increase in prevalence was observed from 3% to 4% in early 1960s to 11% to 15% in mid-1990s.[6]

Earlier studies reported lower prevalence of hypertension in rural populations in India. However, there has been a significant increase of hypertension in these populations as well, from less than 1% in early 1960s to 5–7% in late 1990s. It has been reported that at the turn of the century hypertension prevalence in India was much more in urban as compared to rural populations.[7] Recent reviews in urban and rural populations of India have reported persistent urban-rural gradient.[8] It is observed that more than one-third of adult urban subjects and a quarter of rural adults have hypertension in India.[8] Trend analysis reveals that in the last 20 years (1995-2015) there has been a convergence of hypertension prevalence in urban and rural populations.[9] While the prevalence of hypertension has remained stable at 28-33% among Indian urban subjects, in rural subjects it increased significantly from 10-12% at turn of the century to 24-27% by 2010s.[9,10]

Two recent studies have used proper nationwide sampling and uniform tools to determine the true prevalence of hypertension in India and have been reviewed recently.[10] NFHS-4 (National Family Health Survey) evaluated hypertension prevalence in younger men (15-54 years) and women (15-49 years) and reported hypertension in 13.8% men and 8.8% women with an overall prevalence of 11.3%.[11] Further age-representative data from the District Level Household Study-4 (DLHS-4) documented presence of hypertension in 25.3% of the adults. The prevalence was greater in men (27.4%) in comparison to the women (20.0%), the urban-rural difference being narrow.[12]

These proportions would translate into a large number of hypertensive males and females in the country. Total Indian population is 1.34 billion; out of this 61% are above 18 years (n = 819 million). This age group, with an age-adjusted prevalence of 25.3%, would translate into 207.1 million people (males 112.2 million, females 94.9 million) with hypertension in the country.[10] There was a suggestion in recent US hypertension guidelines to lower the threshold to define hypertension as BP >130 mm Hg and/or >80 mm Hg.[13] If

this new definition were to be applied to the Indian subcontinent, the prevalence of hypertension will increase steeply. The European hypertension guidelines, however, maintain the older criteria for diagnosis of hypertension.[14]

◼ AWARENESS, TREATMENT AND CONTROL OF HYPERTENSION

Though there is a high prevalence of hypertension in India, treatment, awareness, and control status are low in rural as well as urban populations of India.[8] Hypertension awareness status has improved in India over the past 30 years, but remains very low, particularly among rural areas. There is an increase in awareness about hypertension from less than 30% among urban areas in the 1980s to around 60% at present and from less than 10% in rural regions in the 1980s to 35-40% at the present.

Anchala et al.[8] reviewed hypertension awareness, treatment and control status including all the recent studies in India. Overall estimates (95% UI) for awareness of hypertension in India were 42% (UI 35-49%) for urban and 25% (UI 21-29%) for rural populations. The awareness levels for hypertension were consistently above 35% in almost all studies from urban areas. In urban populations the treatment and control status of those with known hypertension was 38% (UI 24-51%) and control in 20% (UI 12-29%). While in rural populations, the treatment status for those with known hypertension was 25% (17-33%), and control status was in 11% (6-15%) (Fig. 1). In the urban parts of India, treatment status showed variation by location with percentage treated for the hypertension ranging from low 19% to high 80%. The percentage of patients who received treatment for hypertension showed high variability in rural southern parts of India, varying from 1% to 47% compared to urban parts. Overall,

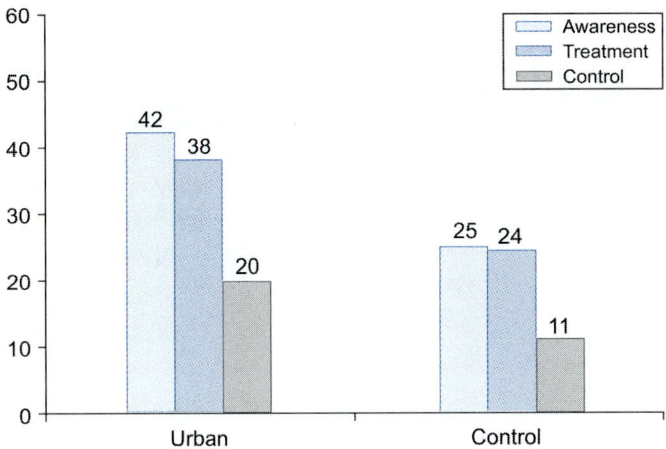

Fig. 1: Meta-analysis of hypertension awareness, treatment and control in Indian urban and rural populations.

nearly 38% of hypertensive urban Indians are receiving treatment. The control of BP among both the rural areas and the urban areas has been very poor ranging from 12% to 29% in urban and 6% to 15% in rural populations. No data on hypertension awareness, treatment and control are available from the NFHS-4 and DLHS studies so far.

The India Heart Watch study on urban populations reported prevalence of awareness, treatment, and control of hypertension in middle class sites in 11 cities in India and enrolled more than 6,000 subjects.[15]

An age-adjusted analysis revealed that there was awareness of hypertension in 53.8% of males and 57.3% of females. Among hypertensive subjects, there were 37.9% of the men and 34.5% of the women who were undergoing treatment. Among subjects with hypertension, in 25.6% of the men and 31.6% of the women (total 28.2%), controlled BP was present (systolic BP <140 mm Hg and diastolic BP <90 mm Hg). There was an increase in awareness of hypertension with age in both the men and the women; less than a quarter of men and women with age less than 30 years were aware of hypertension in comparison to two-thirds of those more than 60 years of age. There was also an increase in treatment status with age; less than 20% of those below age 40 years but more than 50% of those above age 60 years were undergoing treatment. No significant change was noted in hypertension control status with age. Among the subjects who were aware of having hypertension, 78.6% of males and 76.1% of females underwent treatment. Among subjects who received treatment for hypertension, <50% (41.5% of males and 41.6% of females) had controlled BP. This study indicated that there is a low treatment and control status of hypertension even among the urban middle class.

In India, the only long-term prospective cross-sectional hypertension and other cardiovascular risk factor epidemiology study is Jaipur Heart Watch (JHW).[16] Gupta R et al. (2018) studied trends in hypertension awareness, treatment and control over a 25-year period in a series of cross-sectional studies in Jaipur (Rajasthan, India). While the crude prevalence of hypertension has varied from 30% to 50% in these studies, awareness of hypertension has increased significantly (Table 1). In these studies, crude prevalence of hypertension showed variation from 30% to 50%, but there is a significant increase in

TABLE 1: 25-year trends in age and sex-adjusted hypertension prevalence and awareness in among urban subjects in India according to serial Jaipur Heart Watch (JHW) studies.

	JHW-1 (n = 2,212)	JHW-2 (n = 1,123)	JHW-3 (n = 458)	JHW-4 (n = 1,127)	JHW-5 (n = 739)	JHW-6 (n = 1,781)
Years of study and reporting	1992–1994; 1995	1999–2001; 2002	2003–2004; 2004	2005–2006; 2007	2010–2011; 2012	2012–2013; 2015
Age-adjusted prevalence rate (%)	30	30	37	42	34	36
Awareness (% of total hypertensives)	13	33	49	44	49	56
Treatment (% of total hypertensives)	9	22	38	34	41	36
Control (BP <140/90 mm Hg as % of total hypertensives)	2	14	13	18	21	22

awareness of hypertension (Table 1). In early 1990s, the awareness of hypertension was 40%. Presently, it has increased to more than 55%. However, there is a tremendous need to enhance the diagnosis of hypertension via screening and awareness in India so that we can achieve the level of awareness of more than 70% of developed countries.[3] In JHW studies, the reasons for increased awareness of hypertension are not evident; further studies are needed. Better health literacy as a result of public health campaigns could be crucial. Another important finding in this study is increasing treatment and control status (Table 1). However, both these rates are low. At this rate hypertensive people in urban India are unlikely to achieve the WHO and UN Sustainable Development Goal targets of more than 50% hypertension control by the year 2030.[16]

SOCIOLOGY OF HYPERTENSION CONTROL

Socioeconomic factors are important drivers of cardiovascular diseases including hypertension.[17,18] It is well documented in high-income countries that cardiovascular disease and risk factors, comprising hypertension, tend to cluster in the people of low social classes having less education and low income. However, it is less evident why this is the case and several explanations have been proposed for this. Often, adverse social factors are related with poor lifestyle, along with less exercise, less healthy diet, more smoking, and thus an enhanced preponderance of the abdominal obesity and metabolic syndrome. This will lead to an increase in the risk of development of hypertension among susceptible individuals. More explanations were also suggested. In many settings, influence of psychosocial stress on the regulation of BP has been evaluated. As reported by a population-based study from Sweden, there can be an increase in BP because of job strain at the workplace; it was found to be more in men as compared to women.[11] It has been reported by other studies that psychosocial stress can be linked to enhanced levels of cardiovascular risk by a number of biochemical pathways, which include activation of the sympathetic nervous system.[19,20]

Adverse social factors, such as less education, could also affect self-help knowledge and how patients seek and receive medical care for different medical needs, along with control of risk factors. For instance, this could imply that individuals from the population's less socially privileged strata might have less chance of engaging in hypertension screening activities or get less healthcare. Furthermore, compliance with medical treatment in these topics could also be suboptimal and thus control of the risk factor less effective. This is affected not only by the accessibility of healthcare resources, but also by the economy and the level of knowledge of people, which will affect awareness and understanding of risk, affecting the motivation to remain on prescribed medication or adhere to lifestyle advice.

Even the factors present in early life have the potential impact on these relationships.[21] For instance, it has been shown that a poor fetal growth pattern [small for gestational age (SGA) babies] combined with enhanced weight development during postnatal growth (mismatch hypothesis) could be harmful for enhanced cardiovascular risk, including hypertension, and type 2 diabetes mellitus and metabolic syndrome. These relationships are not only affected by social, genetic and nutritional factors, but also by the mother's medical condition, such as hypertension in pregnancy. Thus, in the view of life course, adverse influences from early life like an adverse social environment during childhood, adolescence, and adulthood may increase programming on biology and health. This is a fertile zone for further studies given the huge incidence of low birth babies in India.

Recently, a more controversial research line has been defined as the study of cognitive epidemiology and its health effects.[22] This basically includes analyzing connections between results of early life cognitive function measurements (e.g. IQ, intellectual capacity, or mental ability in particular), academic accomplishments, and negative health outcomes in adult life. In fact, in studies from the UK and Sweden, but also from other nations, it has been shown repeatedly that a reduced than average early-age intellectual ability, based on college grade assessment, is an independent risk factor for adverse health outcomes, even adjusted for personal characteristics and social background. It has been suggested that factors in early life, such as in utero nutrition, may be important for the development of mental and cognitive functions. It was shown in one study that stress susceptibility at conscript testing in young males, as assessed by trained military psychologists, was inversely related with low birth weight, adjusted for gestational age (poor fetal growth), as well as for family social class.[21] Other explanations focused on the problems of adjusting exposures to poor mental stimulation during the childhood and other psychosocial correlates of poor cognitive function.

This remains to be elucidated in more rigorous studies on the importance of genetic predictors of hypertension in a putative relationship with both fetal growth patterns and cognitive function. In a large study, influence of adverse social factors on the development of hypertension in a large cohort of 27,207 women working as health professionals was evaluated.[23] The finding in general was that a lower educational level was associated with an increased risk of hypertension after follow-up. Educational level, but not income, remained significantly associated with BP progression and incident hypertension.

There is, thus, in developed countries, a large evidence that risk of hypertension is greater in those with low educational status.[24,25] This demonstrates that negative social factors are not mediated by income alone for public health. These negative patterns for provoking disease cannot be treated with drugs provided to the people. Instead, they should be the goals of public health initiatives to improve educational accessibility for all and counteract social inequities. Hopefully, this will lead to risk factors like hypertension that are less common. An evidence of this perspective is the steady decline in mean BP in the population that has been defined in Western populations over recent decades.[26] One explanation for this might be that conditions in early life during the latter half of the 20th century have gradually improved in consecutive birth cohorts. This is a promising prospect for less common cardiovascular morbidity and hypertension in the population's middle-aged strata even though there will be no absolute reduction in the number of patients with cardiovascular disease manifestations or hypertension owing to enhanced longevity and an increasing percentage of elder people.

■ INDIAN SCENARIO

In India there is limited evidence of association of social and economic factors with hypertension. The authors for the first time, reported greater prevalence of hypertension in illiterate rural populations in Rajasthan in 1994.[27] Subsequently many studies have reported on greater prevalence of multiple lifestyle risk factors and some have reported greater hypertension in illiterate and poor communities.[28] Low status of hypertension, awareness and control has been reported among less educated participants in the India Heart Watch study.[29] Greater cardiovascular and hypertension-related mortality has been reported in the Mumbai Cohort Study.[30,31]

Poor status of hypertension awareness, treatment and control of high BP has been attributed to variety of socioeconomic factors. These factor include lack of political will, bureaucratic apathy, no focus in national programs, poorly developed healthcare system and primary healthcare, rural residence, cost of therapy and affordability as well as individual factors such as women gender, low educational status and poverty (Table 2).

There have been only a few studies in India that determined determinants of hypertension awareness, treatment and control. The Indian Women Health Study was conducted on middle-aged (35–70 years) low and low-middle socioeconomic status of women in India at various urban and rural sites.[32] Prevalence of known hypertension was reported to be low. Among the urban females, only 56.8% were aware of the condition and in rural women 24.6% were familiar about the disease. Among the women aware of hypertension, only 38.6% received drug therapy (rural 46.5%; urban 38.6%). Hypertension control as defined by systolic BP less than 140 mm Hg and diastolic BP less than 90 mm Hg, among the women who received treatment, was extremely low; only 28.3% of the urban women and 10.2% of the rural women had controlled values of BP. In total, out of the 1,672 hypertensive women (urban 926, rural 746), only 18.3% received treatment (urban 22.5%; rural 13.1%). Control to target was achieved in 3.9% women (urban 5.9%; rural 1.3%) (p <0.05, for rural-urban difference). Significant lifestyle determinants of hypertension awareness, treatment and control revealed that the most important risk factor for low awareness was rural location [age-adjusted odds ratio (OR) 3.13, confidence interval (CI) 2.49–3.93], treatment (1.59, 1.18–2.13), and control (5.11, 2.22–11.74). Low educational level and educational status of spouse have insignificant association respectively with awareness (age- and location-adjusted OR and 95% CI 1.39, 0.92–2.09 and 1.14, 0.75–1.74), treatment (0.62, 0.38–1.03 and 1.74, 0.94-3.25), and control

TABLE 2: Factors associated with treatment and control of low hypertension.

Individual patient	Health systems related	Healthcare providers
• Old age • Female gender • Low socioeconomic status • Social isolation (particularly in elders) • Lack of commitment and motivation • Lack of realization of the seriousness of the issue • Lack of quality information • Finance-related factors and costs • Comorbid conditions which are significant • Failure to sustain lifestyle changes • Confusing multistakeholder messages • Not covered by insurance • Factors related to distance and geography	• Government policies related to tobacco and food • Lack of health-friendly infrastructure • Low perceived need by healthcare managers and bureaucrats • Low access and availability of medicines and medical staff • Media apathy and conflicting messages • Constraints of resource and cost of equipment and drugs, in particular for noncommunicable diseases • Lack of advocacy • Not covered by insurance for management of cardiovascular disease • Frequent changes and use of nonstandardized formulary • Less focus of undergraduate medical education on noncommunicable diseases • Overburdening of healthcare system with communicable diseases	• Less continuity of care • Fixed clinician perception • Lack of motivation and proper education • Overburdened due to large number of patients • Lack of continuing medical education programs • Less understanding of needs of patients • Costs • Prescription of complex regimens • Lack of referrals to clinician • Overtreatment • Avoiding to involve patients in choices • Lack of explanation of benefits and side effects • Less focus on lifestyle changes

(0.55, 0.21–1.42 and 0.60, 0.20–1.80). In most of the developed countries, hypertension awareness, treatment and control is more among women in comparison to men.[3] The Indian Women Health Study showed that in India in both urban and rural women there is low awareness, treatment and control of hypertension.

In India Heart Watch study 6,198 men and women in 11 cities of India, were studied.[15] Educational status was inversely associated with hypertension awareness, treatment and control.[29] Age-adjusted and sex-adjusted prevalence (%) of hypertension in low, medium, and high educational status groups was 31.8, 29.5 and 34.1%, respectively. Significantly increasing trends with low, medium and high educational status were observed for hypertension awareness (30.7, 37.8 and 47.0%), treatment (24.3, 29.2 and 35.5%) as well as control (7.8, 11.6 and 15.5%) (Fig. 2). The authors concluded that in India low educational status subjects have lower awareness, treatment and control of hypertension as well as other cardiovascular risk factors, e.g. diabetes, hypercholesterolemia and smoking quit rates. Clearly, there is a need to focus on low educational status subjects for improving hypertension treatment and control.

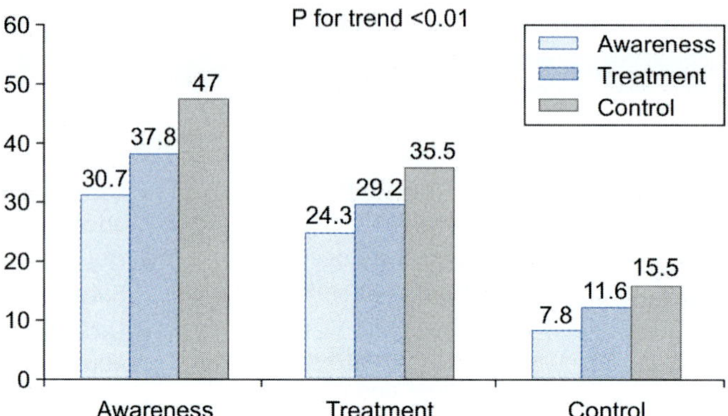

Fig. 2: Educational status and hypertension awareness, treatment, and control in India Heart Watch study.

In a qualitative study to evaluate sociological determinants of low hypertension treatment and control in rural women the authors performed a study in Rajasthan.[33] The authors interviewed 30 women (age-range 20–70, mean age 56.1 years). Majority of women were from low socioeconomic status households and were illiterate (63.3%) and were housewife. Adherence using Morisky scale was determined as low, observed in 12 (36.7%) and medium in 10 women (30.0%). The most commonly prescribed drugs were angiotensin receptor blockers and calcium channel blockers while low-cost drugs such as diuretics and beta blockers were used in low proportions. Although all these patients had access to a medical college hospital only a third had visited a community health center. More than half used public transport system for travel to hospital. All the patients had to pay for medicines out-of-pocket and only two women had some sort of insurance or social security. A large proportion of women borrowed money from relatives or friends to reach the hospital and pay for medicines. Awareness of hypertension and its risk factors was adequate in very few women. Thus, the authors found that a low adherence to medicines as well as healthy lifestyles was observed in Indian rural women with hypertension. Reasons for these include low awareness of complications of hypertension, poor access to care, out-of-pocket payments, borrowing money, lack of insurance, prescriptions of more expensive medicines, and low use of combination pharmacotherapy. Similar situation is likely to be prevalent in other parts of the country.

Association of macrolevel sociodemographic factors with hypertension prevalence has not been well studied in India. To determine association of prevalence of hypertension in different states in India with various social determinants the authors performed a macrolevel analysis. They used data on hypertension prevalence available from the DLHS-4 and correlated it with various social determinants of health, healthcare availability, and other factors and reported the results in a recent review.[10]

The sociodemographic factors include state-level urbanization index, human development index and social development index. Results show that there is a significant positive association (R^2) of state-level hypertension prevalence with urbanization (men 0.17, women 0.08) and human development index (men 0.36, women 0.26) while relationship of social development

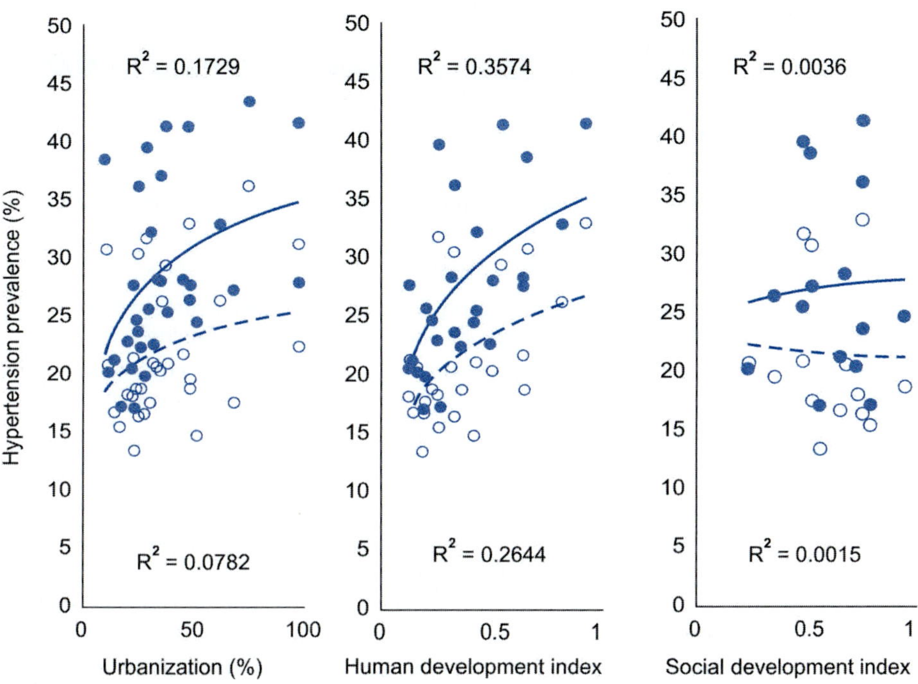

Fig. 3: Association of macrolevel socioeconomic factors with hypertension prevalence in Indian states.

index with hypertension is not significant (Fig. 3).[34] These findings are also similar to results from 11-city India Heart Watch study where it was reported that hypertension prevalence was greater in cities with greater human and social development indices.[35] The authors also determined the association of hypertension with healthcare access and healthcare quality indices. There is poor association of hypertension prevalence with healthcare availability although there is positive association with healthcare access and quality.[34] These findings suggest that healthcare access is to be improved for hypertension management including its detection, treatment and control.

CONCLUSION

It is difficult to eradicate socially patterned risk factors and adverse health outcomes, but based on favorable development in age-adjusted trends of cardiovascular disease in developed countries, it appears that better conditions in childhood could reduce the impact of other negative circumstances in adult life for most people. Thus, in studies on the impact of adverse social factors on adult health, a life course perspective should be implemented.[36] Although people may vary in personal characteristics such as cognitive function and academic achievement, equal healthcare resources need to be provided and customized to personal requirements for better hypertension control.

By improvement in detection and management of hypertension, thousands of premature deaths, heart attacks and strokes can be prevented every year. Hypertension can be better managed by innovative systems-based strategies; these are outlined in Table 3. For lowering risk, a combined approach with changes in lifestyle and use of antihypertensive

TABLE 3: Preventive health measures to improve control of hypertension in India.

Strategy	Examples
Lifestyle changes	• Reduction in high salt in diet, decreasing consumption of alcohol, weight reduction, and more physical activity should be focused • Cessation of use of smoking/tobacco should be done for overall risk reduction
Patient empowerment	• Lifelong commitment to antihypertensive therapy and lifestyle changes in hypertensive patients • Self-monitoring of blood pressure
Opportunistic screening	• Hypertension screening by physicians or other healthcare workers among all adults at all levels of care (universal opportunistic screening) • Measurement of blood pressure once a year in adults by trained nonphysician healthcare workers in rural and urban regions during home visits
Control of vascular risk factors	• Focus should be on the management of all vascular risk factors (such as high cholesterol, smoking, diabetes, other lipids—in every hypertensive) • Polypharmacy approach in high-risk people
Public education	• Hypertension is one of the major cardiovascular risk factors and an important cause of heart disease and strokes • It is most often silent; regular checking of blood pressure is necessary in all adults (>35 years) • It can be prevented and controlled by adopting prudent lifestyle along with safe, simple, and not expensive medications
Low-dose combination pharmacotherapy	• Low doses of two or more individual drug combination as initial therapy should be used • Evidence-based combinations should be used
Physician education	• More focus should be shifted toward noncommunicable diseases in undergraduate education. Hypertension should be focused in public health curriculum • Hypertension should be focused as a primary care issue. Knowledge about the proper management and long-term care should be given. Physician inertia should be managed • Importance of ambulatory blood pressure measurement, home monitoring, and combination therapy should be understand. Focus on vascular risk management should be given

and lipid lowering therapy in combination can decrease the risk of cardiovascular by as much as 75%.[37] We need improved healthcare systems for extensive hypertension screening in order to detect it. Once identified, adequate pharmacotherapy with good compliance will best achieve efficient BP control and decreased cardiovascular disease risk. Such an approach to public health will lead to major modifications in India's clinical outcomes of hypertension.

■ REFERENCES

1. GBD 2016 Risk Factors Collaborators. Global, regional, and national comparative risk assessment of 84 behavioral, environmental and occupational, and metabolic risks or clusters of risks, 1990-2016: a systematic analysis for the Global Burden of Disease Study 2016. Lancet. 2017;390:1345-422.

2. Gupta R, Xavier D. Hypertension: the most important non-communicable disease risk factor in India. Indian Heart J. 2018;70:565-72.

3. World Health Organization. Global Status Report on Non-Communicable Diseases 2014. Geneva: World Health Organization. 2014.

4. Farouzanfar MH, Ng M, Biryukov S, et al. Global burden of hypertension and systolic blood pressure of at least 110 to 115 mm Hg, 1990-2015. JAMA. 2017;317:175-82.

5. NCD Risk Factor Collaboration (NCD-RiSC). Worldwide trends in blood pressure from 1975 to 2015: a pooled analysis of 1479 population-based measurement studies with 19.1 million participants. Lancet. 2017;389:37-55.

6. Gupta R, Al-Odat NA, Gupta VP. Hypertension epidemiology in India: Meta-analysis of fifty-year prevalence rates and blood pressure trends. J Human Hypertens. 1996;10:465-472.

7. Gupta R. Trends in hypertension epidemiology in India. J Human Hypertens. 2004;18:73-8.

8. Anchala R, Kannuri NK, Pant H, et al. Hypertension in India: a systematic review and meta-analysis of prevalence, awareness, and control of hypertension. J Hypertens. 2014;32:1170-7.

9. Gupta R. Convergence in urban-rural prevalence of hypertension in India. J Human Hypertens. 2016;30:79-82.

10. Gupta R, Gaur K, Ram CVS. Emerging trends in hypertension epidemiology in India. J Human Hypertens. 2019;33(8):575-87.

11. National Family Health Survey. Available from http://rchiips.org/nfhs/abt.html. [Last accessed August, 2019].

12. Geldsetzer P, Manne-Goehler J, Theilmann M, et al. Diabetes and hypertension in India: a nationally representative study of 1.3 million adults. JAMA Intern Med. 2018;178:363-72.

13. Whelton PK, Carey RM, Aronow WS, et al. 2017 ACC/AHA/AAPA/ABS/ACPM/AGS/APhA/ASH/ASPC/NMA/PCNA guideline for the prevention, detection, evaluation and management of high blood pressure in adults: executive summary. J Am Coll Cardiol. 2018;71:2199-269.

14. Williams B, Mancia G, Spiering W, et al. 2018 ESC/ESH guidelines for the management of arterial hypertension. Eur Heart J. 2018;39(33):3021-104.

15. Gupta R, Deedwania PC, Achari V, et al. Normotension, prehypertension and hypertension in Asian Indians: prevalence, determinants, awareness, treatment and control. Am J Hypertens. 2013;26:83-94.

16. Gupta R, Gupta VP, Agrawal A, et al. 25-year trends in hypertension prevalence, awareness, treatment and control in an urban population in India. Indian Heart J. 2018;70(6):802-7.

17. Fuster V, Kelly BB, Board for Global Health. Promoting cardiovascular health in developing world: a critical challenge to achieve global health. Washington: Institute of Medicine; 2010.

18. Kaplan GA, Keil JE. Socio-economic factors and cardiovascular disease: a review of the literature. Circulation. 1993;88:1973-98.

19. Öhlin B, Nilsson PM, Nilsson J-Å, et al. Self-reported psychosocial stress predicts cardiovascular morbidity and mortality in middle-aged subjects—a long-term follow-up. Eur Heart J. 2004;25:867-73.

20. Bairey Merz CN, Dwyer J, Nordstrom CK, et al. Psychosocial stress and cardiovascular disease: pathophysiological links. Behav Med. 2002;27:141-7.

21. Gluckman PD, Hanson MA. Developmental plasticity and human disease: research directions. J Intern Med. 2007;261:461-71.

22. Deary IJ, Batty GD. Cognitive epidemiology: Glossary. J Epidemiol Comm Health. 2007;61:378-84.

23. Conen D, Glynn RJ, Ridker PM, et al. Socioeconomic status, blood pressure progression, and incident hypertension in a prospective cohort of female health professionals. Eur Heart J. 2009;30:1378-84.

24. Rozanski A, Blumenthal JA, Davidson KW, et al. The epidemiology, pathophysiology, and management of psychosocial risk factors in cardiac practice: the emerging field of behavioural cardiology. J Am Coll Cardiol. 2005;45:637-51.

25. Rozanski A. Behavioural cardiology: current advances and future. J Am Coll Cardiol. 2014;64:100-10.

26. Danaei G, Finucane MM, Lin JK, et al. National, regional and global trends in systolic blood pressure since 1980: systematic analysis of health examination surveys and epidemiological studies with 786 country-years and 5.4 million participants. Lancet. 2011;377:568-77.

27. Gupta R, Gupta VP, Ahluwalia NS. Educational status, coronary heart disease and coronary risk factor prevalence in a rural population of India. BMJ. 1994;309:1332-6.

28. Prabhakaran D, Jeemon P, Reddy KS. Poverty and cardiovascular disease in India: do we need more evidence for action? Int J Epidemiol. 2013;42:1431-5.

29. Gupta R, Sharma KK, Gupta BK, et al. Education status related disparities in awareness, treatment and control of cardiovascular risk factors in India. Heart Asia BMJ. 2015;7:1-7.

30. Pednekar M, Gupta R, Gupta PC. Illiteracy, low educational status and cardiovascular mortality in India. BMC Public Health. 2011;11:e568.

31. Pednekar MS, Gupta R, Gupta PC. Association of blood pressure and cardiovascular mortality in India: Mumbai Cohort Study. Am J Hypertens. 2009;22:1076-84.

32. Gupta R, Pandey RM, Misra A, et al. High prevalence and low hypertension awareness, treatment and control in Asian Indian women. J Hum Hypertens. 2012;26:585-93.

33. Gupta S, Dhamija JP, Mohan I, et al. Barriers for adherence to anti-hypertensive medicines among rural women in

India: a qualitative study. Indian Heart J. 2018;70(Suppl 2):S10.

34. Gupta R, Gaur K. Epidemiology of hypertension in India: the real scenario. In: Goswami KC (Ed). Cardiological Society of India: Cardiology Update 2018. New Delhi: Jaypee Brothers Medical Publishers; 2019. p. 103-12.

35. Gupta R, Sharma KK, Gupta BK, et al. Geographic epidemiology of cardiometabolic risk factors in urban middle-class residents in India: A cross sectional study. J Global Health. 2015;5:10411.

36. Olson MH, Angell SY, Asma S, et al. A call to action and a lifecourse strategy to address the global burden of raised blood pressure on current and future generations: the Lancet Commission on hypertension. Lancet. 2016;388:2665-712.

37. Gupta R, Yusuf S. Towards better hypertension control in India. Indian J Med Res. 2014;139:657-60.

Etiological and Pathophysiological Aspects (Pathogenesis)

Overview of Various Pathogenic Mechanisms in Essential Hypertension

Chandni Radhakrishnan, Jinu Johnson

■ INTRODUCTION

Pathogenic mechanisms in essential hypertension (EH) are not fully elucidated. This understanding is slowly evolving over the course of time. It is a complex interplay of genetic and environmental factors.

Robert Sterling Palmer,[1] in 1955 in his review, beautifully explained the proposed causes of elevated blood pressure (BP), various treatments with their sites of action, and the same could be contributing to EH as well. Much has changed in the understanding and management of EH over the years. This paper describes the current knowledge about the pathogenic mechanisms in EH.

■ NORMAL BP REGULATION

Blood pressure is the pressure exerted by circulating blood upon the walls of blood vessels. The major determinants of mean arterial pressure (MAP) are cardiac output (CO) and total peripheral arterial resistance (systemic vascular resistance) and it is the product of CO and total peripheral resistance (TPR). CO in turn is determined by stroke volume (SV) × heart rate (HR). That means MAP = SV × HR × TPR. SV is dependent on preload, afterload and myocardial contractility. Systemic vascular resistance or peripheral resistance is decided by functional and anatomical changes in small arteries and arterioles. MAP can be estimated by using the formula diastolic blood pressure (DBP) + one-third of pulse pressure where pulse pressure is the difference between the systolic and DBP.

As MAP is the product of CO and systemic vascular resistance, in simple terms systemic hypertension could be either due to an increase in CO and/or TPR. Normal BP regulation helps to maintain the perfusion of vital organs in varied situations.

■ PATHOGENIC MECHANISMS IN ESSENTIAL HYPERTENSION

The pathogenic mechanisms of EH are supposed to be multifactorial including genetic and environmental factors along with the sympathetic nervous system (SNS), renin–angiotensin–aldosterone system (RAAS) and renal regulation. Obesity, physical inactivity and excessive salt intake are some of the identified environmental factors associated with hypertension.

Autonomic Nervous System

Sympathetic nervous system plays a major role in the regulation of normal circulatory hemodynamics. Our knowledge about the role of SNS in EH dates back to 1900s. The literature shows treatment with splanchnicectomy and lumbar sympathectomy for EH is useful modality of treatment, but with disabilities and inconveniences.[2] Sympathetic system is activated consistently in patients with hypertension along with decreased parasympathetic activity compared to normotensives. Sympathetic hyperactivity is relevant to both the generation and maintenance of hypertension. Some of the causes of increased sympathetic activity in EH include genetic factors, obesity and psychosocial stress. Psychosocial stress increases plasma epinephrine (E) in EH subjects and is accompanied by sodium retention and enhanced vascular reactivity.

Elevations of plasma norepinephrine (NE), epinephrine (E) and dopamine (DA) are seen in EH. Activation of SNS is associated with increase in HR, CO and peripheral vascular resistance affecting BP. Sympathetic activation leads to direct α-receptor–mediated vasoconstriction and vascular remodeling. Apart from this, many trophic factors, including transforming growth factor, insulin-like growth factor 1 and fibroblast growth factors are released which again cause increased vascular resistance.

Increased SNS activity is shown to alter baroreflex and chemoreflex pathways at peripheral and central levels. Baroreceptors are reset to higher pressure resulting in suppression of sympathetic inhibition after activation of aortic baroreceptor nerves. There is exaggerated chemoreflex function resulting in enhanced sympathetic activation in response to stimuli like hypoxia.[3]

Dopamine inhibits aldosterone secretion and enhances sodium excretion. Renal sympathetic stimulation can also contribute to hypertension. In animal models, direct renal nerve stimulation resulted in renal sodium and water retention increasing intravascular volume.[4] Increased sympathetic activation of the kidney is identified to have its role in the pathogenesis of hypertension. Renal sympathetic stimulation is also increased in hypertensive patients compared with normotensive controls.[3]

Centrally, acting sympatholytic agents and α- and β-adrenergic antagonists have proved to be very effective in reducing BP in patients with EH. The clinical utility of these centrally acting agents and of the α-adrenergic antagonists in treating hypertension is reduced over the years due to problems with adverse effects of these agents and not due to lack of antihypertensive efficacy.

Genetic Basis of Essential Hypertension

It has been well known that hypertension clusters within families. Recent studies have shown that one-third to one-half of BP variation may have a genetic basis. Main candidate genes possibly involved in EH are identified and hypertension is caused when it is exposed to a variable compilation of environmental factors.[5] For identifying genetic variants contributing to EH, the methods adopted were candidate gene approach and genome-wide scanning.[6] Genetic studies were successful in finding genetic determinants of secondary hypertension, but not in EH. EH is probably caused by the combination of small quantitative changes in the expression of many genes associated with a variable collection of environmental factors. It was proposed that the regulation of "youth and aging proteins"—GDF11, GDF15, JAM-A/1 and CCL11—can be target object of EH therapy.[7]

Age, Gender and Essential Hypertension

The prevalence of hypertension and so the incidence of arterial stiffness and related cardiovascular disease (stroke, myocardial infarction and pulmonary veno-occlusive disease) increases with age.[8] Many cross-sectional studies have shown that BP particularly systolic arterial pressure increases with age. Though there is some increase in diastolic pressure, it levels off by the age of 60 years and may tend to fall slightly. This is being modified by various factors like gender, obesity and physical activity.[9] Aging is a powerful cardiovascular risk factor associated with endothelial dysfunction. Physiological aging shows a progressively reduced nitric oxide (NO) availability, and with advanced age some degree of oxidative stress emerges.[10] Aging is also associated with increased inflammation and inflammatory markers like interleukin-6 and tumor necrosis factor-α. This leads to vascular endothelial dysfunction and arterial stiffening, thus contributing to the pathogenesis of hypertension.[8]

Studies show that men have higher BP than women through much of life regardless of race and ethnicity[11] and so the cardiovascular complications. Coronary events are twice common in men than women.[12] Age associated increase in BP is more in women than in men after their fifties.[13] This may be the impact of menopause and the related hormonal changes. Estrogens decrease systemic vascular resistance, restore and improve vascular endothelial function. Estrogen loss is associated with accelerated atherosclerosis.[14] Androgens may contribute to vasoconstriction and hypertension by up-regulation on thromboxane A2 expression, NE, angiotensin II (AT II) expression and endothelial action. Thus males have higher BP than females.[15] In males the estradiol—testosterone ratio modulates the atherosclerotic effect of androgen. This is due to the effect of estradiol on vasculature, which is formed by aromatization of testosterone.[16]

Role of Diet in Essential Hypertension

Studies have shown that salt intake has a role in pathogenesis of hypertension. In INTERSALT study; 24-hour urinary sodium was significantly associated with BP as well as the increase in BP with age.[16] The INTERMAP (International Study on Macro/Micronutrients and Blood Pressure) showed that a lower salt intake and smaller sodium or potassium ratio resulted in lower population BP.[17]

In the normal state, increased sodium intake causes an increase in extracellular volume and BP resulting in an increased excretion of sodium and water. These small increases in BP produce natriuresis that restores sodium balance and returns BP to normal. In EH, this pressure natriuresis is impaired.

The alteration in BP with changes in dietary salt intake is variable; dividing people into salt sensitive and insensitive groups. According to "salt sensitivity" trait, BP response with salt reduction is also variable. In salt sensitive persons, rise of BP with salt intake is high contrary to salt insensitive persons who have little or no change. This may be related to the underlying genetic variability in natriuresis. It is estimated that about 50–60% of hypertensives are salt sensitive.

In the DASH (Dietary Approaches to Stop Hypertension) sodium trial, the combination of reduced salt along with DASH diet (rich in fruits vegetables, low fat diet) lowered systolic BP in patients with prehypertension and stage 1 hypertension, which is seen best in black patients, middle- and old-aged and in patients with severe hypertension.[18]

Potassium supplementation, 40–80 mEq/day lowers BP. The benefit of potassium supplementation was significant in hypertensives who does not restrict sodium and also in blacks with hypertension. Higher magnesium intake also has been associated with lower BP. Proposed mechanism is calcium antagonistic action of magnesium on smooth muscle tone, causing vasorelaxation. Other protective factors are fish intake, high fiber diet and increased consumption of fruits and vegetables.

Obesity, Insulin Resistance and Hypertension

Obesity not only forms a component of metabolic syndrome along with insulin resistance, dyslipidemia, hypertension and hyperglycemia, but can itself lead to hypertension.[19]

Insulin resistance occurs from insensitivity of muscle tissues to insulin, which results in compensatory hyperinsulinemia leading to increase in sympathetic activity and development of hypertension.[19] Insulin resistance leads to increased lipolysis and increased concentration of free fatty acids, which can cause vascular dysfunction and accelerated atherosclerosis. Other actions of insulin that increase BP are increased renal sodium reabsorption (antinatriuretic effect of insulin), alteration of transmembrane ion transport, augmented responses to endogenous vasoconstrictors and stimulation of vascular growth by insulin resulting in hypertrophy of vessels.

Sympathetic nervous system activity is increased in obesity particularly of the kidney and of the skeletal muscle. Causes for activation of the SNS in obesity remain uncertain and may be multiple. Increased levels of plasma renin activity, plasma angiotensin II and aldosterone values were observed in humans with obesity.[20]

Renin–Angiotensin–Aldosterone System

Renin–angiotensin system (RAS) has got a crucial role in hypertension. Renin is synthesized in juxtaglomerular cells and released in response to hypovolemia and sympathetic activation. Renin cleaves angiotensinogen to angiotensin I (AT I), which in turn is converted to AT II by angiotensin converting enzyme. AT II by its action on AT I receptor is a potent arteriolar vasoconstrictor increasing peripheral resistance and enhancing reabsorption of sodium and water, increasing BP. AT II stimulates secretion of adrenal aldosterone augmenting the above mentioned action.

High RAS activity may be contributing to EH and high renin levels are seen in patients with EH. But the plasma renin level is not correlated with the magnitude of hypertension. Apart from circulating RAAS, tissue RAAS is involved in maintenance of hemodynamics by its proliferative and hypertrophic effects, potentially resulting in vascular hypertrophy and enhanced atherosclerosis. Cardiovascular complications like myocardial infarction are also more common in patients with increased plasma renin, and show beneficial effect with the use of angiotensin-converting enzyme (ACE) inhibitor and angiotensin receptor II blocker (ARB) in reducing these cardiovascular complications.[21]

Vascular Mechanisms in Essential Hypertension

Vascular endothelium plays an important role in maintaining vascular homeostasis, by the production of the relaxing factor nitric oxide (NO). NO is produced in response to flow-induced shear stress. Beyond vasodilatation, NO has other vasoprotective effects like inhibition of platelet adhesion and aggregation, leukocyte adhesion and migration, and smooth muscle cell proliferation. Decrease in NO production is the major factor responsible for endothelial dysfunction with advancing age and hypertension. In addition to this, excess production of reactive oxygen species

(ROS) reducing NO availability by binding of super oxide to NO contributes to endothelial dysfunction resulting in accelerated atherosclerosis and cardiovascular events.[10] Endothelin-1 (ET-1) is an endothelial cell product that causes vasoconstriction through endothelin receptor type A in vascular smooth muscle. In hypertension, there is increased sensitivity to the vasoconstrictor effects of ET-1. Other vasoregulatory substances include prostacyclin causing vasodilation and thromboxane A2 and prostaglandin A2 causing vasoconstriction. EH is associated with increased risk of arterial thrombotic disease like myocardial infarction and ischemic stroke. This is attributed to the prothrombotic state in hypertension and is contributed by many factors.[22]

Other Factors in Essential Hypertension

Some earlier studies have proposed that hyperuricemia may have a key causal role in the onset of primary hypertension, with increased uric acid (UA) levels resulting in endothelial dysfunction, vasculopathy, and elevated BP.[23] Serum UA is independently associated with nondipper circadian pattern in young patients with newly diagnosed EH.[24]

Vitamin D insufficiency is associated with a higher risk of hypertension. Vitamin D is a potent endocrine suppressor of renin biosynthesis. There is some proof of an inverse correlation between serum vitamin D status and prevalence of EH in epidemiological studies.[4]

CONCLUSION

The pathogenic mechanisms of EH are multifactorial. It involves interplay of genetics, SNS, RAAS along with other factors including diet, vitamin D, psychological stress and factors related to vascular mechanisms and many more. It is an interaction of these various mechanisms, which is contributing to EH and this knowledge is important in prevention and appropriate timely interventions.

REFERENCES

1. Palmer RS. Essential hypertension: a selected review and commentary. N Engl J Med. 1955; 252(22):940-7.
2. Grimson KS, Orgain ES, Anderson B, et al. Results of treatment of patients with hypertension by total thoracic and partial to total lumbar sympathectomy, splanchnicectomy and celiac ganglionectomy. Ann Surg. 1949;129:850-71.
3. Oparil S, Zaman MA, Calhoun DA. Pathogenesis of Hypertension. Ann Intern Med. 2003;139:761-76.
4. Ullah MI, Uwaifo GI, Nicholas WC, et al. Does vitamin d deficiency cause hypertension? Current evidence from clinical studies and potential mechanisms. Int J endocrinology. 2010;2010:579640.
5. Puddu P, Puddu GM, Cravero E, et al. The genetic basis of essential hypertension, Acta Cardiologica. 2007;62:3:281-93.
6. Timberlake DS, O'Connor DT, Parmer RJ. Molecular genetics of essential hypertension: recent results and emerging strategies. Curr Opin Nephrol Hypertens. 2001; 10(1):71-9.
7. Kuznik BI, Davydov SO, Smolyakov YN, et al. The role of «Youth and aging proteins» in essential hypertension pathogenesis. Adv Gerontol. 2018;31(3):362-7.
8. Sun Z. Aging, arterial stiffness, and hypertension. Hypertension. 2014;65:252-6.
9. Freis ED. Studies in hemodynamics and hypertension. Hypertension. 2001;38:1-5.
10. Bruno RM, Masi S, Taddei M, et al. Essential hypertension and functional microvascular ageing. High Blood Press Cardiovasc Prev. 2018;25(1):35-40.
11. Vokonas PS, Kannel WB, Cupples LA. Epidemiology and risk of hypertension in the elderly: the Framingham Study. J Hypertens Suppl. 1988;6:S3-9.
12. Pencina MJ, D'Agostino RB, Larson MG, et al. Predicting the 30-year risk of cardiovascular disease: the framingham heart study. Circulation. 2009;119:3078-84.
13. Burt VL, Whelton P, Roccella EJ, et al. Prevalence of hypertension in the US adult population. Results from the Third National Health and Nutrition Examination Survey, 1988-1991. Hypertension. 1995;25:305-13.
14. Vitale C, Mendelsohn ME, Rosano GM. Gender differences in the cardiovascular effect of sex hormones. Nat Rev Cardiol. 2009;6:532-10.
15. Saxena S, Ali AO, Saxena M. Pathophysiology of essential hypertension: an update. Expert Rev Cardiovasc Ther. 2018;16(12):879-87.

16. Intersalt Cooperative Research Group. Intersalt: an international study of electrolyte excretion and blood pressure: results for 24 h urinary sodium and potassium excretion. BMJ. 1988;297:319-28.

17. Stamler J, Elliott P, Dennis B, et al. INTERMAP: background, aims, design, methods, and descriptive statistics (nondietary). J Hum Hypertens. 2003;17:591-608.

18. Juraschek SP, Miller ER 3rd, Weaver CM, et al. Effects of sodium reduction and the dash diet in relation to baseline BP. J Am Coll Cardiol. 2017;70(23):2841.

19. Kotchen TA. Obesity-related hypertension: epidemiology, pathophysiology, and clinical management. Am J Hypertens. 2010;23(11)1170-8.

20. Jiang SZ, Lu W, Zong XF, et al. Obesity and hypertension. Exp Ther Med. vol. 2016;12(4):2395-9.

21. Allikmets K, Parik T, Viigimaa M. The renin-angiotensin system in essential hypertension: associations with cardiovascular risk. Blood Press. 1999;8(2):70-8.

22. Gkaliagkousi E, Passacquale G, Douma S, et al. Platelet activation in essential hypertension: implications for antiplatelet treatment. Am J Hypertens. 2010;23(3):229-36.

23. Reynolds T. Serum uric acid, the endothelium and hypertension: an association revisited. J Hum Hypertens. 2007;21(8):591.

24. Giallauria F, Predotti P, Casciello A, et al. Serum uric acid is associated with non-dipping circadian pattern in young patients (30–40 years old) with newly diagnosed essential hypertension. Clin Exp Hypertens. 2016;38(2);233-7.

The Renin–Angiotensin–Aldosterone System

Mangesh Tiwaskar

■ INTRODUCTION

The renin–angiotensin–aldosterone system (RAAS) is a hormonal deluge that portrays the homeostatic control of arterial pressure, systemic vascular resistance (SVR), tissue perfusion, and extracellular volume impacting cardiac output and blood pressure. RAAS has attracted augmented attention of medical fraternity in last three decades chiefly due to the advent of the pharmacological therapies for management of hypertension. Dysregulation of RAAS plays an importunate role in the causation of the cardiovascular and renal disorders. RAAS serves as an exceptional endocrine spindle which is initiated by highly regulated renin secretion to form the angiotensinogen (II) which governs the pivotal cascade in blood pressure regulation with the help of aldosterone—a mineralocorticoid. In this chapter we will attempt to especially decrypt the nexus of RAAS and blood pressure regulation and will try and get a bird's eye view of the role of various pharmacological interventions to channelize the dysregulated RAAS homeostasis in a quest to control hypertension.

■ RAAS: HISTORICAL PANORAMA

The discovery of the renin–angiotensin system retracts to 1898 from the studies done by Tigerstedt and Bergman, who reported the vasopressor effect of renal extracts; they christened the extract—*Renin* based on its origin. They demonstrated the existence of a heat-labile substance in crude extracts of rabbit renal cortex that caused a sustained increase in arterial pressure.[1] But this concept was ignored and criticized widely until in 1934; when Goldblatt and colleagues validated that the renal ischemia induced by ligation of the renal artery cajoled hypertension.[1] Shortly thereafter it was also established along with the renin, ischemic kidney also released a heat-stable, short-lived pressor substance and it was proved that renin's vasopressor effect was indirect due to its proteolytic effect on a plasma substrate which got eventually baptized as "*Angiotensinogen*—(initially got labeled as Angiotonin or Hypertensin)". In 1950s, while endeavoring the purification of angiotensinogen, Skeggs and team invented two forms of this peptide "*Angiotensin (Ang)*" which are eventually titled as "*Ang I*" and "*Ang II*".[2] Later they also realized that in presence of another plasma enzyme—angiotensin-converting enzyme (ACE)—Ang I gets cleaved to Ang II.[3] Thereafter as the interest of researchers globally sored up and the huge work performed in this field also revealed that it's this angiotensinogen II also stimulated the release of *Aldosterone* from adrenal cortex—a major governor of Sodium (Na^+) and Potassium (K^+) regulation.[4] These benchmark discoveries ultimately establi-shed the concept of "*Renin-Angiotensin-Aldosterone System*" popularly epitome as "*RAAS*" which regulates both blood pressure and fluid—electrolyte fulcrum.

■ RAAS—COMPONENTS SIMPLIFIED

The RAAS cascade initiated with biosynthesis of angiotensinogen in liver and renin in juxtaglomerular (JG) cells lining the afferent arterioles of renal glomeruli. Renin gets synthesized from preprohormone which gets divorced to pro-renin—a precursor of renin. Mellowed renin gets stored in granules of JG cells and gets secreted by exostosis in kidneys and systemic circulation of stimulation (Fig. 1).

Renin secretion is governed by four mechanisms:[5]

1. Renal baroreceptors which sense the pressure changes in the renal blood circulation
2. Sodium chloride (NaCl) delivery to macula densa cells in distal convoluted tubules
3. Sympathetic stimulation through β-1 adrenergic receptors
4. Negative feedback through Ang II.

Renin secretion is stimulated by a decrease in perfusion pressure or in NaCl delivery and by sympathetic overactivity. Renin is also synthesized in other tissues, including brain, adrenal glands, ovaries and visceral adipose

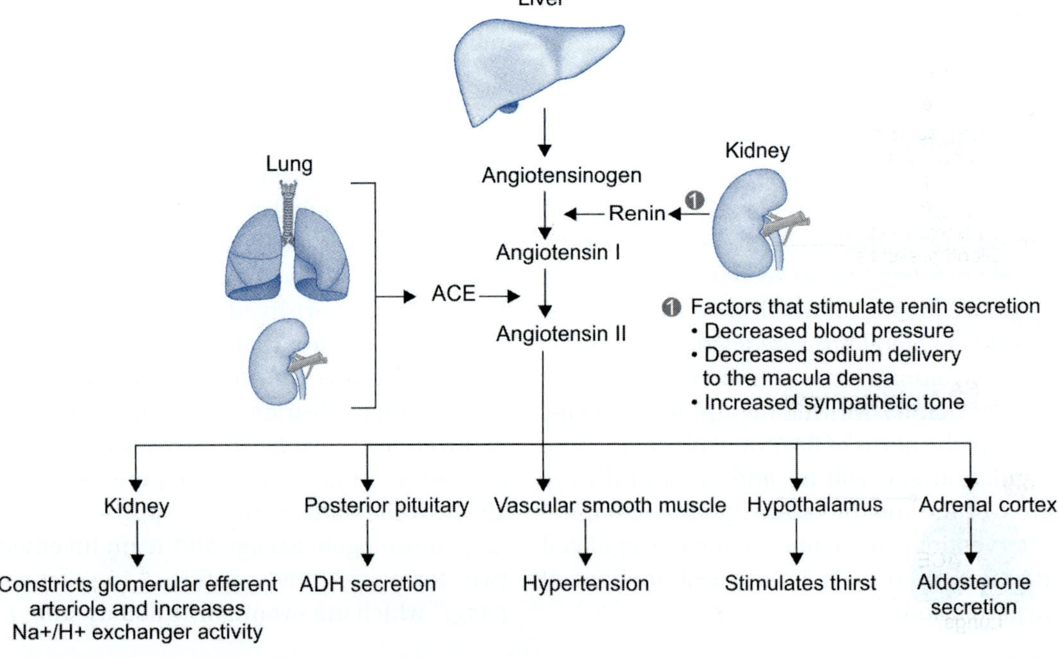

(ACE: angiotensin-converting enzyme; ADH: antidiuretic hormone)

Fig. 1: Renin–angiotensin–aldosterone system.

tissue, and perhaps heart and vascular tissue also. The factors regulating synthesis and possible actions of renin in these other tissues are poorly understood and not well documented.

Renin is the prime determinant of RAAS activity—it regulates RAAS by its cleaving action on "angiotensinogen"—a large molecular weight globulin, primarily secreted continuously from liver. Angiotensinogen is also encountered in other organs like kidney, brain, heart, vascular, adrenal gland, ovary, placenta and adipose tissue (Fig. 2).[6] Angiotensinogen can get influenced by steroids, thyroid hormones, inflammatory cytokines (e.g. interleukin-1 and tumor necrosis factor-α), and Ang II. Angiotensinogen gets chopped to Ang I by renin which is an inactive decapeptide. Ang I loses its C-terminal dipeptide by process of hydrolysis executed by an enzyme—ACE to get converted to an active octapeptide Ang II which is a potent vasoconstrictor.

Angiotensin-converting enzyme, membrane-bound exopeptidase, is localized on the plasma membranes of various cell types, including vascular endothelial cells, microvillar brush border epithelial cells, neuroepithelial cells, etc. ACE primarily dissects Ang I, but it also rips bradykinin and kallikrein—the vasodilator polypeptides to inactive metabolites.[7] Thus, effectively, the lytic actions of ACE potentially result in increased vasoconstriction and decreased vasodilation.

Angiotensin II gets further cleaved to Ang III, and Ang III gets cleaved Ang IV by losing one amino acid from their N-terminals.[8] Preclinical studies have suggested a cooperative effect of Ang IV in Ang II signaling. For instance, it appears that in the brain, Ang IV increases blood pressure by cooperating

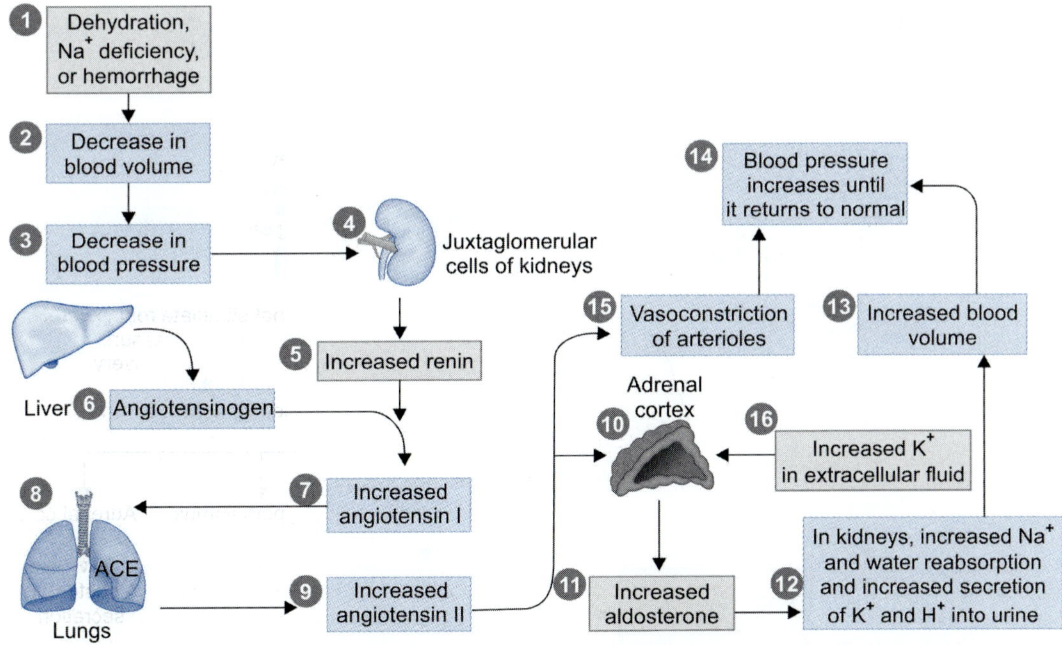

(ACE: angiotensin-converting enzyme)

Fig. 2: Regulation of aldosterone secretion by the Renin–angiotensin–aldosterone pathway.

with Ang II on angiotensin II type 1 (AT1)-receptor signaling (Fig. 3).

As has been noted earlier, Ang II is the primary effector of a diverse set of RAAS-induced physiological and pathophysiological actions. There are at least four angiotensin receptor subtypes been described.[9]

- *Type 1 (AT1) Receptor*: It is widely distributed on many cell types in Ang II target organs. Most of the established physiological and pathophysiological effects of Ang II have been mediated by AT1 receptor. These include actions on the cardiovascular system (vasoconstriction, elevated blood pressure, raised cardiac contractility, vascular, and cardiac hypertrophy), urinary system (renal tubular Na^+ reabsorption, inhibition of renin release), sympathetic nervous system, and adrenal cortex (aldosterone synthesis stimulation). Other effects of Ang II on cell growth and proliferation,

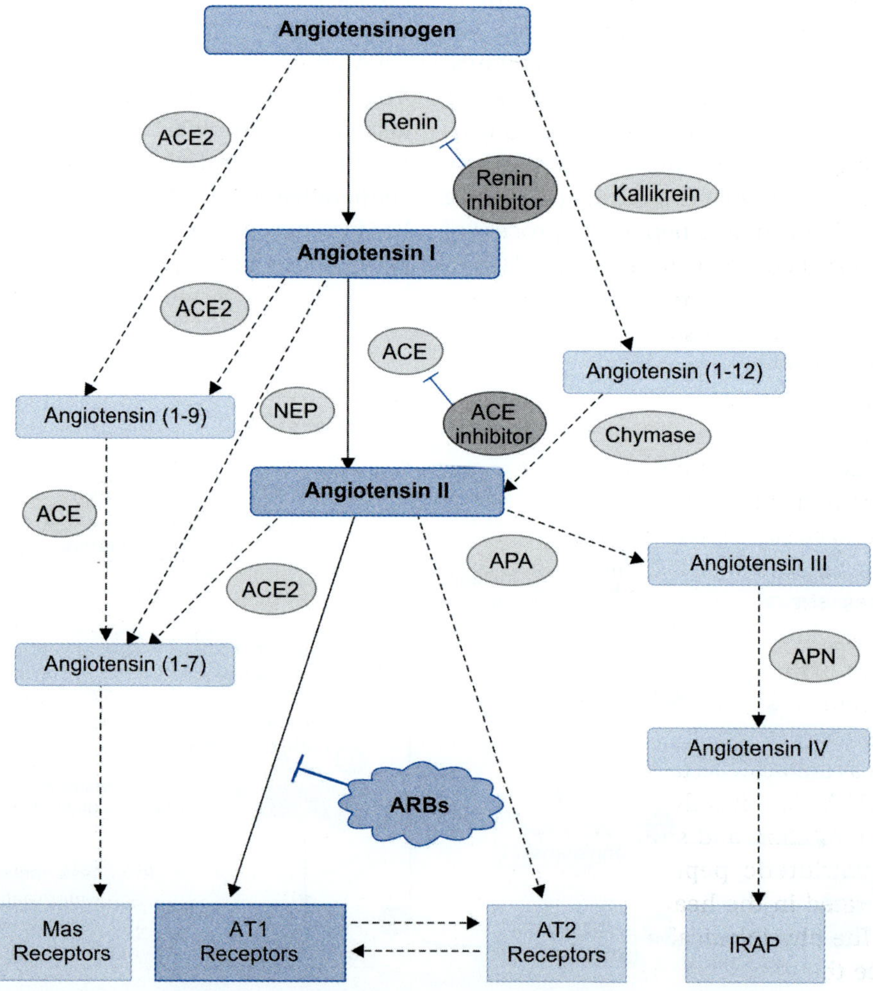

(ACE: angiotensin-converting enzyme; APA: aminopeptidase A; APN: aminopeptidase N; ARB: angiotensin receptor blocker; IRAP: insulin-regulated aminopeptidase; NEP: neutral endopeptidase)

Fig. 3: Renin–angiotensin system and the associated antihypertensive drugs.

oxidative stress, and inflammatory responses are also mediated by the AT1 receptor

- *Type 2 (AT2) Receptor*: It is abundant during fetal life in the brain, kidney, and other sites, and its levels decrease markedly in the postnatal period. There is some evidence that, despite low levels of expression in the adult, the AT2 receptor might mediate vasodilation and antiproliferative and apoptotic effects in the vascular smooth muscles (VSMs). However, the importance of any of these AT2-mediated actions remains uncertain
- *Type 3 (AT3) receptor*: The exact action is still desolate and undiscovered fully
- *Type 4 (AT4) receptor*: They are thought to mediate the release of plasminogen activator inhibitor-1 (PAI-1).

Zona glomerulosa, the outermost zone of the adrenal cortex, is also acted upon by the Ang II, via the AT1 receptor, to stimulate the production of aldosterone. Aldosterone plays a major role in regulating extracellular volume since it is a major regulator of Na^+ and K^+ balance. It acts to increase the reabsorption of Na^+ and water in the distal tubules and collecting ducts (as well as in the colon and salivary and sweat glands) and thus promotes excretion of K^+ (and hydrogen ion).[10] It stimulates the release of vasopressin or [antidiuretic hormone (ADH)] that enhances the fluid retention capacity of the kidneys. Thirst is stimulated due to the amount of Na^+ being reabsorbed. In addition, aldosterone stimulates cardiac hypertrophy.

The RAAS is not only modulated by the internal inhibition and stimulation but also by the natriuretic peptides (NPs), which are generated in the heart, brain and other organs. The physiological function of NPs is to reduce the blood volume and resistance in the systemic vasculature. NPs increase the glomerular filtration rate that results into increased natriuresis (sodium excretion) and increased fluid excretion (diuresis). Moreover, they impede release of renin and reduce circulating levels of Ang II and aldosterone. This results in systemic vasodilation.

■ SICK RAAS AND ITS AFTERMATH

Dysregulation of the RAAS is involved in the pathogenesis of several hypertensive and cardiovascular disorders. Glitched RAAS plays a pivotal role in causation of essential hypertension. It is well-known that plasma renin levels differ widely in patients with "Essential" hypertension.[11] Around 15% patients with essential hypertension have mild-to-moderate rise in the plasma renin activity (PRA), with several postulated mechanisms, that includes increased sympathetic activity and mild volume depletion. This kind of high-renin essential hypertension is mostly prevalent among the younger males. Most of the of essential hypertensive patients (50–60%) have PRA within the "normal" range, while the fact that a normal renin level in the face of hypertension (which ought to suppress renin secretion) may be inappropriate, is debated upon. Also, it has been indicated by the therapeutic responses to RAAS blocking agents that the maintenance of normal renin levels may indeed have a say in increasing the blood pressure, which suggests that renin-dependent mechanisms may be held responsible in more than 70% of patients with essential hypertension.

The RAAS also plays a significant vital role in several nonhypertensive conditions, and in particular in congestive heart failure (CHF) and the other edematous disorders. Additionally, with respect to CHF, Ang II contribution to the increased peripheral vascular resistance (cardiac afterload) plays an important role in the progressive ventricular dysfunction.

There is additional clear confirmation (again from responses to the blockade of RAAS) is that Ang II is involved in the development of both vascular and cardiac hypertrophy and remodeling, as well as on mechanisms contributing to damage in the vasculature and atherosclerosis and also effects that possibly are highly responsible for morbidity and mortality, beyond cardiovascular disease progression. The causes for these pathologic effects of Ang II are vague since they often happen in the absence of any perturbation of the circulating RAAS. It has been thus concluded that there may be dysregulation of some component(s), for example ACE levels, AT-receptor subtypes balance, or even local synthesis of renin or angiotensinogen, that is accountable for such phenomena, but clear-cut evidence of such derangements is mostly unavailable.[12]

RAAS INHIBITION

Because renin is the initial and rate-limiting step in the RAAS cascade, it has long been considered the logical therapeutic target for blocking the system. Renin inhibition induced decreases in plasma renin levels, Ang I, Ang II, and aldosterone, along with decreases in blood pressure.[13]

DIRECT RENIN INHIBITOR

This compound differs from the angiotensin-converting enzyme inhibitors (ACEIs) and angiotensin receptor blockers (ARBs) in that, by blocking the catalytic activity of renin at the point of activation of the RAAS, it blocks the synthesis of all angiotensin peptides and prevents the compensatory increase in renin activity. Aliskiren, is available for use, but it lost its popularity after its worsened side effect profile especially after using it in combination with ACE inhibitors or ARBs. This combination therapy is no more advocated (Flowchart 1).[14]

ANGIOTENSIN-CONVERTING ENZYME INHIBITORS

These inhibitors were discovered, in 1960s, from the peptides isolated from the venom of Brazilian arrowhead viper (*Bothrops jararaca*) which were shown to inhibit the ACE. Synthetic analog of the peptide fraction of snake venom is captopril—first ACE inhibitor to be approved for the use of treating hypertension. Because many of the unacceptable side effects of captopril, such as proteinuria, skin rashes, and altered taste, were attributed to the sulfhydryl group, subsequent work led to the development of ACEIs with carboxyl group (e.g. lisinopril, benazepril, quinapril, ramipril, perindopril, cilazapril and trandolapril) or phosphoryl group (fosinopril).[15] In general, pharmacodynamic responses to decrease in Ang II through inhibition of ACE include dose-dependent reductions in cardiac preload and afterload, with lowering of systolic and diastolic blood pressure.

Angiotensin-converting enzyme inhibitors decrease circulating and local levels of Ang II by competitively blocking the action of ACE and thus the conversion of Ang I to Ang II. ACEIs also reduce secretion of aldosterone and vasopressin and sympathetic nerve activity. However, some evidence suggest that over the long term, inhibition of ACE may be associated with a return of Ang II and aldosterone toward baseline levels (called as "ACE escape"), perhaps, as proposed, through the so-called alternate pathways activation. But its relevance is still unclear. On the other side, since ACEIs competitively inhibit the enzyme, it is possible that increased levels of Ang I (evoked by the compensatory enhancement in PRA due to the loss of negative feedback inhibition) is likely to overcome the blockade partially.[16]

Angiotensin-converting enzyme inhibitor-induced reductions in total peripheral

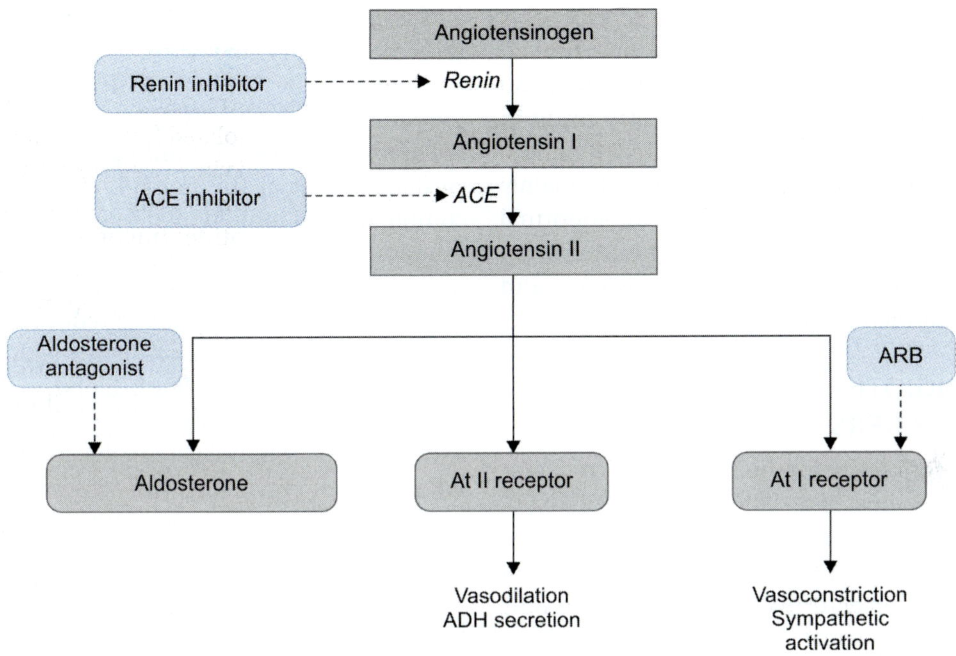

Flowchart 1: Combination therapy.

vascular resistance can take place without a significant alteration in the heart rate. ACEIs also reduce renal vascular resistance, promote renal blood flow, and enhance excretion of Na⁺ and water. Moreover, ACEIs may interfere with the progression of micro-albuminuria to proteinuria, decrease proteinuria in patients with established glomerular disease, and delay or prevent the progression of renal insufficiency to end-stage renal disease, and these effects are mediated mainly through cellular effects in the kidney and through alterations in glomerular hemodynamics. ACEI monotherapy produces a satisfactory decrease in blood pressure in 40–60% of patients with mild-to-moderate hypertension.[17] In patients with CHF, ACEIs relieve pulmonary congestion by a balanced reduction in cardiac preload and afterload. They appear to induce venous vasodilation, which increases peripheral venous capacitance and reduces right atrial pressure, pulmonary arterial pressure, capillary wedge pressures, and left ventricular filling volumes and pressures. ACEIs also induce arterial vasodilation, which reduces peripheral vascular resistance (afterload) and increases cardiac output in this patient population. ACEIs have also been shown to improve endothelial dysfunction in patients with heart failure, as well as in patients with coronary artery disease and type 2 diabetes. Several large-scale studies of various ACEIs have shown a reduction in incidence of new-onset diabetes in association with ACEI therapy. The details of these pharmacotherapies are beyond the scope of this chapter.

Though ACEI therapy is usually well-tolerated in most of the patients, some significant side effects do come along. A dry cough is the most frequent among these, which has been attributed to substance P accumulation (which is normally degraded by kininase II). More serious side effects that are common to all ACEIs are angioedema (potentiated by reduced catabolism of kinins), fetal abnormalities, and mortality. ACE inhibition may also result in hypotension, worsening of renal function, and hyperkalemia. Lastly, toxic effects, mainly related with captopril, include an abnormal (metallic or salty) taste, neutropenia, appearance of rash, hepatic toxicity, and proteinuria (membranous nephropathy).[18]

ANGIOTENSIN RECEPTOR BLOCKERS

As described beforehand, the AT1 receptor regulates most of the known actions of Ang II. Hence, along with the discovery of different receptor subtypes, specific antagonism of Ang II action at the AT1 receptor had certainly become a logical therapeutic target. They were thought to be ARBs being more specific than ACEI. The development of orally active, nonpeptide, selective AT1 receptor blockers initiated in the 1990s with the losartan synthesis. Since that time, various other ARBs have been developed, including valsartan, irbesartan, candesartan, eprosartan, telmisartan, olmesartan, and now the latest azilsartan.

Angiotensin receptor blockers act by blocking action of Ang II at the receptor level, and not by inhibiting its synthesis, they antagonize AT1-mediated effects of Ang II, irrespective of how its synthesis occurs. It can be said that significant Ang II synthesis in tissues by alternate pathways can limit the efficacy of ACEIs , but not of ARBs. A mechanism that contributes to the "escape" phenomenon following long-term ACE inhibition plays a role in that.[19] ARB therapy actually causes an increase in Ang II levels,[20] which is freely able to bind to AT2 or other receptor subtypes. This action is in contrast to the ACEIs. It has been suggested by the earlier preclinical studies that the AT2 receptor activation might mediate

additional beneficial actions on the heart, vasculature, and kidneys.

Similar to the ACEIs, ARBs decrease blood pressure by reducing SVR; but heart rate is not affected and there is minimal effect on the cardiac output in the nonfailing heart.[20] A combination of inhibition of Ang II-mediated vasoconstriction, decreased sympathetic nervous system activity, and decreased extracellular volume result in a reduced SVR. It is noteworthy that monotherapy with ARB leads to a satisfactory decline in blood pressure in 40–60% of patients with mild-to-moderate hypertension. It has been shown that markers of inflammation in patients with atherosclerosis are reduced by the use of ARB therapy that suggests an anti-inflammatory effect, and the reversal of endothelial dysfunction in patients with hypertension, denoting the chances of significant antiatherogenic effects. ARB therapy has also been shown to improve arterial compliance independent of the blood pressure-lowering effect in patients with hypertension. This observation suggests that ARB therapy may have a role in the reversal of vascular wall damage. A number of recent large trials suggest that the ARB class may confer benefits related to the protection of target organs besides blood pressure lowering per se.

Similar to ACEIs, ARBs are contraindicated in pregnancy because of the association of RAAS blockade with increased fetal morbidity and mortality, associated with exposure during the second and third trimester in particular. The ARB therapy is otherwise usually well tolerated, even in many patients who discontinue ACEI therapy due to the side effects.

FUTURE POSSIBILITIES

Angiotensin-converting enzyme inhibitors and ARBs have been currently implicated in the treatment of hypertension, diabetic nephropathy, post myocardial infarction left ventricular dysfunction, and chronic heart failure. Their use has been shown to improve survival and considerable cardiovascular and renal benefits in the high-risk group. These outstanding benefits have been obtained even though RAAS blockade with the currently available agents may be incomplete, raising the possibility that further slow progression of cardiovascular and renal disease can result through additional therapeutic modalities for RAAS blockade. The clinical potential of parallel intervention at various sites of the RAAS is persuasive including the ACE2, Ang III, Ang IV, Ang (1-7) targeted therapies, the possibility of molecular approaches such as antisense gene therapy, targeting, for instance, renin, angiotensinogen, the AT1 receptor, or ACE, will also likely be explored in the not too distant future.

■ REFERENCES

1. Piepho RW, Beal J. An overview of antihypertensive therapy in the 20th century. J Clin Pharmacol. 2000;40:967-77.
2. Ferrario CM. Role of angiotensin II in cardiovascular disease— therapeutic implications of more than a century of research. J Renin Angiotensin Aldosterone Syst. 2006;7:3-14.
3. Skeggs LT Jr, Kahn JR, Lentz K, et al. The preparation, purification, and amino acid sequence of a polypeptide renin substrate. J Exp Med. 1957;106:439-53.
4. Sealey JE, Laragh JH. Renin-angiotensin-aldosterone system and the renal regulation of sodium, potassium, and pressure homeostasis. In: Windhager EE (ed.). Handbook of Physiology–Section 8: Renal Physiology. Volume II. New York: Oxford University Press; 1992. pp. 1409-541.
5. Brown MJ. Direct renin inhibition—a new way of targeting the renin system. J Renin Angiotensin Aldosterone Syst. 2006;7(suppl 2):S7-S11.
6. Morgan L, Broughton PF, Kalsheker N. Angiotensinogen: molecular biology, biochemistry and physiology. Int J Biochem Cell Biol. 1996;28:1211-22.
7. Carey RM, Siragy HM. Newly recognized components of the renin-angiotensin system: potential roles in cardiovascular and renal regulation. Endocr Rev. 2003;24:261-71.
8. Reudelhuber TL. The renin-angiotensin system: peptides and enzymes beyond angiotensin II. Curr Opin Nephrol Hypertens. 2005;14:155-9.
9. Stanton A. Therapeutic potential of renin inhibitors in the management of cardiovascular disorders. Am J Cardiovasc Drugs. 2003;3:389-94.
10. Funder JW. New biology of aldosterone, and experimental studies on the selective aldosterone blocker eplerenone. Am Heart J. 2002;144:S8-11.
11. Laragh J. Laragh's lessons in pathophysiology and clinical pearls for treating hypertension.
12. Am J Hypertens. 2001;14:186-94.
13. Schmidt RJ, Soman SS. Renovascular Hypertension. Available from http://www.eMedicine.com. [Last accessed August, 2019].
14. Staessen JA, Li Y, Richart T. Oral renin inhibitors. Lancet. 2006;368:1449-56.
15. Pool JL. Direct renin inhibition: focus on aliskiren. J Manag Care Pharm. 2007;13(8) (Suppl b): S21-S33.
16. Lopez-Sendon J, Swedberg K, McMurray J, et al.; for the Task Force on ACE-inhibitors of the European Society of Cardiology. Expert consensus document on angiotensin converting enzyme inhibitors in cardiovascular disease. Eur Heart J. 2004;25:1454-70.
17. Atlas SA, Case DB, Yu ZY, et al. Hormonal and metabolic effects of angiotensin converting enzyme inhibitors: possible differences between enalapril and captopril. Am J Med. 1984;77:13-7.
18. Ibrahim MM. RAS inhibition in hypertension. J Hum Hypertens. 2006;20:101-8.
19. Wong J, Patel RA, Kowey PR. The clinical use of angiotensin-converting enzyme inhibitors. Prog Cardiovasc Dis. 2004;47:116-30.
20. Ruilope LM, Rosei EA, Bakris GL, et al. Angiotensin receptor blockers: therapeutic targets and cardiovascular protection. Blood Press. 2005;14:196-209.

Molecular Basis of Hypertension

Role of Cell Membrane (Red Blood Cells and Platelets) in Essential Hypertension

Amit A Saraf, Viplav Deogaonkar

■ INTRODUCTION

Hypertension has been looked upon in various perspectives by scientists, clinicians, researchers and students of medicine from the pathophysiology to molecular medicine. From the early-on days wherein reasons for hypertension were ranging from salt and water retention to endocrine causes, the researchers have left no "stone unturned" for finding the correct treatment and possible cure for hypertension. In the same context there comes a very important and integral part of the human milieu interior, which is the cell membrane. It is the cover of virtually every living cell of the human body and hence forms the core of diagnosis and treatment of any pathological process.

This chapter helps to elucidate the role of cell membrane not only in the pathophysiology of hypertension, but also in its treatment.

■ NORMAL PHYSIOLOGY OF CELL MEMBRANE

The human cell membrane is composed of proteins, which are enclosed in a lipid bilayer. These proteins are the crux of the cell membrane, consisting of ion transport channels, receptors for various chemicals and also maintain the integrity of the cell membrane. They also play an important role in the regulation of vascular smooth muscle contraction.[1]

■ PATHOPHYSIOLOGY

The steep gradient in the concentration of sodium ions across the membrane of cells are maintained by a cation-dependent ATPase which is called a co-chemiporter. The enzyme is embedded in the cell membrane, splits ATP and transports three sodium ions from the interior in exchange for two potassium ions from the exterior. This contributes to the resting membrane potential, and the resulting ion gradients are a source of energy, driving the other cation transport mechanisms. At least three of these transporters are relevant in hypertension—bidirectional Na^+/K^+ co-transport, Na^+/Ca^{2+} counter-transport and Na^+/Li^+ counter-transport.[1,2]

In animal studies, it has been postulated that abnormal ion permeability of the cell membrane and incorrect calcium handling leads to instability of the cell membrane. This defective calcium handling leads to reducing the excitability of the membrane which has been considered the reason to increase the vascular reactivity, thereby leading to a higher peripheral vascular resistance and hence rise in the blood pressure.[1] Abnormalities in the cell membranes of platelets, red blood cells and lymphocytes have been shown to contribute especially essential hypertension. In these patients, it has been shown that these membranes are less "fluid" and hence more "stiff", leading to less permeability of the cell membrane and thereby contributing to hypertension.[3] For example, red blood cells are required for oxygen transportation. If their permeability is compromised, it leads to less oxygen delivery to the peripheral tissues and hence it can be one of the genetic causes for hypertension. Also, less "fluidity" of the red blood cells affect microcirculation and hence again causes rise in the pressures.[3] This is not seen in patients with a secondary cause for hypertension.

Calcium plays an important role in vaso-constriction. Membrane fluidity is inversely correlated to membrane stiffness, thus lack of calcium influx leads to rise in chances of high blood pressure.[3] The cell membrane regulates cytoplasmic calcium ion concentration, which in turn governs smooth muscle contractility. Patients with hypertension possess high membrane excitability and increased intracellular calcium. This increased cytoplasmic calcium also contributes to cell growth and vascular hypertrophy, which in turn leads to increased peripheral vascular resistance.[4] Thus membrane mechanics play a significant role in the calcium metabolism and thereby contribute to primary hypertension.[5]

Insulin is concerned with ionic trans-portation of various systems such as Ca-ATPase, Na-K-ATPase and the Na-Ca exchange system. Insulin is associated with lower fluidity of red blood cell membranes, hence implicated in essential hypertension.[3]

Similarly, high-salt diet decreases membrane fluidity and thereby contributes to rise in blood pressure. Hence patients of high blood pressure are asked to have low sodium diet.

Dyslipidemia has been shown to cause membrane abnormalities and hence contribute to rise in the blood pressure.[6]

A role of Na-K-ATPase and decreased RBC deformability has been seen. The triggering factor for changes of RBC deformability during hypercholesterolemia seems to be the increased content of cholesterol in erythrocyte membranes. This pathological process is seen both in diabetes and hypertension.[7]

Epithelial sodium channels (ENaC) are present in the membranes of the tubular cells of the kidney. Their function is to reabsorb sodium from the lumen of the tubule, thereby regulating total body sodium. Total body sodium reflects extracellular fluid (ECF) volume which in turn reflects the blood pressure. Abnormalities in this ENaC cause errors in sodium metabolism and are associated with high blood pressure.[8]

Intracellular magnesium has been shown to have some role in blood pressure control.[9] This was confirmed in a study where patients of mild-to-moderate hypertension were subjected to oral magnesium (600 mg/day). About 40% of the patients who took magnesium supplements showed significant reductions in the blood pressure (more than 10 mm Hg drop in the mean blood pressure). This was attributed to decreased intracellular sodium which was due to the magnesium ion flux at the cell membrane level.[9]

Like all the physiological processes in the human body, cell membrane too is governed by the genetic makeup of the individual. Research into the *ATP2B1* gene has shown a link to essential hypertension.[10] The absence of this gene leads to rise in the intracellular calcium and subsequently rise in the blood pressure. Further studies are on to elaborate the gene therapy to overcome this potentially treatable condition.

Structural integrity of the cell wall is autoregulated by the sympathetic system. It has been proven that altered sympathetic response will alter the cell wall:lumen ratio, thereby increasing vascular resistance, contributing to hypertension.[11]

Reactive oxygen species (ROS) contribute to a large extent to vascular cell membrane damage, which leads to oxidative stress in hypertension-associated vascular damage. This area has been extensively looked at as a potentially treatable cause of high blood pressure.[12]

Thus, in summary, there is a "physio-chemical" alteration in the cell membrane which affects the intracellular ionic balance, affects the smooth muscle contractility leading to vasospasm and cell hypertrophy leading to increased peripheral vascular resistance.[13] All these factors ultimately lead to rise in blood pressure.

■ TREATMENT MODALITIES OF HYPERTENSION (CELL MEMBRANE-BASED MODALITIES)

Antihypertensive drugs available in the market presently have been categorized in the following classes:
- Diuretics
- Sympathetic blocking agents (sympatholytics)
- Vasodilators
- Angiotensin-converting enzyme (ACE) inhibitors
- Calcium channel blockers
- Angiotensin II receptor antagonists.

All of these classes of drugs are known to act on the cell membrane of their respective target organ. For example, diuretics will cause lowering of blood pressure by primarily acting on the cell membranes of the tubules, vasodilators such as calcium channel blockers act by inhibiting the cell membrane calcium channels and thereby causing vasodilatation, etc. The mechanism of action of all these drugs has been elucidated and elaborated quite extensively. Calcium channel blockers, in vivo, have shown to modify favorably the fluidity of the red cell membranes and hence control blood pressure, but more studies are needed to quantify the same.[3] Treatment of dyslipidemia has been shown to improve the membrane stability and hence control the high blood pressure.[6]

Flowchart 1 depicts the target cellular membrane and its receptors wherein the antihypertensive work.

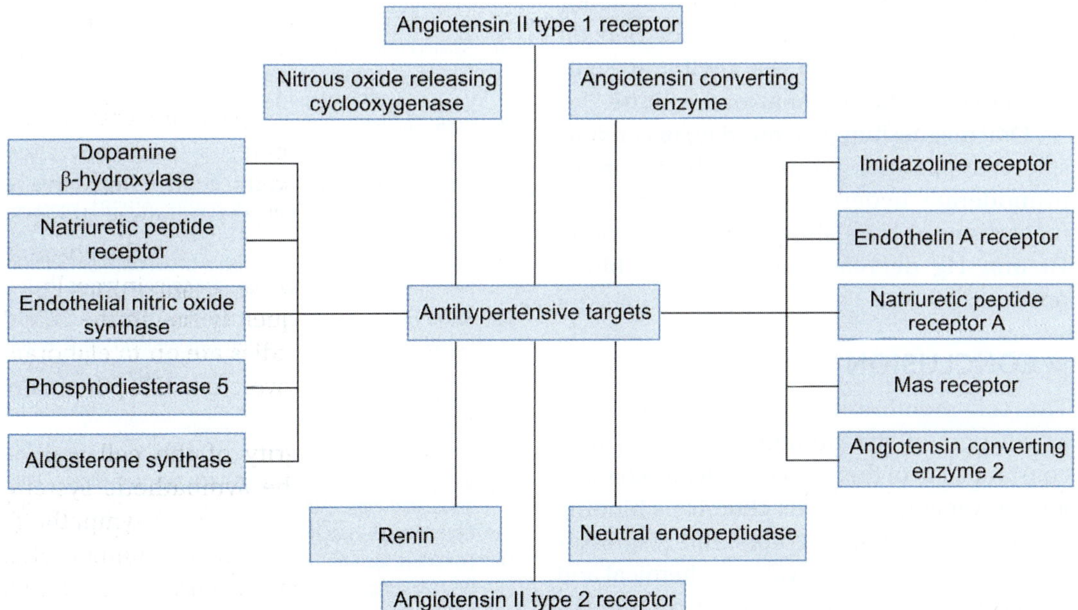

Flowchart 1: Target cellular membrane and its receptors.

Treatment of hypertension is possible on all the pathophysiological mechanisms at work on the cell membrane, right from calcium ion influx to oxidative damage to the cell wall.

RECENT ADVANCES IN TREATMENT OF HYPERTENSION (CELL MEMBRANE-BASED MODALITIES)

Eicosapentaenoic acid has been recently proven to lower the systolic blood pressure (SBP) in patients of essential hypertension. Eicosapentaenoic acid has been shown to decrease intracellular sodium concentration by altering the membrane sodium ion transportation and hence decrease SBP.[14]

Ion channels are ubiquitous in their presence. They have shown to have a role in blood pressure control. In the years to come they provide potential in newer therapeutic agents such as antisense nucleotide technology and gene therapy for hypertension.[15]

In order to deliver antihypertensive drugs to target cell membranes more effectively and thereby decrease the chances of systemic side effects, a novel mode of nanocarriers for antihypertensives is on the anvil and holds major therapeutic potential for the future.[16]

Oral magnesium (600 mg/day) in carefully selected patients (young patients, mild-to-moderate hypertension, no underlying renal disease) have shown to cause around 10 mm Hg decrease in the mean blood pressure.[9]

CONCLUSION

The cell membrane is metabolically very active part of the human body. It is in a constant state of flux with electrically charged ions traversing it, various chemicals binding to its innumerable receptors and responses of the cell membrane to various chemical and hormonal stimuli. All these in turn affect the blood pressure regulation and are all potential sites of medications of blood pressure control. The cell membrane has been successfully targeted for therapeutic purposes in modern medicine and will be continued in doing so for future therapies for optimal control of hypertension.

REFERENCES

1. Rinaldi G, Bohr D. Plasma membrane and its abnormalities in hypertension. Am J Med Sci. 1988;295(4):389-95.
2. Semple PF, Lever AF. Glimpses of the mechanisms of hypertension. Br Med J (Clin Res Ed). 1986;293(6552):901-2.
3. Tsuda K, Nishio I. Membrane fluidity and hypertension. Am J Hypertens. 2003;16(3):259-61.
4. Dominiczak AF, Bohr DF. Cell membrane abnormalities and the regulation of intracellular calcium concentration in hypertension. Clin Sci (Lond). 1990;79(5):415-23.
5. Kosch M, Hausberg M, Barenbrock M, et al. Increased membraneous calcium concentrations in primary hypertension: a causal link to pathogenesis? J Hum Hypertens. 2001;15(1):37-40.
6. Zicha J, Kunes J, Devynck MA. Abnormalities of membrane function and lipid metabolism in hypertension: A review. Am J Hypertens. 1999;12(3):315-31.
7. Radosinska J, Vrbjar N. The role of red blood cell deformability and Na,K-ATPase function in selected risk factors of cardiovascular diseases in humans: Focus on hypertension, diabetes mellitus and hypercholesterolemia. Physiol Res. 2016;65(Suppl 1):S43-54.
8. Soundararajan R, Pearce D, Hughey RP, et al. Role of epithelial sodium channels and their regulators in hypertension. J Biol Chem. 2010;285(40):30363-9.
9. Sanjuliani AF, de Abreu Fagundes VG, Francischetti EA. Effects of magnesium on blood pressure and intracellular ion levels of Brazilian hypertensive patients. Int J Cardiol. 1996;56(2):177-83.
10. Okuyama Y, Hirawa N, Fujita M, et al. The effects of anti-hypertensive drugs and mechanism of hypertension in vascular smooth muscle cell-specific ATP2B1 knockout mice. Hypertens Res. 2018;41(2):80-7.
11. Swales JD. Functional disturbance of the cell membrane in hypertension. J Hypertens Suppl. 1990;8(7):S203-11.
12. Touyz RM. Reactive oxygen species, vascular oxidative stress, and redox signaling in hypertension: what is the clinical significance? Hypertension. 2004;44(3):248-52.
13. Swales JD. Membrane transport of ions in hypertension. Cardiovasc Drugs Ther. 1990;4(Suppl 2):367-72.
14. Miyajima T, Tsujino T, Saito K, et al. Effects of eicosapentaenoic acid on blood pressure, cell membrane fatty acids, and intracellular sodium concentration in essential hypertension. Hypertens Res. 2001;24(5):537-42.
15. Baker EH. Ion channels and the control of blood pressure. Br J Clin Pharmacol. 2000;49(3):185-98.
16. Alam T, Khan S, Gaba B, et al. Nanocarriers as treatment modalities for hypertension. Drug Deliv. 2017;24(1):358-69.

Matrix Metalloproteinases and the Extracellular Matrix

B Khandelwal, Chamma Gupta

■ INTRODUCTION

The multifaceted nature of complications that accompany hypertension (HTN) makes it challenging to develop a molecular model for HTN and its target organ damage. Cardiac and vessel remodeling, atherosclerosis and diabetes mellitus is present in patients with family history of HTN even before they develop HTN. The varied pathophysiological phenomenon has not been conclusively defined under a common molecular basis. However, extracellular matrix (ECM) and its regulation by matrix metalloproteinase (MMPs) have been documented extensively in the pathogenesis of HTN. There are still unanswered questions pertaining to MMPs being involved in the early stages of hypertension and whether they are mediators of hypertension and associated complications.

Vascular Remodeling in Hypertension

Both large (conductance) arteries (i.e. aorta and large arteries) and small (resistance) arterioles are involved in the pathophysiology of HTN. The structure of the conductance arteries helps in serving as a blood reservoir and to stretch or recoil corresponding with the contractile activity of heart. The arterioles,

which is the major site of resistance has more smooth muscle cells and less elastic fibers in their walls. Minor changes in the caliber of the arterioles lead to large changes in the total peripheral resistance. Several types of remodeling, i.e. eutrophic, hypertrophic and hypotrophic are identified in the vasculature depending on the decrease or increase of cellular components of the wall or in its absence.

Thickening of the medial layer leads to reduction of the lumen of the vessel and increased ratio of wall/lumen of the vessel. This is known as eutrophic inward remodeling. This is observed in the initial stage of mild hypertension. Increase in the lumen of the vessel without alteration of its cross sectional area is characteristic of eutrophic outward remodeling. Increased ratio of wall/lumen of the vessel caused by thickening of the medial layer is observed in hypertrophic inward remodeling. This has been observed in renovascular hypertension and in well-established HTN. Hypotrophic outward remodeling is characterized by an increase in the lumen of the vessel wall with decrease in its cross sectional area. Increased intravascular pressure or reduced blood flow results in concentric (inward) vascular remodeling while increased blood flow leads to eccentric (outer) remodeling. However, multiple factors may work simultaneously in a patient and so the effect of antihypertensive drugs on the remodeling of medial layer is also variable.

Rearrangement of the existing cellular and extracellular components of the arterial wall leads to remodeling.[1] Hypertension-induced maladaptive remodeling is improved by inhibition of ECM proteolysis by MMPs. The hypertrophic remodeling mainly in conductance arteries is associated with increased proliferation of vascular smooth muscle cells (VSMC), thickening of arterial media and resynthesis of many ECM components. Resistance arteries undergo eutrophic modeling due to rearrangement of VSMC. MMP-2 degrades collagen type IV thus facilitating migration, proliferation, vascular wall thickening and thus further remodeling. There is a rise in synthesis of collagen type I, tenascin and elastin in VSMC as a compensation to MMP-2 degradation of collagen IV; leading to further increase in the vascular wall thickening. The cleavage products of collagen degradation bind to different integrins in VSMC leading to synthesis of new ECM components. Increased apoptosis and/or atrophy of some layers of vascular wall further contribute to the remodeling.[2]

Cardiac Remodeling in Hypertension

The increased wall pressure in heart results in increase in wall tension and stress leading to excess accumulation of ECM components which in turn raises myocardial stiffness, thus compromising diastolic function. Further accumulation impairs myocardial contraction and systolic function. In postmortem human hearts and endomyocardial human biopsies an increase in the amount of fibrillar collagen in the myocardium of patients with hypertensive heart disease was observed.[3] An increase in the proteoglycan biglycan, and the adhesive proteins fibronectin and laminin are also reported.[4] The increase in wall stress itself is the initial stimulus for excessive collagen deposition which starts as a physiological process but later becomes maladaptive and leads to fibrosis.

■ MATRIX METALLOPROTEINASES

The matrix metalloproteinases are members of metzincins, an ubiquitously expressed family of multi-domain zinc (II)—dependent endopeptidases. The first MMP, interstitial collagenase was identified in 1962 as the protease responsible for the degradation of fibrillar collagen in tadpole tail during metamorphosis which was subsequently named as MMPI after identification of similar collagenase in human skin.[5] The versatile MMP family with wide physiological functions consists of 23 distinct proteases which share structural domains but have variable substrate specificity, cellular sources, tissue localization, membrane binding and transcriptional regulation. There are several conserved domains in the excreted MMPs. The prodomain shields the catalytic domain in the inactive form of the enzyme. The gelatinases (MMP-2 and MMP-9) additionally contain a series of three fibronectin type II inserts in the catalytic domain, which helps binding of gelatine and collagen (Fig. 1).[6]

■ EXTRACELLULAR MATRIX

Extracellular matrix is broadly classified into three major types—structural proteins such as collagen and elastin, specialized and adhesive proteins such as fibronectin and laminin, and proteoglycan and glycosaminoglycan. Type I and type III collagen form 60% and 30% of vascular collagens, respectively and are found in intima, media and adventitia. They are the major source of tensile strength. Elastin in the ECM provides elasticity and

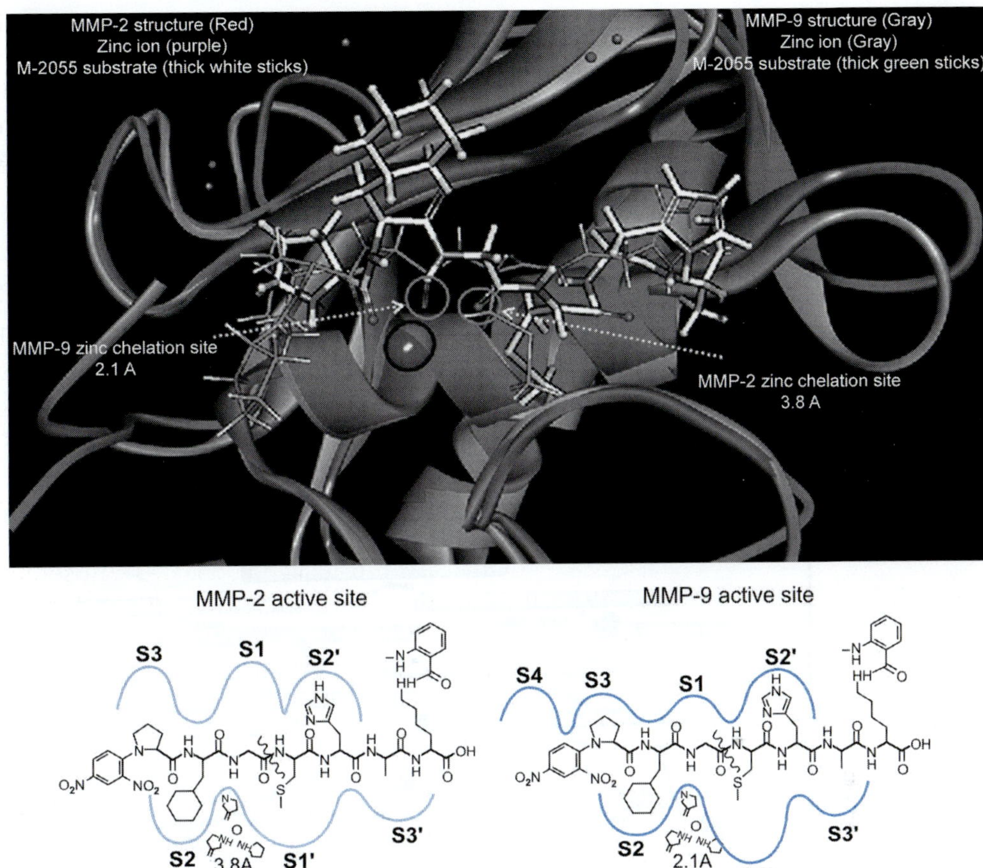

Fig. 1: Docked complexes of 1 substrate and the catalytic domain of human MMP-2 (PDB code 1QIB) and MMP-9 (PDB code 1GKC). The MMP-substrate docked complexes are merged with zinc as the same point of view. MMP-2 structure is shown in red, zinc as purple and 1 substrate (white sticks) docked within MMP-2 active site. MMP-9 is shown in gray, zinc as green and 1 substrate (thin green sticks) docked within its active site. (Bottom) Schematic representation of 1: active site binding interaction in human MMP-2 and MMP-9. MMP-2 and MMP-9 enzyme binding pockets are shown in red and green, respectively. Substrate chemical structure and its scissile bond are shown in black. The zinc ion is indicated in blue. *(For color version, see Plate 1)*.

is present in the large arteries as well as the resistance arteries (Fig. 2).

Matrix Metalloproteinases Regulation

Regulation of MMPs is mediated through gene transcription, zymogen activation, posttranslational modification and TIMP inhibition. The tissue inhibitors of metalloproteinases (TIMPs), four distinct ones, have broad MMP inhibitory activities. They are unique with some similar characteristics. The binding of N-terminal region of TIMP to the catalytic domain of MMPs leads to inhibition of their activity. The inhibitory complex is stabilized by the binding of C-terminal to the hemopexin domain of MMPs. TIMP-1 predominantly inhibits MMP-9, TIMP-2 inhibits MMP-2, TIMP-3 inhibits almost all MMPs in ECM and is an important marker of cardiac hypertrophy. TIMP-4 inhibits MMP-2

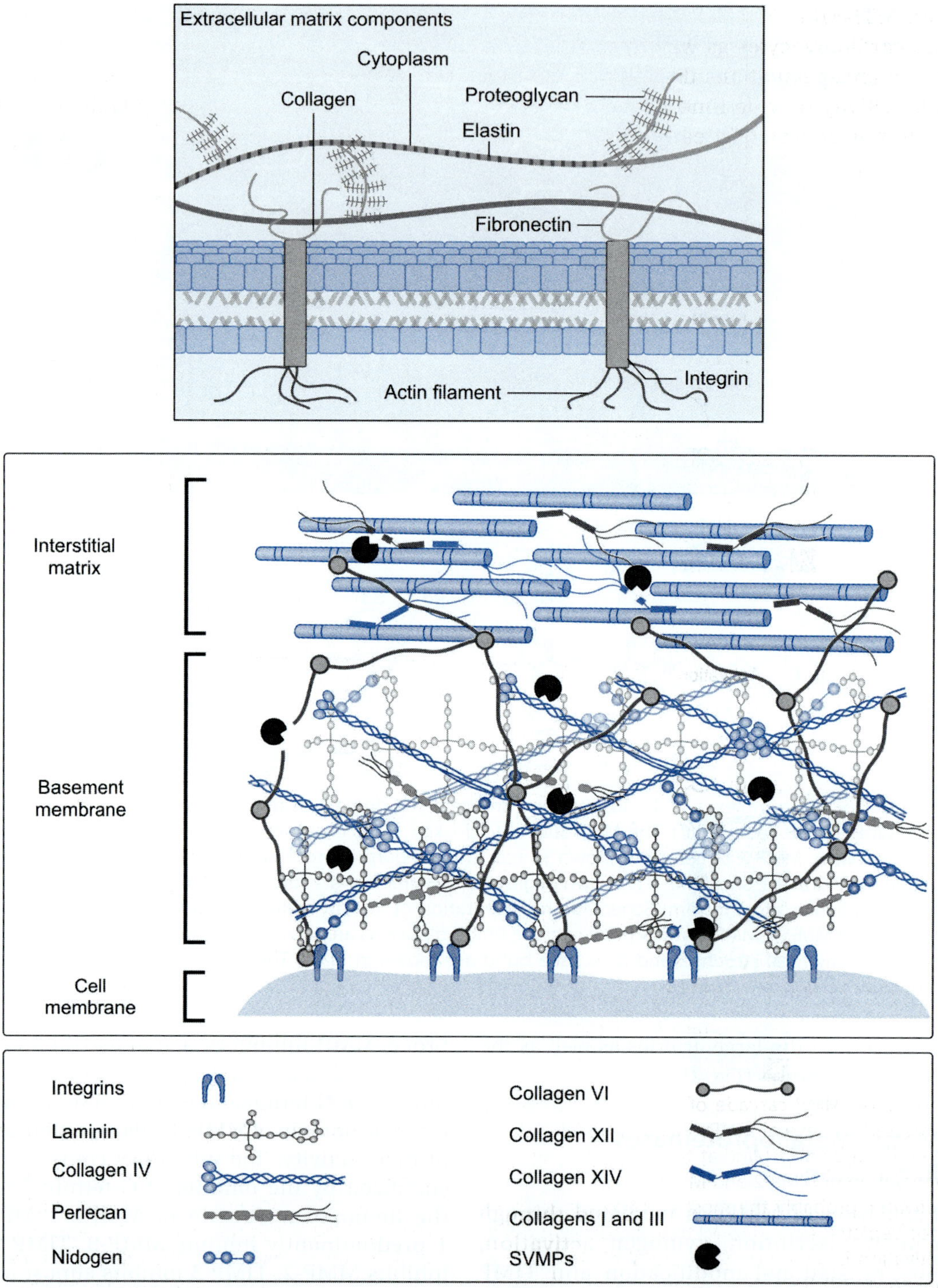

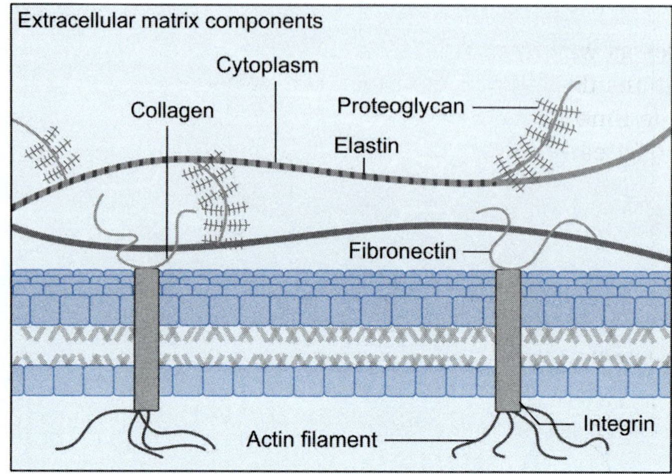

Fig. 2: Extracellular matrix and its component.

and MTI–MMP.[7,8] TIMP-4 is present inside the cardiomyocytes as well as in the ECM. There are speculations that MMP synthesis and activity may be time dependent. MMP system is activated in early phrase of HTN to allow smooth muscle cells migration and vessel wall restructuring. With disease progression there is suppression of MMP system causing ECM deposition and fibrosis (Fig. 3).

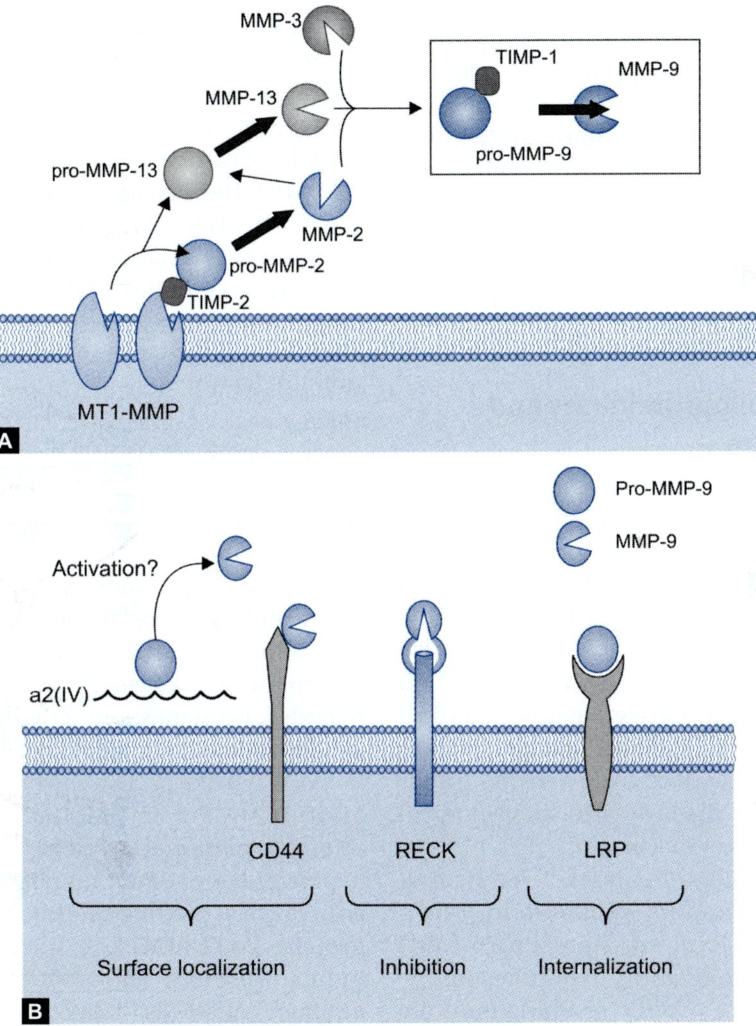

Fig. 3: (A) MMP cascade of zymogen activation involved in pro-MMP-9 activation. Pro-MMP-9 can be activated by several MMPs including MMP-3, MMP-2 and MMP-13. This cascade of zymogen activation is initiated by MT1-MMP at the cell membrane and requires the action of TIMP-2. It culminates with the generation of MMP-2 and MMP-13, which in turn can activate pro-MMP-9. MMP-3 is another pro-MMP-9 activator, probably the most efficient, but is activated by plasmin via uPAR and uPA on the cell surface (not depicted here). Pro-MMP-9 can be found in a complex with TIMP-1 but the role of this complex on activation is unknown. How pro-MMP-9 can be in proximity to this potential activation cascade is also unknown; (B) Reported proteins involved in pro-MMP-9/MMP-9 cell surface association. These diverse proteins play distinct roles in MMP-9 function including surface localization, inhibition and internalization. In the case of a2(IV) and CD44, it is unknown whether the interaction is associated with zymogen activation or inhibition. However, CD44-bound MMP-9 was shown to be in the active state.

Extracellular Matrix Regulation

Extracellular matrix metabolism is regulated by MMP and natural tissue endogenous inhibitors. Interstitial collagenase MMP-1 degrades structural and fibrillar collagens (types I–III). Gelatinase-A (MMP-2) and MMP-9 are two enzymes that mainly digest denatured collagen (gelatins), elastin, fibronectin, laminin as well as collagens types IV and V (found predominantly in the subendothelial basement membrane of the vessel wall). Proteoglycans also indirectly regulate ECM synthesis and degradation. Apart from fibroblasts, other cellular components of cardiovascular system and infiltrative cells may also synthesize ECM components.

Matrix Metalloproteinases and Hypertension

Regulation and modulation of ECM by direct proteolytic degradation of the ECM proteins (e.g. collagen, proteoglycans and fibronectin) are the principal physiological function. MMPs are not just ECM modeling protease. Major complications of HTN also have alterations in their levels.[9,10] All members of MMP family have been linked to disease development ranging from chronic inflammation, hypertension, other cardiovascular disease and neurological disorders to cancer metastasis.

Matrix metalloproteinases-2 is a neutral endopeptidase and its inhibitors may help in maintaining local adrenomedullin (AM) levels and in mitigating hypertension.[11,12] AM is a fragment peptide resulting from the degradation of the vasodilator peptide by MMP-2 and has vasoconstrictive properties. AM, apart from being a vasodilator also inhibits myocardial fibrosis expressed in endothelium and vascular smooth muscle. Due to both the properties, it has direct impact on the vascular tone in arteries and arterioles.[13] Whether MMP-2 mediated HTN has differential signalling in the arterial wall of Angiotensin II induced HTN and cardiac remodeling has conflicting evidence. MMP-2 exerts its effects on ECM as well as within the cardiomyocytes and VSMC thus leading to cell hypertrophy, proliferation and migration. It was observed that expression of MMP-9 is greatly increased in MMP-2 null mice which led to the hypothesis that MMP-2 function maybe interchangeable with other MMPs.[14]

Matrix metalloproteinases--7 also modulates cardiac hypertrophy via activation of MMP-2. The increase in the MMP expression and activity is a compensatory mechanism to limit excess ECM accumulation.

Matrix metalloproteinases-9 does not cause direct proteolysis of collagen I. It releases vascular endothelial growth factor (VEGF) which has an important role in angiogenesis and neovascularization. Plasma concentration of MMP-2 and MMP-9 share similar substrate specificity (collagen type IV and V) related to vascular remodeling and are depressed in essential hypertension. MMP-2 due to its ability to cleave ECM and other intracellular targets in the cardiomyocytes affects the contractile ability and contributes to structural changes also. Other vasoactive peptides, cytokines and growth factors such as TGF-β also mediate the process.

AEV Portik, et al. reported decrease in MMP-1, MMP-2 and MMP-9 activity in the internal mammary artery specimens of hypertensive patients undergoing coronary artery bypass grafting surgery. MMP activator protein (MTI–MMP), extracellular matrix inducer protein (EMMPRIN) and tissue inhibitors of MMPs (TIMP-1 and TIMP-2), all had decreased tissue levels in hypertensive patient thus indicating that in HTN not only MMP levels, but also their inducer and activator proteins are downregulated. Thus, MMP/TIMP ratio is critical for coordinating matrix production and degradation.[15]

Decreased baseline values of MMP-2 and MMP-9 ($p = 0.01$ and 0.002, respectively) was observed in patients with HTN compared to normotensives. Among the hypertensive patients also, those with systemic vascular resistance (SVR) less than 1,440 dyn s/cm^5 had higher values of MMP-2 (p = 0.005) and MMP-9 (p = 0.001) compared to those with SVR >1440 dyn s/cm.^{5} However, the study did not evaluate the plasma concentration of TIMP.[1]

TARGETS OF MATRIX METALLOPROTEINASES OTHER THAN EXTRACELLULAR MATRIX

Other nonECM targets such as big endothelin-1 may also be degraded which leads to production of a potent vasoconstrictor peptide. MMPs can also degrade inflammatory targets. Increased MMPs activate cytokines and in turn increased cytokines and oxidative stress increase the MMP activity and the proteolytic actions in the vasculature.

EXTRACELLULAR MATRIX AND HYPERTENSION

Hypertension related accumulation of ECM proteins in the myocardium and arteries is modulated by altered MMP and/or TIMP activity. Cytoskeletal rearrangement of the vessel wall also occurs (via integrin mediated signalling) due to ECM modulation by MMP. Abnormal degradation of collagen type I (the major form of collagen in hypertensive myocardial fibrosis) is observed in patients with essential HTN. The three dimensional spatial arrangement responsible for the metabolic function and integrity of the tissue in extracellular space is dependent on the ECM. Alterations in the density of ECM components, ECM architecture and cell ECM attachments (both in myocardium and vessel) are evident in HTN. ECM requires constant synthesis and degradation.

Vasoactive hormones and mediators, together with local growth factors and cytokines play a key intermediary role in converting changes in blood pressure to the adaptive changes in the ECM. Multiple systemic and local factors such as vasoactive substances (angiotensin II, aldosterone, adrenergic stimuli, natriuretic peptides, endothelin, adrenomedullin, prostanoids nitric oxide), growth factors, cytokines and other mediators (transforming growth factor beta, platelet-derived growth factor, fibroblast growth factor, insulin-like growth factor 1, bone morphogenetic proteins, tumor necrosis factor-α, connective tissue growth factor hepatocyte growth factor, interleukins, interferons, plasminogen activator inhibitor-1) may be involved in the processes of ECM remodeling in HTN.

Structural changes involving myocyte hypertrophy and excessive accumulation of ECM are important component of cardiac remodeling which is associated with arterial HTN. Accumulation of ECM leads to fibrosis thus influencing myocardial stiffness and promoting arrhythmias.

Serum Markers of Cardiovascular Extracellular Matrix Regulation in Hypertension

New noninvasive assays have been used for collagen fragment peptides by several groups for assessment of cardiovascular collagen synthesis and degradation in hypertensive patients. The measurement of type 1 procollagen carboxy-terminal peptide (PIP) and type III collagen amino-terminal peptide (PIIIP) produced during the synthesis of collagen fibrils components have been utilized to estimate cardiovascular production of these collagens and the carboxy-terminal telopeptide of collagen type I (CITP) is a marker of degradation of type I collagen. Increased levels of PIP, PIIIP, CITP and TIMP-1a and reduced MMP-1 have been reported in hypertensive patients compared to normotensives.[16-19] Whether the changes seen in the serum accurately reflect the situation in the heart and vessel needs further evidence. In future they could be potential serum markers for ECM metabolism.

■ CONCLUSION

The role of ECM and MMP in the pathogenesis of HTN and its comorbidities have ample evidence but unexplored domains still exist. Other MMP—specific signalling cascades, for example MMP-14 (MT-1 MMP) is involved in cell migration (through ECM) and in fibroblast proliferation. MMP not only contributes to the maladaptive vascular and cardiac alterations in HTN by ECM degradation but also affects the non-ECM and inflammatory components in cardiomyocytes and VSMC thus having intracellular effects leading to cell hypertrophy and associated dysfunction. As MMPs are a major contributor to tissue repair and their activity and endogenous inhibitors are not only member specific but also organ specific, hence a broader understanding of the genetic as well as environmental cause of MMP activation is a necessity before therapeutic interventions can be targeted towards it as a molecular culprit with certainty. However, the fact that ECM has a pivotal role in vascular, cardiac and renal remodeling, which results in deterioration of tissue structure, function and perfusion and thus to the morbidity and mortality related to HTN makes it an important target.

■ REFERENCES

1. Zervoudaki A, Economou E, Stefanadis C, et al. Plasma levels of active extracellular matrix metalloproteinases 2 and 9 in patients with essential hypertension before and after antihypertensive treatment. J Hum Hypertens. 2003;17(2):119-24.
2. Page-McCaw A, Ewald AJ, Werb Z. Matrix metalloproteinases and the regulation of tissue remodeling. Nat Rev Mol Cell Biol. 2007;8(3):221-33.
3. Grimm D, Kromer EP, Böcker W, et al. Regulation of extracellular matrix proteins in pressure-overload cardiac hypertrophy: effects of angiotensin converting enzyme inhibition. J Hypertens. 1998;16(9):1345-55.
4. López B, González A, Díez J. Role of matrix metalloproteinases in hypertension-associated cardiac fibrosis. Curr Opin Nephrol Hypertens. 2004;13(2):197-204.
5. Gross J, Lapiere CM. Collagenolytic activity in amphibian tissues: a tissue culture assay. Proc Natl Acad Sci USA. 1962;48:1014-22.
6. Brinckerhoff CE, Matrisian LM. Matrix metalloproteinases: a tail of a frog that became a prince. Nat Rev Mol Cell Biol. 2002;3(3):207-14.
7. Nagase H, Visse R, Murphy G. Structure and function of matrix metalloproteinases and TIMPs. Cardiovasc Res. 2006;69(3):562-73.
8. Schulze CJ, Wang W, Suarez-Pinzon WL, et al. Imbalance between tissue inhibitor of metalloproteinase-4 and matrix metalloproteinases during acute myocardial [correction of myoctardial] ischemia-reperfusion injury. Circulation. 2003;107(19):2487-92.
9. Rodriguez JA, Orbe J, Martinez de Lizarrondo S, et al. Metalloproteinases and atherothrombosis: MMP-10 mediates vascular remodeling promoted by inflammatory stimuli. Front Biosci. 2008;13:2916-21.
10. Rosell A, Lo EH. Multiphasic roles for matrix metalloproteinases after stroke. Curr Opin Pharmacol. 2008;8(1):82-9.
11. Nawarskas J, Rajan V, Frishman WH. Vasopeptidase inhibitors, neutral endopeptidase inhibitors, and dual inhibitors of angiotensin-converting enzyme and neutral endopeptidase. Heart Dis. 2001;3(6):378-85.
12. Corti R, Burnett JC Jr, Rouleau JL, et al. Vasopeptidase inhibitors: a new therapeutic concept in cardiovascular disease? Circulation. 2001;104(15):1856-62.
13. Martinez A, Oh HR, Unsworth EJ, et al. Matrix metalloproteinase-2 cleavage of adrenomedullin produces a vasoconstrictor out of a vasodilator. Biochem J. 2004; 383(Pt. 3):413-8.
14. Esparza J, Kruse M, Lee J, et al. MMP-2 null mice exhibit an early onset and severe experimental autoimmune encephalomyelitis due to an increase in MMP-9 expression and activity. FASEB J. 2004;18(14):1682-91.
15. Ergul A, Portik-Dobos V, Hutchinson J, et al. Downregulation of vascular matrix metalloproteinase inducer and activator proteins in hypertensive patients. Am J Hypertens. 2004; 17(9):775-82.
16. Diez J, Laviades C, Mayor G, et al. Increased serum concentrations of procollagen peptides in essential hypertension. Relation to cardiac alterations. Circulation. 1995;9195):1450-6.
17. Laviades C, Varo N, Fernández J, et al. Abnormalities of the extracellular degradation of collagen type I in essential hypertension. Circulation. 1998;98(6):535-40.
18. Lindsay MM, Maxwell P, Dunn FG. TIMP-1: a marker of left ventricular diastolic dysfunction and fibrosis in hypertension. Hypertension. 2002;40(2):136-41.
19. Timms PM, Wright A, Maxwell P, et al. Plasma tissue inhibitor of metalloproteinase-1 levels are elevated in essential hypertension and related to left ventricular hypertrophy. Am J Hypertens. 2002;15(30):269-72.

Arterial and Venous Function in Hypertension (Mitochondrial)

T Ravikumar

■ INTRODUCTION

Hypertension (HT) is viewed as a multifactorial disease with genetic, environmental, anatomical, adaptive neural, endocrine, humeral and hemodynamic causes having "oxidative stress" as a common denominator. The latter implies an imbalance between the systemic manifestation of reactive oxygen species (ROS) and the cells ability to counteract the reactive intermediates or to repair their damages. Mitochondria are the main source of cellular ROS although their pathophysiological roles in HT are still incompletely understood. The common opinion is that mitochondria have a core position in cellular homeostasis by their function as essential powerhouses of cells. Mitochondria utilize nutrients to generate adenosine triphosphate (ATP) via the electron transport chain coupled with oxidative phosphorylation, supporting cells survival and normal function.

■ VASCULAR REMODELING

Understanding the physiology of the resistance vasculature aids in explaining the pathogenesis of nonhypertrophic changes that are seen in HT. At normal blood pressure, myogenic tone is independent of neurohormonal influences and it is the innate vascular tone of the smaller resistance arteries. Distinctly the smaller resistance arteries have myogenic response, which is the ability to respond by constriction or dilatation in relation with the pressure changes in the upstream vasculature, thereby autoregulating the blood flow and maintaining the capillary pressure, leading to an adequate supply of oxygenated blood at a constant flow and pressure to the downstream vasculature. Increase in pressure leads to myogenic constriction of the smaller resistance arteries. But the same may lead to hypertrophy in those vessels which do not possess myogenic response. In untreated hypertensives, there will be prolonged myogenic constriction as the resistance vasculature strives to protect the target organs downstream, from pressure-induced damage induced by an increase in blood flow.[1] Prolonged vasoconstriction will lead to inward eutrophic remodeling and/or a reduced arterial dispensability. The structural differences among the large conduit, medium-sized arteries and resistance vessels is evident in many models [e.g.—chronic nitric oxide synthase (NOS) inhibition-induced HT model]. The duration and intensity of the alteration in intraluminal pressure determine the remodeling response of these vasculatures.

■ MOLECULAR MECHANISMS IN EUTROPHIC REMODELING

Eutrophic inward remodeling is a process of structural adaptation observed in most stages of HT. HT independent of the renin–angiotensin system (RAS) (An animal model: BPH-2 mice) demonstrates hypertrophy as the predominating structural change. Eutrophic inward remodeling is a functional adaptation observed after prolonged vasoconstriction, so as to preserve a lumen diameter for long periods, thus maintaining the vasomotor tone and normalizing the stress on the vessel walls. Studies involving the use of well-characterized TGR (mREN2) 27 rats have demonstrated that integrin aVβ3, a multifunctional extracellular matrix receptor is crucial for eutrophic inward remodeling. These integrins are cross-linked by molecular complexes to the cytoskeleton thereby aiding in transmission of the tensile forces across the cell membrane. Using peptides and specific antibodies, it has been shown that integrins αVβ3 and α5β1 indirectly regulate the myogenic response by influencing the control of calcium flow through icon channels; α5β1 is responsible for the initial calcium influx required to establish vascular tone and αVβ3 mediates force maintenance by calcium sensitization of contractile components. These integrins can form complexes, which regulate cytoskeletal dynamics and maintain a vascular myogenic force at a given pressure. This is ameliorated if there is cytoskeletal disruption. Cytoskeletal proteins such as heat-shock protein 27 activated by RhoA kinases have been shown to regulate myogenic tone. It is now clear that RhoA signaling plays a central role in both calcium sensitization and regulation of actin dynamics in small artery remodeling.

Systemic HT increases heart workload, expose luminal vascular endothelium to shear stress, and alters cardiomyocytes structure and function. To fulfill cellular energetic demands, mitochondria generate ATP through the electron transport chain located on the inner mitochondrial membrane. This chain generates also ROS (functioning as secondary messengers in signal transduction and metabolism) and imbalances the redox signaling, as key intracellular mechanisms implicated in HT onset and progression. The current overview presents and discusses novel issues in HT-related mitochondrial dysfunction focusing on—(1) cardiomyocytes, and emphasizing the decline in mitochondrial biogenesis, the energetics deficiency regulated by the dynamic processes of fusion and fission, the ROS overproduction, and the augmented mitochondrial degradation by mitophagy, and on (2) arterial smooth muscle cells mitochondrial defects. The review is concluded by outstanding research themes compulsory for filling the gaps on mitochondria-targeted strategies in HT.[2,3]

An example is mitochondrial cardio-myocytes that supply ATP for fulfilling the energetically demanding function of the heart.[4] The novel uncovered roles of mitochondria are related to control of cellular functions and metabolism, by several mechanisms—(1) contribution to maintenance of calcium homeostasis, (2) intervention in cell signaling (via ROS) and modulation of redox signaling, (3) generation of nitric oxide (NO) by mitochondrial NOS, (4) interaction with other cellular organelles, nucleus included, and (5) release of mitochondrial constituents [proteins, lipids, mitochondrial DNA (mtDNA)] that can function as signaling molecules; these are known as "mitochondrial damage-associated molecular patterns" (DAMPs) considered to be potential biomarkers. It is obvious that pathological defects in mitochondrial function, known as "mitochondrial dysfunction" are connected to reduced levels of generated ATP, to excessive ROS production, and diminished antioxidant defense. The latest data demonstrate that cardiac mitochondria cope with energetic deficiency by changing morphology through fission and fusion processes in an attempt to maintain their functionality. Thus, mitochondrial energetic potential and morphology appear as both causal and resultant to excess ROS generation. The overproduction of ROS irreversibly damages the cellular molecules and promotes the intrinsic apoptotic pathway conducting to mitochondria-related cell death. Among the pathologies associated with "mitochondrial dysfunction", the review is focused on systemic HT, as portal and pulmonary HT deserve distinct approaches. The following part examines the novel data on HT-related "mitochondrial dysfunction" in cardiomyocytes and resistance arteries smooth muscle cells.

■ MITOCHONDRIAL MODIFICATIONS IN THE HYPERTENSIVE HEART

There are several modifications of cardio-myocytes mitochondria in HT, such as the decline in biogenesis, reduced energetic efficiency, the overproduction of ROS, and the augmented degradation via mitophagy.

- *The decline of mitochondrial bio-genesis* results from the inability of cardiomyocytes to support the increasing energy demand under pressure overload conditions. Briefly, mitochondria bio-genesis develops in response to ener-getic deficits, and is characterized by increase in cells mitochondrial mass. At molecular level, the mitochondrial biogenesis process is regulated by specific coactivators and transcription factors that control expression of components of the nuclear and mitochondrial genome. In this context, the author quote peroxisome proliferator-activated receptor β/δ (PPAR β/δ), transcription factor per-oxisome proliferator-activated receptor

coactivator 1 α (PGC-1α, a known target gene of PPAR β/δ), sirtuins, and adenosine monophosphate (AMP)-activated protein kinase (AMPK) signaling cascades. To promote mitochondrial biogenesis, several pharmacological strategies exist, such as the use of bezafibrate to activate PPAR-PGC-1α axis, of quercetin or resveratrol as Sirt1 agonists, and of resveratrol to activate AMPK. Recently, activation of cardiac AMPK was recognized as essential for accelerating ATP generation and repair of cardiomyocyte's function, ensuing protection of myocardium against cardiac dysfunction and apoptosis. Another promoter of mitochondrial biogenesis is the prolonged laminar shear stress associated with aerobic exercise. The alleviation of biogenesis decline is expected to increase the mitochondrial mass, oxidative metabolism and bioenergetics capacity under pressure overload conditions

- *The deficient mitochondrial energetics,* i.e. the deficiency in ATP synthesis conducting to impaired heart contractility. The ATP deficit results from the complex interplay between mitochondrial ATP synthase and induction of the permeability transition pore (PTP), an inner membrane channel and key effector of cell death. Reports indicate that dimers of the ATP synthase form PTP. The malfunctioning cardiomyocyte mitochondria cope with energetic deficiency by fusion with "healthy" organelles, resulting information of elongated structures that survive under a lower energy outcome; moreover, normal mitochondria that locally display a modified membrane potential or the dysfunctional elongated organelles are subjected to fragmentation (fission) followed by removal of the dysfunc-tional part by autophagic degradation (mitophagy), while the "healthy" part of the organelle is committed to new fusions. The dynamic processes of fusion and fission engage the interfibrillar mitochondria packed between sarcomeres, while the subpopulations of mitochondria located subsarcolemmal and perinuclear are not subjected to such sequences. Another form of mitochondrial dynamics is the close contact "the kissing" of the outer membranes in adjacent mitochondria; zones with high density of mitochondria are common in the heart, and the "kissing" between them allows local intermitochondria communication. Mitochondrial abnormalities have been identified in experimental models of HT. Thus, in the left ventricle of spontaneously hypertensive rats mitochondrial dynamics are imbalanced, and are characterized by decreased levels of mitochondrial fission protein, dynamin-related protein 1 (Drp1, localized to the outer mitochondrial membrane) and increased expression of fusion protein optic atrophy protein 1 (OPA1, localized to the inner mitochondrial membrane), along with decreased SirT1/AMPK-PGC-1αsignaling (involved in mitochondrial biogenesis). Among the strategies aiming energy recovery in HT, the author quote activation of cardiac AMPK that accelerates ATP generation, attenuates ATP reduction, and protects the myocardium against cardiac dysfunction and apoptosis, and the control of glutathionylation reactions mediated by glutaredoxin-2 (Grx2). Taken together, the novel results support the opinion that in cardiomyocytes, the impairment in energy generation is regulated, at least in part, by dynamic processes such as mitochondrial fusion, fission and "kissing"

- *The overproduction of mitochondrial ROS*: Inhuman HT, excess generation of mitochondrial ROS, the exacerbated response to ROS, and the reduced efficiency of endogenous mitochondrial protective antioxidant defines mechanisms are issues under in depth scrutiny at present. The common perception is that oxidative stress amplifies blood pressure elevation in the presence of prohypertensive factors (such as salty diet, activation of RAS) causing HT-related target organ damage. Moreover, there is a genetic link between mitochondrial proteins and HT. Thus, polymorphisms in cytochrome c gene (a subunit of complex IV) and in *OPA-1* and mitofusin-2 (*Mfn-2*) genes are correlated with blood pressure. The ROS cause an increased number of mtDNA deletions; in turn, damaged mtDNA codes for mutated polypeptides including those responsible for loss of the integrity of the respiratory chain, aggravating oxidative stress and damaging both nuclear and mtDNA. Among the adaptive mechanisms induced in HT in response to increased production of mitochondrial ROS, the author quote— (1) overexpression of major scavengers of mitochondrial O_2 and H_2O_2, such as superoxide dismutases 2 (SOD2) and glutathione peroxidase, (2) increased expression of antioxidant enzymes (such those involved in glutathione synthesis), by induction of redox sensitive transcription factor NF-E2-related factor 2 (NRF2), (3) attenuation of angiotensin II-induced cytoplasmic and mitochondrial O_2 production, by mitochondrial reverse electron transfer inhibition with malonate, malate, or rotenone, (4) inhibition of Nox, by NAPDH-oxidase inhibitor apocynin, (5) in vivo treatment of mice with mitochondrial targeted antioxidant, mitoTEMPO, and (6) stimulation of mitochondrial uncoupling protein 2 (UCP2). Interestingly, according to the new concept of "mitochondrial hormesis" or "mitohormesis" low levels of ROS induce an adaptive response, improving systemic defense mechanisms. The above achievements demonstrate the advancement in our understanding since the earlier hypothesis according to which mitochondrial dysfunction may be involved in the development of systemic HT.

- *The augmented mitochondrial degradation*: The last step in mitochondrial turnover is their degradation by autophagy (mitophagy), considered the hottest topic in mitochondrial biology. Specifically, the damaged mitochondria resulting from the fission process are sequestered within autophagosomes and degraded after fusion with the lysosomal compartment. Mitophagy is a novel uncovered process of central role in cellular metabolism, as sustained by the following achievements— (1) it ensures cellular bioenergetics capacity and cellular homeostasis, by balancing biogenesis process, (2) preserves a healthy population of mitochondria, by removal of damaged ones, (3) promotes mitochondrial biogenesis under basal conditions, and (4) it is a player in mitochondrial "quality control", involving transcriptional activation of nuclear genes during mitochondrial-nuclear communication via mitochondrial unfolded protein response. In hypertensive hearts, mitophagy is enhanced in obesity and renovascular HT, and dysfunctional mitochondria are mentioned as contributors to this pathology. At present, research is focused on procedures or compounds that maintain structural integrity of mitochondria. In this context valsartan (an angiotensin II receptor blocker) appears as a therapeutic option ameliorating myocardial autophagy and mitophagy.

■ MITOCHONDRIAL MODIFICATIONS IN THE ARTERIAL SMOOTH MUSCLE CELLS

Hypertension causes changes in the structure and function of the large and small resistance arteries. Besides inducing endothelial dysfunction, HT modifies vascular smooth muscle cells (VSMCs) phenotype. Recent results demonstrate that mitochondrial dysfunction is implicated in the regulatory control of VSMCs phenotype and illustrates the conversion of the SMCs contractile phenotype into a secretory one in mesenteric resistance arteries; the switch of phenotype is assessed by the presence of rough endoplasmic reticulum, the site of protein synthesis. Mitochondrial dysfunction is illustrated by the occurrence of less electron dense mitochondria of rather small size, by reduced cristae density/mitochondrion, and by altered morphology of cristae organization. The small size mitochondria could be the result of a fission process involved in cells migration, as VSMCs express the mito-chondrial fission protein Drp1; literature data assess that in VSMCs Drp1 is regulated by resistin, an adipocyte-specific hormone and an important link between obesity, insulin resistance, and diabetes.

Vascular smooth muscle cells express also Mfn-2, a mitochondrial outer membrane fusion protein that causes mitochondria assemble into tubular networks and their attachment to the endoplasmic reticulum. The reduced cristae density/mitochondrion, and the altered morphology of cristae organization entail impeded oxidative phosphorylation associated with reduced bioenergetics capacity; at present it is estimated that VSMCs mitochondrial respiration is an incompletely deciphered subject. In metabolic syndrome, accumulation of synthetic and proliferating VSMCs was associated with augmented expression of miR-21 and with coronary collateral growth. Additionally, in diabetes VSMCs dysfunction is characterized by mitochondrial membrane hyperpolarization, impaired mPTP opening, and alterations in the balance of fission and fusion processes; the final results are enhanced VSMCs migration and impaired vasoreactivity.[6] The latter is particularly important for hypertensive resistance arteries, that expose to the blood flow a more constricted vascular wall.

■ OUTSTANDING QUESTIONS ON MITOCHONDRIA-TARGETED STRATEGIES IN HYPERTENSION

The starting point in less understood HT-mitochondria interaction is the fact that the latter possess both a functional RAS and vitamin D receptors, and HT has an increasing prevalence at old age people. In this context, investigation of the interaction between mitochondria-targeted antioxidants and inhibitors of the RAS system appears as necessary. There are several topics under intense investigation, such as—(1) the mitochondria-associated mcmbranes that entails the physical connection between mitochondria and endoplasmic reticulum, a site for the intracellular signaling, (2) the mitophagy, (3) the mitochondria delivery (by nanotechnology-based carriers), (4) the contribution of inflammation-induced mitochondrial dysfunction to intracellular signaling, and (5) the activation of the innate immune system via toll-like receptor 9 (TLR9) in HT. Moreover, a complex of factors, such as aberrant signal transduction, augmented ROS generation, impaired response to ROS, and decreased antioxidant reserve contribute to increased oxidative stress, inflammation and autoimmune vascular dysfunction in human HT. At the horizon, the rapidly advancing field of mitochondrial pharmacology has great potential for clinical application. The novel

therapeutic strategies should address the following biological relevant open issues—(1) the quality control function of mitochondria (by mitochondria mass regulation and bioenergetics capacity maintenance), (2) the regulation of mitochondrial fission, with the intent to decrease VSMCs migration and limit intimal hyperplasia, (3) the protection against mtDNA damage, aiming improvement in mitochondrial function, (4) the use of mitochondria-specific therapies (such the antioxidant MitoTEMPO, a superoxide and alkyl scavenger, and (5) the adequate analytical methods to accurately assess oxidative stress in the clinic. Taken together, the above results illustrate the endeavors in understanding the correlation between mitochondrial dysfunction and HT, point toward the present gaps, and direct toward the potential strategies to ameliorate the dysfunctional condition. According to a study at the New University of Colorado Boulder research, consuming the novel antioxidant that specifically targets the cellular mitochondria, they observed within 6 weeks of usage of the medications, the age-related vascular changes were reversed to equivalent of 15–20 years younger. There is an emerging evidence suggesting nutraceuticals could play an important role in preventing heart disease. The author says, it also resurrects the notion that oral antioxidants, which have been broadly dismissed as ineffective in recent years, could reap measurable health benefits if properly targeted.

According to Matthew Rossman, "This is the first clinical trial to assess the impact of a mitochondrial-specific antioxidant on vascular function in humans". "It suggests that therapies like this may hold real promise for reducing the risk of age-related cardiovascular disease".

For the study, the investigators recruited 20 healthy men and women, aged 60–79 years, from the Boulder area. Of these, 50% of the subjects were prescribed with 20 mg/day of a supplement called MitoQ, a chemically altered naturally-occurring antioxidant coenzyme Q10 for binding the cellular mitochondria. And for the other group, a placebo was given. After 6 weeks, investigators assessed the functioning of the endothelium, by measuring how much subjects' arteries dilated with increased blood flow.

A 2-week no medication/placebo "washout" period was followed. Subsequently the two groups were switched, with the placebo group taking the supplement, and vice versa. Later, on repeating the tests, the investigators found that dilation of subjects' arteries improved by 42%, making their blood vessels resembling those of someone 15–20 years younger.[8] Authors concluded that sustained improvement of that magnitude is associated with about a 13% reduction in heart disease. The study also showed that the improvement in dilation was due to a reduction in oxidative stress.

In participants who, under placebo conditions, had stiffer arteries, supplementation was associated with reduced stiffness.

In younger age, optimal levels of antioxidants will be produced to quench the free radicals. But with ageing, the balance tips, as mitochondria and other cellular processes, produce excess free radicals outweighing the body's antioxidant defenses. These free radicals result in oxidative stress, damaging the endothelium leading to fibrosis, stiffness, and functional impairment of the vasculature.

Studies showed that oral antioxidant supplements like vitamin C and vitamin E to be ineffective and hence they fell out of favor as supplements.

"This study breathes new life into the discredited theory that supplementing the diet with antioxidants can improve health",

said Seals. "It suggests that targeting a specific source—mitochondria—may be a better way to reduce oxidative stress and improve cardiovascular health with aging".

The same laboratory published another study recently, showing that a compound called nicotinamide riboside may also be able to reverse vascular aging in healthy subjects.

◾ CONCLUSION

"Exercise and eating a healthy diet are the most well-established approaches for maintaining cardiovascular health", said Seals. "But at the public health level, not enough people are willing to do that. We are looking for complementary, evidence-based options to prevent age-related changes that drive disease. These supplements may be among them".

◾ REFERENCES

1. Rossman MJ, Santos-Parker JR, Chelsea AC Steward, et al. Chronic Supplementation With a Mitochondrial Antioxidant (MitoQ) Improves Vascular Function in Healthy Older Adults. Hypertension. 2018;71:1056-63.
2. Popov D. Mitochondria revisited: Hypertension-related alterations and perspectives for therapy. J Hypertens Res. 2015;1(2):81-7.
3. Dikalov SI, Ungvari Z. Role of mitochondrial oxidative stress in hypertension. Am J Physiol Heart Circ Physiol. 2013;305(10):H1417-27.
4. Manucha W, Ritchie B, Ferder L. Hypertension and insulin resistance: implications of mitochondrial dysfunction. Curr Hypertens Rep. 2015;17(1):504.
5. Cheng Z, Ristow M. Mitochondria and metabolic homeostasis. Antioxid Redox Signal. 2013;19(3):240-2.
6. Galloway CA, Yoon Y. Mitochondrial Dynamics in Diabetic Cardiomyopathy. Antioxid Redox Signal. 2013;19(4):415-30.
7. Hill S, Van Remmen H. Mitochondrial stress signaling in longevity: a new role for mitochondrial function in aging. Redox Biol. 2014;2:936-44.
8. Williams D, Venardos KM, Byrne M, et al. Abnormal mitochondrial L-arginine transport contributes to the pathogenesis of heart failure and reoxygenation injury. PLoS One. 2014;9(8):e104643.

Role of Calcium Channel in Hypertension

E Dhandapani

■ INTRODUCTION

Calcium channel function is essential for vascular muscle membrane excitation and provides the significant voltage sensitivity to the small blood vessels. The actions of the electrogenic sodium pump on the membrane potential and therefore on the calcium channels can define perturbations, which could be conceived alternatively as acting on the other mechanisms. The evidence of the altered calcium channel function in high blood pressure indicates that insufficiency in calcium channel function as such exists at the root of changed membrane function. The disease can be comparable in this regard to at least one form of the skeletal muscle dysgenesis.

For normal excitation-contraction coupling in the skeletal muscle, heart and different kinds of smooth muscle comprising vascular smooth muscle cells (VSMCs), voltage-dependent Ca^{2+} channels are needed. Earlier purification studies utilizing skeletal tissue reported that the voltage-gated Ca^{2+} channels were multisubunit complexes, comprising of a central pore-forming $\alpha 1$ subunit and extra β, $\alpha 2\delta$, and γ subunits (Curtis and Catterall, 1984, 1985; Hosey et al., 1987; Ice et al., 1987; Leung et al., 1987; Vaghy et al., 1987). Presently, it is known that the large (about 190–240 kDa) $\alpha 1$ subunit gives the CaL channel most of the functional properties, comprising Ca^{2+} permeability, voltage sensing, Ca^{2+} channel blocker (CCB) inhibition, and Ca^{2+}-dependent inactivation.[1] The $\alpha 1$ subunit structure consists of four repeat domains (I, II, III and IV), each domain consisting of six transmembrane segments (Catterall, 2000; Jurkat-Rott and Lehmann-Horn, 2004). Intracellular binding domains for signaling molecules comprising protein kinase A and protein kinase C enable the modulation of channel behavior by phosphorylation. Additionally, in modulating channel phenotype and expression, the amino (N)- and carboxy (C)-termini play particular roles. As an example, the C-terminus was involved in Ca^{2+}-dependent signal transduction consisting of the constitutive calmodulin binding to allow Ca^{2+}-dependent channel inactivation[2] (Kobrinsky et al., 2005; Lee et al., 1999; Liang et al., 2003; Peterson et al., 1999; Qin et al., 1999; Zuhlke et al., 1999).

■ ROLE OF CALCIUM CHANNEL IN PATHOGENESIS OF HYPERTENSION

Abnormalities of Ca^{2+} channels are regarded as part of the extensive biological and morphological adaptations that characterize the vasculature during the pathogenesis of hypertension. Initially, during acute increase in blood pressure, small arteries and arterioles show an immediate "stretch-dependent" depolarization and constriction commonly referred to as the "myogenic" response. The myogenic response relies on the opening of CaL channels in the VSMCs for contraction (Nelson et al., 1990; Wang et al., 1999). In fact, the requisite role of CaL channels in mediating pressure-induced contraction is evident by the absence of myogenic tone in the arteries of mice in which the CaL channel (CaV1.2) gene is inactivated (Moosmang et al., 2003). Importantly, the myogenic response may be viewed as either a contributing or protective influence in hypertension (Cox and Rusch, 2002). On the one hand, the myogenic response of the small arteries and arterioles may amplify the initial rise in blood pressure and further elevate peripheral vascular resistance and blood pressure levels. Alternatively, in the cerebral, coronary and renal circulations that are primarily involved in the autoregulation of local blood flow, the myogenic response is postulated to dampen the transmission of the high systemic pressure to the microvasculature of the brain, heart and kidneys, respectively, thereby preventing pressure-induced damage to the capillary beds. Indeed, the loss of myogenic tone in the renal circulation has been linked to renal injury in animals and in humans with hypertension (Dworkin and Feiner, 1986; Feld et al., 1977; Gebremedhin et al., 1990; Hayashi et al., 1992, 1996; Olson et al., 1986), and also appears to precede the occurrence of hemorrhagic stroke in rats that are genetically predisposed to develop hypertension (Smeda and King, 2003). The myogenic response of the different vascular beds continues to play a central role in regulating blood pressure levels and organ blood flow during the progression of hypertension. However, if blood pressure is not restored to normal levels by compensatory neural and renal mechanisms, the VSMCs of the arterial circulation appear to "electrically remodel" as an adaptive response to sustain the higher levels of voltage-gated Ca^{2+} influx required for persistent arterial contraction. This adaptation is postulated to rely, at least in part, on the development of a "disease-specific" profile of vascular ion channels that promote arterial contraction and Ca^{2+} influx (Cox and Rusch, 2002). To date, two fundamental events have been implicated as the cellular mechanisms that evolve to sustain an elevated level of voltage-gated Ca^{2+} influx and contractile activation in VSMCs exposed to chronic increases in intravascular pressure (Fig. 1). First, a loss of resting membrane K^+ conductance resulting in depolarization-induced opening of CaL channels has been observed in VSMCs from several rat models of hypertension (Harder et al., 1983; Harder et al., 1985; Stekiel et al., 1986; Stekiel et al., 1993). Second, even short-term exposure to high intravascular pressures appears to upregulate the $\alpha 1C$ subunit and the number of functional CaL channels in VSMCs (Lozinskaya and Cox, 1997; Martens and Gelband, 1996; Pesic et al., 2004; Simard et al., 1998; Wilde et al., 1994). Interestingly, new evidence suggests that depolarization per se promotes $\alpha 1C$ subunit expression in the VSMCs of small arteries, suggesting that this "myogenic stimulus" may both activate existing CaL channels and increase the number of CaL channels in VSMCs during the evolution of hypertension (Pesic et al., 2004).

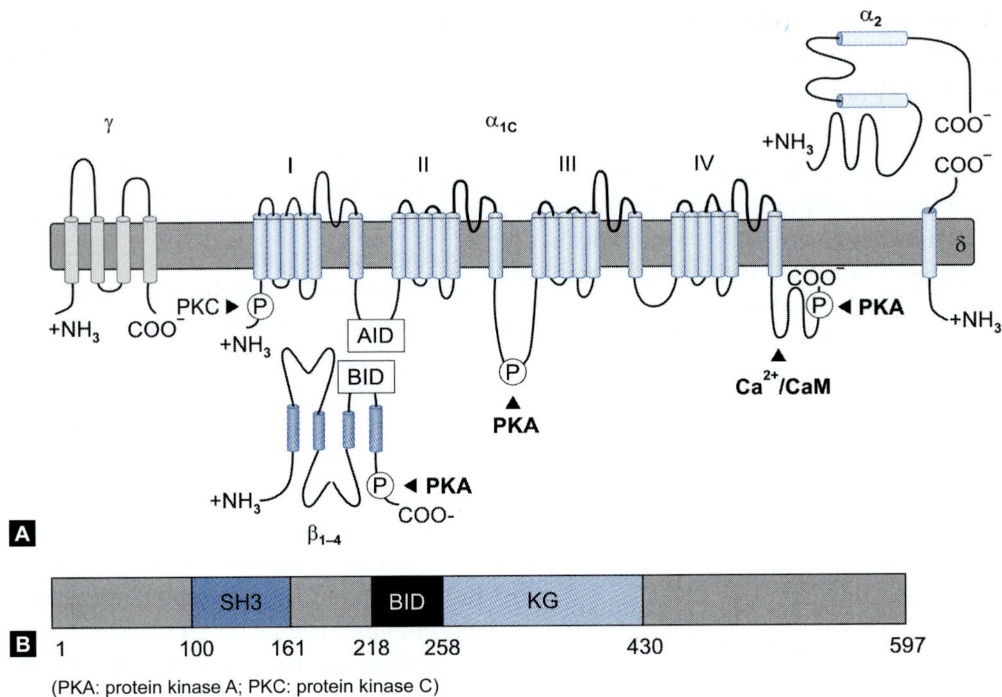

(PKA: protein kinase A; PKC: protein kinase C)

Fig. 1: Voltage-gated calcium channel.

UPREGULATION OF CAL CHANNELS IN RESPONSE TO HIGH BLOOD PRESSURE

An increase in voltage-gated Ca^{2+} current due to an enhanced number of CaL channels has been found in the cerebral, mesenteric, and renal VSMCs of spontaneously hypertensive rat (SHR), which manifest a genetic form of hypertension.[3] The increased CaL current was noted early in the hypertension development and does not seem to correspond to the channel's altered voltage sensitivity (Lozinskaya and Cox, 1997; Ohya et al., 1993). Rather, single-channel recordings have found an increase in number of CaL channel openings without the evidence of altered open-time distribution or single-channel conductance (Ohya et al., 1998). All of these results are compatible with the hypothesis that an enhanced number of the functional CaL channel proteins other than altered channel properties can account for the increase in CaL current in the VSMCs of the SHR. In this respect, it is confirmed by western blots that there is an enhanced expression of the pore-forming α1C subunit of the CaL channel in the arteries of adult SHR as compared to the age-matched Wistar-Kyoto (WKY) rats with normal levels of blood pressure (Pratt et al., 2002). Indeed, it is indicated by a panel of arteries from the two rat strains that there is an overabundance of α1C subunits in the SHR's femoral, mesenteric, and renal circulations, which implies that this abnormality extends to at least many vascular beds. In particular, the increased expression of α1C subunits in the renal, mesenteric, and skeletal muscle circulations corresponds to higher CaL current density and anomalous vascular tone development (Cox and Lozinskaya, 1995; Lozinskaya and Cox, 1997; Ohya et al., 1993,

1998; Pesic et al., 2004; Pratt et al., 2002). For instance, increased expression of $\alpha1C$ subunits in renal arteries of the adult SHR is correlated with an increased Ca^{2+} current and an accentuated Ca^{2+}-dependent spontaneous tone, which is reversed by treatment with nifedipine—a CaL channel blocker.

In VSMCs, the membrane density of CaL current from either the SHR or the WKY rat strain seems to be proportional to levels of blood pressure. This suggests that CaL channel overexpression does not require the genetic background of the SHR. For instance, in VSMCs isolated from the small mesenteric arteries of either WKY rats or SHR during natural development, there is a close linear correlation between systolic blood pressure and Ca^{2+} current density (Lozinskaya and Cox, 1997). Moreover, the use of angiotensin-converting enzyme inhibitor, e.g. ramipril for treatment of SHR, is associated with a reduction in both systolic blood pressure and Ca^{2+} current density concurrently in mesenteric VSMCs (Cox et al., 2002). A strong, positive relationship is indicated by these data between the blood pressure and the number of functional CaL channels in the vasculature in vivo and increase the intriguing likelihood that elevated blood pressure as such may enhance $\alpha1C$ subunit expression in the arterial circulation.

Recently, in the renal circulation of the aortic-banded rat, the hypothesis that high blood pressure can lead to stimulation of vascular CaL channel expression has been directly tested. The aorta is surgically banded between the right renal (RR) arteries and the left renal (RR) arteries in this model of hypertension. This leads to the selective elevation of the blood pressure in the RR circulation that is situated proximal to the banded site. While these animals right and left renal circulations were given exposure of the similar neuroendocrine and genetic influences, the expression of the $\alpha1C$ subunit was profoundly higher in the right kidney vasculature subjected to an elevated blood pressure level for 4 weeks. Patch-clamp recordings, in the same animals, verified that the appearance of the $\alpha1C$ subunit was related with an enhanced CaL current in the RR circulation VSMCs and the accompanying small arteries developed spontaneously vascular tone which was reversed by nifedipine. Interestingly, if the right kidney circulation is exposed for as little as 2 days to high levels of blood pressure of approximately 150 mm Hg, it was found to cause an enhanced expression of the $\alpha1C$ subunit in the affected arteries (Pesic et al., 2004). Strong evidence is provided by these latest findings that upregulation of the $\alpha1C$ subunit by higher levels of blood pressure in vivo enhances the accessibility of functional CaL channels in renal VSMCs, and even short-term elevation in blood pressure can quickly increase the expression of the CaL channel.[4,5]

IMPLICATIONS FOR ANTIHYPERTENSIVE THERAPIES

It is suggested by latest evidence that during raised blood pressure, the development of anomalous arterial tone is related with enhanced expression of vascular CaL channels, which at the minimum consist of subunits $\alpha1C$, β, and $\alpha2\delta$. Notably, for all of the three classes (phenylalkylamines, dihydropyridines (DHPs) and benzothiazepines) of organic CCBs, which are used for the treatment of essential hypertension in humans, the $\alpha1C$ subunit is the binding site. The open-state probability of the CaL channel is decreased by the interaction between these drugs and the $\alpha1C$ subunit and thus it attenuates the voltage-gated Ca^{2+} influx needed for vascular activation.[6,7] Fortuitously, during hypertension, more binding sites for CCBs can be provided by the enhanced abundance of vascular $\alpha1C$ subunits, thus amplifying their vasodilator action proportional to the elevation of blood pressure. This can help in explaining why CCBs efficiently reduce blood pressure in case of hypertensive humans and animals, but only mildly decrease blood pressure levels in normotensive people (Godfraind et al., 1991; Miyamori et al., 1987; Narita et al., 1983; Takata and Hutchinson, 1983).

■ CALCIUM CHANNEL BLOCKER

Calcium channel blockers bind to L-type calcium channels located on the vascular smooth muscle, cardiac myocytes, and cardiac nodal tissue (sinoatrial and atrio-ventricular nodes). These channels are responsible for regulating the influx of calcium into muscle cells, which in turn stimulates smooth muscle contraction and cardiac myocyte contraction. In cardiac nodal tissue, L-type calcium channels play an important role in pacemaker currents and in phase 0 of the action potentials. Therefore, by blocking calcium entry into the cell, CCBs cause vascular smooth muscle relaxation (vasodilation), decreased myocardial force generation (negative inotropy), decreased heart rate (negative chronotropic), and decreased conduction velocity within the heart (negative dromotropy), particularly at the atrioventricular node.

Different Classes of Calcium Channel Blockers

There are three chemical classes of CCBs. They differ not only in their basic chemical structure but also in their relative selectivity toward cardiac versus vascular L-type calcium channels. The most smooth muscle selective class of CCBs is the *dihydropyridines*. Because of their high vascular selectivity, these drugs are primarily used to reduce systemic vascular resistance and arterial pressure, and therefore are used to treat hypertension.

Extended-release formulations or long-acting compounds are used to treat angina and are particularly effecting for vasospastic angina; however, their powerful systemic vasodilator and pressure lowering effects can lead to reflex cardiac stimulation (tachycardia and increased inotropy), which can offset the beneficial effects of afterload reduction on myocardial oxygen demand.

Calcium channel blockers comprise of three chemical classes. They vary in their basic chemical structure as well as in their relative selectivity toward vascular versus cardiac L-type calcium channels. DHPs are the most smooth muscle selective class of CCBs. These drugs are mainly used to decrease systemic vascular resistance and arterial pressure due to their high vascular selectivity and are therefore used in treating hypertension. Long-acting compounds or extended-release formulations are used for angina treatment and are especially effective for vasospastic angina. However, reflex cardiac stimulation (increased inotropy and tachycardia) can be caused by their powerful systemic vasodilator and pressure lowering effects that can offset the useful effects of afterload reduction on the myocardial oxygen demand.

Dihydropyridines comprise of the specific drugs as following—amlodipine, felodipine, isradipine, nicardipine, nifedipine, nimodipine and nitrendipine.

Third-generation DHP Ca^{2+} antagonist is barnidipine because it exerts a slow onset but strong and long-lasting vasodilatory effect without baroreflex activation.[8,9] It has preferential effects on renal and mesenteric vasodilation, barnidipine also significantly decreased both blood pressure and plasma NE level, indicating that it lowered the blood pressure by sympathoinhibition possibly via the central nervous system due to their more lipophilic property allowing them easily to cross the blood-brain barrier.

The *fourth-generation cilnidipine* (L/N-type CCB) and *lercanidipine* are highly lipophilic DHPs.

Nondihydropyridines comprise two classes of CCBs. *Verapamil* (phenylalkylamine class), is relatively selective for the myocardium and is less effective as a systemic vasodilator drug. This drug has a very important role in treating angina (by reducing myocardial oxygen demand and reversing coronary vasospasm) and arrhythmias. *Diltiazem* (benzothiazepine class) is intermediate between verapamil and DHPs in its selectivity for vascular calcium channels. By having both cardiac depressant and vasodilator actions, diltiazem is able to reduce arterial pressure without producing the same degree of reflex cardiac stimulation caused by DHPs.

■ CONCLUSION

It is concurred through reports from a number of laboratories that in VSMCs voltage-gated Ca^{2+} influx through CaL channels is increased. It appears that in the VSMC membrane, the expression of CaL channels is promoted by high blood pressure. Even short-term increase in the blood pressure in vivo can increase the number of CaL channels in the small resistance arteries.[10-12] As suggested by a recent study, pressure-induced depolarization of VSMCs that takes place during the development of hypertension can give an electrophysiological signal, which can trigger vascular CaL channels upregulation. Therefore, in the arterial circulation, blood pressure appears to represent an endogenous promoter of CaL channel expression.[13-15] Latest attempts are centerd on recognizing the molecular mechanisms that mediate this event.

■ REFERENCES

1. Arikkath J, Campbell KP. Auxiliary subunits: essential components of the voltage-gated calcium channel complex. Curr Opin Neurobiol. 2003;13:298-307.

2. Avila G, O'Connell KM, Groom LA, et al. Ca^{2+} release through ryanodine receptors regulates skeletal muscle L-type Ca^{2+} channel expression. J Biol Chem. 2001;276: 17732-8.

3. Balijepalli RC, Lokuta AJ, Maertz NA, et al. Depletion of T-tubules and specific subcellular changes in sarcolemmal proteins in tachycardia-induced heart failure. Cardiovasc Res. 2003;59:67-77.

4. Ball SL, Powers PA, Shin HS, et al. Role of the β2 subunit of voltage-dependent calcium channels in the retinal outer plexiform layer. Invest Ophthalmol Visual Sci. 2002;43:1595-603

5. Beguin P, Nagashima K, Gonoi T, et al. Regulation of Ca^{2+} channel expression at the cell surface by the small G-protein kir/Gem. Nature. 2001;411:701-6.

6. Berjukow S, Marksteiner R, Sokolov S, et al. Amino acids in segment IVS6 and β-subunit interaction support distinct conformational changes during Cav2.1 inactivation. J Biol Chem. 2001;276:17076-82.

7. Berrou L, Bernatchez G, Parent L. Molecular determinants of inactivation within the I–II linker of α1E (CaV2.3) calcium channels. Biophys J. 2001;80:215-28.

8. Berrow NS, Campbell V, Fitzgerald EM, Brickley K, Dolphin AC. Antisense depletion of β-subunits modulates the biophysical and pharmacological properties of neuronal calcium channels. J Physiol. 1995;482:481-91.

9. Birnbaumer L, Qin N, Olcese R, et al. Structures and functions of calcium channel β subunits. J Bioenerg Biomembranes. 1998;30:357-75.

10. Bogdanov Y, Brice NL, Canti C, et al. Acidic motif responsible for plasma membrane association of the voltage-dependent calcium channel β1b subunit. Eur J Neurosci. 2000;12:894-902.

11. Bowles DK, Maddali KK, Ganjam VK, et al. Endogenous testosterone increases L-type Ca^{2+} channel expression in porcine coronary smooth muscle. Am J Physiol. 2004;287:H2091-8.

12. Brice NL, Berrow NS, Campbell V, et al. Importance of the different β subunits in the membrane expression of the α1A and α2 calcium channel subunits: studies using a depolarization-sensitive α1A antibody. Eur J Neurosci. 1997;9:749-59.

13. Bunemann M, Gerhardstein BL, Gao T, et al. Functional regulation of L-type calcium channels via protein kinase A-mediated phosphorylation of the β2 subunit. J Biol Chem. 1999;274:33851-4.

14. Canti C, Bogdanov Y, Dolphin AC. Interaction between G proteins and accessory β subunits in the regulation of α1B calcium channels in Xenopus oocytes. J Physiol. 2000;527:419-32.

15. Catterall WA. Structure and regulation of voltage-gated Ca^{2+} channels. Annu Rev Cell Dev Biol. 2000;16:521-55.

Role of Cytokines and Inflammation in Hypertension

JPS Sawhney, Prashant Wankhade, Simran Sawhney

■ INTRODUCTION

Hypertension is one of the most common cardiovascular risk factors contributing to widespread morbidity and mortality worldwide. Around 90% of cases are classified as essential hypertension and only minority have secondary causes such as primary aldosteronism, obstructive sleep apnea, renal and renovascular disease, etc.

Clinical studies have shown that elevated serum C-reactive protein (CRP) is a risk factor for the development of hypertension. Several studies have also suggested that vascular and renal abnormalities can predict the development of hypertension but none has demonstrated that inflammation contributes to the development of hypertension by inducing vascular or renal abnormalities.[1,2]

Plasma levels of proinflammatory cytokines have shown to correlate with increased blood pressure in certain forms of human hypertension.[3] Several studies have shown that chronic increase in plasma levels of cytokines in preeclampsia result in significant and sustained increases in arterial pressure. But still the quantitative role of endogenous cytokines in various forms of hypertension remains unclear.

Sympathetic nervous system (SNS) plays an important role in this aspect by serving as a source of cytokines and stimulating the release of proinflammatory cytokines.[4] Another important system, i.e. renin–angiotensin–aldosterone system (RAAS) contributes to inflammation by enhancing the synthesis of various cytokines like tumor necrosis factor-α (TNF-α) and interleukin-6 (IL-6) via angiotensin II (Ang II) and also by stimulating chemokine monocyte chemoattractant protein-1 (MCP-1) and nuclear factor-κB (NF-κB).[5] Ang II also plays a role in development of oxidative stress induced inflammation via the production of reactive oxygen species (ROS).

Though the relation between hypertension and inflammation has now been clearly demonstrated, it is presently unclear whether inflammation is the cause or effect of hypertension.

■ ROLE OF CYTOKINES IN THE DEVELOPMENT OF HYPERTENSION

Activated immune cells produce cytokines that determine the local inflammatory response. Chemokines are chemoattractants that direct migration of immune cells into tissues. Some of the inflammatory cytokines and chemokines like TNF-α, IL-17, MCP-1 and IL-6 have been studied for their involvement in hypertension.

Tissue Necrosis Factor-alpha

Animal models of Ang II-induced hypertension, lupus, metabolic syndrome and preeclampsia have demonstrated contribution of TNF-α to the development of high blood pressure by pharmacological or genetic approaches.[6] In these cases, blockade of the TNF-α pathway led to decreased blood pressure and inflammation. However, DOCA-salt hypertension or a human Ang/renin double transgenic rat model of Ang II hypertension has shown contrasting results.[6] The reason behind these opposite observations may be related to the different type of TNF-α receptor that is activated in each model.

To date two different TNF-α receptors have been described, i.e. tumor necrosis factor receptor 1 (TNFR1) and TNFR2, but their detail understanding is still lacking. There are contrasting reports regarding the function of both these receptors and hence further investigation on the role of TNF-α and its receptors in hypertension is needed to develop better therapies. In humans, high serum TNFR1 levels strongly correlate with diseases associated with hypertension, like end-stage renal disease and type 2 diabetes mellitus whereas other reports indicate that genetic deletion of TNFR1 leads to increase in blood pressure in response to Ang II.[7]

Studies have reported that a two-fold elevation in the plasma levels of TNF-α has significantly increased arterial pressure and renal vascular resistance in pregnant rats.[5]

Interleukin-6

Levels of IL-6, a proinflammatory cytokine are also elevated in hypertensive conditions. Activation of the JAK/STAT3 pathway by IL-6 plays a key role in the development of Ang II-induced hypertension.[8]

Experimental study has demonstrated that mice with knockout of IL-6 had significantly lower mean arterial pressure of approximately 30 mm Hg as compared to wild-type mice during the 2 weeks of Ang II infusion.

The TNF-α and IL-6 have been shown to induce structural as well as functional changes in endothelial cells by enhancing the formation of a number of endothelial cell substances, such as endothelin, reducing acetylcholine-induced vasodilatation and by destabilizing the mRNA of endothelial nitric oxide synthase.[5]

Interleukin-17

Interleukin-17, a proinflammatory cytokine, has also shown some role in the development of hypertension. It is produced by Th17 cells, macrophages, dendritic cells and natural killer cells in response to immune activation. Elevated IL-17 has shown correlation with hypertension in subjects with type 2 diabetes and in patients with preeclampsia and lupus.[7] Madhur et al.[9] reported that IL-17 is required for the maintenance of Ang II-induced hypertension and vascular dysfunction. This effect of IL-17 on vascular function is mediated by promotion of NOS3 phosphorylation, thus decreasing enzyme activity and nitric oxide (NO) production in endothelial cells.

Recent studies indicate that naïve T-cells increase expression of serum/glucocorticoid-regulated kinase 1 (SGK1; a known salt-sensor protein) and polarize to Th17 cell phenotype in the presence of high salt indicating the role of this cytokine in salt-sensitive hypertension. These studies demonstrate the importance of SGK1 for the induction of Th17 cells, and hint toward the mechanism by which high salt may trigger Th17 development, IL-17 production, and promote tissue inflammation.[7]

Monocyte Chemoattractant Protein-1

Angiotensin II and endothelin-1 stimulate the production of chemokine MCP-1 (also known as CCL2) which leads to the activation and migration of monocytes and leukocytes to sites of inflammation by activating the CCR2 receptor. The use of ANG receptor blockers has shown to reduce MCP-1 levels both in experimental models and in hypertensive patients.[10] Genetic deletion of the MCP-1 axis or blockade of CCR2 in experimental models has demonstrated decrease in blood pressure and reduces vascular and renal inflammation,[11] highlighting the potential of MCP-1 axis inhibition for treating hypertension.

CD40L

The CD40L, a part of TNF superfamily, derived from activated platelets, acts by promoting cytokine and chemokine release. Role of CD40L has been implicated in thrombosis. Research suggests that Ang II promotes and augments the inflammatory activity of the CD40/CD40L system in human vascular cells.[12] Genetic deletion of CD40L has shown to improve endothelial dysfunction and decrease in aortic inflammation and oxidative stress. Hypertensive patients have increased levels of soluble CD40L (sCD40L) and these levels decrease significantly after anti-hypertensive treatment. Thus, CD40L could be a valuable biomarker of cardiovascular disease and a potential therapeutic target.[7]

■ ROLE OF INFLAMMASOMES IN HYPERTENSION

The nucleotide-binding oligomerization domain (Nod)-like receptor containing pyrin domain 3 (NLRP3, also known as NALP3 or cryopyrin) inflammasome is the member of the nucleotide-binding domain leucine-rich repeats (NLR) family of pattern recognition receptors (PRRs). Activation of the NLRP3 inflammasome is responsible for the maturation of inactive proinflammatory cytokine precursors like pro-IL-1β or pro-IL-18 via activation of a subclass of inflammatory caspases. NLRP3 inflammasome formation controls the activation of innate immune system in response to danger signals including pathogen-associated molecular patterns (PAMPs) and DAMPs derived from disease and infection.[7]

Recent literature suggests an important role of NLRP3 inflammasomes in humans and animal models of kidney disease and hypertension. Role of NLRP3 inflammasome has been implicated in glomerular and tubulointerstitial injury as suggested by significantly increased levels of NLRP3 mRNA in renal biopsies of patients with various types of nondiabetic kidney disease, including acute tubular necrosis, focal segmental glomerulosclerosis, etc. NLRP3 deficient mice have shown attenuated glomerular injury, renal leukocyte infiltration, and T-cell activation associated with nephrotoxic serum nephritis.[13] The inflammasome has also been shown to contribute to IgA nephropathy, hyperhomocysteinemia-induced glomerular sclerosis and ischemia-reperfusion injury.[7]

■ INFLAMMATION IN HUMAN HYPERTENSION

Antihypertensive therapy reduces the risk of total major cardiovascular events and this benefit has linear correlation, i.e. greater the reduction in blood pressure, the greater the reduction in cardiovascular risk.[14] While most of the patients respond to routine antihypertensive therapy, there is a group of patients who are resistant to such treatment. It has been observed that even after achieving the optimum blood pressure target, many hypertensive patients remain at risk for a

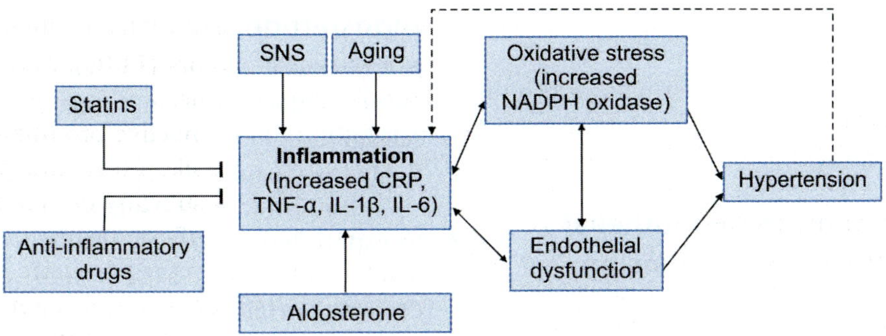

(CRP: C-reactive protein; IL: interleukin; SNS: sympathetic nervous system; TNF-α: tumor necrosis factor-α; NADPH: nicotinamide adenine dinucleotide phosphate)

Flowchart 1: Schematic diagram illustrating the relationship between inflammation and hypertension.

cardiovascular event, which may be due to underlying inflammation.

Though inflammation is a protective response to injury or infection, excessive inflammation can have detrimental effects and contribute to the progression of chronic and/or prolonged diseases such as atherosclerosis, rheumatoid arthritis, etc.[15] Various factors including aging, oxidative stress, sympathetic nervous system, etc. have their role in inflammatory process and development of hypertension (Flowchart 1).

C-reactive Protein

C-reactive protein is involved in innate immune responses and has role in activating the complement system and enhancing phagocytosis. It can also stimulate endothelial cells to express intercellular adhesion molecule (ICAM)-1 and vascular cell adhesion molecule (VCAM)-1 which further promotes inflammation.[15]

Among inflammatory markers, CRP is considered to have the strongest association with hypertension. Numerous clinical trials have demonstrated that CRP levels are commonly increased in hypertensive patients.[16] Prehypertensive patients usually have higher plasma CRP levels than normotensive patients, and higher baseline levels of CRP have been shown to

be associated with a higher risk of developing overt hypertension.[17] Studies revealed that nonhypertensive offspring of hypertensive parents tend to have higher serum CRP levels than offspring of nonhypertensive parents. This suggests that systemic low-grade inflammation may precede overt hypertension. Studies have also demonstrated higher plasma levels of IL-6, IL-1β and TNF-α in hypertensive patients compared to normotensive ones.[15]

Immune System and Hypertension

Evidence suggests involvement of immune cells in human hypertension. Patients with hypertensive nephrosclerosis have higher infiltration of CD4+ and CD8+ T cells in renal tissue than normotensive control patients. Circulating levels of CXC chemokine receptor type 3 (CXCR3), a tissue-homing chemokine for T cells, have been reported to be elevated in hypertensive patients. Acquired immunodeficiency syndrome (AIDS) patients have reduced CD4+ T cells and the incidence of hypertension has been reported to be lower in these patients. The highly active antiretroviral therapy which can raise T-cell levels increases the incidence of hypertension in AIDS patients. It is becoming increasingly recognized that prenatal environment is linked with subsequent neonatal and childhood health and disease. Indeed, infants born following intrauterine inflammation are at increased risk of perinatal morbidity and mortality as compared to infants born to healthy mothers.[15]

Inflammation and Endothelial Dysfunction in Hypertension

Inflammation may promote hypertension by causing endothelial dysfunction. Endothelium is involved in regulation of vascular tone and structure. NO derived from endothelial nitric oxide synthase (eNOS) is a signaling molecule important for regulation of vascular tone and causes smooth muscle relaxation and subsequent vasodilation. Endothelial dysfunction may lead to impaired endothelium dependent vasodilation due to an imbalance between vasoconstrictors and vasodilators which subsequently results in increased systemic vascular resistance and thus leads to the development of hypertension.[18] Inflammation can alter the rates of synthesis and degradation of vasoconstrictors and vasodilators including NO, and the resultant impaired bioactivity of NO is associated with hypertension.

Aging and Chronic Inflammation

The prevalence of hypertension increases with age and more than half of the elderly (above 65 years of age) have hypertension. Chronic low-grade inflammation commonly occurs with aging and is termed as "inflammaging". Inflammaging is characterized by an imbalance of proinflammatory and anti-inflammatory markers. Levels of proinflammatory markers such as IL-6, TNF-α and CRP are elevated, whereas those of anti-inflammatory cytokines such as IL-10 are reduced.[19] Thus, there may be a possible role of inflammation in the elderly hypertensive population.

Aldosterone and Inflammation

It is now well understood that in addition to kidney, aldosterone can target other tissues relevant to blood pressure control including the brain, vasculature and the heart.

Administration of exogenous aldosterone to experimental animals results in elevated levels of ICAM-1, MCP-1 and TNF-α in coronary arteries, and increased vascular infiltration of macrophages and lymphocytes. Association between aldosterone and inflammation has been reported in essential hypertension, where high plasma aldosterone levels are correlated with high levels of circulating CRP and leukocytes.[20]

The Sympathetic Nervous System and Inflammation in Hypertension

Sympathetic nervous system activation can contribute to the development of hypertension, and inflammation may also promote SNS activation. Patients with essential hypertension have increased renal sympathetic outflow. Renal sympathetic nerves have shown to play a role in renal inflammation. Experimental rats undergoing renal sympathetic denervation have reduced renal macrophage levels and cortical TNF expression.

Increased sympathetic drive to the kidneys causes the release of renin, subsequently raising blood pressure. Catheter-based renal denervation is an evolving therapeutic approach to treat resistant hypertension. However, the SYMPLICITY HTN-3 clinical trial has concluded that renal denervation does not result in a significant reduction in systolic blood pressure in resistant hypertensive patients when compared to sham control.[21]

Inflammation and Oxidative Stress in Hypertension

Chronic inflammation can trigger oxidative stress, which has been associated with hypertension. Innate immune cells, such as neutrophils and macrophages, produce ROS such as superoxide and hydrogen peroxide in the process to kill pathogens. Presence of sustained inflammation can lead to an overproduction of ROS. Oxidative stress is defined as an imbalance between the production and breakdown of ROS and is a major cause of endothelial dysfunction. This phenomenon occurs primarily through reducing NO bioavailability via the direct chemical reaction of superoxide with NO which subsequently results in the formation of peroxynitrite. This peroxynitrite formation may result in further impairment of NO levels by inhibiting eNOS activity through oxidation of 4-tetrahydrobiopterin (BH4), a cofactor of eNOS. Excessive ROS levels can induce cellular damage by interacting with DNA, lipids and proteins, which may further impair vascular structure and function. CRP levels also have been shown to correlate with the level of oxidative stress in inflammatory cells from hypertensive patients.[15]

ANTI-INFLAMMATORY DRUGS AND HYPERTENSION

Till date, anti-inflammatory drugs are not used to treat hypertension. Of the various classes of anti-inflammatory agents, immunosuppressant drugs could potentially be used to treat hypertension, e.g. mycophenolate mofetil, which blocks T-cell and B-cell proliferation by inhibiting inosine monophosphate dehydrogenase, has shown to reduce hypertension in various rodent hypertensive models like spontaneously hypertensive rats (SHR) and in Dahl salt-sensitive rats, and also in patients with psoriasis and rheumatoid arthritis.[22,23] Tacrolimus, a calcineurin inhibitor and blocker of T-cell activation is reported to reduce hypertension in Dahl salt-sensitive rats.[24] Chronic kidney disease patients with hypertension who were also on immunosuppressant drugs were found to require less antihypertensive medications compared to those who were not taking immunosuppressant drugs. These studies suggest that T cells may be a potential target in treating hypertension. Ang II and aldosterone have proinflammatory effects and Ang II has demonstrated to stimulate T-cell proliferation; hence, targeting the RAAS could simultaneously target inflammation in hypertension.

The CYT006-AngGb vaccine targeting Ang II has reported to reduce blood pressure in patients with mild to moderate hypertension without any serious safety issues in a phase IIa clinical trial.[25] The ATRQβ-001 vaccine targeting the AT1R was found to be successful in lowering blood pressure in Ang II-induced hypertensive mice and SHR. Contrary to this, one of the earlier vaccines developed which targeted renin was found to cause fatal autoimmunity; hence, further studies are required to establish their role as therapeutic agents.[26]

CONCLUSION

It is unclear whether inflammation is a cause or effect of hypertension, but as discussed above there is evidence from human and animal studies which suggest that inflammation can lead to the development of hypertension. Oxidative stress and endothelial dysfunction are associated with inflammation and can contribute to hypertension. Other factors contributing to hypertension such as SNS activation, aging, and aldosterone have also shown to be associated with inflammation. It is still in the experimental stage to know whether anti-inflammatory drugs are beneficial in reversing hypertension or not.

■ REFERENCES

1. Wang TJ, Gona P, Larson MG, et al. Multiple biomarkers and the risk of incident hypertension. Hypertension. 2007;49(3):432-8.

2. Chen W, Li S, Fernandez C, et al. Temporal relationship between elevated blood pressure and arterial stiffening among middle-aged black and white adults: The bogalusa heart study. Am J Epidemiol. 2016;183(7):599-608.

3. LaMarca BB, Bennett WA, Alexander BT, et al. Hypertension produced by reductions in uterine perfusion in the pregnant rat: role of tumor necrosis factor-alpha. Hypertension. 2005;46(4):1022-5.

4. Zhang ZH, Wei SG, Francis J, et al. Cardiovascular and renal sympathetic activation by blood-borne TNF in rat: the role of central prostaglandins. Am J Physiol Regul Integr Comp Physiol. 2003;284(4):R916-27.

5. Granger JP. An emerging role for inflammatory cytokines in hypertension. Am J Physiol Heart Circ Physiol. 2006; 290(3):H923-24.

6. Ramseyer VD, Garvin JL. Tumor necrosis factor-α: regulation of renal function and blood pressure. Am J Physiol Renal Physiol. 2013;304(10):F1231-42.

7. De Miguel C, Rudemiller NP, Abais JM, et al. Inflammation and hypertension: new understandings and potential therapeutic targets. Curr Hypertens Rep. 2015;17(1):507.

8. Brands MW, Banes-Berceli AK, Inscho EW, et al. Interleukin 6 knockout prevents angiotensin II hypertension: role of renal vasoconstriction and janus kinase 2/signal transducer and activator of transcription 3 activation. Hypertension. 2010;56(5):879-84.

9. Madhur MS, Lob HE, McCann LA, et al. Interleukin 17 promotes angiotensin II-induced hypertension and vascular dysfunction. Hypertension. 2010;55(2):500-7.

10. Fliser D, Buchholz K, Haller H. European Trial on Olmesartan and Pravastatin in Inflammation and Atherosclerosis (EUTOPIA) Investigators. Antiinflammatory effects of angiotensin II subtype 1 receptor blockade in hypertensive patients with microinflammation. Circulation. 2004;110(9):1103-7.

11. Chan CT, Moore JP, Budzyn K, et al. Reversal of vascular macrophage accumulation and hypertension by a CCR2 antagonist in deoxycorticosterone/salt-treated mice. Hypertension. 2012;60(5):1207-12.

12. Ruef J, Browatzki M, Pfeiffer CA, et al. Angiotensin II promotes the inflammatory response to CD40 ligation via TRAF-2. Vasc Med. 2007;12(1):23-7.

13. Andersen K, Eltrich N, Lichtnekert J, et al. The NLRP3/ASC inflammasome promotes T-cell-dependent immune complex glomerulonephritis by canonical and non-canonical mechanisms. Kidney Int. 2014;86(5):965-78.

14. Turnbull F. Blood Pressure Lowering Treatment Trialists' Collaboration. Effects of different blood-pressure-lowering regimens on major cardiovascular events: results of prospectively-designed overviews of randomised trials. Lancet. 2003;362(9395):1527-35.

15. Dinh QN, Drummond GR, Sobey CG, et al. Roles of inflammation, oxidative stress, and vascular dysfunction in hypertension. Biomed Res Int. 2014;2014:406960.

16. Xu T, Ju Z, Tong W, et al. Relationship of C-reactive protein with hypertension and interactions between increased C-reactive protein and other risk factors on hypertension in Mongolian people, China. Circ J. 2008;72(8):1324-8.

17. Niskanen L, Laaksonen DE, Nyyssönen K, et al. Inflammation, abdominal obesity, and smoking as predictors of hypertension. Hypertension. 2004;44(6):859-65.

18. Chrissobolis S, Faraci FM. The role of oxidative stress and NADPH oxidase in cerebrovascular disease. Trends Mol Med. 2008;14(11):495-502.

19. Esler MD, Krum H, Schlaich M, et al. Symplicity HTN-2 Investigators. Renal sympathetic denervation for treatment of drug-resistant hypertension: one-year results from the symplicity HTN-2 randomized, controlled trial. Circulation. 2012;126(25):2976-82.

20. Tzamou V, Vyssoulis G, Karpanou E, et al. Aldosterone levels and inflammatory stimulation in essential hypertensive patients. J Hum Hypertens. 2013;27(9):535-8.

21. Bhatt DL, Kandzari DE, O'Neill WW, et al. SYMPLICITY HTN-3 Investigators. A controlled trial of renal denervation for resistant hypertension. N Engl J Med. 2014;370(15):1393-401.

22. Rodríguez-Iturbe B, Quiroz Y, Nava M, et al. Reduction of renal immune cell infiltration results in blood pressure control in genetically hypertensive rats. Am J Physiol Renal Physiol. 2002;282(2):F191-201.

23. Herrera J, Ferrebuz A, MacGregor EG, et al. Mycophenolate mofetil treatment improves hypertension in patients with psoriasis and rheumatoid arthritis. J Am Soc Nephrol. 2006;17(12 Suppl 3):S218-25.

24. de Miguel C, Guo C, Lund H, et al. Infiltrating T lymphocytes in the kidney increase oxidative stress and participate in the development of hypertension and renal disease. Am J Physiol Renal Physiol. 2011;300(3):734-42.

25. Tissot AC, Maurer P, Nussberger J, et al. Effect of immunization against angiotensin II with CYT006-AngQb on ambulatory blood pressure: a double-blind, randomised, placebo-controlled phase IIa study. Lancet. 2008; 371 (9615):821-7.

26. Michel JB, Guettier C, Philippe M, et al. Active immunization against renin in normotensive marmoset. Proc Natl Acad Sci USA. 1987;84(12):4346-50.

Natriuretic Peptides in Hypertension

Tiny Nair

INTRODUCTION

Incorporation of natriuretic peptide (NP) as an essential cardiac biomarker in the diagnostic algorithm of heart failure, followed by understanding of the beneficial role of angiotensin receptor-neprilysin inhibitor (ARNI) therapy in the treatment of the failing heart, made NPs come into the limelight; a quick transition from bench-to-bedside. Essential hypertension, being a major driver of vascular disease, is a vexing therapeutic problem, waiting to see newer drugs for its treatment.

This narrative review takes a look at the current understanding of NPs in pathophysiology, diagnosis and treatment of hypertension and hypertensive heart disease.

TYPES OF NATRIURETIC PEPTIDES—NOMENCLATURE AND DISCOVERY

Natriuretic peptides are a family of small molecules secreted by the atria or ventricle of the heart that has autocrine, endocrine and paracrine functions. The existence of such a peptide was suspected long back when diuresis was noted following conversion of atrial tachyarrhythmias to sinus rhythm.

Atrial natriuretic peptide (ANP), discovered in 1984, is secreted from the atrial muscles where it is stored as granules (pro-ANP). Pro-ANP is stripped up into an "omega"-shaped ANP with 28 amino acids and a linier "n" terminal (NT) pro-ANP with 98 amino acids.

"B"-type natriuretic peptide (BNP), discovered in 1988, is secreted from the ventricular myocardium in response to stretch. Stored pro-BNP is further cleaved out into NT-pro-BNP with 75 amino acids and BNP with 36 amino acids.

Subsequently, in 1990, a third NP, C-type natriuretic peptide (CNP) was isolated from pig brain.[1,2]

NATRIURETIC PEPTIDE RECEPTORS

There are three kinds of receptors for NPs—(1) Natriuretic peptide receptor-A (NPR-A); (2) Natriuretic peptide receptor-B (NPR-B) and (3) Natriuretic peptide receptor-C (NPR-C). NPR-B is biologically least active, main effects being carried out by A and C.

Receptor types A and B are "G-coupled" receptor system meaning that they are the first step of a two-step messenger system.

Generally, NPR-A and NPR-C are active. NPR-A acts as a stimulatory receptor, which regulates most of actions of both ANP and BNP. In contrast, the NPR-C is associated with destruction of the ANP and BNP.

It is now understood that the receptor system (NPR-C) is not the only system that regulate the destruction and neutralization of NPs. One other mechanism by which NPs are neutralized and inactivated are by a "endopeptidase system" called neprilysin, which incidentally has come under intense clinical interest in view of the clinical improvement of heart failure patients by its modulation by ARNI.

"Natriuretic peptide receptor-C" receptors are located in adipose tissue and kidney while neprilysin is seen in high concentrations in vascular endothelium, cardiomyocytes as well as fibroblasts.

Both NPR-C and neprilysin play an important role in deciding the role of NPs in the body by controlling their degradation.[3-5]

EFFECT OF NATRIURETIC PEPTIDES ON BLOOD PRESSURE

High blood pressure (BP) is mediated by volume change, sodium retention, sympathetic nervous system (SNS) tone as well as activity of renin-angiotensin system (RAS). NPs seem to have effect on all these factors.[6] It has been shown that NPs exert protective effect on counterbalancing the RAS in controlling BP. NPs produce vasorelaxation, reduce renin–angiotensin–aldosterone system (RAAS) activity and SNS tone as well as show antiatherosclerotic effects in hypertension. In clinical trials of ARNI, the BP reduction had been consistently better as compared to RAAS inhibition alone.[7] In the long term, upregulation of ANP gene transcription is thought to be a protective factor in hypertension. Circulating ANP levels have also shown to have close relationship with corin levels as well as levels of Proprotein convertase subtilisin/kexin type 9 (PCSK9), a lipid modulating target. This opens up an exciting possibility of combining ARNI with PCSK9 inhibition for better cardioprotection in chronic hypertension.[8]

Natriuretic peptide levels are also known to increase in presence of left ventricular hypertrophy (LVH) whether it represents the result of cardiac stress or if this protects the heart from deleterious effects of hypertensive cardiac effects is not clear. Data shows that in early hypertension, there is substantial reduction of NPs (loss of counterbalance) while in late hypertension, there is increased levels of NPs.[9]

Higher NP levels have shown to have a positive correlation with ischemic stroke, and that makes NPs an important predictor of neurovascular ischemic events.[10] It is now known that a subset of isolated systolic hypertension of the elderly population with low diastolic BP has a higher propensity of vascular events. This subset tends to have more often an elevated BNP, making NPs an important marker of high risk in this subset.[11]

In a meta-analysis of 25,000 patients, increased cardiovascular (CV) events and mortality seem to relate well to NP levels, in a general population, opening up the possibility of NPs being used as a screening biomarker. In this analysis, those with the highest quartile of NPs seem to have a 2.7 times higher CV mortality and 2.4 times higher all-cause mortality.[12]

EFFECT OF NATRIURETIC PEPTIDES ON HYPERTENSION WITH DIABETES

The insulin resistance in a typical metabolic syndrome (MS) shows a high level of glucose as well as a high level of insulin. Experimental data have shown that such a combination of high glucose and high insulin causes overexpression of NPR-C resulting in excess destruction and consequent lowering of NP levels driving the progression of the disease. Elevation of insulin levels or glucose levels in isolation has not shown such suppressive effects on NPR-C.

Decades back, fasting and calorie restriction were used as standard therapy for the treatment of diabetes. The improvement was thought to be because of loss of body weight and carbohydrate restriction. Present data indicate that fasting results in downregulation of NPR-C in adipose tissue with possible upregulation of NPR-A. This results in increase in net circulatory levels of NP causing natriuresis of fasting.[13]

■ EFFECT OF NATRIURETIC PEPTIDES ON HYPERTENSION WITH OBESITY AND METABOLIC SYNDROME

Perhaps the most overwhelming information connection between deranged NP with altered and hyperactive RAAS comes from study of MS and adiposity. It is postulated that while RAAS activation can produce hypertension, alteration of NPs play a major role in altered fat metabolism and adipocyte derangement. Altered adiponectin and ghrelin resulting from a decreased NP levels might be important in MS. It is also theorized that in an attempt to correct the abnormal adipocytes, the body increases sympathetic activity to expend more energy "internal metabolic exercise" resulting in increased heart rate and elevated systolic BP.

The NPR-C null mouse with high levels of NP tends to be leaner, less adipocytes and also more brown fat in contrast to its normal siblings. Short-term infusion of BNP reduces hunger by reduction of adiponectin and ghrelin levels.[14]

■ EFFECTS OF NATRIURETIC PEPTIDES ON TARGET ORGANS IN HYPERTENSION

Kidneys

Atrial natriuretic peptide tends to have more physiological effects on the kidney, heart and blood vessels, making it a "physiological" tool for supporting the delicate cardiorenal balance. In contrast, BNP tend to get activated in pathological situations like "myocardial" stress; the classic example being stretched, failing myocardium, as happens in heart failure.

The affinity of NPR-C to ANP is much higher compared to BNP, resulting in a longer half-life of circulating BNP compared to ANP. NT-pro-BNP has 6 times longer half-life as compared to BNP.[2]

The effect of NPs on kidney are opposite of RAAS activation. In fact, the NPs seem to protect against RAS-induced kidney damage. Increased natriuresis was the first observed effect, but increased glomerular filtration rate (GFR) perhaps is the most defining effect of NPs on kidney.

Adipose Tissue

Natriuretic peptide receptor-C, the major receptor system that clears circulating NPs, is abundant in kidneys and adipose tissues. In the adipose tissue, NPs produce a host of physiological effects. Increased lipolysis and energy utilization seem to be the principal effect. Decreased adiponectin and ghrelin levels are involved in the mechanism, though the effects are not entirely clear.

Natriuretic peptides tend to alter lipolysis efficiently. The browning of white fat converts the fat into more energy efficient adiposity. Such alteration seems to have beneficial effect in altering sympathetic tone and improves CV status.[15]

> **Box 1: Cardiovascular effects of natriuretic peptides.**
>
> **Cardiovascular effects**
> *Heart:*
> - Decreased atherosclerosis
> - Decreased myohypertrophy
> - Decreased myocardial fibrosis
> - Improved myocardial relaxation
>
> *Peripheral vessels:*
> - Vasodilation
> - Volume reduction

Cardiovascular System

Natriuretic peptides relax vascular smooth muscles of the arterial system and tend to lower BP and peripheral resistance. In long term, NPs seem to counter effects of atherosclerosis. In the heart, it reduces afterload, reduces myohypertrophy as well as myocardial interstitial fibrosis. These effects combine together to improve myocardial function, especially in presence of heart failure (Box 1).

Natriuretic peptides counterbalance the effects of SNS activation.[6]

All these actions are good and favorable for the CV system. There is very clear proof that a higher NP levels are beneficial for the physiologic function of the CV system.

Many physiological effects of NPs are not well-understood. Estradiol, the female hormone, tends to upregulate NPR-A while downregulate NPR-C, increasing its efficacy in females. This might play a role in the female type body fat distribution and difference of CV disease in women, especially myocardial infarction with normal coronary arteries (MINOCA).

Physiological effects of NP differ distinctly from those happening in pathological conditions like heart failure and myocardial dysfunction. The increased levels of NPs, e.g., during cardiac failure (stretched failing myocardium) tend to produce more NPs. In this background, a higher BNP indicate a poor CV outcome.

■ FUTURE

We are likely to see use of NPs/ARNI in the treatment of severe hypertension. NPR-C receptor blockers looks promising as a treatment modality of hypertension related to obesity, diabetes and full-fledged MS.

■ CONCLUSION

Natriuretic peptides have a complex physiological effect on CV system as well as maintenance of BP. While NPs have a profound role in maintain physiology by counteracting the levels of SNS tone and RAAS activity, severely elevated NPs are pathological markers of cardiac damage in hypertension. Long-term modulation of NPs remains to be a challenging prospect in the management of hypertension.

■ REFERENCES

1. Sudoh T, Minamino N, Kangawa K, et al. C-type natriuretic peptide (CNP): a new member of natriuretic peptide family identified in porcine brain. Biochm Biophys Res Commun. 1990;168(2):863-70.
2. Volpe M. Natriuretic peptides and cardio-renal disease. Int J Cardiol. 2014;176(3):630-9.
3. Waldman SA, Rapoport RM, Murad F. Atrial natriuretic factor selectively activates particulate guanylate cyclase and elevates cyclic GMP in rat tissues. J Biol Chem. 1984;259(23):14332-4.
4. Schlueter N, de Sterke A, Willmes DM, et al. Metabolic actions of natriuretic peptides and therapeutic potential in the metabolic syndrome. Pharmacol Ther. 2014;144(1): 12-27.
5. Mukoyama M, Nakao K, Hosoda K, et al. Brain natriuretic peptide as a novel cardiac hormone in humans. Evidence for an exquisite dual natriuretic peptide system, atrial natriuretic peptide and brain natriuretic peptide. J Clin Invest. 1991;87(4):1402-12.
6. Heymsfield SB, Wadden TA. Mechanisms, pathophysiology, and management of obesity. N Engl J Med. 2017;376(3): 254-66.
7. Ruilope LM, Dukat A, Böhm M, et al. Blood-pressure reduction with LCZ696, a novel dual-acting inhibitor of

the angiotensin II receptor and neprilysin: a randomised, double-blind, placebo-controlled, active comparator study. Lancet. 2010;375(9722):1255-66.

8. Volpe M, Rubattu S. Novel Insights into the Mechanisms Regulating Pro-Atrial Natriuretic Peptide Cleavage in the Heart and Blood Pressure Regulation: Proprotein Convertase Subtilisin/Kexin 6 is the Corin Activating Enzyme. Circ Res. 2016;118(2):196-8.

9. Macheret F, Heublein D, Costello-Boerrigter LC, et al. Human hypertension is characterized by a lack of activation of the antihypertensive cardiac hormones ANP and BNP. J Am Coll Cardiol. 2012;60(16):1558-65.

10. Folsom AR, Nambi V, Bell EJ, et al. Troponin T, N-terminal pro-B-type natriuretic peptide, and incidence of stroke: the atherosclerosis risk in communities study. Stroke. 2013;44(4):961-7.

11. Rubattu S, Volpe M. High natriuretic peptide levels and low DBP: companion markers of cardiovascular risk? J Hypertens. 2014;32(11):2142-3.

12. Geng Z, Huang L, Song M, et al. N-terminal pro-brain natriuretic peptide and cardiovascular or all-cause mortality in the general population: a meta-analysis. Sci Rep. 2017;7:41504.

13. Dessì-Fulgheri P, Sarzani R, Serenelli M, et al. Low calorie diet enhances renal, hemodynamic, and humoral effects of exogenous atrial natriuretic peptide in obese hypertensives. Hypertension. 1999;33(2):658-62.

14. Engeli S, Negrel R, Sharma AM. Physiology and pathophysiology of the adipose tissue renin-angiotensin system. Hypertension. 2000;35(6):1270-7.

15. Sarzani R, Dessì-Fulgheri P, Paci VM, et al. Expression of natriuretic peptide receptors in human adipose and other tissues. J Endocrinol Invest. 1996;19(9):581-5.

Multiple Roles of Eicosanoids in Blood Pressure Regulation

Mrinal Kanti Das

■ INTRODUCTION

Eicosanoids, a group of oxygenated C20 unsaturated fatty acids that mediate both cellular and humoral responses, include prostaglandin, leukotriene and epoxyeicosatrienoic acid (EET), and are usually produced from arachidonic acid (AA: 5,8,11,14-eicosatetraenoic acid) by cyclooxygenase, lipoxygenase and epoxygenase.[1-3] AA is rich in phospholipids and released by the catalytic activity of phospholipase A2 (PLA2).[4] Hypertension contributing to about one-third population with noncommunicable disease burden is a complex interaction between a host of blood pressure regulatory factors mediated through various mechanisms, one of them being renin–aldosterone–angiotensin-neprilysin system. They envisage sympathetic nervous system, aldosterone, endothelin, nitric oxide (NO), kinins, neprilysins and various eicosanoids. Eicosanoids take part as both prohypertensive and antihypertensive agents.[5] There is now enough documentation regarding the occurrence of cyclooxygenases, lipoxygenases, and cytochrome P450 (CYP) oxygenases in renal as well as vascular tissues.[1,6-8] Being very promising and interesting molecules, it is worthwhile to keep abreast of the latest happenings especially in the light of hypertension being a major cardiovascular risk factor with very high mortality and morbidity if not properly controlled.

■ BEGINNING OF THE HISTORY

Lee et al. reported the isolation of two blood pressure lowering lipids from rabbit renal medulla in 1965.[9] The development of pharmacological, genetic and biochemical tools have allowed for detailed studies to determine the contribution of CYP metabolites of AA to renal microvascular function. Renal microvessels can generate CYP hydroxylase metabolites including 20-hydroxyeicosatetraenoic acid (20-HETE), 12-HETE, etc. and CYP epoxygenase metabolites, epoxyeicosatrienoic acids, combiningly known as eicosanoids. EETs have cardioprotective, vasodilatory, angio-genic, anti-inflammatory and analgesic effects, which are diminished by EET hydrolysis yielding biologically less active dihydroxyeicosatrienoic acids (DHETs) by EPHX2, also known as soluble epoxide hydrolase (sEH).[10,11] While 12-HETE has been found to be an inhibitory regulator of renin secretion (antihypertensive effect), but it along with 15-HETE has been associated with inhibition of prostacyclin synthase, an action which may lower the antihypertensive effect of prostacyclin (PGI2).[1,12,13] 20-HETE constricts afferent arterioles and contributes to renal blood flow autoregulation. EETs act as endothelium-dependent hyperpolarizing factors (EDHFs) on the renal microcirculation. 20-HETE inhibits whereas EETs activate renal microvascular smooth muscle cell large-conductance calcium-activated K^+ channels (K_{Ca}). Likewise, 20-HETE actions on renal microvascular are prohypertensive and EET actions are antihypertensive. These findings in the renal microvasculature and those of others have provided impetus for the development of enzymatic inhibitors, agonists and antagonists for 20-HETE and EETs to determine their potential therapeutic value. Initial genetic studies and experimental studies with soluble epoxide hydrolase inhibitors to increase EETs, EET analogs and 20-HETE inhibitors have demonstrated improved renal microvascular function in hypertension. These findings have demonstrated the important contributions that 20-HETE and EETs play in the regulation of renal microvascular function. The recognition that CYP enzymes had the capacity to metabolize AA and generate EETs and HETEs ignited curiosity to determine their biological actions.[10,11] Flowchart 1 shows the metabolic pathway of AA.

As the identification of the CYP enzymes that catalyzed the reactions were being identified and further characterized in the 1980s, there was slower progress with the determination of the physiological actions for EETs and HETEs. The reason for selecting the renal vasculature for studies was guided by the early studies demonstrating that kidneys had significant expression of CYP enzymes and that EETs and HETEs had actions on epithelial cells to alter sodium transport.[14,15] So, it is considered to be one of the cornerstone mechanisms of genesis of hypertension. Vascular actions for EETs as dilators were first attributed toward the end of 1980s.[16] During the same period, NO got detected as an endothelial-derived relaxing factor.[17] and the endothelial cells were detected to release a hyperpolarizing factor (EDHF) that was thought to be a noncyclooxygenase AA metabolite.[18] A number of researchers continued with this idea on EETs during the 1990s. 20-HETE got recognized as a vasoconstrictor in the early 1990s. It was intriguing to note that the 20-HETE had antihypertensive effect on the epithelial cells, whereas prohypertensive actions on the vascular.[19,20] Thus, the biological curiosity on CYP generated EETs and HETEs gave rise to a metabolic pathway that influenced not only the physiological mechanisms but also pathophysiological states. The importance

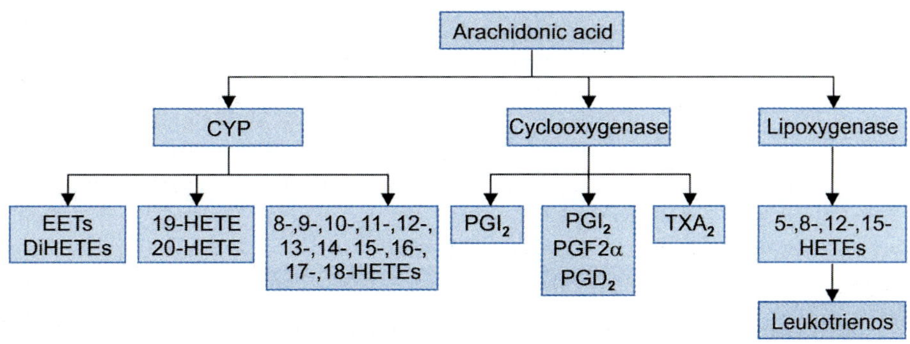

(CYP: cytochrome P450; EET: epoxyeicosatrienoic acid; HETE: hydroxyeicosatetraenoic acid; PG: prostaglandin; DiHETEs: dihydroxyeicosatetraenoic acids)

Flowchart 1: The metabolic pathway of arachidonic acid.[1]

of CYP AA metabolites got established with the advent of pharmacological, molecular, biological and different analytical tools to determine biological actions attributed to CYP enzymes, EETs and 20-HETE. Jorge Capdevila and John Falck have been pioneers in this journey of finding out the all-important metabolic pathway. These works surged a number of experimental studies on the influence of CYP enzymes, EETs and 20-HETE on renal microvascular function and their actions on the contribution to hypertension.

ACTIONS OF ARACHIDONIC ACID METABOLITES

The CYP metabolites of AA have been found to not only regulate renal function, but also vascular tone. It is already known that vascular smooth muscle (VSM) cells generate 20-HETE which acts as second messenger playing an important role[1] in the myogenic responses, tumor growth factor (TGF) and hypertrophy and[2] in the vascular responses to the vasoconstrictors and dilators by modulating the K^+ channel activity. The CYP metabolites of AA are produced in the proximal tubules and distal Loops of Henle of the kidney. They inhibit the active Na^+ transport and thereby modulate the hypertension.

Epoxyeicosatrienoic acids produced by the endothelial cells on the other hand, hyperpolarize the VSM cells and open up the K_{Ca}-channels and thus act as vasodilator or EDHF on the coronary arteries and other vascular beds.[20]

The 20-hydroxyeicosatetraenoic acid has its role in the myogenic response of renal, cerebral, mesenteric and skeletal muscle arterioles raising transmural pressure and autoregulation of renal and cerebral blood flow in rat models.[18,20,21]

These influences of the CYP metabolites of AA on the vascular tone may be associated with the genesis of the various kinds of experimental and genetic models of hypertension, diabetes mellitus, cyclosporin/cisplatin-induced nephrotoxicity, hepatorenal syndrome and pregnancy and there is huge scope of the metabolites and the drugs modifying the EETs and HETEs in management of the various disorders. Flowchart 2 highlights the various metabolites of EETs and HETEs mediated by cyclooxygenase, epoxide hydrolase and β-oxydation. Each of them has influences on hemodynamics of blood pressure—either prohypertensive or antihypertensive.

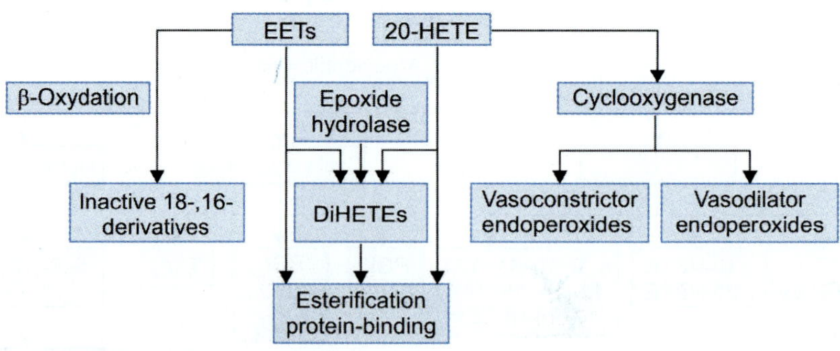

(EET: epoxyeicosatrienoic acid; HETE: hydroxyeicosatetraenoic acid; DiHETEs: dihydroxyeicosatetraenoic acids)

Flowchart 2: Highlights of the various metabolites of EETs and HETEs.[20]

ROLE OF ENDOPEROXIDES[1,22]

- Prostaglandin E2 acts on multiple receptor subtypes at renal tubules that inhibit Na^+ transport and the vasculature that elicit dilation and increase medullary blood flow. In concert, they result in diuresis-natriuresis due to elevation of renal perfusion pressure and/or volume overload caused by sodium retention
- TxA2 receptors are responsible for angiotensin-dependent hypertension. In experimental models in spontaneously hypertensive rats, increased TxA2 production precipitated hypertension
- 20-hydroxyeicosatetraenoic acid causes vasoactivity and modulation of transport in different nephron segments and thus regulates the renal autoregulation and tubuloglomerular feedback as well as sodium excretion by cotransporter and Na^+ pump inhibition, which directly influences the regulation of blood pressure
- The variety of activities of 20-HETE is also caused by prostaglandin analogs consequent to cyclooxygenase-2–dependent transformation of 20-HETE in the renal vasculature
- Activating adenosine A2A receptors in response to salt loading results in raised blood pressure is done by the inhibition of EET (antipressor) synthesis which stimulates generation of CYP450 epoxygenase isoform 2C23
- Monogenic form of hypertension is a rare condition caused by 11,12-EET deficiency. These EETs are responsible for endogenous regulation of epithelial Na^+ channel in cortical collecting ducts.

TANGO BETWEEN EETS AND HETES

Intricate relationship of the various biological molecules in the VSM and the endothelium has been highlighted in the cartoon below (Fig. 3). Membrane stretch and vasoactive agents like angiotensin II (ANG II), norepinephrine (NE) activate the phospholipase C (PLC) and releases the inositol triphosphate (IP_3) and diacylglycerol (DAG). IP_3 triggers the release of intracellular Ca^{2+}-sensitive phospholipase A_2 (PLA) and DAG lipase to release AA and stimulate the generation of 20-HETE which blocks the large–conductance, calcium-activated potassium (K_{Ca}) channel in VSM cells. This leads to fall in membrane potential (E_m) that enhances the Ca^{2+} influx through L-type voltage-sensitive Ca^{2+}-channels. EETs are produced by the endothelium and act as vasodilator which also hyperpolarizes the VSM cells by increasing the activity of the K_{Ca}-channel. Acetylcholine and bradykinin stimulate the release of EETs from the endothelium, and they act as the endothelial-derived hyperpolarizing factor (EDHF) in cerebral and renal arteries. NO, a small membrane permeable signal molecule, is synthesized from L-arginine by NO synthase (NOS) released from the endothelium.[23] It activates guanylyl cyclase to increase cGMP levels which activate the protein kinase-G that enhances Ca^{2+} reuptake of intracellular stores and decreases the Ca^{2+} sensitivity of the contractile mechanisms. NO inhibits the formation of 20-HETEs, the fall of which increases the activity of the K_{Ca}-channel. This hyperpolarizes the cells and reduces the Ca^{2+} influx through voltage-sensitive channels. NO also directly activates K^+ channels and thus maintains the homeostasis of blood pressure. NO mediates both cellular and humoral immune responses using eicosanoids as a downstream signal.[17] Some of the mechanisms are shown in Figure 1 which highlights the complex interaction between various endocrine and paracrine molecules derived from endothelium and smooth muscle.

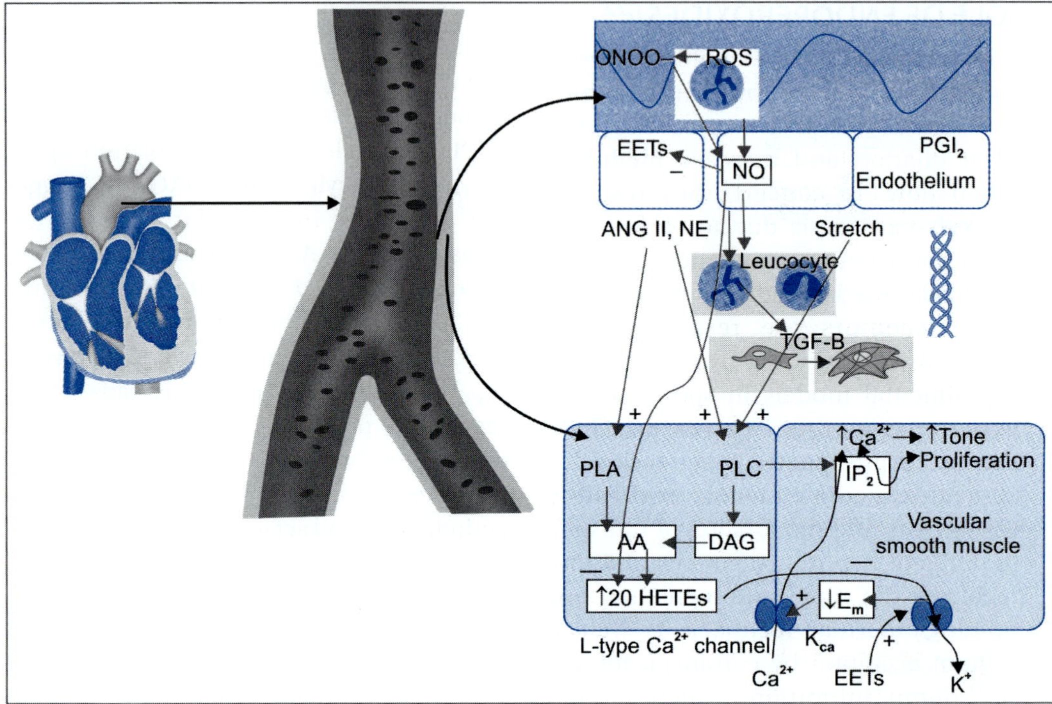

(EET: epoxyeicosatrienoic acid; HETE: hydroxyeicosatetraenoic acid; DAG: diacylglycerol; PLC: phospholipase C; PLA: phospholipase A$_2$; AA: arachidonic acid; TGF: tumor growth factor; PG: prostaglandin; NO: nitric oxide; ROS: reactive oxygen species.

Fig. 1: Complex interactions of cytochrome P-450 metabolites of arachidonic acid and control of the vascular tone.

HYPOTENSIVE–PROHYPERTENSIVE CONUNDRUM

This is to re-emphasize that autoregulation of blood pressure is an intricate balance between two CYP metabolites of AA namely EETs and HETEs. They act as second messengers regulating the renal function and the vascular tone. However, these metabolites have both hypotensive and prohypertensive effects and may have differential roles in different tissues. On proximal renal tubules and thick ascending loop of Henle, 20-HETEs inhibit sodium transport and increase the volume overload generating hypertension. On the other hand, same 20 HETEs promotes vasoconstriction in the renal vasculature and glomeruli causing sodium retention and hypertension.

In the peripheral vasculature also it causes vasoconstriction and hypertension. EETs on the other hand having vasodilator properties inhibit generation of hypertension. The activities of the 20-HETEs are shown in the Flowchart 3. Future advances will better define the cellular mechanisms by which CYP metabolites control renal and other microvascular function and determining their significance in hypertension, coronary, and peripheral vascular diseases as well as in renal diseases.

PHARMACOANALYTICAL WORKS

The interest with the eicosanoids is not only ever-increasing, both in terms of determining their exact biological roles but also in terms

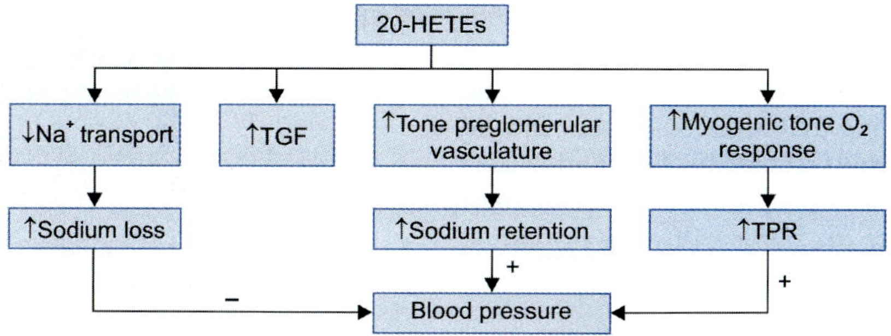

(HETE: hydroxyeicosatetraenoic acid; TGF: tumor growth factor; TPR: total peripheral resistance)

Flowchart 3: Pro- and antihypertensive effects of 20-HETEs.[2]

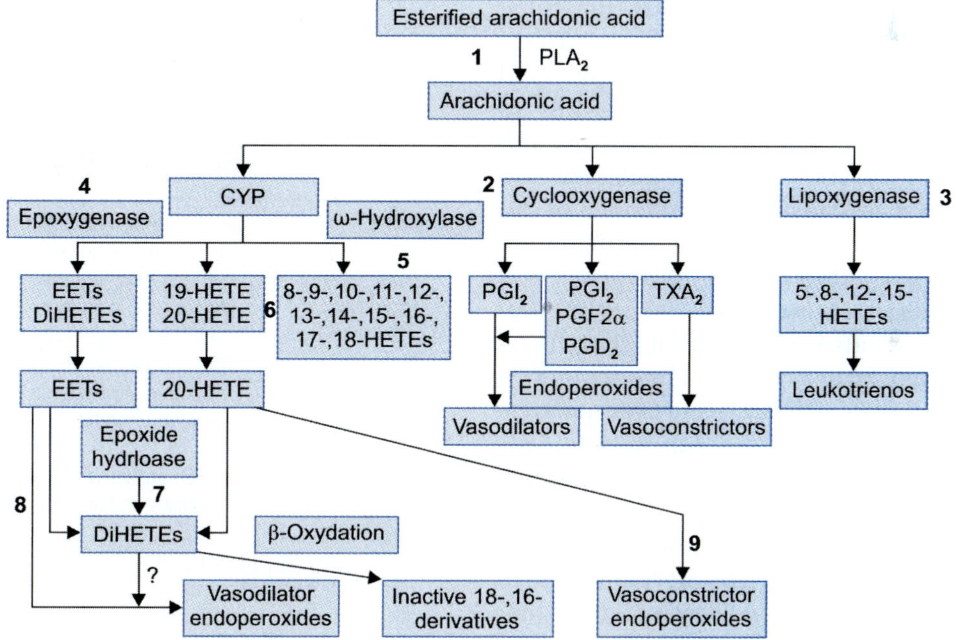

1→AACFCF3 (–); 2→ETYA, indomethacin, meclofenamate (–);3→Baicalein, CDC, ETYA (–); 4→β-naphthoflavone, phenobarbital (+) miconazole, ketoconazole PPOH, PPOMS (–); 5→Fibrate(+) DDMS, DDBB, HET0016 (–); 6→ABT,17-ODYA, SKF-525,NO, ETYA (–); 7→TCPO, 4PCO, DCU (–); 8→EET analog (–); 9→5-,15-,19-HETE (–) 6-,15-,20-HEDE (WIT 002) (–).

(CYP: cytochrome P450; EET: epoxyeicosatrienoic acid; HETE: hydroxyeicosatetraenoic acid; PG: prostaglandin; PLA: phospholipase)

Flowchart 4: Metabolic pathway of the arachidonic acid with the sites of action of various agents or drugs acting by inhibition or induction. The numbers in bold are suggestive of the various molecules.[20]

of finding out different therapeutic tools. The various drugs or molecules are shown in Flowchart 4 with their sites of action with numbers.

The list earlier depicts the molecules or drugs, some of which are already commercially available and some are in the laboratories and so they are code-named. The +ve within the bracket implies induction and –ve within bracket implies inhibition. The advent of these drugs have a tremendous influence on the understanding the mechanisms and sites of action of various metabolites (AA) and is likely to create and sustain further interest amongst the workers pursuing with this intriguing molecules.

CONCLUSION

The past 15 years have resulted in great advances in our understanding of the microvascular actions and functions for cytochrome P metabolites of AA. The initial descriptions of 20-HETE as a constrictor and EETs as dilators of afferent renal arterioles initiated series of studies to determine cell-signaling mechanisms and their contribution to autoregulatory and hormonal responses. The influence of 20-HETE on calcium influx and participation in afferent autoregulatory responses was established. Meanwhile, experimental evidences also established that EETs activated large conductance calcium-activated K^+ (K_{Ca}) channels to hyperpolarize renal microvascular smooth muscle cells inhibiting the Ca^{2+} influx, a mechanism responsible for antipressor effect and thus was labeled as an EDHF. These new findings resulted in surge in the development of genetic and pharmacological tools to further define the physiological and pathological importance of 20-HETE and EETs in not only renal micro-vascular function, but also other vasculature. The results of these experimental studies have now reached a point where novel therapeutic agents targeting 20-HETE and EETs are being tested. The pharmacotherapeutic information and the ongoing research projects related to therapy are beyond the scope of the present article.

REFERENCES

1. Imig JD. Epoxyeicosatrienoic acids and 20-hydroxyecosa-tetraenoic acid on endothelial and vascular function. Adv Pharmacol. 2016;77:105-41.
2. Bonventre JV. Phospholipase A2 and signal transduction. J Am Soc Nephrol. 1992;3(2):128-50.
3. Stanley DW. Eicosanoids in Invertebrate Signal Transduction Systems. Princeton: Princeton University Press; 2000. pp. 1-292.
4. Dennis EA, Cao J, Hsu YH, et al. Phospholipase A2 enzymes: Physical structure, biological function, disease implication, chemical inhibition and therapeutic intervention. Chem Rev. 2011;111(10):6130-85.
5. Mistry M, Nasjletti A. Prostanoids as mediators of prohypertensive and antihypertensive mechanisms. Am J Med Sci. 1988;295(4):263-7.
6. Stein N, Nozawa K, Kisch E, et al. Tonic inhibition of rennin secretion by the 12-lipoxygenase pathway: augmentation by high salt intake. Endocrinology. 1996;137(5):1878-84.
7. McGiff JC. Cytochrome P-450 metabolism of arachidonic acid. Ann Rev Pharmacol Toxicol. 1991;31:339-69.
8. Harder DR, Campbell WB, Roman RJ. Role of cytochrome P-450 enzymes and metabolites of arachidonic acid in the control of vascular tone. J Vasc Res. 1995;32(2):79-92.
9. Lee JB, Corvino BG, Takman BH, et al. Renomedullary vasodepressor substance, medullin: isolation, chemical characterization and physiological properties. Circ Res. 1965;17:57-77.
10. Edin ML, Hamedani BG, Gruzdev A, et al. Epoxide hydrolase 1 (EPHX1) hydrolyzes epoxyeicosanoids and impairs cardiac recovery after Ischemia. J Biol Chem. 2018;293(9):3281-92.
11. Morisseau C, Hammock BD. Impact of soluble epoxide hydrolase and epoxyeicosanoids on human health. Annu Rev Pharmacol Toxicol. 2013;53:37-58.
12. Lin L, Balazy M, Pagano PJ, et al. Expression of prosta-glandin H2-mediated mechanism of vascular contraction in hypertensive rats. Relation to lipoxygenase and prostacyclin synthase activities. Circ Res. 1994;74(2): 197-205.
13. Saito F, Hori MT, Ideguchi Y, et al. 12-lipoxygenase products modulate calcium signals in vascular smooth muscle cells. Hypertension. 1992;20(2):138-43.
14. Spector AA, Norris AW. Action of epoxyeicosatrienoic acids on cellular function. Am J Physiol Cell Physiol. 2007;292(3):C996-1012.
15. Larsen BT, Miura H, Hatoum OA, et al. Epoxyeicosatrienoic and dihydroxyeicosatrienoic acids dilate human coronary arterioles via BK(Ca) channels: implications for soluble epoxide hydrolase inhibition. Am J Physiol Heart Circ Physiol. 2006;290(2):H491-9.

16. Václavíková R, Hughes DJ, Souček P. Microsomal epoxide hydrolase 1 (EPHX1): Gene, structure, function, and role in human disease. Gene. 2015;571(1):1-8.

17. Sadekuzzaman M, Kim Y. Nitric oxide mediates antimicrobial peptide gene expression by activating eicosanoid signaling. PLoS One. 2018;13(2):e0193282.

18. Gebremedhin D, Harder DR, Pratt PF, et al. Bioassay of an endothelium-derived hyperpolarizing factor from bovine coronary arteries: role of cytochrome P450 metabolite. J Vasc Res. 1998;35(4):274-84.

19. Mitchell JA, Kirkby NS. Eicosanoids, prostacyclin and cyclooxygenase in the cardiovascular system. Br J Pharmacol. 2018. [Epub ahead of print].

20. Roman RJ. P-450 Metabolites of arachidonic acid in the control of cardiovascular function. Physiol Rev. 2002;82(1):131-85.

21. Gebremedhin D, Lange AR, Lowry TF, et al. Production of 20-HETE and its role in autoregulation of cerebral blood flow. Circ Res. 2000;87(1):60-5.

22. Edin ML, Wang Z, Bradbury JA, et al. Endothelial expression of human cytochrome P450 epoxygenase CYP2C8 increases susceptibility to ischemia-reperfusion injury in isolated mouse heart. FASEB J. 2011;25(10):3436-47.

23. Rivero A. Nitric oxide: an antiparasitic molecule of invertebrates. Trends Parasitol. 2006;22(5):219-25.

Accuracy of Blood Pressure Measurements

Importance of Out-of-office Blood Pressure Monitoring

Ravi R Kasliwal, Anusha Singh

■ INTRODUCTION

Hypertension is the most common, readily identifiable and reversible risk factor for myocardial infarction, stroke, heart failure, atrial fibrillation, aortic dissection, peripheral arterial disease and cognitive decline and yet it often remains undetected and undertreated. The asymptomatic nature of systemic hypertension delays diagnosis.

In India, hypertension alone is directly responsible for 57% of all stroke deaths and 24% of all coronary heart disease deaths.[1] Studies show that about 33% urban and 25% rural Indians are hypertensive. Of these, 25% rural and 42% urban Indians are aware of their hypertensive status and only 25% rural and 38% of urban Indians are being treated for hypertension.[2] Moreover, only 25.6% of treated patients have their blood pressure (BP) under control.[3]

Effective treatment of hypertension requires accurate measurement of BP. There are four approaches to BP measurement:

1. Conventional office BP recording
2. Automated office BP (AOBP) recording
3. Home BP monitoring (HBPM)
4. Ambulatory BP monitoring (ABPM).

■ CONVENTIONAL OFFICE BLOOD PRESSURE MEASUREMENT

Conventional office BP readings are measured by the auscultatory method by medical personnel. However, these readings are often inaccurate because of common measurement errors, the white coat reaction and factors that influence BP outside the medical office. More recently, oscillometric semiautomatic and automatic sphygmomanometers are becoming the preferred method for measuring BP in the doctor's office but even these devices should be validated according to standardized conditions and protocols.

The recent American College of Cardiology (ACC) or American Heart Association (AHA) and European Society of Cardiology (ESC) or European Heart for Children (EHC) guidelines have placed major emphasis on proper measurement of BP, beginning with preparation of the patient to appropriate data collection. Although measurement of BP in office settings is relatively easy, errors are common and can result in a misleading estimation of an individual's true level of BP.

Box 1 summarizes the recommendations for accurate office BP measurements as directed by latest guidelines.

Box 1: Recommendations for office blood pressure (BP) measurement.

- Patients should be seated comfortably in a quiet room for 5 min before BP measurement
- Patients should avoid caffeine, exercise, and smoking for at least 30 min before measurement
- Ensure patients have emptied his/her bladder
- An appropriate size cuff and a validated measurement device should be used to measure BP
- The cuff should be positioned at the level of the heart, with patients arm and back supported
- At least three BP measurements should be recorded, 1–2 min apart and BP is recorded as the average of the last two BP readings
- Measure BP in both arms and use the arm with higher value as the reference
- Additional measurements may be performed in patients with unstable BP, arrhythmias such as atrial fibrillation
- Always measure heart rate while recording BP
- In older persons and those with diabetes or conditions with autonomic insufficiency, BP should also be measured after 1 min and 5 min of standing from a seated position to exclude significant postural fall in BP

Limitations of Conventional Office Blood Pressure Monitoring

- White-coat hypertension (WCH) and white-coat effect
- Masked hypertension
- Detection of hypotension in untreated and treated patient
- Resistant hypertension, patients with autonomic dysfunction
- Exaggerated BP response to exercise
- Assessment of nocturnal hypertension.

White-coat Hypertension

White-coat hypertension was first described by Thomas Pickering in the year 1984.[4] WCH refers to the untreated condition in which BP is elevated in the office, but is normal when measured otherwise. If a patient who is not receiving any antihypertensive treatment has office BP more than 140 mm Hg systolic and more than 90 mm Hg diastolic but ambulatory daytime BP less than 135/85 mm Hg, the patient has office-only or white-coat hypertension.[5]

However, white-coat hypertension and white-coat effect are different entities. White-coat effect is rise of BP that occurs in medical environment, regardless of daytime ABPM levels or use of antihypertensive drugs.[6]

White-coat hypertension is caused by a transient adrenergic response to the measurement of BP only in the doctorgsn measured otherwise. It accounts for 30-40% of people with an elevated office BP. It is benign if global cardiovascular disease (CVD) risk is low especially if the mean awake and sleep BP are optimal. The incidence of WCH converting to sustained hypertension is 1–5% per year. It is more common with increasing age, in women and in nonsmokers. Compared with normotensive people, WCH is associated with an increased prevalence of dysmetabolic risk factors and asymptomatic organ damage.[7,8]

Masked Hypertension

In 2002, Pickering et al. found that hypertension in patients may get masked in office because of sympathetic overactivity in daily life, which gets dissipated when they come to doctor's office.[9,10] This phenomenon was called masked hypertension and was attributed to sympathetic overactivity caused by job or home stress, tobacco abuse or other adrenergic stimulation like obstructive sleep apnea (OSA). When referring to untreated persons, the term masked hypertension is appropriate. When referring to persons receiving antihypertensive treatment, however, by definition, the diagnosis of masked hypertension is known, and therefore the term "masked uncontrolled hypertension" is preferred and implies that further treatment is necessary for optimal BP control.

Masked hypertension can be found in approximately 15% of patients with a normal office BP. It is a common phenomenon in patients with diabetes mellitus, chronic kidney disease (CKD) and African Americans. In contrast to WCH, masked hypertension is associated with a CVD and all-cause mortality risk twice as high as that seen in normotensive individuals, with a risk range similar to that of patients with sustained hypertension. Hypertension may also get masked when a patient has only nocturnal hypertension.

Nocturnal Hypertension

The BP normally decreases during sleep. Patients with a reduced night-time dip in BP (i.e. <10% of the daytime average BP or a night-to-day ratio >0.9) have an increased cardiovascular risk. Recognized reasons for an absence of nocturnal BP dipping are sleep disturbance, OSA, obesity, high salt intake in salt-sensitive subjects, orthostatic hypotension, autonomic dysfunction, CKD, diabetic neuropathy and old age. Nocturnal hypertension is known to aggregate hemodynamic load on the cardiovascular system and it predicts CVD outcomes better than either daytime ambulatory BP or conventional office measurement.

■ AUTOMATED OFFICE BLOOD PRESSURE MEASUREMENT

The term "automated office blood pressure (AOBP)" refers to BP measurements obtained using a fully automated electronic sphygmomanometer that records multiple BP readings with the patient resting undisturbed in a quiet place without medical staff being present. It was first attempted by Myers et al. in 1997 to eliminate white-coat effect and later validated my various studies. The Systolic Blood Pressure Intervention Trial (SPRINT) used AOBP in determining the optimum target BP for antihypertensive drug therapy.[11,12]

The AOBP measurement of BP includes BP measurements at 1 minute intervals once patient has been sitting in the examination room for 5 minutes unaccompanied using an oscillometric monitor. Average of five or three such readings is taken in account. On average, AOBP is 15/10 mm Hg lower than conventional office BP. There is abundant evidence to support the replacement of conventional BP measurement with AOBP since its readings are more accurate, correlate better with home and awake ambulatory BP, and eliminates digit preference and white-coat effect.

■ HOME BLOOD PRESSURE MEASUREMENT

Office BP can both overestimate and underestimate a person's ambulatory BP evidence to support the replacement of HBPM values are lower, more reproducible and more closely related to target organ damage particularly left ventricular hypertrophy.[13] Self-measurement of BP at home can accomplish several advantages such as greater number of readings, avoidance of white-coat effect and when automated devices are used, an absence of observer bias. Also patients self-monitoring of BP have shown beneficial effect on BP control, adherence to medications, and reduced number of visits required to diagnose and treat hypertension.

The HBPM can only be useful if the application of the technique is well standardized and meets the quality criteria. Before taking BP measurement at home, patient should receive training under medical supervision regarding selection of equipment, technique and interpretation of results.

Instructions on HBPM Procedures

- Avoid smoking, caffeinated beverages air exercise within 30 minutes before BP measurements
- Ensure more than 5 minutes of quiet rest before BP measurements
- Sit with back straight and supported
- Sit with feet flat in the floor and legs uncrossed
- Keep arm supported on a flat surface with the upper arm at heart level
- Patients should take at least two readings 1 minute apart in morning before taking medications and in evening before meals
- Patient should measure BP for at least 3 days in a week or 6–7 consecutive days before each visit to doctor medication.

◼ AMBULATORY BLOOD PRESSURE MEASUREMENT

Ambulatory BP Monitoring is the gold standard, it provides automated measurements of BP during a 24 hours or 48 hours period while patients are engaged in their usual activities, including sleep. Over the last 50 years, ABPM has evolved from a research device to a valuable tool for assessment and management of hypertension. At first, its role was only focused on identifying patients with WCH but now various cross-sectional evidences have proven that ABPM has valuable prognostic significance as well in determining target organ damage and cardiovascular outcomes.

Various out-of-office BP measurements can be obtained using ABPM data, including morning, daytime, night-time, and average 24-hour ambulatory BP. ABPM demonstrates the circadian pattern of BP which includes early morning BP surge, lower BP levels in evening, and a BP dip during sleep.[14] Thus, ABPM helps to identify periods of uncontrolled BP and also excessive BP reductions.[15] Also, ABPM can be used to determine duration of effect of antihypertensives and BP profile

TABLE 1: Definitions of hypertension according to office, ambulatory and home BP levels.[5]

Category	SBP (mm Hg)		DBP (mm Hg)
Office BP	>140	and/or	>90
Ambulatory BP:			
Daytime/ awake mean	>135	and/or	>85
Night-time/ asleep mean	>120	and/or	>70
24 h mean	>130	and/or	>80
Home BP mean	>135	and/or	>85

(BP: blood pressure; DBP: diastolic blood pressure; SBP: systolic blood pressure)

Source: Adapted from 2018 ESC/ESH Guidelines for the management of arterial hypertension.

associated with drug treatment.[16] Studies show that ABPM predicts fatal and nonfatal MI and stroke better than standard office measurement does and is the only way to detect nocturnal hypertension.

Out-of-office hypertension is defined as average daytime BP of 135/85 mm Hg or higher, night-time BP 120/70 mm Hg or higher, or 24-hour BP 130/80 mm Hg or higher. Table 1 summarizes the definitions of hypertension according to various methods of BP measurements.

The ABPM provides the average of BP readings over a defined period, usually 24 hours. The device is conventionally programmed to record BP at 15–30 min intervals and average BP values are provided.[17] At least 14 readings must be taken to confirm the diagnosis of hypertension. A record of patient's activities and sleep time should also be maintained.

◼ IMPORTANCE OF OUT-OF-OFFICE BP MEASUREMENT

Out-of-office BP measurement refers to the use of either HBPM or ABPM (Table 2). It provides a larger number of BP measurements

TABLE 2: Comparison between ambulatory BP monitoring and home BP monitoring.

ABPM	HPBM
Can identify white-coat and masked hypertension	Can identify white-coat and masked hypertension
Stronger prognostic evidence	Measurement in a home setting, which is more relaxed than doctor's office
Night-time readings	No nocturnal readings
Measurement in real-life settings	Patient engagement in BP measurement
Additional prognostic BP phenotypes	Easily repeated and used over longer periods to assess day-to-day BP variability
Abundant information from a single measurement session, including short term BP variability	Only static BP is available
Expensive and sometimes limited availability	Cheap and widely available
Can be uncomfortable	Potential for measurement error

(BP: blood pressure; ABPM: ambulatory blood pressure monitoring; HBPM: home blood pressure monitoring)

than conventional office BP in conditions that are more representative of daily life.

Clinical Indications for Out-of-office BP Monitoring

- Grade I hypertension on office BP measurement
- Marked office BP elevation without end-organ damage
- Normal office BP in individuals with end-organ damage or high total cardiovascular risk
- Evaluation of resistant hypertension
- Evaluation of BP control in high-risk patients on antihypertensives
- Evaluation of BP response to exercise
- Evaluation of symptoms consistent with hypotension during treatment
- Postural and postprandial hypotension in untreated and treated patients
- Assessment of nocturnal BP values
- Patients suspected with autonomic dysfunction, endocrine hypertension and sleep apnea.

■ CONCLUSION

Out-of-office BP monitoring, particularly ABPM is the best method to diagnose hypertension. It prevents unnecessary treatment of patients of patients with WCH, able to screen high-risk patients with masked hypertension and in diagnosing suspected treatment-related hypotension. ABPM and HBPM are better predictors of CVD risk due to elevated BP than are office BP measurements, with ABPM being the preferred measurement option. If ABPM resources are not readily available, HBPM provides a reasonable but less desirable alternative to screen for hypertension. In summary, both HBPM and ABPM are necessary procedures beyond in-office BP recordings to identify patients needing antihypertensive treatment and how best to treat them.

■ REFERENCES

1. Gupta R. Trends in hypertension epidemiology in India. J Hum Hypertens. 2004;18:73-8.
2. Raghupathy A, Nanda K, Hira P, et al. Hypertension in India: a systematic review and meta-analysis of prevalence, awareness, and control of hypertension. J Hypertens. 2014;32(6):1170-7.
3. Hypertension Study Group. Prevalence, awareness, treatment and control of hypertension among the elderly in Bangladesh and India: a multicentre study. Bull World Health Organ. 2001;79:490-500.
4. Kleinert HD, Harshfield GA, Pickering TG, et al. What is the value of home blood pressure measurement in patients with mild hypertension? Hypertension. 1984;6:574-8

5. William B, Mancia G, Spiering W, et al. 2018 ESC/ESH Guidelines for the management of arterial hypertension. European Heart J. 2018;39:3021-104.

6. Verdecchia P, Staessen JA, White WB, et al. Properly defining white coat hypertension. Eur Heart J. 2002;23: 106-9.

7. Afsar B. Comparison of demographic, clinical, and laboratory parameters between patients with sustained normotension, white coat hypertension, masked hypertension, and sustained hypertension. J Cardiol. 2013;61: 222-6.

8. Afsar B. Comparison of demographic, clinical, and laboratory parameters between patients with sustained normotension, white coat hypertension, masked hypertension, and sustained hypertension. J Cardiol. 2013;61(3):222-6.

9. Cushman WC, Whelton PK, Fine LJ, et al. SPRINT trial results. Latest news in hypertension management. Hypertension. 2016;67:263-5.

10. Cushman WC, Whelton PK, Fine LJ, et al. SPRINT Trial Results: Latest News in Hypertension Management. Hypertension. 2016;67(2):263-5.

11. Verdecchia P, Schillaci G, Borgioni C, et al. White-coat hypertension and white-coat effect. Similarities and differences. Am J Hypertens. 1995;8:790-8.

12. Wright JT Jr, Williamson JD, Whelton PK, et al. A randomized trial of intensive versus standard blood pressure control. N Engl J Med. 2015;373:2103-16.

13. Pickering TG, Davidson K, Gerin W, et al. Masked hypertension. Hypertension. 2002;40:795-6.

14. Bliziotis IA, Destounis A, Stergiou GS. Home versus ambulatory and office blood pressure in predicting target organ damage in hypertension: a systematic review and meta-analysis. J Hypertens. 2012;30:1289-99.

15. Bliziotis IA, Destounis A, Stergiou GS. Home versus ambulatory and office blood pressure in predicting target organ damage in hypertension: a systematic review and meta-analysis. J Hypertens. 2012;30(7):1289-99.

16. Pickering T. Ambulatory blood pressure monitoring: an historical perspective. Clin Cardiol. 1992;15:II3-5.

17. Parati G. Blood pressure variability: its measurement and significance in hypertension. J Hypertens Suppl. 2005; 23:S19-25.

Correct Methodology of Blood Pressure Measurements

Shraddha More, Milind Y Nadkar

■ INTRODUCTION

Blood pressure (BP) measurement is one of the most commonly performed day-to-day procedures by all physicians. "Practice makes one perfect". But in day-to-day practice, we often tend to take accuracy of BP measurement for granted or is ignored, which definitely has influence on patient's management. BP is quantitative trait with tremendous variability secondary to observer, patient, instrument, environment and procedure-related factors. As accurate measurement of BP is fundamental for diagnosis, treatment and management aspects, patterns of individual's BP behavior are more important than isolated reading, which may be influenced by multiple factors as mentioned above. This fact and need of today's time have led to changing trends in BP measurements from the time of Riva-Rocci and Korotkoff of using conventional methods to aneroid, automatic, and semi-automatic devices and newer methods like ambulatory blood pressure monitoring (ABPM). Emerging methods like central aortic blood pressure (CABP) measurements are future of hypertension management. Increasing awareness in community and availability of newer devices day by day with increased use of such newer devices by healthcare professional and by patients for self-monitoring and home-based monitoring have lead to need for this monograph writing. The purpose of this monograph is to give our readers source of information regarding accurate methodology for BP measurements.

■ METHODS AND DEVICES FOR BLOOD PRESSURE MEASUREMENTS

Accurate device used is most important when it comes to BP measurement. If device used is inaccurate, however correct methodology is used or observer, patient and environment-related factors are improved it is of little relevance. Standardization and validation of whichever device used have to be according to protocols led by the European Society of Hypertension (ESH) and British Society of Hypertension.[1]

Various devices available for BP measurements are:
- Mercury column sphygmomanometer
- Aneroid manometer
- Electronic semi-automatic devices
- *Automatic devices*:
  - Upper arm devices
  - Finger devices
  - Wrist devices.

- Ambulatory BP measuring devices
- Central aortic BP measuring devices.

Conventional mercury column sphygmomanometer works on auscultatory principle. It is still the most common type of device used by physicians of developing countries. This device mainly works on inflation-deflation system with occluding bladder encased in cuff and nonelectronic stethoscope for auscultation. Environmental hazard secondary to mercury is of concerns and in future, Hg manometers will be banned all over the world.

Aneroid manometers have same system of inflation-deflation, bladder in cuff and stethoscope as mercury manometer, but it works on oscillatory method and register pressure through bellows and lever system, which may become inaccurate with chronic use and can give rise to false low readings and hence underestimation of BP. Aneroid manometers are also widely used by patients but they require skill and training.

Automated electronic BP measuring devices are especially used by patients for SBPM tremendously in view of increased health awareness, easy availability and affordable cost. Considering tremendous use of such automated machines by community without physician's consultation may be hazardous and hence advice regarding buying good independently validated machine as per standard ESH protocols is must. Automated devices use oscillometric technique and are of different categories such as finger devices, wrist devices and upper arm devices. Finger devices are not recommended as measurements at finger level, are not accurate due to very distal site of recording, and effects of peripheral vasoconstriction and limb position on BP measurements are unignorable. Wrist devices have to be used with caution though they are more accurate than finger devices but still positional variation and distal site of recording are important factors for distorted readings.

Upper arm devices are recommended ones among above all automated category of devices. They measure pressure at brachial artery level. General recommendations to any BP measuring device are applicable to these devices, also such as cuff size, position of arm, environmental factors, etc. which are discussed further ahead in detail. Ideal device should be able to take accurate measurements with capacity of storing readings for future use, printout facilities and telephonic connections to physicians.

Ambulatory BP monitoring method gives profile of BP of patient rather than single recording, which may be influenced by multiple factors. Details of information of recommended ABPM devices are available on www.dableducational.org website.

■ ASPECTS OF BLOOD PRESSURE MEASUREMENTS COMMON TO MOST OF THE TECHNIQUES

This section is further divided into subsections:
- Individual/subject/patient-based aspects
- Equipment-based aspects
- Observer-based aspects
- Procedure-based aspects
- Environment-based aspects.

Individual/Subject/Patient-based Aspects

While recording BP, patient must be relaxed. Anxiety, exercise, stimulants (tea, coffee) and overdistended bladder will definitely impair BP reading. After explaining patient of what is going to be done, patient should not talk for few minutes before and during the actual measurement procedure. Position of patient should be sitting, upright with back support, uncrossed legs and arm supported on table at level of heart. Unsupported arm will give rise to high BP whereas arm below heart level gives overestimation and above heart level gives underestimation of BP. In case patient has giddiness secondary to postural hypotension component, then supine position is ideal.

Observer/Doctor-based Aspects

Observer must make patient comfortable and should not make hurry in measurements. He should also sit in comfortable and relaxed position. Explaining the procedure to patients is utmost important before proceeding with actual recording. After explaining procedure, he should not communicate with patient either. Hurrying while measurements may lead to forget the readings and hence they should be noted down immediately by observer.

Equipment-based Aspects

Individually validated device should be used as per standard protocols. Cuff with enclosed inflatable bladder is encircled around arm with Velcro tapes or by wrapping or rarely by hooks. Velcro cuffs need monitoring in view of their tendencies to loose adhesiveness, whereas, tapering type of cuffs should be long enough such that they can encircle arm multiple times. Ideally, full length of cuff should extend 25 cm beyond the end of inflatable bladder and then it should gradually taper in width for another 60 cm. Undercuffing, i.e. using too narrow or too short bladder leads to cuff hypertension due to overestimation of BP whereas using too wide or too long bladder leads to overcuffing, i.e. underestimation of BP. Hence, too long cuffs misdiagnose patients with high BP to be normotensives and too short cuffs can overdiagnose normotensive patients with hypertension. Length of tubings between cuff and manometer should be at least 70 cm and between inflating pump and cuff is advised to be 30 cm.

According to the British Hypertension Society (BHS), recommendations for standard cuff sizes are given in Table 1.

TABLE 1: Recommendations for standard cuff sizes according to the British Hypertension Society (BHS).[2]

Types of adult	Bladder size
Standard cuff for majority of adults	12 × 26 cm
Large cuff for obese adults	12 × 40 cm
Small cuff for lean adults and children	12 × 18 cm

TABLE 2: Guidelines for cuff size according to the American Heart Association (AHA).[3]

Types of adult	Arm circumference	Bladder size
Small adult	22–26 cm	10 × 24 cm
Average adult	27–34 cm	13 × 30 cm
Large adult	35–44 cm	16 × 38 cm
Adult thigh cuff	45–52 cm	20 × 42 cm

Guidelines for cuff size from the American Heart Association (AHA) are different and it depends on arm circumference (Table 2).

For BP measurement in children, three cuffs with bladder size of 4 × 13 cm, 8 × 18 cm and adult cuff of 12 × 26 cm are commonly available.

Procedure-based Aspects

Explanation of procedure is very important before starting actual measurements to eliminate false high recordings secondary to anxiety components. Inflation of cuff with occlusion of artery may give rise to tingling sensation, which can elevate anxiety and hence BP readings. At least 5–10 minutes of rest before measurements should be given to patient. Proper relaxed sitting position with back rest and arm support and position of arm at heart level is ideal, otherwise isometric exercise-dependent false high BP may occur due to unsupported arm. Few patients may require supine position in view of giddiness secondary to orthostatic hypotension/postural hypotension. Ideally, first reading should be measured in both arms. Difference of 20 mm Hg in systolic blood pressure (SBP) and 10 mm Hg in diastolic blood pressure (DBP) in both arms is considered significant and needs further workup to rule out arterial occlusive pathologies. Subsequently, arm with higher BP should be used for further readings. Distance between device and observer should not exceed 1 m for better visuals of readings. Cuff should be wrapped around the arm with center of cuff over brachial artery. Few cuff has brachial artery arrow marking, which ensures proper placement of bladder and cuff. Rubber tubings can be placed superiorly, posteriorly or horizontally around bladder such that cubital fossa becomes easily available for auscultation of Korotkoff's sounds.

Palpatory method is ideal to start with followed by auscultatory. While measuring SBP with palpatory method, cuff is inflated to pressure almost 30 mm Hg above the point of disappearance of radial pulse and then slow deflation of cuff at 2–3 mm/s is made to the point of return of radial pulse, which is documented as SBP. Palpatory method of BP measurement is important in view of auscultatory gap phenomenon where phase 1 Korotkoff's sounds may sometimes disappear and reappear later at lower pressure when cuff is deflated further and hence if auscultatory method is used at first go itself may lead to false underestimation of SBP. After palpatory method, observer should go ahead with auscultatory method by inflating cuff 30 mm Hg above SBP reading gained by palpatory method and slowly deflation at 2–3 mm/s to be done so that the level at which first Korotkoff's sounds, are heard are labeled as SBP and disappearance of Korotkoff's sound are labeled as DBP. After DBP reading, rapid deflation should be done to avoid unnecessary venous congestion and tingling sensation to patient. The AHA recommends use of bell of stethoscope for auscultation of low-pitched Korotkoff's sounds but diaphragm is easier to hold and covers greater area (Table 3). Try avoiding touching clothing, cuff and tubings as it may give friction sounds.

Due to diastolic dilemma of labeling stage 4 versus stage 5 for DBP, it is recommended to take pressure at level 5, i.e. disappearance of Korotkoff's sounds as DBP unless Korotkoff's sounds persists down till 0 when muffling of sounds at stage 4 can be considered as DBP. Finally, while summarizing BP measurements ideally mentioning position of patient, arm side in which BP was recorded, bilateral BP at first visit should be done. Hypertension specialists like to summarize further details like arm circumference, bladder size, auscultatory gap if present, stages IV and V for DBP in view of diastolic dilemma, individuals physical state like anxiety/exercise/rest, etc. and not to miss time of antihypertensive dose ingestion while interpreting the results.

As multiple measurements will be definitely better than one single reading which may be erroneous secondary to multiple factors hence three measurements at different intervals separated over 1–2 minutes could be done. In case of >10 mm Hg difference between first two readings, then additional

TABLE 3: Characteristics of Korotkoff's sounds.

Korotkoff's sounds phase	Characteristics of sound
1	Faint, repetitive clear tapping sounds appear
2	Short period where sounds soften, in some patients they may disappear (silent gap)
3	Sharper sounds are again heard, which may increase in intensity compared to phase 1
4	Muffling of the sounds start abruptly and distinctly
5	All sounds disappear

recordings could be done and average of last two recordings is taken as final BP reading. Alternatively, ABPM, HBPM and SBPM modes are better to give profile of hypertension away from medical office aura. In older patients, diabetics and patients prone to develop orthostatic hypotension such as patients on antihypertensive medications repeat BP measurements after 1 and 3 minutes of standing should be performed, where drop of >20 mm Hg in SBP and >10 mm Hg in DBP within 3 minutes of standing is labeled as orthostatic hypotension and is associated with increased morbidity and cardiovascular (CV) mortality. Along with BP measurements, pulse rate measurement is good practice leading to independent assessment of CV risk.

Environmental-based Aspects

Recording of BP has to be made in quiet, comfortable room with adequate light and ventilation.

■ CONVENTIONAL BLOOD PRESSURE MONITORING/ OFFICE-BASED BLOOD PRESSURE MONITORING

This is the most common setting of BP measurement where patient is assessed by physician at clinic. As it is very common method of BP monitoring, physician must follow the rules before going ahead with actual measurements. All the important factors are discussed in detail already in Section 2 of this monograph. Table 4 gives grades of hypertension as per conventional office-based measurement.

■ UNATTENDED OFFICE BLOOD PRESSURE MEASUREMENTS

To eliminate the white coat hypertension (WCH) effect (described in detail later), BP measurements can be obtained at clinical settings itself with use of automatic device. Here, either patient or doctor's assistant can check BP in absence of physician.

■ HOME BLOOD PRESSURE MONITORING/SELF-BLOOD PRESSURE MONITORING

Automated/semi-automated machines are commonly used for HBPM as they are easily available and affordable. Preliminary requisite of rest, position is same as conventional devices. Studies have shown that HBPM values are usually lower than office-based values and hence >135 mm Hg for SBP and >85 mm Hg for DBP is criteria for defining hypertension in HBPM method. Advanced HBPM devices have storing, printout, and telephonic

TABLE 4: Grades of hypertension as per conventional office-based measurement.

Category	SBP (in mm Hg)		DBP (in mm Hg)
Optimal	<120	And	<80
Normal	120–129	And/or	80–84
High normal	130–139	And/or	85–89
Grade I HTN	140–159	And/or	90–99
Grade II HTN	160–179	And/or	100–109
Grade III HTN	>180	And/or	>110
Isolated systolic HTN	>140	And	<90

(DBP: diastolic blood pressure; HTN: hypertension; SBP: systolic blood pressure)

communication with physician and heart rate assessment facilities. In this as patient himself is monitoring BP more often compared to office-based method, compliance with medications, diet and exercise are seemed to be improved. Patient must know proper method of using HBPM machines and all machines must be individually validated as per standard protocols. Only disadvantage of this methodology over ABPM is night assessment of BP is not done and only one time static BP readings can be available. Masked hypertension and WCH both can be diagnosed by this method.

White Coat Hypertension

Patients with grade I hypertension on office-based visits are candidates to screen for WCH. Such patients with WCH have high office BP and normal home BP or ambulatory BP. Its incidence is 30–40%, which is more commonly seen in elderly people, females and nonsmokers. Hypertension-related end-organ damage and CV risk are less commonly associated with WCH compared to sustained hypertension but more compared to normotensive patients in long term. ABPM/HBPM is choice of modalities to confirm WCH.

White-coat Uncontrolled Hypertension

White-coat uncontrolled hypertension is elevated office BP, but controlled home BP or ambulatory BP in known hypertensive patient on treatment.

Masked Hypertension

Many times we get patients with normal office BP, but simultaneous workup of such patients show end organ damage and associated diseases like impaired glucose control, dyslipidemia especially in population with history of smoking, stress, alcohol intake, obesity, chronic kidney disease (CKD) and family history of hypertension. Such patients are candidates for screening for masked hypertension where office BP is normal but if ABPM/HBPM is done, high BP readings are obtained. Masked hypertension is associated with increased CV risk.

Masked Uncontrolled Hypertension

Masked uncontrolled hypertension is terminology used for hypertensive patients already on treatment with antihypertensive drugs whose office BP is controlled, but home BP/ambulatory BP is high.

◼ AMBULATORY BLOOD PRESSURE MONITORING

Multifactorial influenced single office-based BP reading and hence probable misdiagnosis and mismanagement of patients have led to need of device, which would eliminate these issues. ABPM gives average of multiple BP measurements over 24 hours. Multiple recommended ABPM devices are available in market, list of which can be obtained at www.dableducational.org website. This device is usually programmed such that BP is measured at every 15–30 minutes interval and average values for daytime, nighttime and overall 24 hours are calculated accordingly. Studies have shown ABPM values on an average lower than office values hence cutoff for defining hypertension for ABPM is >130 mm Hg for SBP and >80 mm Hg for DBP over 24 hours or >135 mm Hg for SBP and >85 mm Hg for DBP for daytime average values. For nighttime average value, SBP >120 mm Hg and DBP >90 mm Hg are considered significant (Table 5).

Various parameters assessed by ABPM are daytime recordings, nighttime recordings, nighttime dipping status, ratio of daytime to nighttime BP, daytime average BP value, 24 hours BP variability, morning BP surge and ambulatory arterial stiffness index. Dipping status is normal phenomenon observed during sleep where night BP drops compared

TABLE 5: Cut off values for ambulatory blood pressure monitoring.

Time of the day	SBP (in mm Hg)	DBP (in mm Hg)
24 hours average	>130	>80
Daytime average	>135	>85
Nighttime average	>120	>90

(DBP: diastolic blood pressure; SBP: systolic blood pressure)

to day. Individual with approximately 10% drop in night BP compared to daytime BP is defined as dipper. Studies have shown that nondippers have stronger CV risk. Various etiologies such as obstructive sleep apnea (OSA), autonomic dysfunction could be attributed to nondipping status. ABPM enables diagnosis of WCH and masked hypertension as it gives measurements in real-life settings. Though ABPM is good method for BP measurement but at the same time, it is costly and hence has limited availability.

Indications of ABPM/HBPM are:

- Suspected WCH
- Suspected masked hypertension
- *Refractory hypertension*: Few patients have refractory hypertension despite multiple medications whereas some group of patients have side effects of anti-hypertensive drugs such as hypotension, postural hypotension, and variable BP secondary to autonomic dysfunction, especially elderly population. Such patients are candidates for ABPM/HBPM
- Variable hypertension during regular follow-up of patients. If physician notices extreme variability in BP readings, then ABPM/HBPM should be advised. Postprandial hypotension commonly seen in elderly can be diagnosed with ABPM.

To assess nocturnal dipping, status of BP especially in cases like sleep apnea, CKD, diabetic autonomic neuropathy and endocrine disorders.

Ambulatory BP monitoring device has to be independently validated as per BHS/ESH protocols. Software program used in ABPM device should be user friendly and inexpensive. The functions of software should be chosen as per the requirements for either clinical practice or research work. Data is generally printable like electrocardiogram (ECG). ABPM is generally used for 24 hours with readings at interval of 20–30 minutes, sometimes frequent readings at 15–20 minutes intervals may be done, but it may interfere with patients daily activities. ABPM graph has vertical axis showing BP readings and horizontal axis showing 24 hours time, two horizontal bands indicating normal SBP and DBP values over 24 hours with shaded vertical area depicting nighttime zone to assess dipping status at night.

■ CENTRAL AORTIC BLOOD PRESSURE MONITORING

Measurements of BP in arm have served well as it is convenient, relatively easy and does not require expertise, and is also reliable but it has been noticed that CABP is more sensitive than peripheral BP in brachial artery and is associated with increased CV risk. BP experienced by vitals organs is aortic BP and not brachial BP hence aortic BP gives real estimation of target organ damage. At the starting when CABP was being developed was experimental and required invasive cardiac catheterization, but over time due to rapid development, various noninvasive and much convenient ways have been designed. Basic principle of CABP measurements is applanation tonometry. By using applanation tonometry principle, CABP can be measured by pulse wave analysis (PWA) in noninvasive way. Pulse wave is indirect reflector of CABP. Systole gives rise to generation of BP along with pulse wave—forward wave, this wave comes back to heart as reflected wave—backward wave hence combination of generated wave and reflected wave is used for estimation of CABP. Using PWA, CABP can be estimated in noninvasive manner. There is good correlation between noninvasive and invasive methods of CABP measurements. CABPs are reliable, reproducible and predictors of CV risks. CABP is more sensitive indicator of CV risk than brachial artery BP as per trials including the Strong Heart Study. Augmentation index (AI) correlates with CABP. High AI is suggestive of high CABP and is associated with high CV risk, target organ damage, and premature mortality. Studies have shown that drugs reducing CABP such as angiotensin-converting enzyme (ACE) inhibitors or calcium channel blockers (CCBs), also known as vasoactive drugs, are associated with lesser mortality compared to drugs that reduce only brachial BP. These findings have been noticed in the Anglo-Scandinavian Cardiac Outcomes Trial (ASCOT) as well. Hence, CABP is no more only invasive and research purpose modality but is being used by clinicians for day-to-day practice as well.

■ REFERENCES

1. Available from: http://www.dableducational.org/
2. Available from: https://bihsoc.org/
3. Smith L. New AHA Recommendations for Blood Pressure Measurement. Am Fam Physician. 2005 Oct 1;72(7):1391-1398.

Central Aortic Blood Pressure: An Overview

Rohit Kapoor

■ INTRODUCTION

The conventional method of measuring the blood pressure (BP) has always been the brachial artery measurement by the traditional sphygmomanometer. Since its introduction more than a century ago, brachial artery measurement of BP has been used for the evaluation of hypertension and follow-up of its treatment.[1] This measurement of BP by the sphygmomanometry has been shown to predict cardiovascular (CV) morbidity and mortality. With recent advances in knowledge and technology, newer devices for automatic BP measurement have become available, both for 24-hour recording and for home self-assessment of BP. All these newer automated devices have become quite popular for a wider out-of-office BP assessment; however, they still give a measure of the brachial BP.[2]

In the past 30 years, there has been a growing evidence on the measurement of central (aortic) BP, which is the pressure directly exerted on the vital organs such as the brain, heart and kidneys. This BP is different from the BP measured peripherally (arm), as there is an amplification effect [also known as pulse pressure (PP) amplification] which increases in the central circulation.[1] A number of invasive hemodynamic studies have shown that there is a considerable difference between systolic BP (SBP) when measured in the brachial artery versus in the aorta, underlining the need for evaluating central BP. In addition, there is increasing evidence that central SBP may be a greater predictor of future CV events than brachial pressure.[2]

The two major advantages of long-term usage of brachial BP have been its ease of measurement, and the wide variety of devices available for clinical use. However, current research has demonstrated that brachial pressure is a poor surrogate for aortic pressure, which is invariably lower than corresponding brachial values. In fact, current evidences suggest that central pressure is more strongly related to future CV events than brachial pressure, as well as it responds differently to certain drugs.[2,3] Today, central pressure can be assessed noninvasively as easily as brachial pressure, however, clinicians are unlikely to discard the brachial cuff sphygmomanometer without robust evidence that CV risk stratification and monitoring response to therapy are better when measured through central rather than peripheral pressure.[3]

In this review, the authors are going to discuss the current understanding of the use of central BP measurements, along with the current available methods for central aortic pressure, and their use with important clinical implications, such as improving diagnostic and prognostic stratification of hypertension and providing a more accurate assessment of the effect of treatment on BP.

PHYSIOLOGICAL CONCEPT OF MEASURING CENTRAL BLOOD PRESSURE

In patients with hypertension, there is a reduction in the caliber and number of small peripheral arteries with an increase in mean arterial pressure, which is a product of cardiac output and peripheral vascular resistance. The peripheral arteries are muscular, made up of collagen fibers making them less distensible. In comparison, aortic and carotid arteries are majorly consisting of elastin fibers. During systole, the arterial wall of large arteries will allow filling by distention and during diastole it will push blood forward with a steady flow with recoiling of artery. Hence, elastic ascending and thoracic aorta has the lowest arterial stiffness and distal arteries like tibial artery have highest stiffness. Progressive loss of elasticity is encountered with PP in peripheral arteries. The pressure wave produces from the left ventricle moves down the arterial tree and after that it is reflected back centrally at the arterial-arteriolar junction. Subsequently, the total pressure waveform within aorta becomes

the total sum of the forward moving waveform produced from the left ventricle and the reverse reflected wave generated by peripheral muscular and stiffer arteries. The reversed wave increases central peak SBP, which in turn increases PP. This incremental total aortic PP is identified as augmentation pressure (Fig. 1) which is indicated by percentage of the total pressure in terms of augmentation index (AIx).[1]

There is a continuous variation in the arterial pressure during the cardiac cycle, but in clinical practice only the traditional sphygmomanometric measurements of systolic and diastolic BPs are only reported as routine practice.

These are perpetually measured within the brachial artery using cuff sphyg-momanometry—a routine practice which has seen very few changes over the last 8–10 decades. However, there is continuous change throughout the arterial tree in the shape of the pressure waveform. Systolic pressure can be higher by 40 mm Hg in the brachial artery than it is reported the aorta irrespective of diastolic and mean arterial pressures remaining relatively constant.

Thus, the phenomenon of increased systolic pressure occurs due to increased arterial stiffness which is moving away from the heart. As the pressure wave migrates toward the stiffer brachial artery from the highly elastic central arteries, the upper

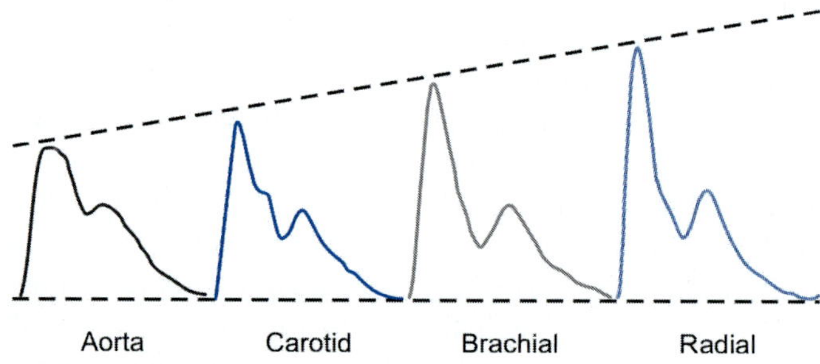

Fig. 1: Amplication of the preassure waveform moving from the arota to the radial artery.

portion of the wave becomes smaller, the systolic peak becomes more prominent increasing the systolic pressure (Fig. 1).[3]

■ TECHNIQUES OF ASSESSING CENTRAL BLOOD PRESSURE (TABLE 1)

There are various methods now available for assessing central pressure. One of the most direct but invasive method is cardiac catheterization, where the BP in the ascending aorta using a pressure-sensing catheter is measured (Fig. 2A). However, this technique is highly invasive, requires a trained technician to perform and clearly unsuitable for use in routine screening of large populations. More recently, a number of noninvasive methods have been developed, where pressure waveforms are recorded from sites distal to the aorta, such as the carotid (Fig. 2B), radial (Fig. 2C) or brachial (Fig. 2D) arteries, and calibrated to BP recorded by cuff sphygmomanometry.[3] Each of these approaches has its strengths and limitations.

Central pressures are inferred from noninvasive procedures of estimation of radial or carotid pulses, and a validated generalized

TABLE 1: Indirect noninvasive methods for measuring central blood pressure.

Method of waveform recording	Device	Company	Method of calibration	Method of estimation	Clinical applicability[†]
Radial tonometry	BPro	HealthSTATS	Brachial- radial cuff BP	GTF (radial-aortic)	++
	SphygmoCor	AtCor medical	Brachial-radial cuff BP	GTF (radial-aortic)	+
				Late systolic shoulder	+
	HEM9000AI	Omron	Brachial cuff BP	Algorithm	++
				Late systolic shoulder	++
Brachial cuff PVP	*ARCsolver		Brachial cuff BP	GTF (brachial-aortic)	+++
	Centron cBP301	Centron diagnostics	Brachial cuff BP	GTF (brachial-aortic)	++++
	Vicorder	Skidmore medical	Brachial cuff BP	GTF (brachial-aortic)	+++
	XCEL	AtCor medical	Brachial cuff BP	GTF (brachial-aortic)	+++
Supras-ystolic brachial cuff PVP	Arteriograph	TensioMed	Brachial cuff BP	Late systolic wave amplitude	+++
	Cardioscope II	Pulsecor	Brachial cuff BP	Algorithm	++++

*Incorporated in Mobil-O-Graph PWA device (IEM GmbH).

[†]Personal view based on experience, operator-dependency, need for computer/software interface, with + indicating limited applicability to routine clinical practice and ++++ indicating high aplicability.

(BP: blood pressure; GTF: generalized transfer function; PVP: pulse volume plethysmography)

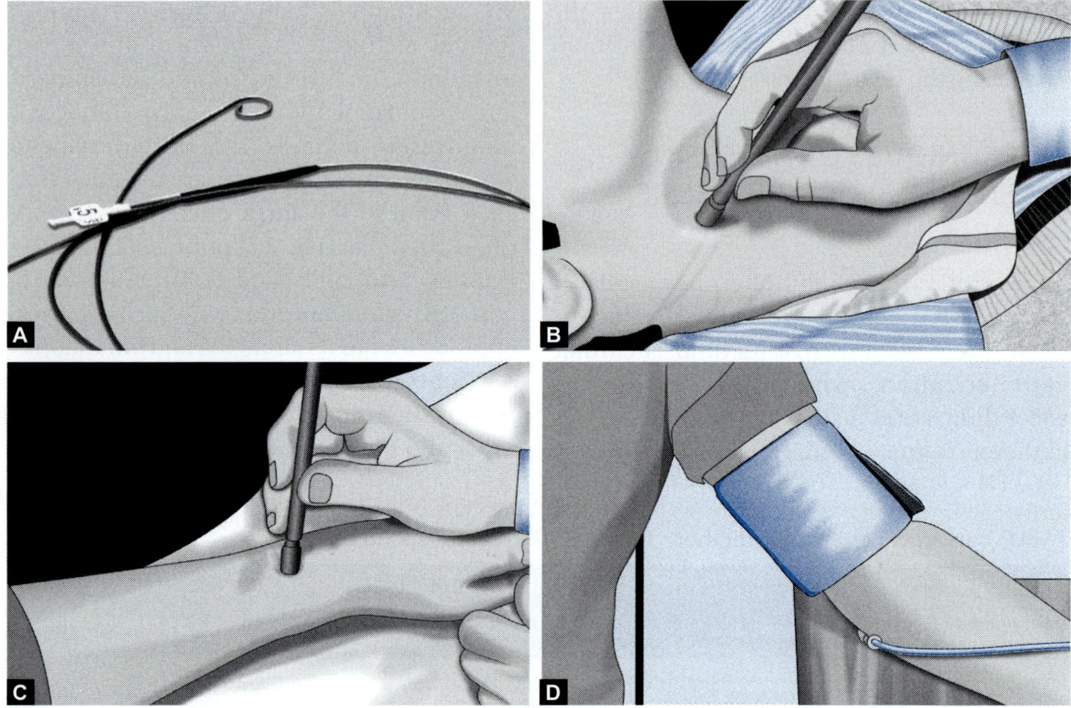

Figs. 2A to D: Techniques for assessing central blood pressure. (A) Invasive cardiac catheterization; (B) Direct applanation tonometry of the carotid artery; (C) Applanation tonometry of the radial artery; (D) Cuff-based oscillometry at the brachial artery.

transfer function is utilized to measure central pressures from the peripheral signal.[4] This process involves applanation tonometry, during which transcutaneous pressure transducer at the probe end gets pressure waveforms that are most similar to those obtained with intra-arterial measurement.[5] This process is appropriate for carotid, radial, as well as femoral arteries. The carotid waveform then can be utilized as a substitute of the aorta. Alternative option is a mathematical description of the charge from the input to output signals to get an aortic waveform based on measurements of the radial artery. Computer-based programs then adjust the values for heart rate, age and height. Thus, central SBP, PP and diastolic BP are measured and arterial stiffness indices like AIx and pulse wave velocity (PWV) are calculated.[6]

The normal transfer function of applanation tonometry is associated with range of error, but the errors are less frequent as compared to standard brachial cuff pressure measured using sphygmomanometer or an oscillometric device.[7] There is a possibility of intrinsic variations in the measurements provided by various instruments and can also be operator dependent. The AIx measurement, which is a quantifying arterial wave reflection on total BP, can differ due to variations in cardiac contractility, heart rate and age. PWV is the measurement of aortic pulse velocity which can be evaluated by estimating the distance between two arteries (mostly carotid and femoral arteries) and dividing it with the transit time. Higher arterial stiffness is an indication of less compliant arteries which will to quick wave traveling to and from the periphery. PWV is an improvised marker for arterial stiffness, due to its relative ease of measurement and reliability of the outcomes, although there are some variabilities in measurements based on types of populations, with age and different BP levels. There is no influence of smoking, dyslipidemia, or sex, but heart rate and diabetes can influence the measurements to some extent.[8]

A prospective study conducted by Mitchell and his colleagues, among 2,232 participants from Framingham Heart Study after a mean follow-up of 7.8 years, reported that the PWV pulsatile hemodynamic measure is the best predictor of a first major CV event for an individual.[9]

A systematic review of 15,877 subjects conducted and Vlachopoulos et al. concluded that the future CV events and all-cause mortality can be better predicted with aortic PWV and have a predictive value independent of traditional CV risk factors and other potential confounders.[10]

The relative risk of total CV events and CV mortality for a high PWV was increased for high-risk populations as compared to populations at low risk. These data confirm that measurement of arterial stiffness can appropriately estimate CV risk from a genetic background and cumulative damage on the arterial wall due to CV risk factors. The reference values for arterial stiffness collaboration group from Europe has recently published PWV reference values.[11]

The mean normal PWV value for younger individuals of age less than 30 years is 6.2 m/s and for older individuals above 70 years of age is 10.9 m/s. Although there can be some overlap between younger and older individuals in normal PWV values, many CV risk factors such as stress and positive family history are not quantifiable.[11]

■ IMPLICATIONS OF CENTRAL BLOOD PRESSURE ON THERAPY

The vital organs of the body such as the heart, kidneys and brain receive blood from the major arteries which are exposed to aortic rather than brachial pressure. Therefore, there is a strong rationale to show that CV events may ultimately be more closely related to central rather than brachial pressure. A plethora of evidences have been published over the last 12 years with regards to the link between central pressure and both surrogate markers of risk and hard endpoints which strongly support this concept.[12] It has been proved in various cross-sectional studies that central pressure strongly linked with widely accepted surrogate measures of CV risk such as carotid intima-media thickness (CIMT) and left ventricular mass (LVM), as compared to brachial pressure.[13,14]

In the REASON study,[15] regression of LVM was more strongly related to change in central compared with brachial pressure and, after adjustment, only central pressure remained predictive. Similar observations were seen in a substudy of ASCOT.[16] Furthermore, on treatment with antihypertensive drugs, the reduction in CIMT relates better to the fall in central pressure. However, recently, it was widely believed that BP reduction per se, matters more than the choice of antihypertensive agent.[17] However, the beta-blocker atenolol was found to be inferior to other major antihypertensive drug classes in preventing CV events. This was demonstrated in two comprehensive meta-analyses,[18,19] along with analysis of large comparison studies including the MRC-Elderly,[20] LIFE[21] and ASCOT[22] trials.

Remarkably, there is now convincing evidence that beta-blockers exert differential effects on brachial versus central pressure.

Such evidence may help to explain the adverse findings with atenolol in outcome studies and provides support for the hypothesis that drugs which lower central pressure the most will be more effective.

CONCLUSION

- Central BP measurements may have better prognostic value as compared to peripheral BP measurements as it estimates core BP to which organs like heart, brain and kidneys are exposed
- Arterial stiffness is a well-established CV risk factor and can be a better risk index of end-organ damage and CV incidences in hypertensive individuals. Investigation of increased vascular stiffness can serve as a marker of inherent atherosclerotic risk as it can predict incident hypertension for high-risk individuals
- After years of research, there is now a substantial body of evidence that antihypertensive drugs, and particularly beta-blockers, exert differential effects on brachial and central pressure
- Thus, future treatment strategies based on central rather than brachial BP measurement would be beneficial and may have important implications in future diagnosis and management of hypertension
- However, cuff measurements are here to stay, and will remain the most accepted method for measuring BP in clinical practice
- Therefore, appropriately powered clinical trials demonstrating that preferential lowering of central pressure improves outcome, will ultimately be required before central pressure becomes an accepted surrogate of CV risk.

REFERENCES

1. Trudeau L. Central blood pressure as an index of antihypertensive control: determinants and potential value. Can J Cardiol. 2014;30:S23-8.
2. Muiesan ML, Salvetti M, Bertacchini F, et al. Central blood pressure assessment using 24-hour brachial pulse wave analysis. J Vasc Diagn Interv. 2014;2:141-8.
3. McEniery MC, Cockroft JR, Roman MJ, et al. Central blood pressure: current evidence and clinical importance. Eur Heart J. 2014;35:1719-25.
4. Siebenhofer A, Kemp CR, Sutton AJ, et al. The reproducibility of central aortic blood pressure measurements in healthy subjects using applanation tonometry and sphygmocardiography. J Hum Hypertens. 1999;13:625-9.
5. Kelly R, Hayward C, Avolio A, et al. Noninvasive determination of age-related changes in the human arterial pulse. Circulation. 1989;80:1652-9.
6. Mancia G, De Backer G, Dominniczak A, et al. 2007 guidelines for the management of arterial hypertension: the Task Force for the management of arterial hypertension of the European Society of Hypertension (ESH) and of the European Society of Cardiology (ESC). J Hypertens. 2007;25:1105-87.
7. O'Brien E, Waeber B, Parati G, et al. Blood pressure measuring devices: recommendations of the European Society of Hypertension. BMJ. 2001;322:531-6.
8. ESH/ESC Task Force for the Management of Arterial Hypertension. 2013 Practice guidelines for the management of arterial hypertension of the European Society of Hypertension (ESH) and the European Society of Cardiology (ESC): ESH/ESC Task Force for the management of arterial hypertension. J Hypertens. 2013;31:1925-38.
9. Mitchell GF, Hwang SJ, Vasan RS, et al. Arterial stiffness and cardiovascular events: the Framingham Heart Study. Circulation. 2010;121:505-11.
10. Vlachopoulos C, Aznaouidis K, Stefanadis C. Prediction of cardiovascular events and all-cause mortality with arterial stiffness. J Am Coll Cardiol. 2010;55:1318-27.
11. Reference Values for Arterial Stiffness' Collaboration. Determinants of pulse wave velocity in healthy people and in the presence of cardiovascular risk factors: 'establishing normal and reference values'. Eur Heart J. 2010;31:2338-50.
12. Laurent S, Cockcroft JR, van Bortel LM, et al. Abridged version of the expert consensus document. Artery Res. 2007;1:2-12.
13. Boutouyrie P, Bussy C, Lacolley P, et al. Association between local pulse pressure, mean blood pressure, and large-artery remodeling. Circulation. 1999;100:1387-93.

14. Wang KL, Cheng HM, Chuang SY, et al. Central or peripheral systolic or pulse pressure: which best relates to target organs and future mortality? J Hypertens. 2009;27:461-7.

15. de Luca N, Asmar RG, London GM, et al. Selective reduction of cardiac mass and central blood pressure on low-dose combination perindopril/indapamide in hypertensive subjects. J Hypertens. 2004;22:1623-30.

16. Manisty CH, Zambanini A, Parker KH, et al. Differences in the magnitude of wave reflection account for differential effects of amlodipine- versus atenolol-based regimens on central blood pressure: an Anglo-Scandinavian Cardiac Outcome Trial Substudy. Hypertension. 2009;54:724-30.

17. ALLHAT Officers and Coordinators for the ALLHAT Collaborative Research Group. Major outcomes in high-risk hypertensive patients randomized to angiotensin-converting enzyme inhibitor or calcium channel blocker vs diuretic: the Antihypertensive and Lipid-Lowering Treatment to Prevent Heart Attack Trial (ALLHAT). JAMA. 2002;288:2981-97.

18. Carlberg B, Samuelsson O, Lindholm LH. Atenolol in hypertension: is it a wise choice? Lancet. 2004;364:1684-9.

19. Lindholm LH, Carlberg B, Samuelsson O. Should beta blockers remain first choice in the treatment of primary hypertension? A meta-analysis. Lancet. 2005;366:1545-53.

20. Medical Research Council trial of treatment of hypertension in older adults: principal results. MRC Working Party. BMJ. 1992;304:405-12.

21. Dahlof B, Devereux RB, Kjeldsen SE, et al. Cardiovascular morbidity and mortality in the Losartan Intervention for Endpoint reduction in hypertension study (LIFE): a randomized trial against atenolol. Lancet. 2002;359:995-1003.

22. Dahlof B, Sever PS, Poulter NR, et al. Prevention of cardiovascular events with an antihypertensive regimen of amlodipine adding perindopril as required versus atenolol adding bendroflumethiazide as required, in the Anglo-Scandinavian Cardiac Outcomes Trial-Blood Pressure Lowering Arm (ASCOT-BPLA): a multicentre randomised controlled trial. Lancet. 2005;366:895-906.

Evaluation of Hypertension

Hypertension: Clinical Approach

M Chenniappan

■ INTRODUCTION

The incidence, prevalence, and complications of hypertension (HT) are increasing in India. This is primarily due to uncontrolled HT. But the complications are also due to late diagnosis, failure to identify secondary causes, missing hypertension-mediated organ damage (HMOD), ignoring other risk factors, as well as comorbidities and their drugs. Most often we rely upon investigations such as ECG, echocardiogram, and laboratory investigations to diagnose above conditions. A good clinical approach which includes good history taking and meticulous physical examination will help us in identifying all the abnormalities mentioned above at the earliest with little or no cost to the patient. In this article we are aiming at exploring this possibility.

■ CLINICAL APPROACH

- History
- Physical examination.
  In both these segments we should concentrate on:
- Identifying secondary causes
- Other risk factors
- Recognition of HMOD
- Comorbidities and their drugs.

History

History Identifying Secondary Causes

Identifying secondary causes in HT is very crucial in the management of HT because most of the secondary HT is curable whereas essential HT is only controllable.

In any new or uncontrolled HT following factors may indicate the possibility of secondary HT (Box 1).

Box 1: History clues to secondary hypertension (HT)
• Any difficult to control HT
• Onset of HT before 30 years
• New onset of diastolic HT after 65 years
• Abrupt onset of HT
• Sudden out of control of blood pressure
• Unprovoked or excessive hypokalemia after diuretics
• Acclerated or malignant HT or any hypertensive crisis
• Dispropotionate HT-mediated organ damage to the degree of HT
• Claudication in young patients
• Unexplained anemia in HT
• Daytime sleepiness or tiredness
• Drugs (other allopathic or other system medicines)

History regarding specific cause:
- Family history of renal disease (polycystic kidney)
- Renal disease, urinary tract infection, hematuria, analgesic abuse (parenchymal renal disease), oral contraceptives (HT due to drugs)
- Episodes of sweating, headache, anxiety (pheochromocytoma)
- Episodes of muscle weakness and tetany (hyperaldosteronism)
- Intermittent claudication in young (coarctation of aorta)
- Intermittent episodes sudden acute dyspnea requiring hospitalization (flash acute pulmonary edema due to renal artery stenosis)
- Snoring and acute breathlessness at night (sleep apnea)
- Increased weight and striae (Cushing's syndrome)
- Weight gain or weight loss with HT (thyroid disorders).

History to Identify Other Risk Factors
- Family and personal history of HT, cardio-vascular disease, stroke, or renal disease
- Family and personal history of associated risk factors (e.g. familial hypercholestero-lemia)
- Smoking history
- Dietary history and salt intake
- Alcohol consumption
- Lack of physical exercise/secondary life-style
- History of erectile dysfunction
- Sleep history, snoring, sleep apnea (information also from partner)
- Polyuria, polydipsia of diabetes mellitus (DM).

History Suggestive of HMOD
- *Brain and eyes*—headache, vertigo, syncope, impaired vision, transient ischemic attack (TIA), sensory or motor deficit, stroke, carotid revascularization, cognitive impairment, or dementia (in the elderly)
- *Heart*—coronary artery disease (CAD)-exertional and rest angina, history of revascularization; heart failure—dyspnea, paroxysmal nocturnal dyspnea and orthopnea for left heart failure; neck pulsation, right hypochondrial tenderness, swelling of abdomen, pedal edema for right heart failure; arrhythmias—palpitation and syncope
- *Kidney*—thirst, polyuria, nocturia, hematuria, and urinary tract infections
- *Peripheral arteries*—cold extremities, intermittent claudication, pain free walking distance, pain at rest, and peri-pheral revascularization.

History Regarding Comorbidities and Drugs
- History of bronchial asthma and drugs like sympathomimetic and steroids
- History of orthopedic diseases and intake of nonsteroidal anti-inflammatory drugs and COX-2 inhibitors
- History of anemia of renal disease and erythropoietin
- History of malignancy and chemo-therapeutic drugs
- History of psychiatric diseases and anti-psychiatric drugs
- Routine use of drugs such as ginseng and herbal medicines.

Physical Examination

Physical examination in HT is divided into general examination and specific examination to identify secondary causes, other risk factors, HMOD, and comorbidities.

General examination includes exami-nation of pulse (arterial and venous), blood pressure (BP), pallor, edema, obesity (general or midsegment), and features suggestive of endocrine disorders (thyroid and Cushing's).

Examination of Arterial Pulse in Hypertension

All pulses should be palpated. Absence of lower limb pulse and radio femoral delay is suggestive of coarctation, asymmetry of pulse in hypertensive emergency is suggestive of aortic dissection, asymmetry of pulse in chronic situations is indicative of peripheral arterial disease, absence of upper limb pulse is suggestive of Takayasu's disease, and absence of individual pulse is suggestive of embolism in a case of atrial fibrillation (AF).

Rate may be fast, slow, regular, or irregular. Tachycardia with HT may occur in hyperthyroidism, pheochromocytoma, and heart failure. Slow pulse with HT is suggestive of hypothyroidism, drugs induced, or complete heart block. Irregular pulse is likely to be due to premature beats or AF.

Volume of the pulse is to be checked which has to be correlated with pulse pressure. The pulse volume is normal if the pulse pressure is normal (30–50 mm Hg.). The volume of the pulse can be normal, high or low in HT. Whenever pulse volume is high, aortic regurgitation (AR), hyperthyroidism, anemia, pregnancy, and high pulse pressure HT should be suspected. In high pulse pressure HT, the systolic BP is high and diastolic BP is low due to aortic stiffening and high pulse wave velocity which is the most dangerous HT. The low volume pulse in HT is rare and if present it is suggestive of arterial disease and end stage hypertensive heart disease due to severe left ventricular (LV) dysfunction.

Character of the pulse can give some clues regarding the basic disease. Collapsing pulse or Corrigan's pulse indicates AR which may produce systolic HT. Bisferiens pulse is the sign of chronic severe AR or aortic stenosis (AS) with AR. Change in volume of pulse for alternate beats, pulsus alternans occurs in LV failure.

Examination of Venous Pulse

Jugular venous pressure (JVP) and pulse should be examined in HT. Elevated JVP and prominent "a" wave are the signs of associated pulmonary HT which may coexist with systemic HT. The JVP is elevated in all volume overloaded conditions which may produce HT such as chronic kidney disease (CKD) and iatrogenic fluid overload. Flat JVP even in lying position is indicative of dehydration which can also produce HT due to increased renin release secondary to hyponatremia which happens in polyuric phase of CKD. Intermittent cannon waves with bradycardia may happen in isolated systolic HT due to complete heart block (CHB).

Measurement Blood Pressure

The first and foremost important prerequisite of correct management of HT is the proper recording of BP (Fig. 1).

Measurement of Blood Pressure (ESC Guidelines 2018) (Box 2)

Steps which should be followed for correct recording of BP is given in Box 2.

Blood Pressure Apparatus, Cuff Size, and Lowering of Column

Mercury BP apparatus is being replaced by aneroid in recent days which should be calibrated every year. As there are no proper calibrating methods in India it is preferable to get a new BP apparatus every year. The width of cuff should be 40% of arm circumference and the length of the cuff is 80% of arm circumference. The cuff width and length for proper measurement of BP is shown in Table 1.

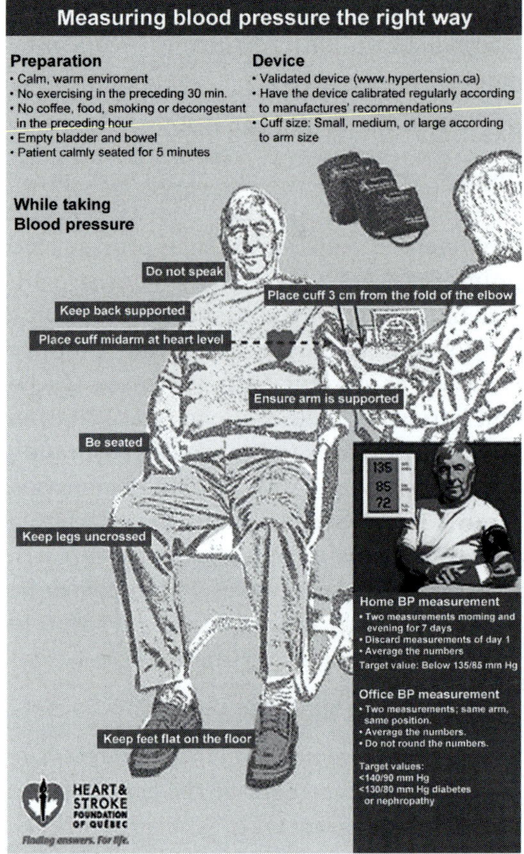

Fig. 1: Diagram shows the steps to be followed for proper recording of blood pressure at office and home.
Courtesy: HEART & STROKE foundation of Quebec.

Large cuff for the small arm will underestimate systolic BP and small cuff for the large arm overestimates systolic BP. Lowering of mercury column or the numbers in aneroid BP apparatus is about 2–3 mm Hg per second. Rapid lowering results in overestimation of diastolic pressure.

Blood Pressure Measurement Methods

- Office (attended, OBPM)—oscillometric (electronic)—preferred method; auscultatory (mercury, aneroid)
- Office Automated (unattended, AOBP)— oscillometric (electronic)

TABLE 1: Required cuff width and length in various groups.

Cuff denomination	Arm circumference (cm)	Cuff width (cm)	Bladder length (cm)
Small adult	22–26	10	24
Adult	27–34	13	30
Large adult	35–44	16	38
Thigh	45–52	20	42

- Ambulatory blood pressure monitoring (ABPM)
- Home blood pressure monitoring (HBPM).

Grade of Hypertension

Once the BP is recorded correctly, the classification of HT is done based on numbers into various grades.

The grades of HT vary according to different guidelines (Table 2).

Specific Physical Examination to Identify Secondary Causes

- Features of Cushing's syndrome (obesity, striae, and facies)
- Skin stigmata of neurofibromatosis (pheochromocytoma)
- Palpation of enlarged kidneys (polycystic kidney)
- Auscultation of abdominal murmurs (renovascular HT)
- Auscultation of precordial or chest murmurs (aortic coarctation)
- Diminished and delayed femoral pulses and reduced leg blood pressure (aortic coarctation)
- Short neck and obesity (sleep apnea)
- Edema, pallor, and facial puffiness (CKD)
- Typical hypothyroid features with bradycardia (hypothyroidism)
- Tachycardia and sweating (pheochromocytoma and hyperthyroidism).

Specific Physical Examination to Diagnose Other Risk Factors

- Features of metabolic syndrome—waist circumference more than 90 cm in men, more than 80 cm in women with other laboratory features—prediabetic, prehypertensive, and precardiovascular disease status
- *External features of DM*—acanthosis nigricans, foot ulcers, and features of metabolic syndrome
- *External features of hypercholesterolemia*—xanthelasma
- Tar staining of fingers—chronic smoker.

Specific Physical Examination to Identify HMOD

Brain

Presence of previous CVA like hemiplegia or paresis, focal neurological deficit, carotid bruit, and motor or sensory defects indicate chronic HMOD. Acute ischemic or hemorrhagic stroke and hypertensive encephalopathy indicate hypertensive emergency.

Eye

There may be various grades of hypertensive retinopathy and objective visual disturbances as HMOD in the eye. Presence of grade III retinopathy indicates accelerated HT and presence of papilledema is malignant HT. Papilledema with loss of vision is hypertensive emergency.

Heart

The abnormalities in arterial pulse and venous pulse indicative of cardiac HMOD are already explained.

Left ventricular hypertrophy (LVH) is indicative of chronic pressure overload due to HT which is an important HMOD determining the prognosis. LVH can be diagnosed clinically by the presence of heaving apical impulse where duration of

TABLE 2: Classification of HT according to recent American and European guidelines.

ESC/ESH vs. ACC/AHA Hypertension guideline							
ESC/ESH 2018 (June)				ACC/AHA 2017 (November)			
Category	Systolic (mm Hg)		Diastolic (mm Hg)	Category	Systolic (mm Hg)		Diastolic (mm Hg)
Optimal	<120	and	<80	Normal	<120	and	<80
Normal	120–129	and	80–84	Elevated BP	120–129	and	<80
High Normal	130–139	and/or	85–89	Stage 1	130–139	Or	80–89
Grade 1	140–159	and/or	90–99	Stage 2	≥140	Or	≥90
Grade 2	160–179	and/or	100–109	Hypertensive crisis	≥180	Or	≥120
Grade 3	≥180	and/or	≥110				
Isolated systolic hypertension: Systolic >140 mm Hg, diastolic <90 mm Hg							

(HT: hypertension; ESC: European Society of Cardiology; ESH: European Society of Hypertension; ACC: American College of Cardiology; AHA: American Heart Association; BP: blood pressure)

apical thrust is prolonged without much altering the position of the apical impulse. Sometimes there may be palpable 4th heart sound in addition to heaving apical impulse. Presence of clinical evidence of LVH and palpable or auscultatory LV 4th heart sound indicate diastolic dysfunction which is the earliest manifestation of cardiac HMOD. In all patients with HT clinical evidence for LVH should be looked for clinically.

Auscultation of the heart includes abnormalities of heart sounds, presence of additional heart sounds, and murmurs.

S1 and S2

S1 may be soft due to increased end diastolic pressure of LV. In HT A2 is loud due to high diastolic pressure in aorta. HT produces paradoxical splitting of S2 due to prolonged LV systole (Figs. 2A and B).

Presence of Additional Sounds

Left-sided 3rd and 4th sounds are low-pitched sounds heard with bell of stethoscope lightly applied to the apex and they give valuable information regarding LV function (Fig. 3).

Left-sided 4th heart sound (LA4) is a low-pitched sound which occurs due to left atrial contraction against raised LV end-diastolic pressure and is heard before 1st heart sound (Fig. 3). Most commonly it is associated with stiff LVH. In patients with dyspnea in HT the presence of LVH and LA4 indicate that dyspnea is probably due to heart failure with preserved ejection fraction. So LA4 is a sign of diastolic dysfunction.

Left-sided 3rd heart sound (LV3) in adults is a low-pitched sound due to exaggerated early diastolic filling due to high LA pressure due to LV systolic dysfunction and is heard after the 2nd sound (Fig. 3). In patients with dyspnea in HT the presence of LV3 indicates that dyspnea is probably due to heart failure with reduced ejection fraction. So LV3 is a sign of systolic dysfunction.

Presence of Murmurs

The two common murmurs in HT are mitral regurgitation (MR) and aortic regurgitation (AR).

Mitral regurgitation can occur due to multiple causes such as LV dilatation, papillary muscle dysfunction, and associated CAD. Thepan systolic murmur of MR is heard over the apex (Figs. 4A and B).

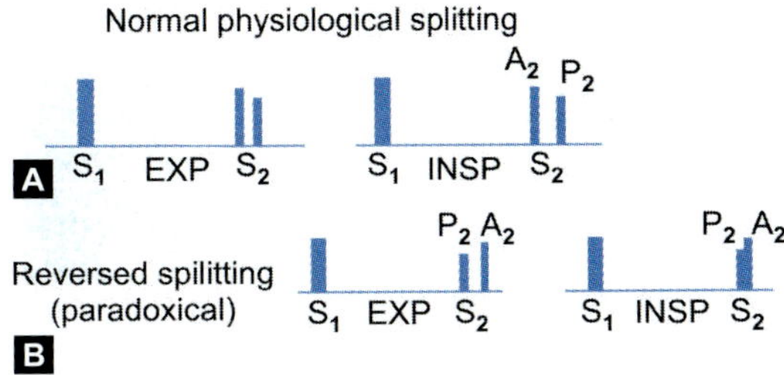

Figs. 2A and B: (A) Normal S2 splitting where single second is heard in expiration and two components are heard in inspiration; (B) In reversed splitting, two components are heard in expiration and single sound is heard in inspiration. Please note that in reversed splitting A2 occurs later than P2 due to delayed left ventricular systole because of hypertension.

Aortic regurgitation is due to increased diastolic pressure in aorta and aortic root dilatation. It is the most common murmur in HT as well as due to congenital bicuspid aortic valve (CBAV) which is the most common association of coarctation of aorta. The early diastolic murmur of AR is heard over left sternal edge as well as in aortic area (Figs. 4A and B).

Peripheral Vessels

Examination of peripheral arteries may show absence, reduction, or asymmetry of pulses, cold extremities, and ischemic skin lesions. Carotids should be auscultated in all patients with HT to detect carotid artery bruit which is the most cost-effective way of detecting HMOD of peripheral arteries.

Specific Physical Examination to Detect Comorbid Conditions

Most of comorbid conditions are identified through good history.

Chronic Obstructive Pulmonary Disease

The patients with chronic obstructive pulmonary disease (COPD) may have mild cyanosis, clubbing, and barrel-shaped chest. During acute episode of asthma it may be mistaken for acute LVF. The differentiating points are the action of accessory muscles, inspiratory collapse of JVP, rhonchi rather than crepitation and more of cyanosis.

Orthopedic Diseases

Deformity of joints, swelling of joints, reduced mobility, and abnormal gait are indicators of joint abnormalities.

Psychiatric Disorders

Abnormal behavior and communication of the patient are suggestive of associated psychiatric disorder such as anxiety and/or depression. Many antipsychotic drugs produce visceral obesity and metabolic syndrome.

Malignancy

Presence of obvious tumors, emaciation, pallor, and external evidence of chemotherapy-induced side effects may indicate associated malignancy.

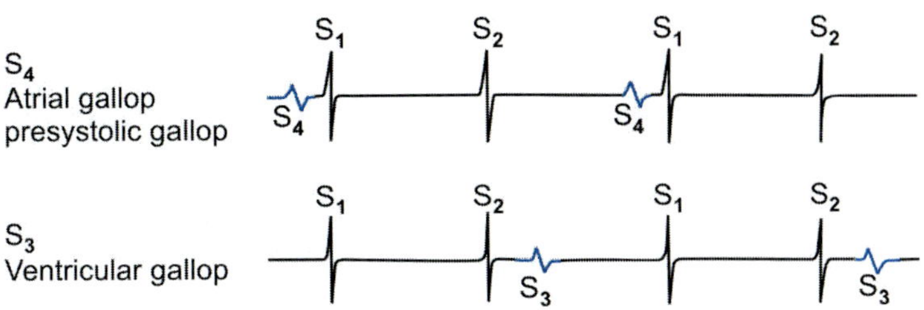

Fig. 3: Diagram shows S4 (LA4) and S3 (LV3).

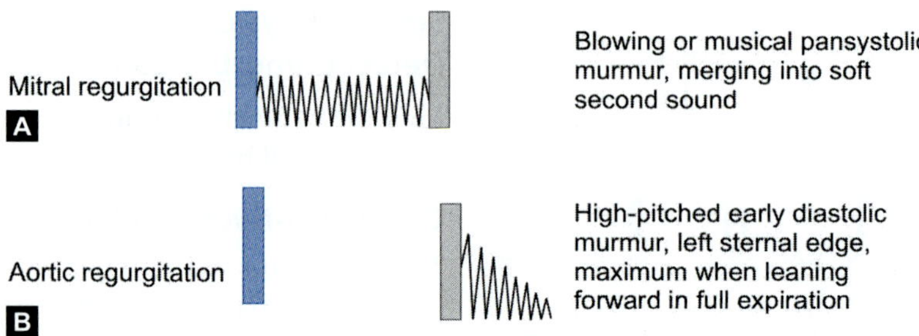

Figs. 4A and B: Murmurs of (A) mitral regurgitation and (B) aortic regurgitation.

■ CONCLUSION

A good clinical evaluation of a patient with HT can reveal secondary causes, unmask other risk factors, expose HMOD and identify comorbid conditions and drugs without sophisticated investigations. So no investigation, however sophisticated it may be, should ever replace a good clinical judgment. We must utilize the advanced investigatory modalities to refine our clinical knowledge rather than replace it. A skillful history taking and meticulous and focused physical examination most often give us many crucial information regarding diagnosis and management of HT without wasting time (of the doctor) and money (of the patient).

■ SUGGESTED READING

1. Leung AA, Daskalopoulou SS, Dasgupta K, et al. Hypertension Canada's 2017 guidelines for diagnosis, risk assessment, prevention, and treatment of hypertension in adults. Can J Cardiol. 2017;33(5):557-76.

2. Pickering TG, Hall JE, Appel LJ, et al. Recommendations for blood pressure measurement in humans and experimental animals: part 1: blood pressure measurement in humans: a statement for professionals from the Subcommittee of Professional and Public Education of the American Heart Association Council on High Blood Pressure Research. Circulation. 2005;111(5):697-716.

3. Mancia G, Fagard R, Narkiewicz K, et al. 2013 ESH/ESC guidelines for the management of arterial hypertension: the task force for the management of arterial hypertension of the European Society of Hypertension (ESH) and of the European Society of Cardiology (ESC). Eur Heart J. 2013;34(28):2159-219.

4. Hubert HB, Feinleib M, McNamara PM, et al. Obesity as an independent risk factor for cardiovascular disease: a 26-year follow-up of participants in the Framingham Heart Study. Circulation. 1983;67(5):968-77.

5. Elliott P, Stamler J, Nichols R, et al. Intersalt revisited: further analyzes of 24 hour sodium excretion and blood pressure within and across populations. Intersalt Cooperative Research Group. BMJ. 1996;312(7041):1249-53.

6. Leary AC, Donnan PT, MacDonald TM, et al. The influence of physical activity on the variability of ambulatory blood pressure. Am J Hypertens. 2000;13(10):1067-73.

7. Devereux RB, Roman MJ. Left ventricular hypertrophy in hypertension: stimuli, patterns, and consequences. Hypertens Res. 1999;22(1):1-9.

8. Devereux RB, Wachtell K, Gerdts E, et al. Prognostic significance of left ventricular mass change during treatment of hypertension. JAMA. 2004;292(19):2350-6.

9. Whelton PK, Carey RM, Aronow WS, et al. 2017 ACC/AHA/AAPA/ABC/ACPM/AGS/APhA/ASH/ASPC/NMA/PCNA guideline for the prevention, detection, evaluation, and management of high blood pressure in adults: A report of the American College of Cardiology/American Heart Association Task Force on Clinical Practice Guidelines. J Am Coll Cardiol. 2018;71(19):e127-e248.

10. Williams B, Mancia G, Spiering W, et al.; 2018 ESC/ESH Guidelines for the management of arterial hypertension. Eur Heart J. 2018;39(33):3021-104.

Hypertension: ECG in Decision Making

M Chenniappan

■ INTRODUCTION

In India, one in three has hypertension and 50% of the population is in high normal range. Mortality and morbidity are quite high in hypertension if not detected early and treated properly. The complications in hypertension depend upon the presence of target organ disease (TOD), secondary causes, comorbidities and complications due to hypertension. Most often we rely upon echocardiography and blood studies to diagnose these issues. The electrocardiogram (ECG) when interpreted skilfully gives valuable information regarding these issues, even when they are not detected by echocardiography. ECG is underutilized in hypertension. The purpose of the chapter is to explore the utilities of ECG in hypertension in detecting causes, complications and to plan the management. To our knowledge, the management of hypertension has not been looked from this ECG angle so far. ECG aids in ECG (**E**xcellent **C**are **G**iving) in patients with hypertension.

■ ELECTROCARDIOGRAM IN HYPERTENSION

Electrocardiogram in hypertension is better utilized in following headings:

- *Role of ECG in detecting TOD[1]*
- *ECG clues for secondary causes*
- *ECG signs of comorbidities*
- *ECG in hypertensive complications.*

This chapter also discusses the selection of antihypertensive drugs under above headings.[2]

Role of Electrocardiogram in Detecting Target Organ Disease

Left Ventricular Hypertrophy

One of the important TODs is left ventricular hypertrophy (LVH). The presence of LVH for the same level of blood pressure (BP) enhances the risk of coronary artery disease (CAD), heart failure and arrhythmias. Although echo is ideal to detect LVH, the ECG remains a cost-effective method of detecting LVH.

ECG Criteria to Detect LVH

- *Limb lead*: R in lead aVL more than 11 mm
- *Chest leads*:
  - R in V5, V6 +S in V1 >35 mm
  - R in V5, V6 more than 26 mm.

Limb lead criteria are used in children and patients with chronic obstructive pulmonary disease (COPD) in whom chest lead criteria may not be reliable. The ECG has high specificity and low sensitivity to diagnose LVH (Fig. 1).

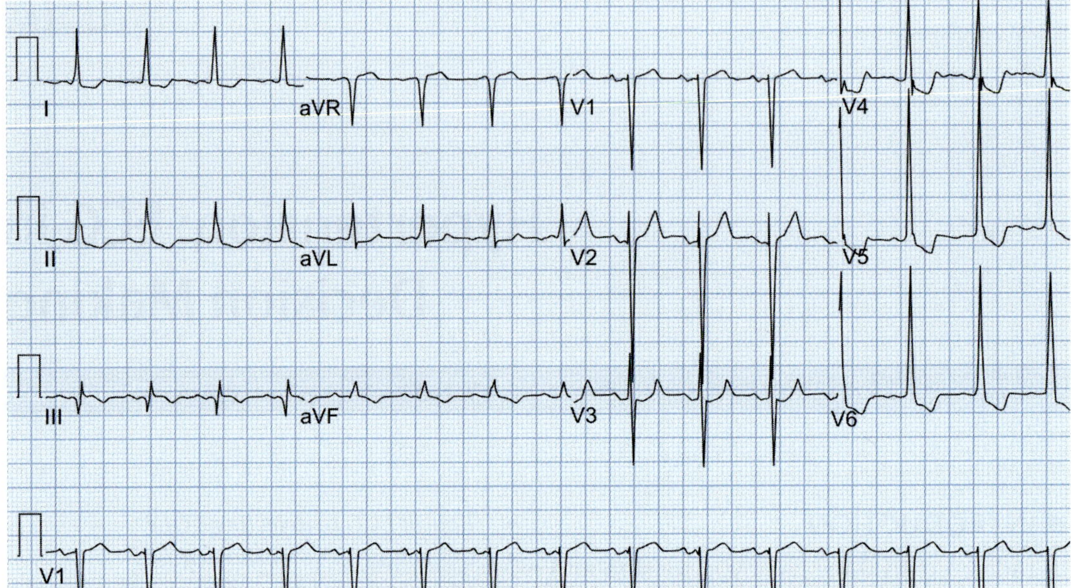

Fig. 1: ECG showing left ventricular hypertrophy: Voltage criteria and secondary ST-T changes.

LVH—Preferred Drugs

- Angiotensin receptor blockers (ARB)
- Angiotensin-converting enzyme (ACE) inhibitors
- Amlodipine
- Indapamide.

LVH—Drugs to be Avoided

- Hydralazine
- Alpha-blockers
- Other diuretics
- Older β-blockers.

Life study had demonstrated that in addition to BP lowering, regression of LVH would reduce clinical events.

Coronary Artery Diseases

Although LVH can produce secondary ST-T changes in hypertension, one should suspect associated CADs if the T-wave inversion is symmetrical with well-formed ST segment (Fig. 2).

CAD—Preferred Drugs

- Beta-blockers (except atenolol)
- ACE inhibitor (ramipril and perindopril)
- ARB (telmisartan)
- Aspirin and statin.

CAD—Drugs to be Avoided

- Short acting Ca antagonists (nifedipine)
- Hydralazine
- Alpha-blockers.

Left Ventricle Dysfunction

Although echo is a gold standard to diagnose left ventricular dysfunction (LVD), ECG as the first investigation gives clue regarding LV dysfunction (systolic and diastolic) (Fig. 3).

LVD—Preferred Drugs

- ACE inhibitor
- ARB (valsartan)
- Beta-blockers (carvedilol, bisoprolol, long-acting metoprolol)
- Aldosterone inhibitors.

LVD—Drugs to be Avoided

- Verapamil
- Diltiazem
- Propranolol
- Atenolol.

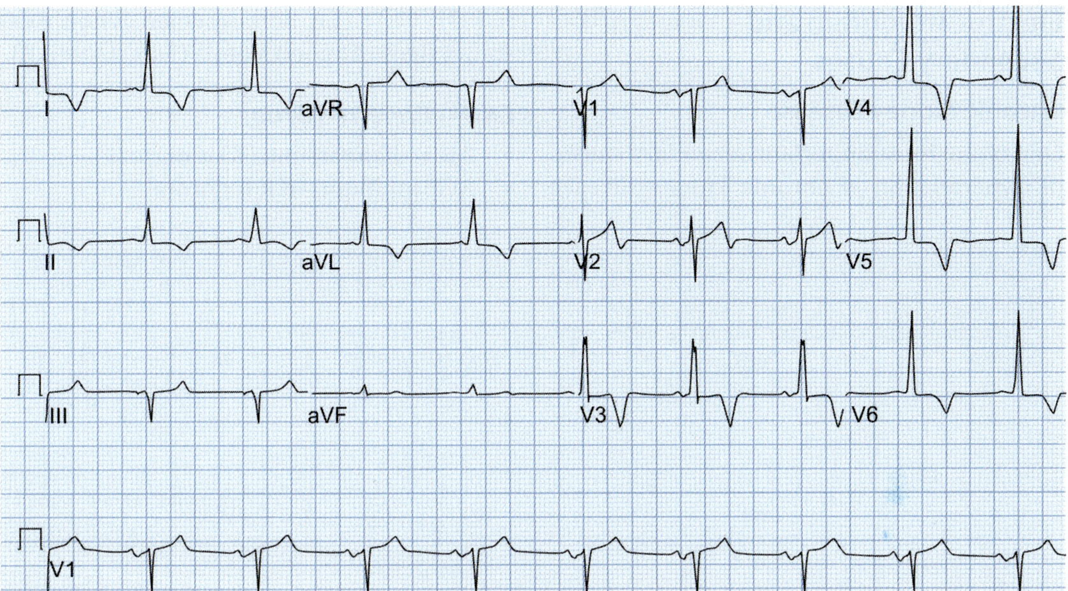

Fig. 2: ECG showing left ventricular hypertrophy and primary ST-T changes (Well-formed ST segment, symmetrical T inversion).

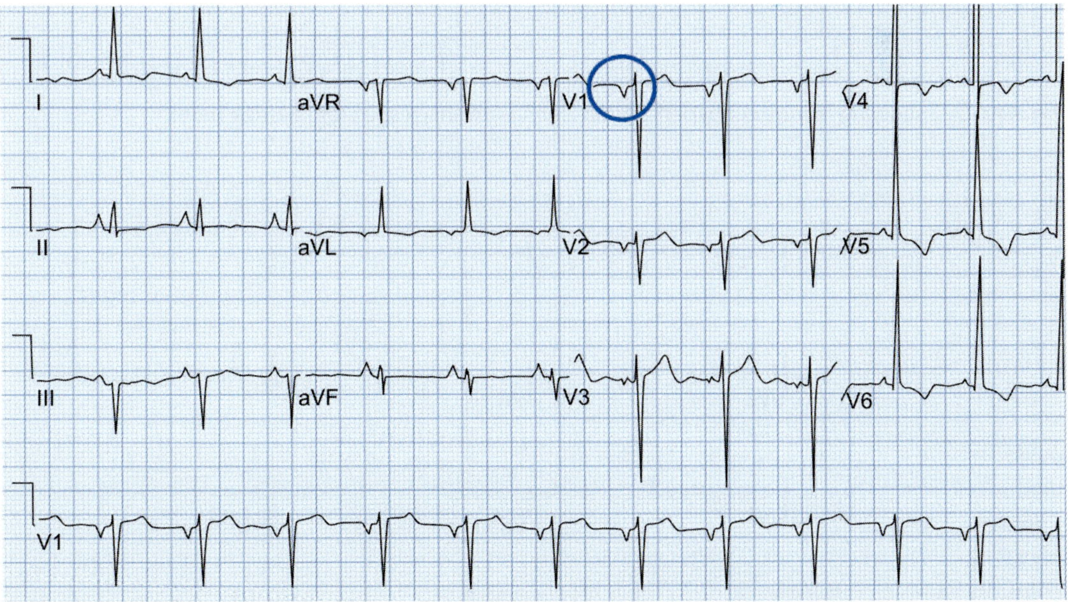

Fig. 3: ECG showing left ventricular hypertrophy as well as deep and wide negative component of P in V1 suggestive of left atrial abnormality—an indirect sign of left ventricular dysfunction.

Electrocardiogram and Secondary Causes

Chronic Kidney Disease

One of the most important secondary causes of hypertension is chronic kidney disease (CKD). CKD can be suspected when ECG shows signs of hyperkalemia (Figs. 4A and B).

CKD—Preferred Drugs

- ARB—if potassium (K) is normal
- ACE inhibitor—if K is normal

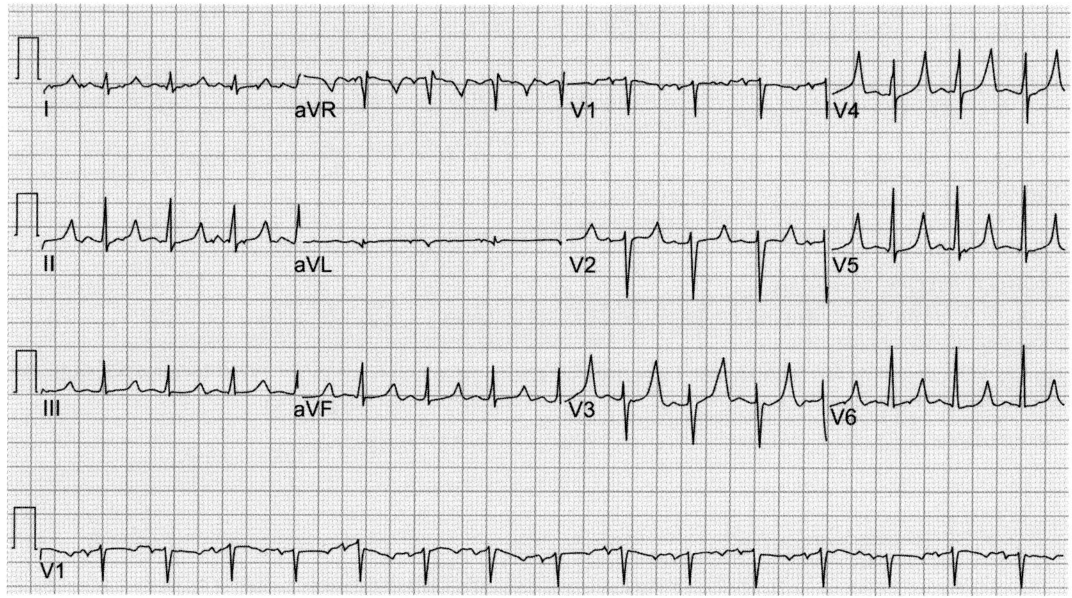

Fig. 4A: ECG showing features of hyperkalemia (Tall T with sharp apex and narrow base).

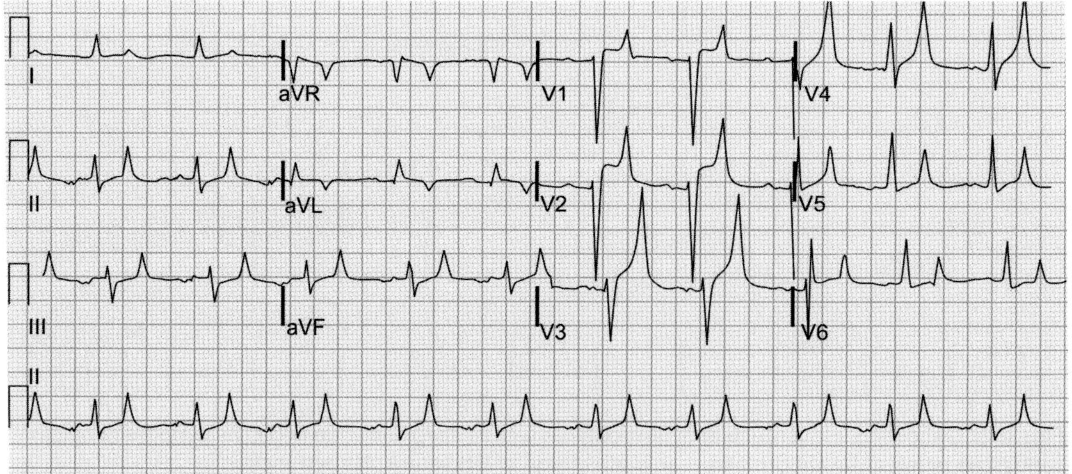

Fig. 4B: ECG showing features of hyperkalemia and hypocalcemia (Tall T due to hyperkalemia with prolonged ST segment due to hypocalcemia)—highly suggestive of chronic kidney disease.

- Amlodipine—if K is raised
- Alpha-blockers—if K is raised.

CKD—Drugs to be Avoided

- Atenolol
- Aldosterone inhibitors (hyperkalemia).

Serial ECGs in patient with CKD on angiotensin inhibitors will help to identify early hyperkalemia.

Hyperaldosteronism

Electrocardiogram changes of hypokalemia are a valuable clue regarding hyperaldosteronism (Fig. 5).

Hyperaldosteronism—Preferred

- Aldosterone inhibitors
- ACE inhibitor
- ARB
- Amlodipine.

Hyperaldosteronism—Not Preferred

- Loop diuretics
- Thiazide diuretics.

Hyperaldosteronism is frequently associated with resistant hypertension.

Cushing's Syndrome and Hypothyroidism

Both of these conditions produce low-voltage QRS in limb and chest leads. One usually expects high-voltage QRS in hypertension. Low-voltage QRS is defined as QRS voltage less than 5 mm in limb leads and 10 mm in chest leads (Fig. 6).

Hypothyroidism—Preferred Drugs

- ACE inhibitor
- ARB

Hypothyroidism—Drugs to be Avoided

- Beta-blockers (bradycardia)
- Calcium antagonists (edema).

Pheochromocytoma

When high BP is associated with unprovoked sinus tachycardia, one should suspect pheochromocytoma (Fig. 7).

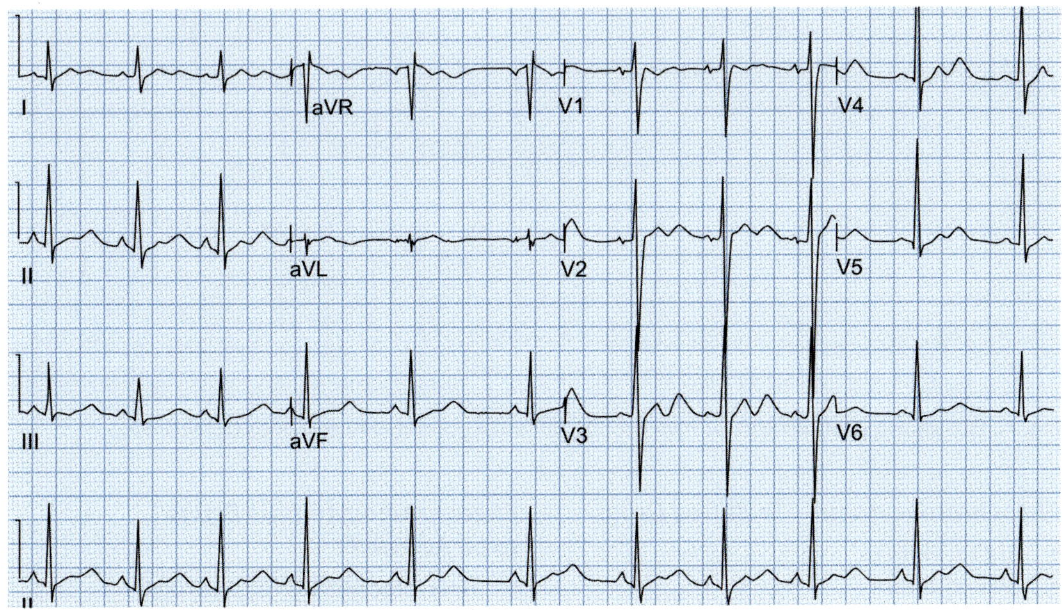

Fig. 5: ECG shows Hypokalemia (low-voltage T wave with prominent U wave).

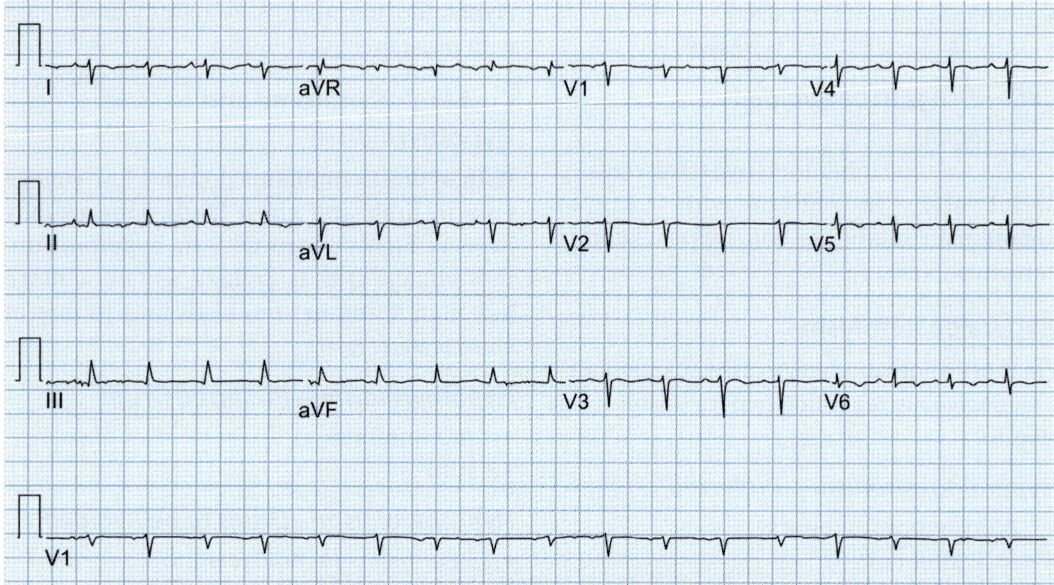

Fig. 6: ECG showing low-voltage QRS complexes in limb and chest leads.

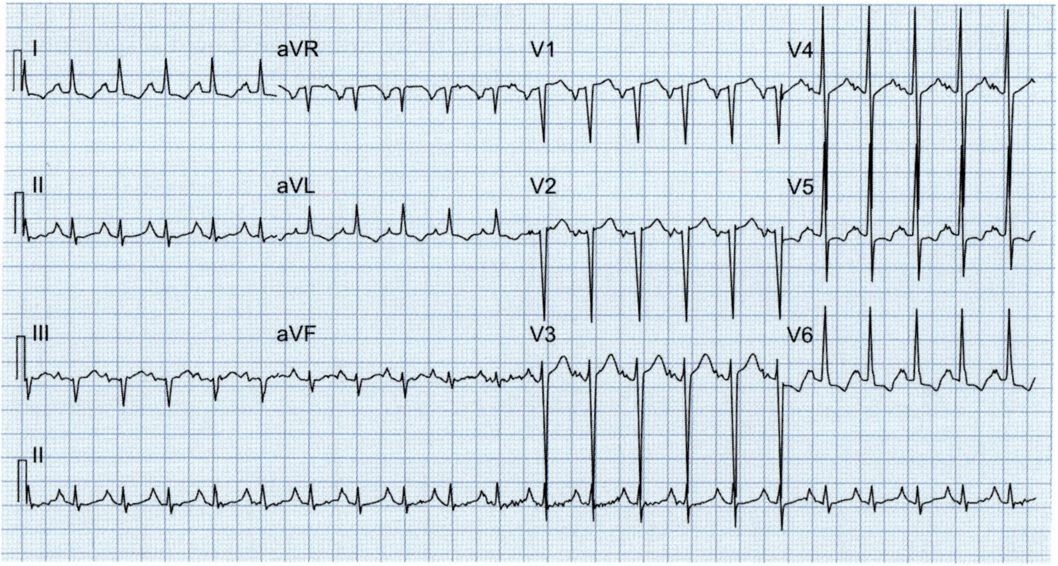

Fig. 7: ECG showing left ventricular hypertrophy, left atrial abnormality and sinus tachycardia.

Pheochromocytoma—Preferred Drugs

- Alpha-blocker
- ACE inhibitor
- ARB.

Pheochromocytoma—Drugs to be Avoided

- Beta-blockers (as initial drugs)
- Hydralazine (tachycardia)

- Short-acting calcium antagonists (nifedipine).

Electrocardiogram Signs of Comorbidities

Pulmonary Hypertension

Usually LVH is expected in systemic hypertension. If there is associated right ventricular hypertrophy (RVH) in ECG, one should suspect associated pulmonary hypertension (PHT) (Fig. 8).

Whenever RVH is present with LVH in hypertension, following conditions should be suspected:

- PHT
- LVD and PHT
- COPD and corpulmonale
- Sleep apnea (PHT).

PHT—Preferred Drugs

- Amlodipine
- Sildenafil
- Aldosterone antagonists (sleep Apnea).

PHT—Drugs to be Avoided

- Beta-blocker (except nebivolol)
- Loop diuretics (in the absence of cardiac failure).

Coronary Artery Disease: Acute Coronary Syndrome

When a patient with hypertension comes with acute coronary syndrome (ACS), ECG plays a crucial role in deciding the mode of management. If the ECG shows ST elevation of sub-epicardial injury, it is suggestive of acute total occlusion of a major epicardial coronary artery with red thrombus (rich in fibrin) and so primary percutaneous intervention or thrombolysis is the best mode of treatment (Fig. 9).

If the ECG shows ST depression, it means that it is a critical occlusion with white thrombus (rich in platelets) and so, the treatment of choice is heparin, dual antiplatelets and high dose statins and in high risk patients early interventional treatment. Thrombolysis is not useful and even harmful (Fig. 10).

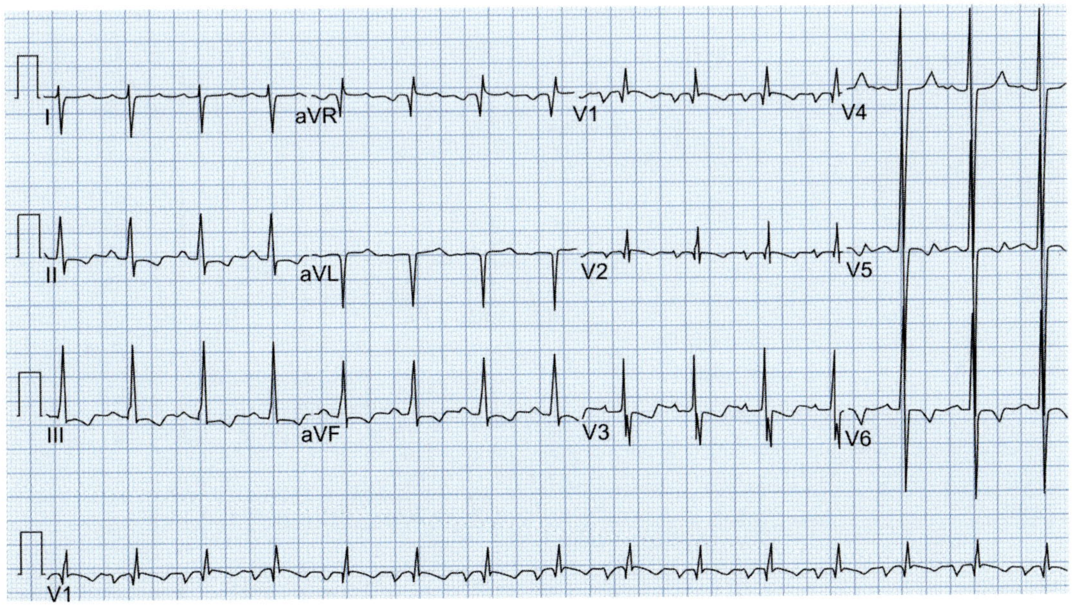

Fig. 8: ECG showing left ventricular hypertrophy and right ventricular hypertrophy (Tall R in V1 with right axis deviation).

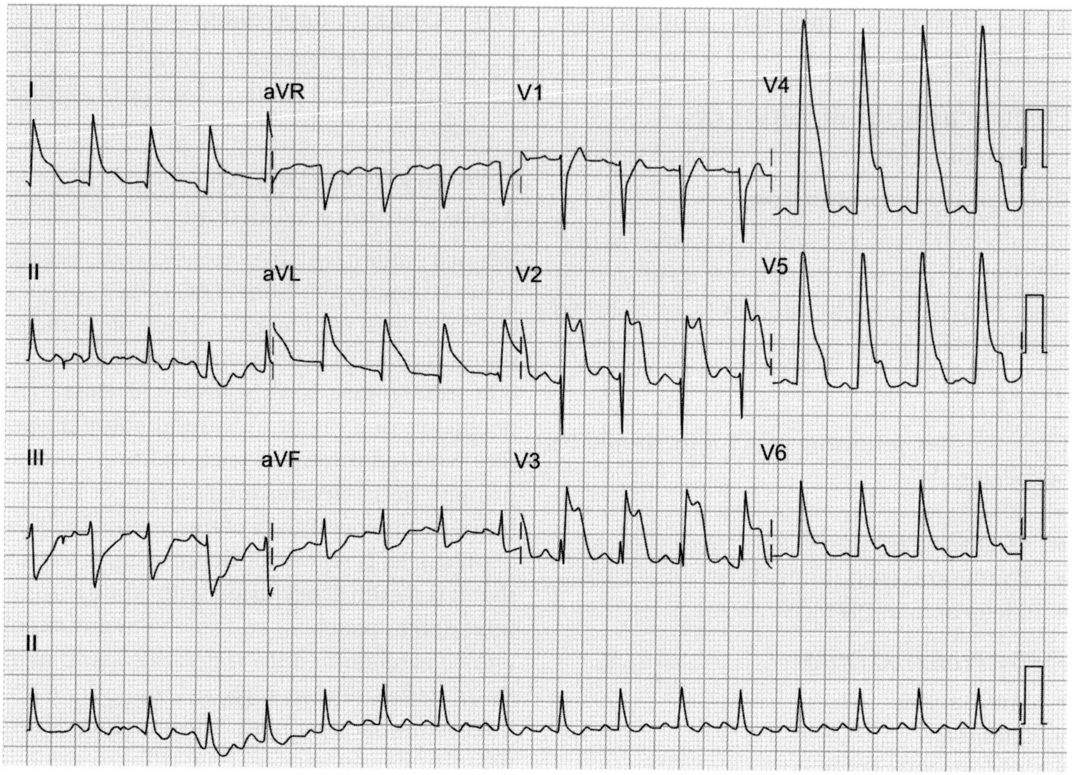

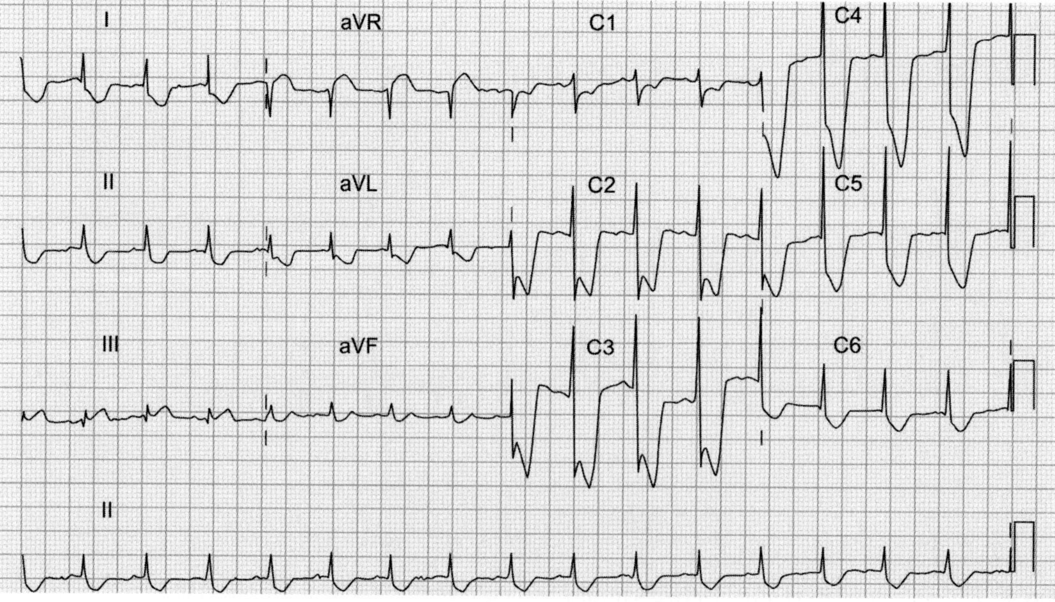

Fig. 9: ECG shows ST elevation (acute total occlusion, red thrombus)—needs primary PCI or thrombolysis.

Fig. 10: ECG showing ST depression (critical occlusion, white thrombus)—thrombolysis is not indicated.

Hypertension with ACS is hypertensive emergency.

Preferred Drugs

- IV β-blockers (metoprolol and esmolol)
- IV enalapril
- IV nitroglycerine.

Drugs to be Avoided

- IV nitroprusside
- Nicardipine.

Hypertension with ACS (Subacute Phase)

Preferred Drugs

- Beta-blockers (metoprolol and carvedilol)
- ACE inhibitors (ramipril and perindopril)
- Dual antiplatelets
- Statins.

Drugs to be Avoided

- Short-acting calcium antagonists
- Calcium antagonists as initial drugs
- Hydralazine
- Alpha-blockers.

Hypertension, Cerebrovascular Accident

When the patient has cerebrovascular accident (CVA), the ECG may show deep broad T inversion with prolonged QT. This has to be differentiated from CAD which shows deep symmetrical T inversion with normal or shortened QT (Fig. 11).

Hypertension with CVA is hypertensive emergency. Parental antihypertensive drugs are to be used depending upon the type of stroke, BP level at which drugs have to be started, target BP and the time frame to achieve the target BP.

Hypertension and CVA (Ischemic)

Preferred drugs—secondary prevention

- ACE inhibitors
- Indapamide
- Amlodipine.

Drugs to be avoided

- Beta-blockers (Brady)
- Alpha-blockers (as initial drugs) (Flowchart 1).

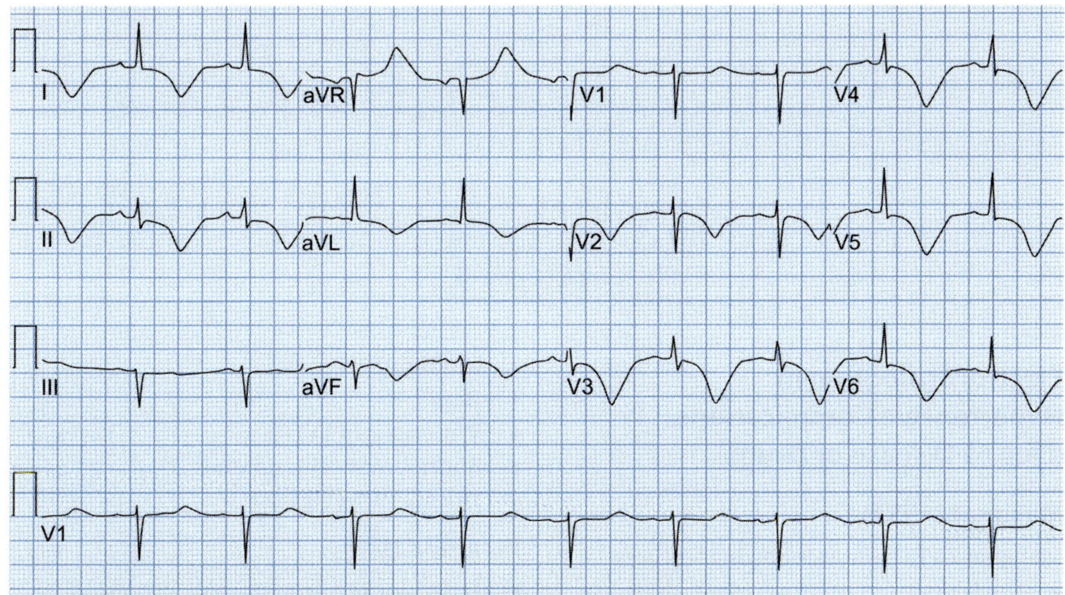

Fig. 11: The ECG shows deep broad T inversion with prolonged QT (CVA).

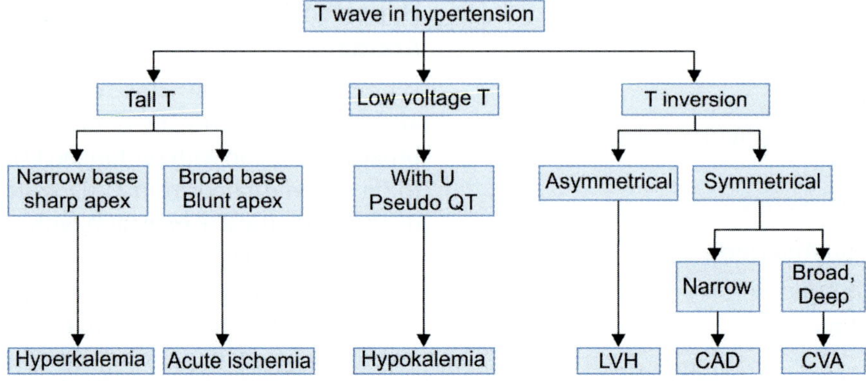

(LVH: left ventricular hypertrophy; CAD: coronary artery disease; CVA: cerebrovascular accident)

Flowchart 1: T-wave in hypertension.

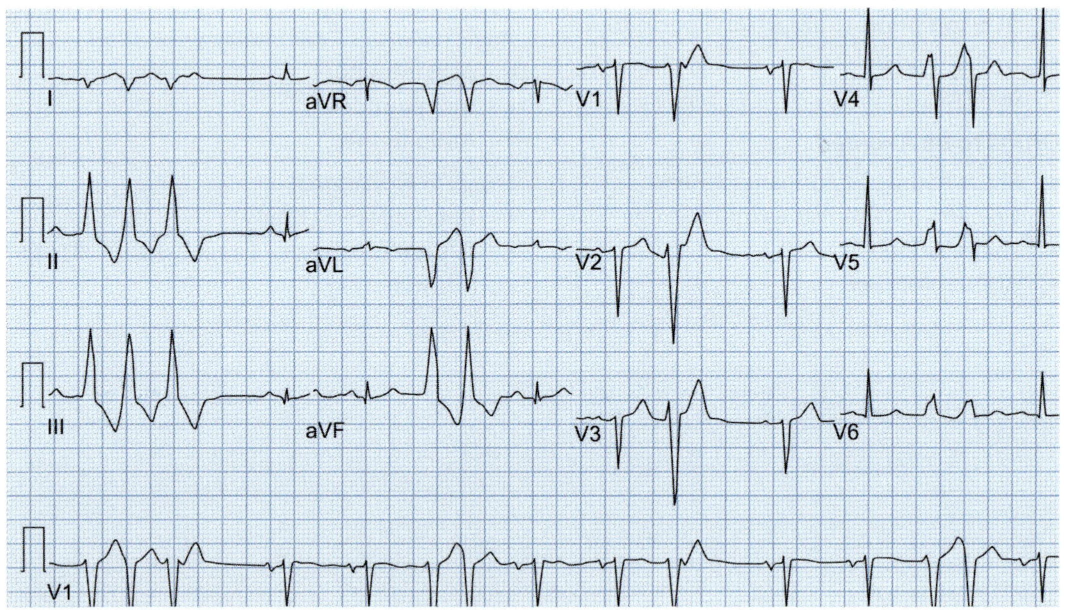

Fig. 12: The ECG showing malignant VPDs (Couplets + Runs).

Electrocardiogram in Hypertensive Complications (Due to Disease or Drugs)

Malignant VPDs

Malignant VPDs show following features:
- Couplets
- Runs
- Multiform
- R on T
- With signs of LVD
- Short, broad with notches
- During ACS (Fig. 12).

Preferred Drugs
- Beta-blockers (metoprolol, carvedilol)
- ACE inhibitor.

Drugs to be Avoided

- Calcium antagonists (nifedipine)
- Alpha-blockers
- Hydralazine
- Alpha-blockers.

Hypertension with Atrial Fibrillation

One of the most common causes of atrial fibrillation (AF) is hypertension. It worsens systolic and diastolic function and precipitates heart failure. It also complicates CAD. As the patient is prone for embolism, the anti-coagulants and their problems are added (Fig. 13).

Hypertension, AF, Fast Ventricular Response (>100/min)

Preferred Drugs

- Beta-blockers
- Verapamil or diltiazem (if LV function is normal)
- Oral anticoagulants.

Drugs to be Avoided (as Initial Drugs)

- Dihydropyridine calcium antagonists (nifedipine, amlodipine)
- Hydralazine
- Alpha-blockers.

Hypertension and Bradycardia

The bradycardia in hypertension may be due to sinus node or AV node (Figs. 14 to 16).

Preferred drugs

- ACE inhibitor
- ARB
- Amlodipine
- Alpha-blockers (add on).

Drugs to be avoided

- Beta-blockers
- Verapamil
- Diltiazem
- Clonidine
- Alpha methyldopa.

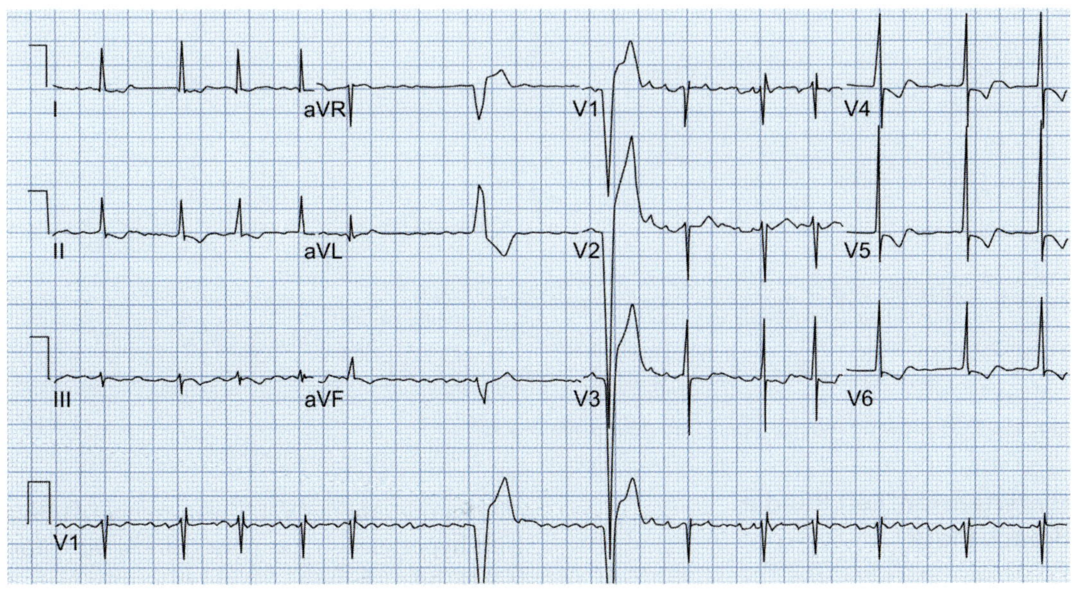

Fig. 13: ECG showing atrial fibrillation (absent P, irregular QRS, presence of fibrillary waves).

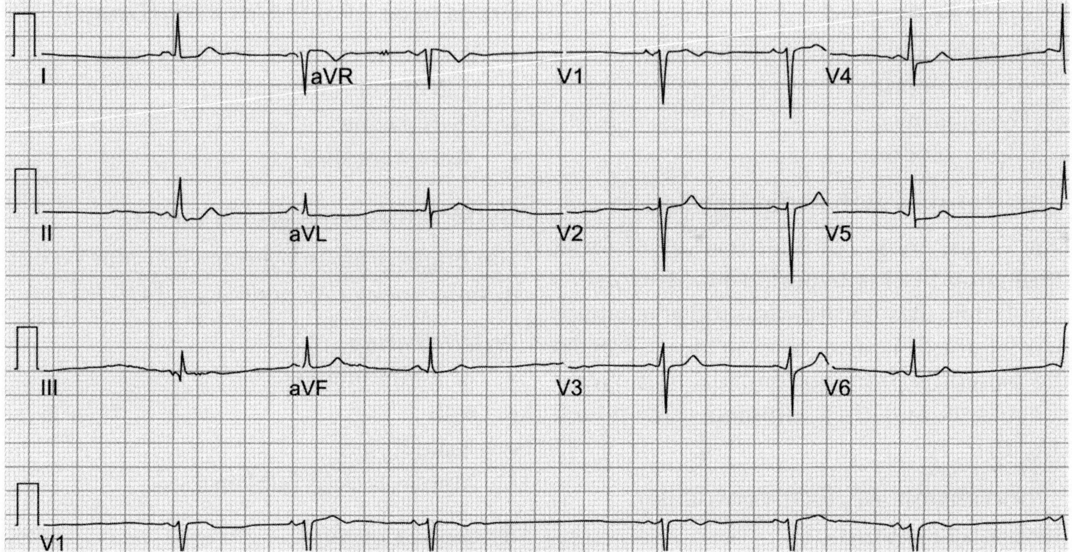

Fig. 14: ECG showing sinus bradycardia and sinus pauses.

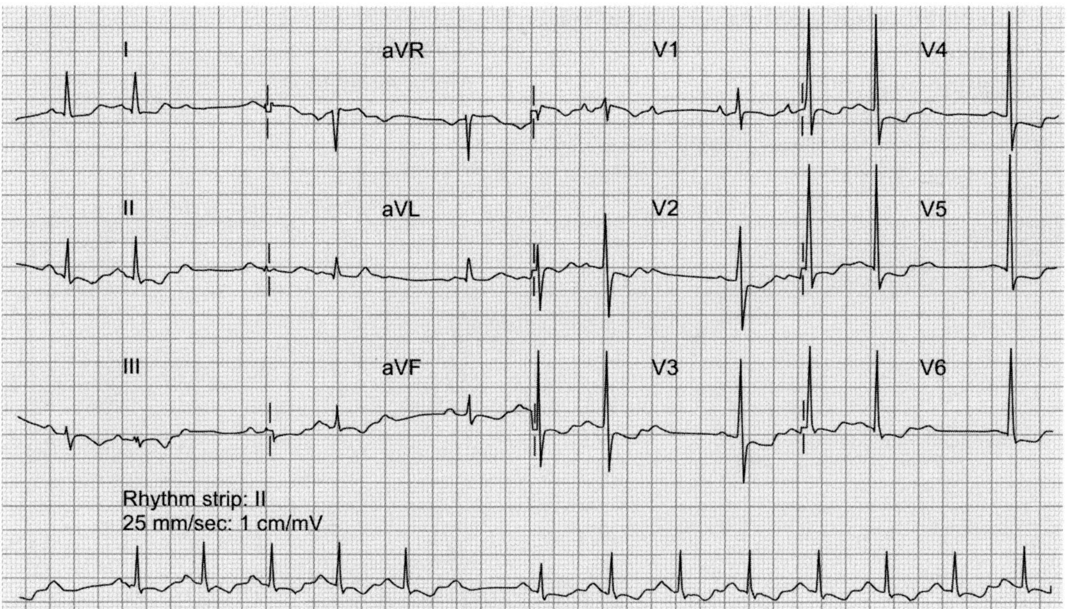

Fig. 15: ECG showing mobitz type II 2nd degree AV block.

Hypertension, Left Bundle Branch Block

Left ventricle hypertension is difficult to diagnose in the presence of left bundle branch block (LBBB). High-voltage LBBB may be a clue for underlying LVH. The presence of LBBB with hypertension has poor clinical outcome (CAD, heart failure). In elderly presence of LBBB indicates advanced and advancing disease (Fig. 17).

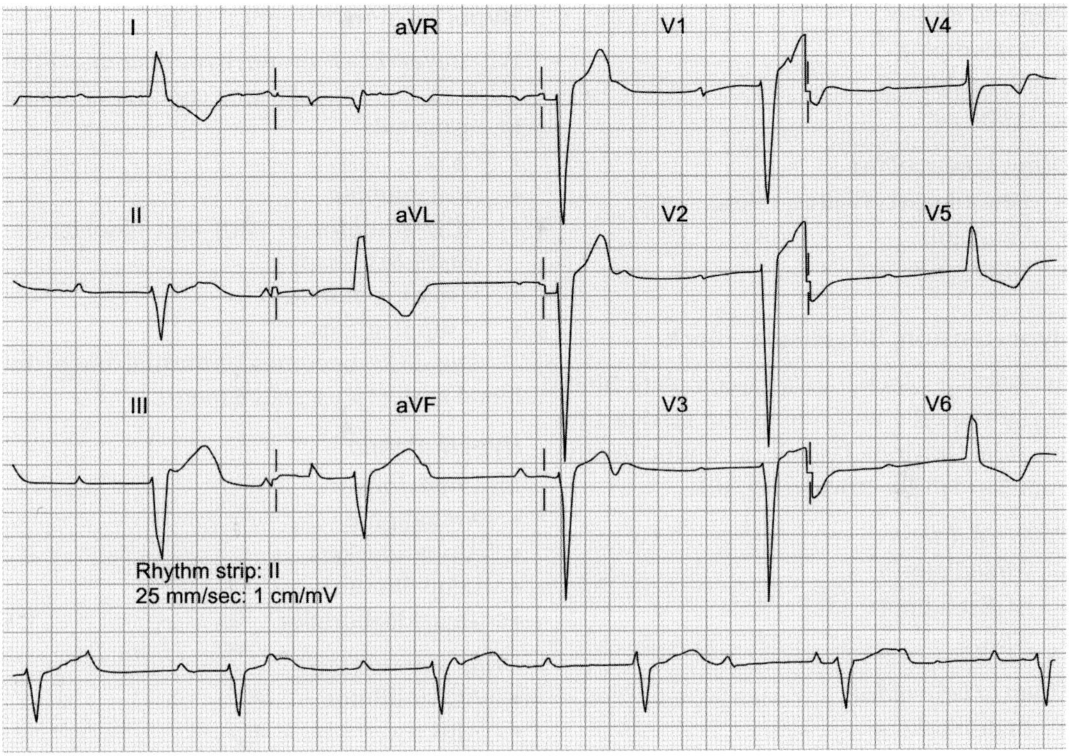

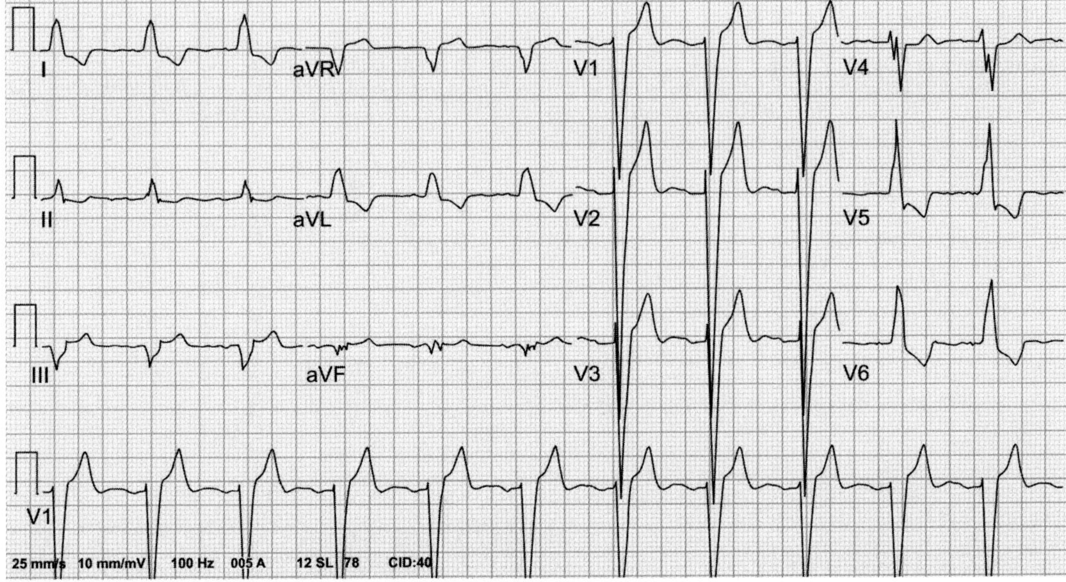

Fig. 16: ECG showing infra-His complete heart block.

Fig. 17: ECG shows high-voltage left bundle branch block.

Preferred drugs
- Amlodipine
- ACE inhibitor
- ARB.

Drugs to be avoided
- Beta-blockers (with caution)
- Verapamil
- Diltiazem.

Hypertension, Bifascicular Block

Bifascicular block indicates complete block of right bundle and one of the fascicles on left side. Only one fascicle is conducting the impulse to the ventricles (Fig. 18).

Preferred drugs
- Amlodipine
- ACE inhibitor
- ARB.

Drugs to be avoided
- Beta-blockers
- Verapamil
- Diltiazem.

Hypertension, Hyperkalemia

Whenever ECG shows hyperkalemia (Tall T-waves, Fig. 19), following conditions should be suspected:
- CKD
- ACE inhibitor
- ACE inhibitor or ARB and aldosterone inhibitor therapy
- K sparing diuretics
- K supplements.

The ECG becomes abnormal once the blood level of K exceeds 6 meq/L

Hyperkalemia

Preferred drugs
- Amlodipine
- Alpha-blockers
- Loop diuretics
- Thiazide diuretics.

Drugs to be avoided
- ACE inhibitor
- ARB
- Older β-blockers
- Aldosterone antagonists.

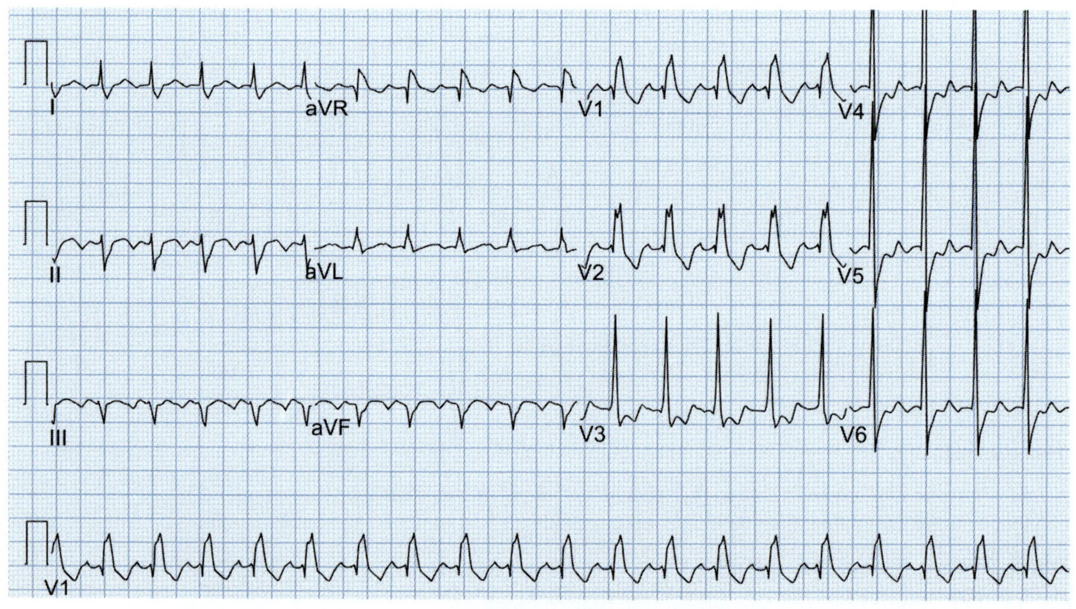

Fig. 18: ECG shows bifascicular blocks (right bundle branch block, LAFB).

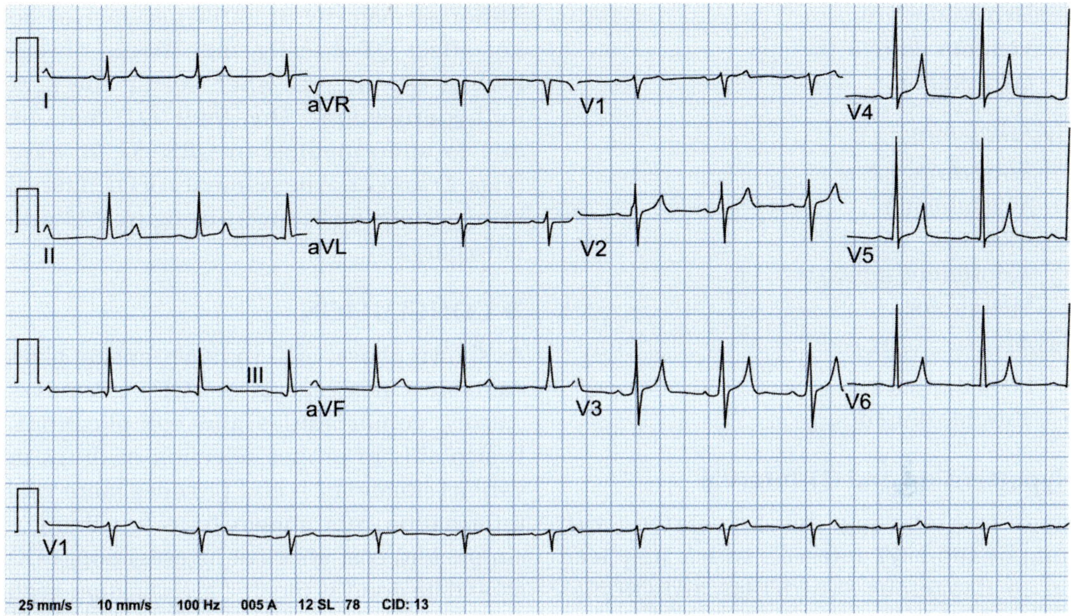

Fig. 19: ECG showing hyperkalemia (Tall T with sharp apex and narrow base).

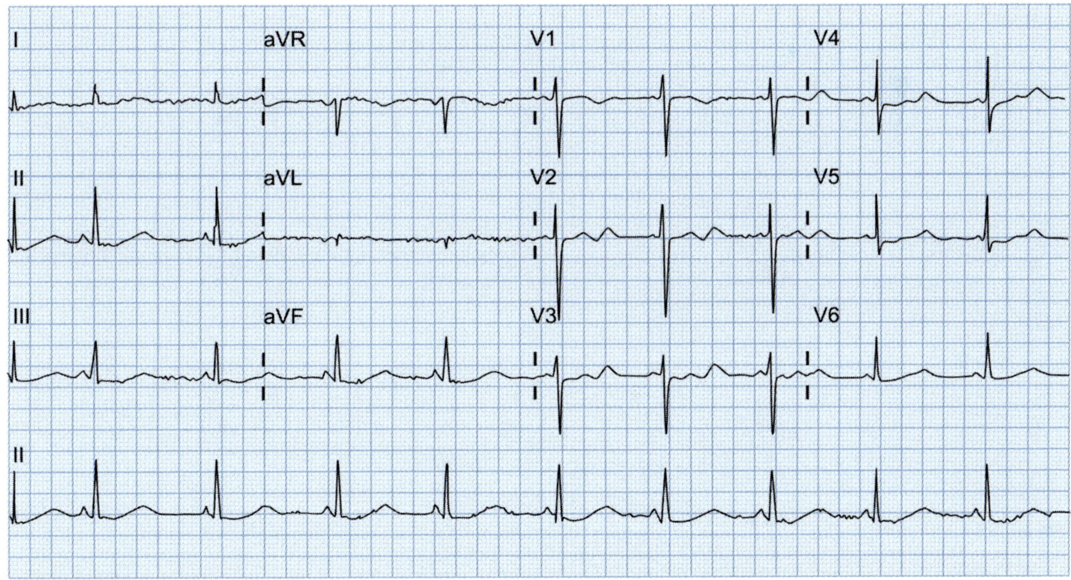

Fig. 20: ECG showing hypokalemia (low-voltage T with prominent U waves, pseudo QT prolongation).

Hypertension, Hypokalemia

ECG signs of hypokalemia happen when K level is below 2.7.

Whenever hypertension is associated with hypokalemia (Fig. 20) following situations should be suspected:

- Hyperaldosteronism
- Vigorous diuretic therapy
- Dehydration.

Hypokalemia:

Preferred drugs
- ACE inhibitor
- ARB
- Aldosterone inhibitors
- Metoprolol.

Drugs to be avoided
- Loop diuretics
- Thiazide diuretics.

Hypertension and QT Interval

Hypertension may be associated with long or short QT intervals which may lead on to dangerous ventricular arrhythmias like polymorphic ventricular tachycardia.

Although majority of antihypertensives do not affect QT directly, one should always look at QT interval when seeing the ECG in hypertension. The long QT may be due to abnormalities in QRS, ST or wave (Figs. 21 and 22). The summary of QT interval in hypertension is given in figures 23 and flowchart 2.

■ CONCLUSION

As shown above, ECG in hypertension gives valuable clues regarding TOD, secondary causes, comorbidities and complications. It also aids in proper selection of drugs in various situations. It also provides more vital information, not shown by echo. Being a simple and cost-effective investigation, ECG should be done as the first investigation in all hypertensive patients.

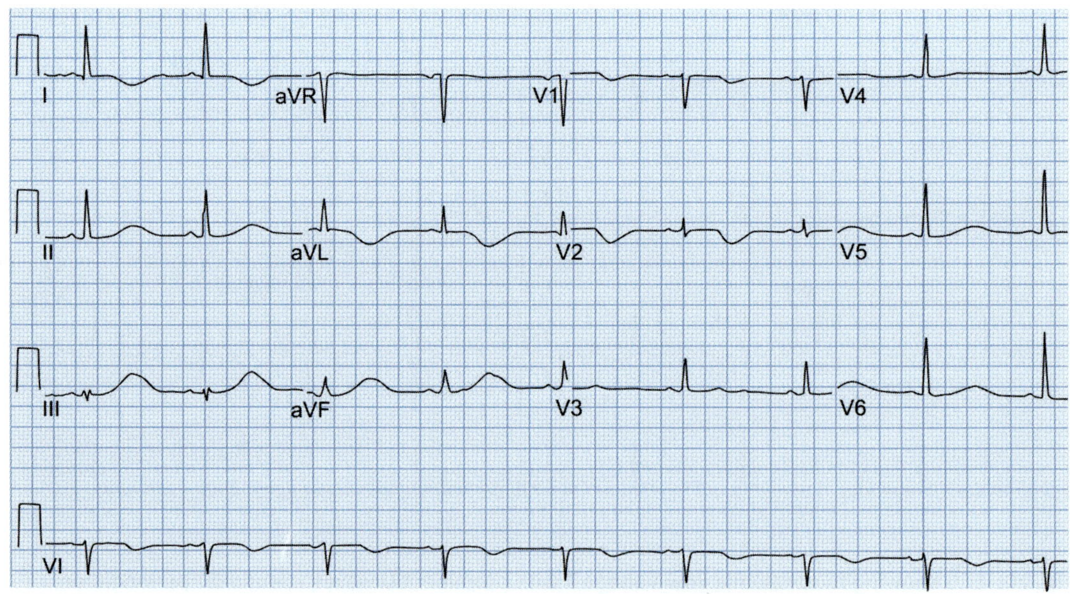

Fig. 21: ECG shows prolonged QT due to T wave.

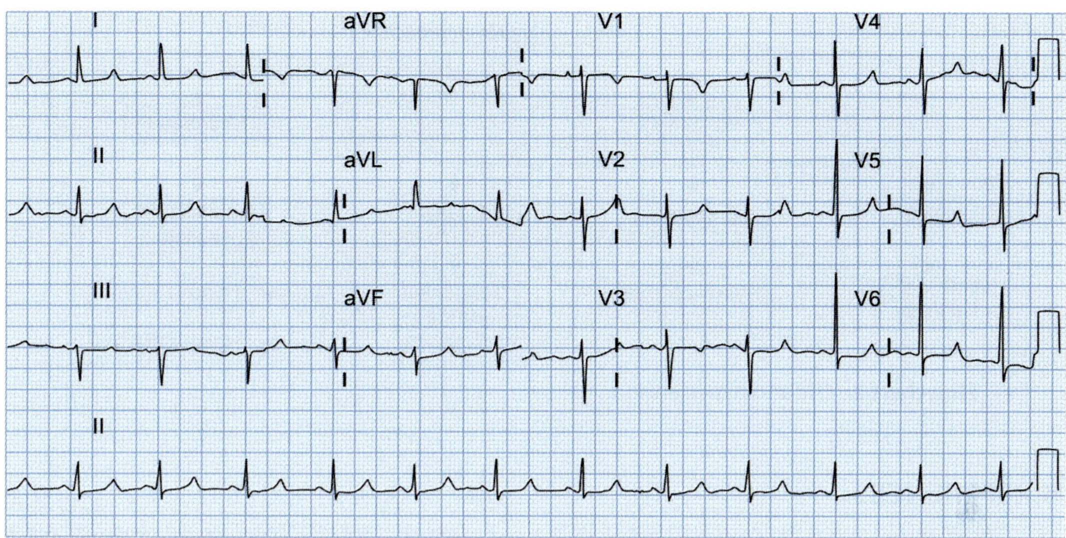

Fig. 22: ECG Shows prolonged QT due to ST segment. This ECG suggests CKD due to hypocalcemic and hyperkalemic (sharp apex T wave) changes.

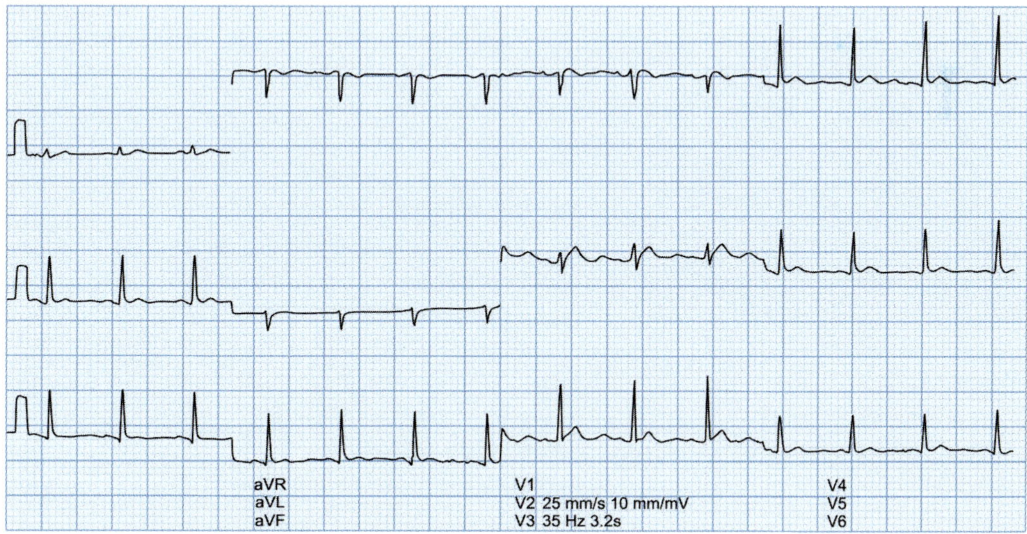

Fig. 23: ECG showing short QT (hypercalcemia/hyperparathyroidism).

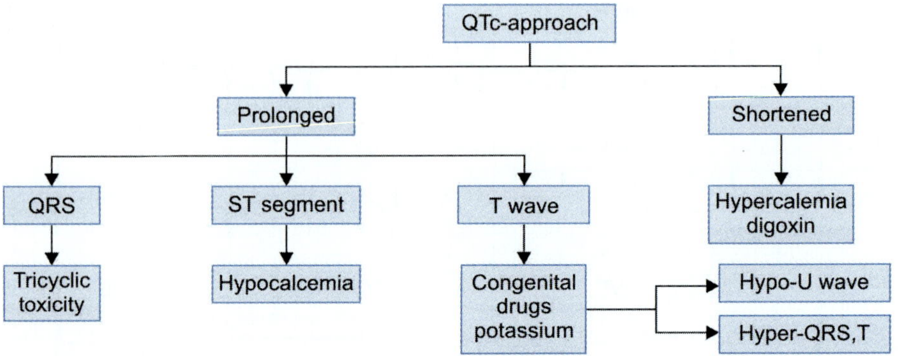

Flowchart 2: QTc and hypertension.

■ REFERENCES

1. Chenniappan M. Practical Cardiology. Echo Club of Trichy (ECG).

2. Opie LH, Gersh BJ. Drugs for the Heart, 8th edition. Saunders; 2013. pp. 1-592

Imaging Studies in Hypertension

Alpa Hemant Bharati

■ INTRODUCTION

Essential hypertension accounts for 95% of the cases of systemic hypertension. Most of these patients are asymptomatic and often identified on regular health check-up or may present with debilitating or life-threatening complications.

Almost 25% of urban and 10% rural Indian population is estimated to be suffering from hypertension across all strata of our society.[1] Many of the educated and affording patients are diagnosed with hypertension on routine health check-ups who can be effectively monitored for future complications. The lower socioeconomic and uneducated patients with poor access to basic health care facilities often present with complications that are often life threatening.

Imaging in systemic essential hypertension can thus be categorized as:
- In regular monitoring to look for and pre-empt future complications
- Imaging complications of hypertension.

Although role of imaging in both these categories is extensive, this chapter will focus on providing an overview of imaging in uncomplicated hypertension and will outline what can be expected in the results of imaging and how it can impact clinical decision making.

■ REGULAR MONITORING IN HYPERTENSION WITHOUT ANY COMPLICATION

A large number of patients who are asymptomatic for hypertension may present to the clinic for either routine health check-up or for an unrelated symptom and get diagnosed with essential hypertension. Based on their age, gender, coexisting morbidities, genetic susceptibility, and various other lifestyle factors they may be considered as high- or low-risk complications. The most life-threatening complications would invariably involve the vascular system which manifest as transient ischemic attack, stroke, coronary artery disease (CAD) with or without myocardial ischemia or infarction and aortic atherosclerotic disease leading to aneurysm or dissections.

Noninvasive imaging along with regular monitoring of blood pressure can play a vital role in avoiding or limiting the adverse prognosis of the complications of hypertension. In association with coexistent diabetes, the risk of the complications is further increased and therefore warrants judicious use of noninvasive imaging techniques to monitor disease progression which can go a long way in maintaining the quality and extent of life.

Noninvasive imaging other than 2D echocardiography would include:

- Ultrasonography (USG) and doppler imaging
- Computed tomography (CT) imaging
- Magnetic resonance imaging (MRI).

Ultrasonography and Doppler imaging

As a screening tool, USG of the neck and renal vessels can provide information about the earliest manifestation of atherosclerotic disease. It is a simple, reproducible surrogate marker of atherosclerosis and age-related vascular degeneration.[2-5]

Ultrasonography of the neck vessels can image the intima-media thickness (IMT) in a simple noninvasive radiation free method. IMT is an important marker for atherosclerosis and is related to subclinical atherosclerosis though it does not directly signify existing atherosclerotic disease. Increase in the carotid IMT has been identified as an independent risk marker for adverse cardiovascular events.[6-9]

As per the European Society of hypertension (ESH) guidelines 2013 score chart, hypertensive individuals with moderate risk should undergo assessment of IMT to look for target organ damage by screening of the carotids by USG. An IMT of >0.9 mm or presence of plaque signifies damage. Guidelines have been provided for the equipment and method of assessment of the IMT for carotid arteries.[10] Normal IMT values vary with age and sex, and show progressive increase in thickness over time.[11-13]

Table 1 shows the normal IMT values for right and left carotid arteries at 25th, 50th (median), and 75th percentiles.[10]

As per the recent ESH/European Society of Cardiology hypertension guidelines (2013) a carotid IMT >0.9 mm is considered indicative of a marker of asymptomatic organ

TABLE 1: Normal IMT values—median (P50), 25th and 75th percentile (P) IMT values for men and women at different age categories, separately for right (A) and left (B) CCA.[10]

Right (A)			
Age	P25	P50	P75
Men <30	0.39	0.43	0.48
Men 31–40	0.42	0.46	0.50
Men 41–50	0.46	0.50	0.57
Men >50	0.46	0.52	0.62
Women <30	0.39	0.40	0.43
Women 31–40	0.42	0.45	0.49
Women 41–50	0.44	0.48	0.53
Women >50	0.50	0.54	0.59
Left (B)			
Age	P25	P50	P75
Men <30	0.39	0.43	0.48
Men 31–40	0.42	0.46	0.50
Men 41–50	0.46	0.50	0.57
Men >50	0.46	0.52	0.62
Women <30	0.39	0.40	0.43
Women 31–40	0.42	0.45	0.49
Women 41–50	0.44	0.48	0.53
Women >50	0.50	0.54	0.59

(IMT: intima-media thickness)

damage, though the threshold for the same may be higher in middle-aged and elderly individuals. In this scenario, an IMT greater than the 75th percentile may be considered as indicative of increased cardiovascular risk as recommended by the American Society of Echography. Correspondingly, values between 25th and 75th percentile can be considered average and below 25th percentile may indicate low risk of cardiovascular disease.[10]

Measurement of IMT can be easily achieved and should be considered an important marker of subclinical atherosclerosis which can help in reclassifying patients with intermediate cardiovascular risk to low or high groups and thereby impact further clinical follow-up and management.

CT Imaging

The proven role of CT in uncomplicated hypertension is for identifying calcium in the CAD. Vascular calcification is a common feature of atherosclerosis secondary to inflammation and metabolic factors and not only secondary to aging.[14] Multi-center studies show definitive and predictable correlation between coronary artery calcium (CAC) and major adverse cardiovascular outcomes in asymptomatic individuals.[15] CAC can help in better risk assessment of asymptomatic individuals and help guide preventive therapies especially as CAC is cost effective testing in asymptomatic population.[16,17] Calcium scoring by noncontrast CT imaging shows that a calcium score of >400 has high correlation with risk of significant CAD. A calcium score of AJ >400 is considered significant and raises the risk status to high in patients who would otherwise be considered moderate cardiovascular risk patients. The CAC score further risk-stratifies subjects considered intermediate risk for CVD by Framingham risk score[18] and those with CAC >400 showed much higher risk compared to those with CAC = 0.[19]

Weber LA et al, mention that in the low-intermediate risk group, based on opinion of experts, a CAC of 300 Agatston units or 75th percentile (for age, sex and ethnicity), risk is suggested to be revised upward, thus lead to clinical decision in these cases to initiate statin treatment.[20] Risk prediction with CAC and guide to statin therapy (Table 2) has been proposed by Greenland et al.[14]

Computed tomography coronary angiography (CTCA) thus plays a role in identifying the otherwise moderate risk population of CAD into low risk or high risk thereby guiding treatment and follow-ups.

Routine screening CTCA is not recommended in asymptomatic patients to exclude CAD.

TABLE 2: Proposed decision-making approach to use coronary artery calcium for risk prediction.[14]

10-year risk for atherosclerotic CVD risk estimate	<5%	5%–7.5%	>7.5%–20%	>20%
Consulting ASCVD risk estimate alone	Statin not recommended	Consider for statin	Recommend statin	Recommend statin
Consulting ASCVD risk estimate + CAC				
If CAC score = 0	Statin not recommended	Statin not recommended	Statin not recommended	Recommend statin
If CAC >0	Statin not recommended	Consider for statin	Recommend statin	Recommend statin
Does CAC modify treatment plan	• No • CAC not effective for this population	• Yes • CAC can reclassify risk up or down	• Yes • CAC can reclassify risk up or down	• No • CAC not effective for this population

(ASCVD: atherosclerotic cardiovascular disease; CAC: coronary artery calcium; CVD: cardiovascular disease)

■ IMAGING COMPLICATIONS OF HYPERTENSION

Imaging of complications of hypertension is extensive and beyond the scope of this textbook. A brief outline of the routinely used and recommended modalities for commonly associated complications is listed in Table 3. Brief uses of CT and MRI in assessment of cardiovascular and neurological complications, respectively is provided below. CT and MRI play a role as first-line imaging modality in stroke and atypical chest pain, respectively.

CT Imaging

CT imaging in primary hypertension is mainly limited to complications of the disease. The common complications associated with hypertension that would require evaluation by cross-sectional imaging are listed in Table 3.

Coronary artery disease is a major complication of long-standing hypertension and is often associated with diabetes. Evaluation of CAD in cases with long-standing hypertension by CTCA has been proven effective in ruling out significant stenosis and guide further management in high-risk patients with atypical symptoms. The role of CTCA is predominantly to establish an absence of significant CAD in patients with atypical symptoms of CAD or inconclusive or doubtful stress test. CTCA has also shown to reduce the need for catheter angiograms and in improving patient selection for catheter angiography in emergency setting when patients present with atypical chest pain. In patients with severe chest pain, where clinical dilemma exists regarding CAD versus aneurysm or dissection, CT angiogram can conclusively identify the two diseases in a single study obtained on faster 128 slice scanners. In patients presenting with dissection, the coronary anatomy and CAD can be detected on the same imaging study which would prove useful in further intervention or surgical planning.

TABLE 3: Imaging modalities recommended in common complications associated with hypertension.

Neurology	
TIA	MRI brain + Angio
Stroke	MRI brain with carotid and brain angiogram
Carotid artery disease	Doppler USD/MRA
Cardiovascular	
Atypical chest pain	CT calcium score with CT angiogram
Suspected dissection/ aneurysm of aorta	• CT aortogram (first cross-sectional imaging) • Postprocedural follow-up–1st imaging CT aortogram, thereafter MRI for assessment of extent of size and leak if any
Renal	
Renal artery stenosis	• USG doppler • CT renal angiogram • Noncontrast MR angiogram especially in patients with renal dysfunction
Peripheral vascular disease	• Peripheral artery—USD doppler/MRA/CT • MRA not advised if excess calcifications

(CT: computed tomography; MRA: magnetic resonance angiography; MRI: magnetic resonance imaging; TIA: transient ischemic attack; USG: ultrasonography)

Atherosclerotic disease can be seen affecting the renal arteries which are very optimally visualized on CT compared to USG or MRI. USG doppler may be limited by overlying bowel shadows or shadowing from dense calcification or poor breath hold and obesity. These factors are not detrimental to CT quality and accurate assessment of the renal arteries on CT imaging can be obtained. CT can evaluate the renal arteries for the extent and nature of plaques as well as give quantitative information regarding the length of stenosis, distance from the ostium and poststenotic dilatation, if any. This information helps in planning intervention procedures.

One of the important advantages of CT over MRI is it is faster and can show plaque morphology. Plaques can be categorized on CT as soft, mixed or calcific. CT will provide comprehensive information regarding the plaque morphology, length, location from the ostium, and the distance from the first branch, all of which can be useful in guiding intervention procedures.

Magnetic Resonance Imaging

Magnetic resonance imaging in hypertension is predominantly limited to evaluation of the carotids and brain angiograms and in identifying ischemic versus hemorrhagic stroke.

Magnetic resonance angiogram of the neck and brain vessels gives comprehensive information with regards to extent of stenosis. Its advantage over CT imaging is that the study can be conducted without radiation and with no contrast. More detailed information can be deciphered regarding fresh or old areas of infarction or hemorrhage. Age of hemorrhage, infarction and the extent of cerebral edema are much better assessed on the MRI compared to CT imaging.

CONCLUSION

Imaging has a predominant role in hypertension keeping in mind the common complications and in assessment of complications when they occur. Hypertension being a systemic disease, regular non-invasive imaging can play an important role in preventive serious and debilitating consequences of hypertension such as stroke. Preventive screening by US doppler and calcium scoring by CT imaging can be considered important tools in identifying high-risk cases and preventing complications in these cases.

REFERENCES

1. Anchala R, Kannuri NK, Pant H, et al. Hypertension in India: a systematic review and meta-analysis of prevalence, awareness, and control of hypertension. J Hypertens. 2014;32(6):1170-7.
2. Tanaka H, Dinenno FA, Monahan KD, et al. Carotid artery wall hypertrophy with age is related to local systolic blood pressure in healthy men. Arterioscler Thromb Vasc Biol. 2001;21(1):82-7.
3. Schmidt-Trucksass A, Grathwohl D, Schmid A, et al. Structural, functional, and hemodynamic changes of the common carotid artery with age in male subjects. Arterioscler Thromb Vasc Biol. 1999;19(4):1091-7.
4. Bianchini E, Bozec E, Gemignani V, et al. Assessment of carotid stiffness and intima-media thickness from ultrasound data: comparison between two methods. J Ultrasound Med. 2010;29(8):1169-75.
5. Wright JT, Williamson JD, Whelton PK, et al; SPRINT Research Group. A randomized trial of intensive versus standard blood-pressure control. N Engl J Med. 2015;373(22):2103-16.
6. Tardif JC, Heinonen T, Orloff D, et al. Vascular biomarkers and surrogates in cardiovascular disease. Circulation. 2006;113(25):2936-42.
7. Lorenz MW, Markus HS, Bots ML, et al. Prediction of clinical cardiovascular events with carotid intima-media thickness: a systematic review and meta-analysis. Circulation. 2007;115(4):459-67.
8. de Groot E, van Leuven SI, Duivenvoorden R, et al. Measurement of carotid intima-media thickness to assess progression and regression of atherosclerosis. Nat Clin Pract Cardiovasc Med. 2008;5(5):280-8.

9. Sehestedt T, Jeppesen J, Hansen TW, et al. Risk prediction is improved by adding markers of subclinical organ damage to SCORE. Eur Heart J. 2010;31(7): 883-91.

10. Intima-media thickness: Appropriate evaluation and proper measurement, described. An article from the e-journal of the ESC Council for Cardiology Practice. E-Journal of Cardiology Practice. 2015;13(21).

11. Tosetto A, Prati P, Baracchini C, et al. Age-adjusted reference limits for carotid intima-media thickness as better indicator of vascular risk: population-based estimates from the VITA project. J Thromb Haemost. 2005;3(6):1224-30.

12. Lorenz MW, von Kegler S, Steinmetz H, et al. Carotid Intima-Media Thickening Indicates a Higher Vascular Risk Across a Wide Age Range. Prospective Data From the Carotid Atherosclerosis Progression Study (CAPS). Stroke. 2006;37(1):87-92.

13. Touboul PJ, Labreuche J, Vicaut E. Country-based reference values and impact of cardiovascular risk factors on carotid intima-media thickness in a French population: the 'Paroi Artérielle et Risque Cardio-Vasculaire' (PARC) Study. Cerebrovasc Dis. 2009;27(4):361-7.

14. Greenland P, Blaha MJ, Budoff MJ, et al. Coronary Calcium Score and Cardiovascular Risk. J Am Coll Cardiol. 2018; 72(4):434-47.

15. Agastston AS, Janowitz WR, Hildner FJ, et al. Quantification of coronary artery calcium using ultrafast computed tomography. J Am Coll Cardiol. 1990;15(4):827-32.

16. van Kempen BJ, Ferket BS, Steerberg EW et al. Comparing the cost-effectiveness of four novel risk markers for screening asymptomatic individual to prevent cardiovascular disease (CVD) in the US population. Int J Cardiol. 2016;203:422-31.

17. Hong JC, Blankstein R, Shaw LJ et al. Implications of coronary artery calcium testing for treatment decisions among statin candidates according to the ACC/AHA cholesterol management guidelines: a cost-effectiveness analysis. JACC Cardiovasc Imaging. 2017;10(8):938-52.

18. Greenland P, LaBree L, Azen SP et al. Coronary artery calcium score combined with Framingham score for risk prediction in asymptomatic individual (published correction appears in JAMA. 2004;231:563). JAMA. 2004;239: 210-15.

19. Arad Y, Goodman KJ, Roth M et al. Coronary calcification, coronary disease risk factors, Creactive protein, and atherosclerotic cardiovascular disease events: the St. Francis Heart Study. J Am Coll Cardio. 2005;4(1):158-65.

20. Weber LA, Cheezum MK, Reese JM, et al. Cardiovascular Imaging for the Primary Prevention of Atherosclerotic Cardiovascular Disease Events. *Curr Cardiovasc Imaging Rep.* 2015;8(9):36. doi:10.1007/s12410-015-9351-z.

Target Organ Damage: Evaluation and Clinical Importance

Hypertensive Retinopathy

Ashraya Nayaka TE, Jatinder Singh, Ramamurthy D

■ INTRODUCTION

Systemic arterial hypertension (SAH) is a major risk factor for cardiovascular disease, which is a leading cause of morbidity and mortality. The effects of arterial hypertension can be directly visualized in the fundus. These changes may manifest as three distinct and independent manifestations—(1) hypertensive retinopathy (HR); (2) hypertensive optic neuropathy; and (3) hypertensive choroidopathy.[1,2] Observation of these fundus changes may lead to a diagnosis of hypertension in a previously undiagnosed patient.

■ RISK FACTORS

Hypertension and HR are more prevalent among the Afro-Caribbean population than the European population. However, the relationship between the prevalence of retinopathy and hypertension is weaker among the Afro-Caribbean versus the European population.[1] The relationship is weakest for the Afro-Caribbean female population and strongest for the European female population.[3] HR is more prevalent among women than in men.[3]

Smoking is another risk factor, which is associated with hypertension and is often confounded by other socioeconomic and lifestyle -related factors.[4]

Individuals with hypertension who are carrying ε4 allele of the apolipoprotein E gene or are homozygous carriers of a point mutation (cytosine to thymidine substitution) in the gene encoding 5,10-methylenetetra-hydrofolate reductase (IT polymorphism) are at higher risk of HR.[5]

■ CLINICAL SYMPTOMS

Mild-to-moderate degrees of hypertension often result in asymptomatic fundus changes. Severe or malignant hypertension may produce fundus changes resulting in blurred or distorted vision. These fundus changes include central macular thickening or lipid deposition from retinal vascular or optic disc leakage. Serous macular detachment secondary to choroidal ischemia may also occur. In addition, transient obscuration of vision may result from hypertension-induced optic disc edema.

■ PATHOGENESIS

Pathogenesis of HR probably begins with failure of retinal vascular autoregulation, leading to endothelial cell alterations and breakdown of the blood-retinal barrier, resulting in leakage of fluid, blood and macromolecules into the retina. The damage caused to tissues by systemic hypertension follows a sequential pattern—the initial phase is vasoconstrictive, followed by the sclerotic and exudative phases.

Vasospasm and vasoconstriction, which are attempts to optimize blood flow, are the initial response to elevated luminal blood pressure (BP).[6] This phase known as the vasoconstrictive phase, is evident on retinal examination by the narrowing of retinal arteries. In the vasoconstriction phase, there is a vascular response to the increase in BP, i.e. made by the myogenic and metabolic mechanisms. This is because, apparently, the retinal arterioles do not present autonomic sympathetic innervation. This phase may evolve differently, if BP is controlled or not. If BP is controlled, vasoconstriction may disappear. Gradually, hypertension then causes endothelial damage and thickening of the intima, with further attenuation of the blood vessels leading to the intermediate phase called "sclerotic" phase. The resulting focal or diffuse arterial wall opacification produces the typical "copper wire" appearance. Arteriovenous nicking which is noted on retinal examination is caused by the pressure of thickened arteries over veins at their crossing junctions, where they share a common adventitial sheath.[7]

Further persistent hypertension then leads to the disruption of the blood-retinal barrier and leakage of plasma material into the retina. Fluid and blood aggregates in multiple layers of the retina, and are the pathognomonic of the "exudative phase". The extravasation of blood, intermingling the nerve fibers gives the appearance of hemorrhages in candle flame. Cotton wool spots appear as a result of noninfusion of nerve fibers. Nerve fiber layer infarcts , the "cotton wool spots" indicating ischemia, may be noted, along with microaneurysms and retinal hemorrhages.[8] Occasionally, optic nerve head edema (papillitis) and optic nerve head damage may also be seen in patients with malignant hypertension or in patients with prolonged systemic hypertension.

■ CLINICAL SIGNS

Arteriolar sclerosis, seen by increased arteriolar reflex, may acquire the appearance of copper wire and silver wire; the arterio-venular crossover; and the narrowing of the arteriolar caliber to varying degrees, retinal hemorrhage, hard exudate, cotton wool spots and papilledema are the classic signs of HR. Rectification and arteriolar tortuosity are added to these as signs of HR.[9] Retinal edema, arterial, and venous obstruction were also cited as signs of HR.[10] In the past, choroid impairment has been described as Siegrist's striae and Elschnig's spots. The lumen reflex, which is traditionally associated with atherosclerosis, is also sensitive to changes in BP,[11] requiring a reassessment in its interpretation and its usefulness for HR classification. Generalized retinal arteriolar narrowing was significantly associated with subsequent 5-year incidence of severe (grade 2 or 3) hypertension.[12] Ischemic optic neuro-pathy is considered by some authors[13-15] to be a form of presentation of HR. Special attention should be given to the care with which BP is reduced in patients with ischemic optic neuropathy, due to the possibility of permanent blindness.[14] Focal intraretinal periarteriolar transudation (focal intraretinal periarteriolar transudates—FIPTs) has been described more recently.[16] This finding is nothing more than retinal perivascular edema that could distort arteriolar narrowing.[17] Alterations in the retinal vascular bed, through analysis of the vascular diameter after its bifurcation, and changes in the angle of bifurcation between vessels have been investigated.[18] These changes were associated with the patient's age and, possibly, with SAH. These authors also questioned the relevance of these findings in the pathogenesis of vascular diseases and hypertension. Retinal hemorrhage and microaneurysms are relatively frequent lesions in the elderly and significantly related to the presence and severity of SAH.[19]

■ KEITH–WAGENER–BARKER CLASSIFICATION

In 1939, a study was presented[20] comparing the alterations of the vascular changes of the retina of 219 untreated hypertensive individuals, to biopsy of the pectoralis major muscle. This muscle was selected because it is the most representative muscle tissue in the human body and also because it is easily accessible. The vascular histological characteristics of this tissue were observed, comparing it to the alterations observed in the retina, which were classified into four groups (Table 1). From group I to group IV, when compared to the histological alterations of the pectoralis major muscle, a more intense vascular impairment was observed, with progressive reduction of

the lumen rate or thickness of the vessel wall, and also the presence of other histological alterations, such as—increase in the number and size of the muscle cells of the vessel wall; increased size of the nucleus in the intima of the arterioles; and thrombi, evidence of arteritis and periarteritis, indicated by the evidence of lymphocytes, and fibroblasts in the middle and adventitial layers of the vessel wall. With this classification, it was possible to observe the progression of HR, as well as to translate the vascular condition of other target organs of SAH, and also to associate them with the classification groups, the severity of SAH, and the patient's survival. It should be noted that the authors themselves suggest a cautious analysis of the findings of the muscle arterioles, since the alterations are not always consistent, and there is no definitive correlation between the division of the four groups with the findings of the muscular arterioles, the clinical severity of the SAH, and retinal arteriolar changes. For example, some patients in the group IV of the Keith–Wagener–Barker classification with characteristic retinal arteriolar alterations had only mild alterations in the muscular arterioles.

■ CLINICAL MANAGEMENT

The treatment of HR should be based on the "simplified classification",[8] which is shown in table 2. This evaluation allows clinicians to assess patients at risk for target organ damage based on the assessment of retinal microvascular changes.

Hypertensive patients with only mild retinopathy signs, according to established guidelines, will in all likelihood require only routine monitoring of BP. It is advisable for patients with moderate retinopathy to undergo further assessment for vascular risk, such as renal damage or left ventricular hypertrophy.

TABLE 1: Stages of hypertensive vascular changes (as described by Keith, Wagener and Barker).

Stages	Clinical features
Stage I	Constricted, tortuous arterioles
Stage II	Severe vascular constriction and Gunn's crossing sign. The column of venous blood is constricted by the sclerotic artery at an arteriovenous crossing
Stage III	Retinal hemorrhages, hard exudates, cotton-wool spots and retinal edema
Stage IV	Papilledema

Note: The WHO distinguishes between hypertensive retinopathy (stages I and II) and malignant hypertensive retinopathy (stages III and IV).

TABLE 2: Simplified classification and management of hypertensive retinopathy.

Retinopathy grade	Description	Treatment
Mild (Fig. 1)	All or any of these signs: Generalized arteriolar narrowing, focal arteriolar narrowing, arteriovenous nicking and silver-wiring of arteries	• Observation
Moderate (Fig. 2)	Mild retinopathy with all or any of these signs: Dot-blot or flame-shaped hemorrhages, hard exudates microaneurysms, cotton-wool spots	• Observation • Control of diabetes • Medical management of hypertension and other risk factors
Malignant (Fig. 3)	Moderate retinopathy signs along with disc edema and macular edema	• Immediate management of hypertension

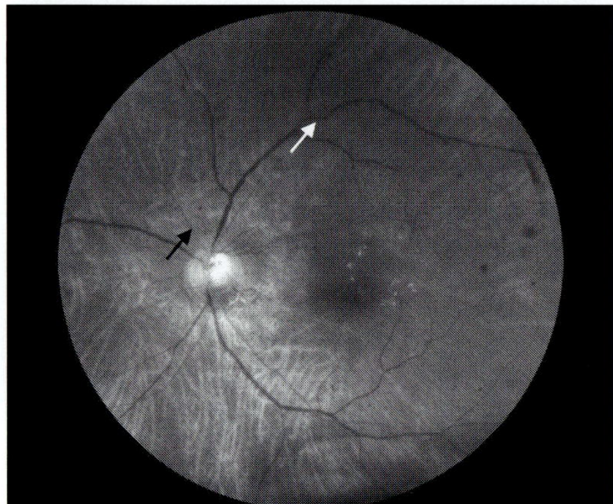

Fig. 1: Mild hypertensive retinopathy: generalized arteriolar attenuation (black arrow) with arteriovenous nicking (white arrow) *(For color version, see Plate 2)*.

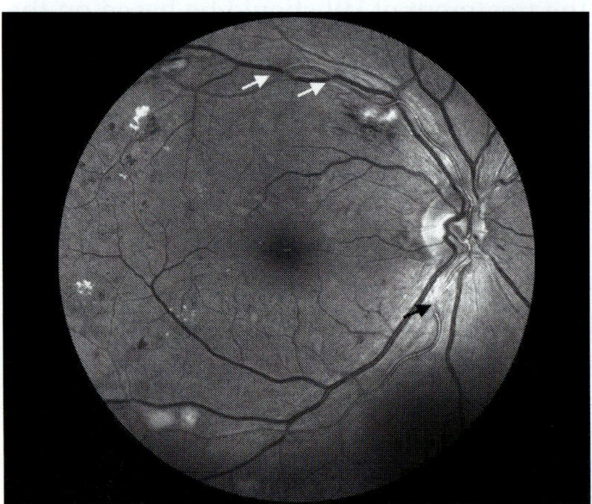

Fig. 2: Moderate hypertensive retinopathy: Arteriolar narrowing (white arrow) with arteriovenous nicking (black arrow) *(For color version, see Plate 2)*.

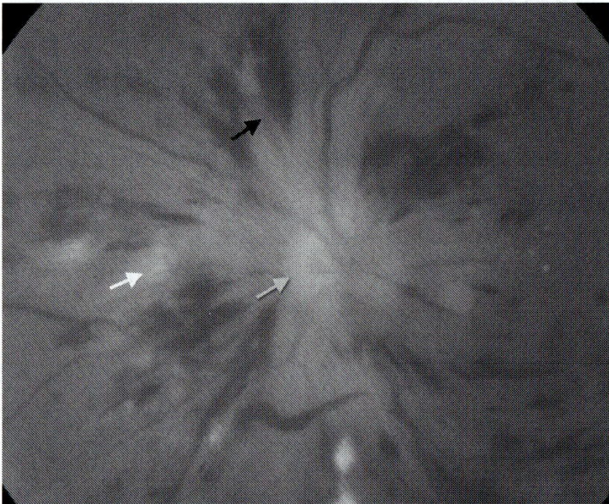

Fig. 3: Malignant retinopathy: Disc edema (yellow arrow) with cotton wool spots (white arrow) and flame shaped hemorrhage (black arrow) *(For color version, see Plate 2)*.

If clinically indicated, these patients can receive appropriate risk reduction therapy. Patients with malignant retinopathy will need urgent antihypertensive management.[8]

The primary treatment for HR is systemic arterial BP control. Control of BP with antihypertensive medication may reverse retinopathy signs, as has been noted in several case series[21,22] showing regression of hemorrhages and cotton-wool spots with control of hypertension.

Newer method of evaluation using computerized analysis color fundus images have shown a reduction in arteriolar attenuation and widening of arteriolar branch angle with control of hypertension.[23]

PROGNOSIS

The visual prognosis is excellent in mild-to-moderate cases of HR. When there is foveal edema and/or lipid deposition, a variable degree of permanent visual loss may occur due to structural changes in the retina and retinal pigment epithelium (RPE).

It is not clear whether different classes of antihypertensive medications produce different effects on retinal signs. A similar degree of regression of retinal vascular signs have been noted with angiotensin antagonists and calcium channel blockers.[23]

However, calcium channels blockers when compared to beta-blockers did show a better response in the remodeling of retinal microvasculature in a single study. This may be attributed to the vasodilatory action of calcium channel blockers.[24]

A fundal examination may also help in screening for patients with "white-coat/masked" hypertension. Masked hypertension which may be seen in 12–30% of elderly women,[25] represents an intermediate group between normotensives and sustained hypertensives, differing in organ damage and cardiovascular risk. The presence of retinal vascular changes in these patients in all likelihood would indicate the need for initiation of antihypertensive medication.[26]

When optic disc edema and macular edema are observed, as in patients with malignant hypertension, ocular treatments aimed at reducing vascular endothelial growth factor (VEGF) activity alongside the management of systemic hypertension are becoming more commonplace.

In eyes with macular edema due to malignant hypertension or vein occlusion, anti-VEGF agents reduce macular edema presumably by reducing vascular permeability. Though good visual outcomes in malignant hypertension have been noted in a few anecdotal reports, further research is necessary before these therapies may be considered the norm.[27-29]

CONCLUSION

The protocols for management of systemic hypertension should include comprehensive dilated retinal examination by an ophthalmologist in hypertensive patients aided by color fundus photography. Using "simplified classification" for management of HR in clinical practice can may enable clinicians to manage cardiovascular risks more effectively.

REFERENCES

1. Hayreh SS. Systemic arterial blood pressure and the eye. Duke–Elder Lecture. Eye (Lond). 1996;10:5-28.
2. Hayreh SS, Servais GE, Virdi PS, et al. Fundus lesions in malignant hypertension: III. Arterial blood pressure, biochemical and fundus changes. Ophthalmology. 1986;93:45-59.
3. Sharp PS, Chaturvedi N, Wormald R, et al. Hypertensive Retinopathy in Afro- Caribbeans and Europeans: Prevalence and Risk Factor Relationships. Hypertension. 1995;25:1322-5.
4. Poulter NR. Independent effects of smoking on risk of hypertension: small, if present. J Hypertens 2002;20:171-2.
5. Yilmaz H, Isbir T, Agachan B, et al. Is epsilon4 allele of apolipoprotein E associated with more severe end-organ damage in essential hypertension? Cell Biochem Funct. 2001;19:191-5.
6. Hsueh WA, Anderson PW. Hypertension, the endothelial cell, and the vascular complications of diabetes mellitus. Hypertension. 1992;20(2):253-63.
7. Ryan SJ. Retina, 4th edition. Philadelphia: Elsevier/Mosby; 2006.
8. Wong TY, Mitchell P. Hypertensive retinopathy. N Engl J Med. 2004;351(22):2310-7.
9. Gelfand M. Hypertensive retinopathy: a suggested modified classification. Cent Afr J Med. 1979;25:110-1.
10. Matas BR. The Optic fundus and hypertension. Med Clin North Am. 1997;61:547-64.
11. Brinchmann-Hansen O, Christensen CC, Myhre K. The response of the light reflex of retinal vessels to reduced blood pressure in hypertensive patients. Acta Ophthalmol. 1990;68:155-61.
12. Parr JC. Hypertensive generalized narrowing of retinal arteries. Trans Ophthalmol Soc NZ. 1974;26:55-60.
13. Ellenberger CJ. Ischemic optic neuropathy as a possible early complication of vascular hypertension. Am J Ophthalmol. 1979;88:1045-51.

14. Kishi S, Tso MO, Hayreh SS. Fundus lesions in malignant hypertension: II. A pathologic study of experimental hypertensive optic neuropathy. Arch Ophthalmol (Copenhagen). 1985;103:1198-206.

15. Hayreh SS, Servais GE, Virdi PS. Fundus lesion in malignant hypertension: V. Hypertensive optic neuropathy. Ophthalmology. 1986;93:74-87.

16. Hayreh SS, Servais GE, Virdi PS. Fundus lesions in malignant hypertension: IV. Focal intraretinal periarteriolar transudates. Ophthalmology. 1986;92:60-73.

17. Hayreh SS, Servais GE, Virdi PS. Retinal arteriolar changes in malignant arterial hypertension. Ophthalmologica. 1989;198:178-96.

18. Stanton AV, Wasan B, Cerutti A, et al. Vascular network changes in the retina with age and hypertension. J Hypertens. 1995;13:1724-8.

19. Yu T, Mitchell P, Berry G, et al. Retinopathy in older persons without diabetes and its relationship to hypertension. Arch Ophthalmol. 1998;116:83-9.

20. Keith NM, Wagener HP, Barker NW. Some different types of essential hypertension: their course and prognosis. Am J Med Sci. 1939;197:332-43.

21. Bock KD. Regression of retinal vascular changes by antihypertensive therapy. Hypertension. 1984;6(Pt 2):158-62.

22. Dahlof B, Stenkula S, Hansson L. Hypertensive retinal vascular changes: relationship to left ventricular hypertrophy and arteriolar changes before and after treatment. Blood Press. 1992;1:35-44.

23. Hughes AD, Stanton AV, Jabbar AS, et al. Effect of antihypertensive treatment on retinal microvascular changes in hypertension. J Hypertens. 2008;26:1703-7.

24. Thom S, Stettler C, Stanton A, et al. Differential effects of antihypertensive treatment on the retinal microcirculation. An Anglo-Scandinavian Cardiac Outcomes Trial substudy. Hypertension. 2009;54:405-8.

25. Karter Y, Curgunlu A, Altinisik S, et al. Target organ damage and changes in arterial compliance in white coat hypertension. Is white coat innocent? Blood Press. 2003;12:307-13.

26. Grosso A, Veglio F, Porta M, et al. Hypertensive retinopathy revisited: some answers, more questions. Br J Ophthalmol. 2005;89:1646-54.

27. Zucchiatti I, Iacono P, Battaglia PM, et al. Intravitreal bevacizumab in a patient with a macular star in malignant hypertension. Eur J Ophthalmol. 2011;21:336-9.

28. Kim EY, Lew HM, Song JH. Effect of intravitreal bevacizumab (Avastin®)) therapy in malignant hypertensive retinopathy: a report of two cases. J Ocul Pharmacol Ther. 2012;28:318-22.

29. Salman AG. Intravitreal bevacizumab in persistent retinopathy secondary to malignant hypertension. Saudi J Ophthalmol. 2013;27:25-9.

SECTION 8

Special Conditions and Situations

Hypertensive Crises

Pritam Gupta, Sunita Aggarwal, Gayathri Ranie AP

INTRODUCTION

Systemic hypertension is the most common chronic medical disorder affecting over 1 billion people worldwide.[1] Among the hypertensive population, it is estimated that about 1–2% of patients ultimately develop hypertensive crisis. There is an urgent need to lower the elevated blood pressure (BP) in these patients to prevent the target organ damage and complications. If left untreated, these hypertensive emergencies have 1-year mortality incidence more than 79% with median survival of 10.4 months.[1]

DEFINITION

Hypertensive crisis is defined as the elevation of systolic BP more than 180 mm Hg or diastolic BP more than 110 mm Hg.[2] Hypertensive crises can be divided further into hypertensive emergencies or hypertensive urgencies.

Hypertensive emergency is characterized by an acute severe elevation of systolic BP more than 180 mm Hg and/or diastolic BP 110 mm Hg associated with the presence of target organ damage.[2]

Hypertensive urgencies are characterized by a similar acute elevation in BP, but are not associated with target organ dysfunction.[2]

Target organ damage can be defined as the acute damage resulting in dysfunction of the eyes, the brain, the heart or the kidneys. The differentiation is useful in clinical practice, as hypertensive emergencies require an immediate BP reduction to prevent irreversible organ damage whereas in hypertensive urgencies, the BP should be reduced within 24–48 hours.[2,3]

EPIDEMIOLOGY

High BP is a major public health problem in India with rapid increase in prevalence among both urban and rural populations. The prevalence of hypertension ranges from 20% to 40% in urban and 12% to 17% among rural area.[4] There is low awareness, treatment and control status of hypertension in India, more among the rural than in urban populations.[4,5] The episodes of hypertensive crisis is seen in 1–2% patients of diagnosed hypertension.[1] Most patients with a hypertensive crisis have previously been diagnosed as hypertensive with inadequate BP control. There is a great need to increase awareness of hypertension in general population to avoid complications related to it.

■ PATHOPHYSIOLOGY

Autoregulation is the ability of organs to maintain a stable blood flow over a wide range of perfusion pressure.[6] It is postulated that a failure in the adaptive autoregulatory mechanisms in the vasculature could be a contributory factor in the pathogenesis of hypertensive emergency and the consequent end-organ damage. As a result of the failure of autoregulation, there is an increase in vascular resistance leading to mechanical stress and endothelial injury.[6] Also, there is activation of the renin–angiotensin system, which causes vasoconstriction and further ischemic insult.[7] The endothelial injury and platelet activation are believed to give rise to a prothrombotic state.[8] Differences in the amount of cardiac output received, total oxygen consumption and autoregulatory capacity explain the differences in the prevalence of individual organ dysfunction.[7]

The flowchart 1 shows pathophysiology of hypertensive emergency.

■ CLINICAL MANIFESTATIONS OF HYPERTENSIVE EMERGENCY

The clinical manifestations of hypertensive crises are related to end-organ dysfunction. Various organs involved are brain, heart, kidney, liver, eye, etc. Cerebral infarction and acute pulmonary edema are the most common clinical manifestation in clinical practice (Table 1).

The symptoms and signs of hypertensive crises vary from patient to patient.

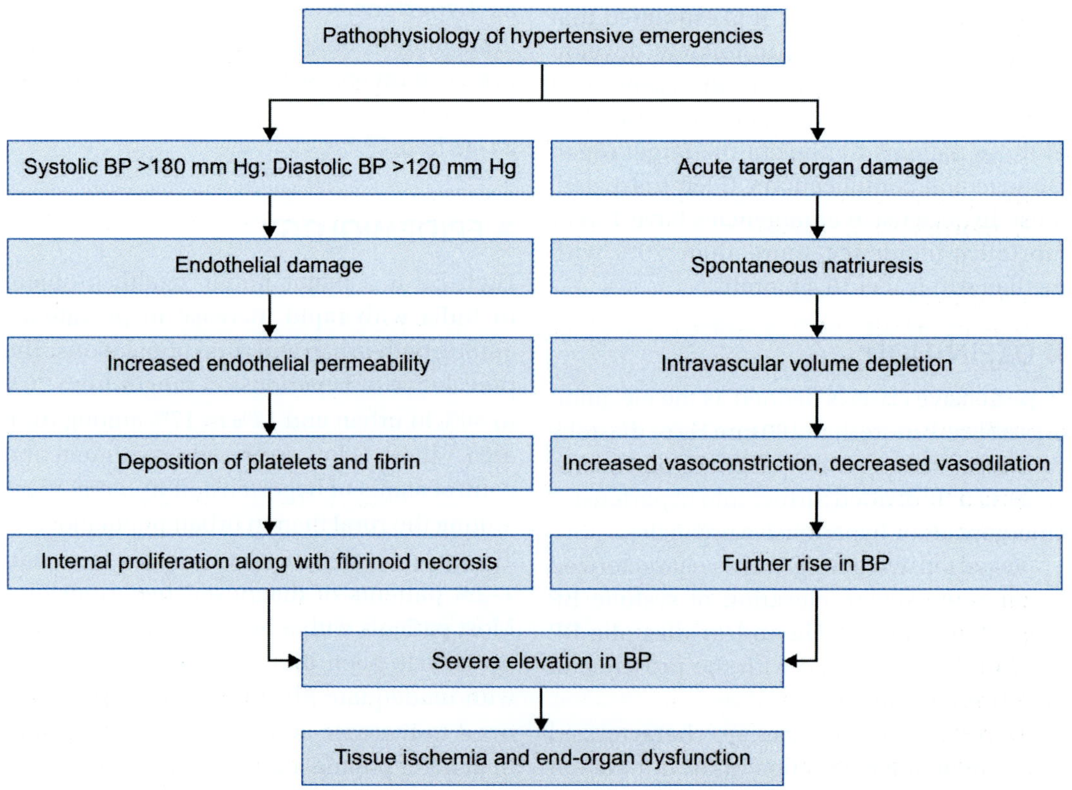

Flowchart 1: Pathophysiology of hypertensive emergency.

TABLE 1: Target organ involvement and their presentation with their prevalence.[9]

Neurologic	Cerebral infarction (24.5 %)
	Hypertensive encephalopathy (16.3%)
	ICH or SAH (4.5%)
Cardio-vascular	Acute pulmonary edema (22.5%)
	Acute coronary ischemia (12%)
Renal	Acute kidney injury/failure (<10%)
Liver	Liver enzyme elevation (HELLP syndrome) (0.1–0.8%)
Eye	Retinal hemorrhage (0.01–0.02%)
Vascular	Eclampsia (4.5%)
	Aortic dissection (2%)

(HELLP: hemolysis, elevated liver enzymes, and low platelet count; ICH: intracerebral hemorrhage; SAH: subarachnoid hemorrhage)

- *Central nervous system:* Headache, altered level of consciousness and/or focal neurologic signs are seen in patients with hypertensive encephalopathy and cerebral infarction or hemorrhage[9]
- *Eye:* Retinopathy with arteriolar changes, hemorrhages, detachment and exudates as well as papilledema
- *Cardiovascular manifestations:* Hypertensive crises may present with angina, acute myocardial infarction or acute left ventricular failure[10]
- *Kidney:* Severe injury to the kidneys may lead to acute renal failure with oliguria and/or hematuria
- *Aortic dissection*: This should be considered in patients presenting to the emergency department with acute chest pain and elevated BP. If left untreated, about three-quarters of patients with type A dissection die within 2 weeks of an acute episode, but with successful initial therapy the 5-year survival rate increases to 75%.[10]

Hence, timely recognition of this entity coupled with urgent and appropriate management is mandatory[9,11]

- *Pregnancy*: In pregnant patients, the acute elevations in BP may range from a mild to a life-threatening disease process. The clinical features vary, but may include visual field defects, severe headaches, seizures, altered mental status, acute cerebrovascular accidents, severe right upper quadrant abdominal pain, congestive heart failure and oliguria.[9]

■ DIAGNOSIS

In patients with sudden uncontrolled hypertension, a detailed clinical history along with thorough diagnostic evaluation is required.

History

- The duration of hypertension
- Compliance to antihypertensives drugs
- Evidence of uncontrolled BP recordings in the past
- Concomitant administration of other drugs which might increase BP (e.g. monoamine oxidase inhibitors) or drug abuse (cocaine and amphetamines)[10]
- History suggestive of sleep apnea syndrome[10]
- Evaluation of cardiovascular risk factors and other comorbidities.

Physical Examination[10]

- Vital signs, including oxygen saturation and pulse rate
- Auscultation of heart sounds/murmurs/abdominal bruit
- Fundoscopy
- Neurological deficit.

Blood pressure should be measured in both the arms preferably, to detect any potential differences.[6]

■ INVESTIGATIONS

- *Electrocardiogram (ECG):* To rule out acute myocardial infarction, left ventricular hypertrophy
- *Chest X-ray:* It shows the presence of cardiomegaly, features of acute pulmonary edema
- *Kidney function test:* Blood urea and serum creatinine levels to assess the renal involvement
- *Urinalysis*: It may reveal significant proteinuria, hematuria, cellular casts or analysis for metanephrines in case of suspected pheochromocytoma[10]
- *Computed tomography or magnetic resonance imaging (MRI) of brain*: To rule out acute cerebrovascular events like infarction or intracerebral hemorrhage
- *Echocardiogram*: To assess the left ventricular function and other cardiac pathology.[10]

■ TREATMENT OF HYPERTENSIVE CRISES

In hypertensive crisis, there is a need of fast acting, rapidly reversible and easily titratable drug with no major side-effects. The choice of drug depends upon the clinical presentation of the patient. Numerous drugs are available in the market but the preferred agents are labetalol, nicardipine, esmolol and fenoldopam.[10]

Hypertensive Urgency

In cases with hypertensive urgency, BP control should be managed with the use of oral hypertensive medications, where a gradual decrease of BP over hours to days is desired. Oral labetalol and clonidine are preferred.[10]

Hypertensive Emergency

In cases with hypertensive emergency, a rapid BP control is required with parenteral

TABLE 2: Treatment goals in hypertensive emergency.[9]

Goal time	BP target
First hour	Reduce MAP by 25% (maintain DBP >100 mm Hg)
2–6 h	SBP 160 mm Hg and or DBP 100–110 mm Hg
6–24 h	Maintain the blood pressure over the same range as in 2–6 hours for 24 hours
24–48 h	Outpatient BP goals according to recent guidelines

(BP: blood pressure; DBP: diastolic blood pressure; MAP: mean arterial pressure; SBP: systolic blood pressure)

antihypertensive medications, with the patient admitted to intensive care unit. The BP should be reduced within minutes to an hour to about 20–25% in the first hour and then to 160/100 mm Hg or 160/110 mm Hg over the next 2–6 hours. However, BP should not be reduced to normal values (Table 2).[12]

It may be dangerous to normalize BP following a cerebrovascular accident as an abrupt decrease in BP to normal values could aggravate ischemia due to abnormal autoregulation in these patients.[10,12] For instance, lowering the BP in patients with ischemic strokes may reduce cerebral blood flow resulting in further ischemic injury.

Conditions like aortic dissection and preeclampsia prove to be exceptions, rapid BP control is crucial in these conditions to decrease mortality.[11]

■ DRUGS

Several drugs are available for the treatment of hypertensive emergencies (Table 3).

Sodium nitroprusside is the first choice for majority of the hypertensive emergencies, and it acts within seconds as a potent arterial and venous dilator.[12] The disadvantage of sodium nitroprusside is thiocyanate toxicity which is especially seen

TABLE 3: The common drugs used in hypertensive emergency with their doses.

Drug	Intravenous doses
Vasodilators	
Hydralazine	10–50 mg at 30 min intervals
Nitroglycerin	Initial 5 µg/min, then titrate by 5 µg/min at 3–5 min intervals; if no response seen at 20 µg/min incremental increases of 10–20 µg/min may be used
Sodium nitroprusside	Initial 0.3 µg/kg/min; usual 2–4 µg/kg/min; maximum 10 µg/kg/min for 10 min
Calcium channel blockers	
Clevidipine	1–6 mg/h; titrate by 1–2 mg/h; max 32 mg/h
Nicardipine	Initial 5 mg/h; titrate by 2.5 mg/h at 5–15 min intervals; max 15mg/h
β-blockers	
Esmolol	Initial 80–500 µg/kg over 1 min, then 50–300 µg/kg/min
Labetalol	2 mg/min up to 300 mg or 20 mg over 2 min, then 40–80 mg at 10 min intervals up to 300 mg total
Metoprolol	5–15 mg every 5–15 min
Others	
Enalaprilat	0.625–1.25 mg over 5 min every 6–8 h; max 5 mg per dose
Phentolamine	1–5 mg, max 15 mg
Fenoldopam	0.03–1.6 µg/kg/min

in patients with hepatic or renal failure and on prolonged administration for more than 48–72 hours.[12,13]

Enalaprilat is usually not recommended as the potential of renal failure in hypertensive emergency is high with this drug.[14]

Diuretics—volume depletion is common in patients with hypertensive crises, and the administration of a diuretic together with a hypertensive agent can lead to a further drop in BP. Diuretics should be avoided except in cases of renal parenchymal disease with coexisting pulmonary edema.[2,15]

Drug of Choice in Specific Conditions

- *Acute pulmonary edema:* The drugs of choice are intravenous nitroglycerine, clevidipine or nitroprusside. Beta-blockers are contraindicated in the treatment of acute pulmonary edema[9]
- *Acute myocardial infarction:* Myocardial infarction with severe hypertension, intravenous esmolol is preferred[16]
- *Cerebrovascular accidents:* In patients with intracerebral hematomas, the intracranial pressure rises due to reflex systemic hypertension. There is no evidence that hypertension provokes further bleeding in patients with intracranial hemorrhage. However, cerebral perfusion will be compromised with precipitous fall in systemic BP. The controlled lowering of the BP is currently recommended only in intracranial bleed when the BP is greater than 200/100 mm Hg[10]
- In acute ischemic stroke, goal of BP should be less than 185/110 mm Hg to avoid complications related to cerebral edema[10]
- *Aortic dissection:* The drug of choice for treating aortic dissection is intravenous esmolol. A target BP of 120 mm Hg of systolic BP is to be maintained. In case the target BP is not attained with beta-blockade, vasodilators such as intravenous nitroglycerin or sodium nitroprusside can be opted for[11]
- *Pregnancy:* Before delivery, it is desirable to maintain the diastolic BP greater than 90 mm Hg because this pressure allows for adequate uteroplacental perfusion. In these patients, intravenous drug therapy is reserved for those patients with BP persistently greater than 180/110 mm Hg. In patients of eclampsia or preeclampsia,

the drugs of choice are hydralazine, labetalol, and nicardipine. Angiotensin-converting enzyme (ACE) inhibitors, angiotensin receptor blockers and direct renin inhibitors are avoided in these patients[17,18]

- *Pheochromocytoma:* Intravenous clevidipine, nicardipine and phentolamine are the drugs of choice[6]
- *Drug induced:* Hypertensive emergency caused by drugs like cocaine, amphetamine, phencyclidine or monoamine oxidase inhibitors or by abrupt cessation of clonidine, intravenous clevidipine, nicardipine, and phentolamine are the drugs of choice.[6]

■ CONCLUSION

Hypertensive crises being associated with significant morbidity and mortality, so it is crucial that the patient be diagnosed promptly and managed appropriately. The prognosis is worse in hypertensive emergencies due to the target organ damage as compared to hypertensive urgencies. Hence, timely recognition and intervention of hypertensive emergency is mandatory to prevent long-term morbidity. Patient education on proper compliance and healthy lifestyle modifications go a long way in avoiding these complications and ensuring a good quality of life.

■ REFERENCES

1. Fields LE, Burt VL, Cutler JA, et al. The burden of adult hypertension in the United States 1999 to 2000: a rising tide. Hypertension. 2004;44(4):398-404.
2. Keith NM, Wagener HP, Barker NW. Some different types of essential hypertension: their course and prognosis. Am J Med Sci. 1974;268:336-45.
3. Chobanian AV, Bakris GL, Black HR, et al. Seventh report of the joint national committee on prevention, detection, evaluation, and treatment of high blood pressure. Hypertension. 2003;42(6):1206-52.
4. Reddy KS. Regional case studies–India. Nestle Nutr Workshop Ser Pediatr Program. 2009;63:15-24;discussion 41-16, 259-268.
5. Fuster V, Kelly BB. Board for Global Health. Promoting cardiovascular health in developing world: a critical challenge to achieve global health. Washington: Institute of Medicine; 2010.
6. Taylor DA. Hypertensive crisis: a review of pathophysiology and treatment. Crit Care Nurs Clin North Am. 2015;27(4):439-47.
7. Papadopoulos DP, Mourouzis I, Thomopoulos C, et al. Hypertension crisis. Blood Press. 2010;19(6):328-36.
8. Van den Born BJ, Löwenberg EC, van der Hoeven NV, et al. Endothelial dysfunction, platelet activation, thrombogenesis and fibrinolysis in patients with hypertensive crisis. Hypertens. 2011;29(5):922-7.
9. American College of Clinical Pharmacy; Hypertensive emergencies. Benken ST (Ed). Medical issues in the ICU. CCSAP Book 2018. Washington: American College of Clinical Pharmacy; 2018:7-30.
10. Varounis C, Katsi V, Nihoyannopoulos P, et al. Cardiovascular Hypertensive Crisis: Recent Evidence and Review of the Literature. Front Cardiovasc Med. 2017;3:51.
11. Khan IA, Nair CK. Clinical, diagnostic, and management perspectives of aortic dissection. Chest. 2002;122:311-28.
12. Rodriguez MA, Kumar SK, De Caro M. Hypertensive crisis. Cardiol Rev. 2010;18(2):102-7.
13. Hall VA, Guest JM. Sodium nitroprusside-induced cyanide Intoxication and prevention with sodium thiosulfate prophylaxis. Am J Crit Care. 1992;1(2):19-25.
14. White WB, Radford MJ, Gonzalez FM, et al. Selective dopamine-1 agonist therapy in severe hypertension: effects of intravenous fenoldopam. J Am Coll Cardiol. 1988;11(5):1118-23.
15. Holzer-Richling N, Holzer M, Herkner H, et al. Randomized placebo-controlled trial of furosemide on subjective perception of dyspnoea in patients with pulmonary oedema because of hypertensive crisis. Eur J Clin Invest. 2011;41(6):627-34.
16. Rosendorff C, Lackland DT, Allison M, et al. Treatment of Hypertension in Patients With Coronary Artery Disease: A Scientific Statement from the American Heart Association, American College of Cardiology, and American Society of Hypertension. J Am Coll Cardiol. 2015;65:1998-2038.
17. Rhoney D, Peacock WF. Intravenous therapy for hypertensive emergencies, part 1. Health Syst Pharm. 2009;66:1687.
18. Marik PE, Varon J. Hypertensive crises: challenges and management. Chest. 2007;131:1949-62.

Difficult to Control Hypertension (Resistance, Pseudoresistance, and Malignant Hypertension)

NN Anand

◾ RESISTANT HYPERTENSION

Resistant hypertension is defined as blood pressure (BP) that remains above goal in spite of the concurrent use of three antihypertensive agents of different classes in adequate doses. One of the three drug classes should be a diuretic. Resistant hypertension is described in order to identify patients who are at high risk of having reversible causes of hypertension. These patients may benefit from special diagnostic and therapeutic considerations.

Prevalence

Exact prevalence of resistant hypertension is unknown. Studies suggest that it is not uncommon.

The proportion of patients with uncontrolled hypertension is even higher among higher risk populations and, particularly, for patients with diabetes mellitus or chronic kidney disease (CKD) with the application of the lower goal BP as recommended in the 7th Report of the Joint National Committee on Prevention, Detection, Evaluation and Treatment of High Blood Pressure (JNC 7).[1]

To accurately determine the prevalence of resistant hypertension, study of a large, diverse hypertensive cohort would be required.

Patient Characteristics Associated with Resistant Hypertension

Blood pressure remains above target range mostly due to persistent elevations in systolic BP. The disparity between systolic and diastolic BP control worsens with increasing age.

Older age had been reported as the strongest predictor of lack of BP control in an analysis of Framingham study data. The participants >75 years were less than one-fourth as likely to have control on systolic BP as compared with participants ≤60 years of age. The other strongest predictors of lack of controlled systolic BP were left ventricular hypertrophy (LVH) and obesity [body mass index (BMI) >30 kg/m^2]. With regards to the controlled diastolic BP, the strongest negative predictor was obesity, with BP being controlled about one-third less often in comparison to the lean participants (BMI <25 kg/m^2). As stated in a prospective analysis of the participants in the Framingham Study not only older age but higher baseline systolic BP was also associated with increased risk of never achieving BP target. The prevalence of resistant hypertension can be further anticipated to increase with an increasingly older and heavier population in association with a growing incidence of diabetes mellitus and CKD.

Following are the patient characteristics associated with resistant hypertension:

- Older age
- High baseline BP
- Obesity
- Excessive dietary salt ingestion
- Chronic kidney disease
- Diabetes
- Left ventricular hypertrophy
- Black race
- Female sex.

Genetics

It is reasonable to predict that genetic factors may play a greater role than in the general hypertensive population. The data on genetic assessments of patients with resistant hypertension are limited. A rare monogenic form of hypertension, Liddle's syndrome, can be caused by the mutations of the β and γ subunits of the epithelial sodium channel (ENaC). The two β ENaC and γ ENaC gene variants show significantly high prevalence in the patients with resistant hypertension in comparison to the normotensive patients. The presence of the gene variants is related with a raised excretion of urinary potassium relative to plasma renin levels. An important role in the metabolism of cortisol and corticosterone is played by the CYP3A5 enzyme (11β-hydroxysteroid dehydrogenase type 2) in particular in the kidneys. Identifying genetic influences on resistance to current therapies might also promote the growth and development of new therapeutic targets.

Lifestyle Factors

Obesity

Obesity is related with more severe hypertension. In addition, the need for an increased number of antihypertensive medications is also linked with obesity. In fact, obesity is a common attribute of patients with resistant hypertension. The mechanisms of hypertension induced by obesity are complex and not fully elucidated. However, impaired sodium excretion, elevated sympathetic nervous system activity, and activation of the renin-angiotensin-aldosterone system are amongst the few that are included.

Dietary Salt

Excessive intake of sodium in the diet contributes to the development of resistant hypertension. This occurs by both a direct increase in BP and blunting of the BP-lowering effect of most classes of antihypertensive agents. In typical salt-sensitive patients, which include the elderly, these effects are more pronounced. Excessive dietary sodium is though fairly widespread, it has been explicitly accepted as being common in patients with resistant hypertension.

Alcohol

Heavy alcohol intake is linked with an increased risk of hypertension along with a treatment-resistant hypertension. As per study conducted in a Finnish hypertension clinic, heavy drinkers, as suggested by increases in liver transaminase levels, were much less likely to have control on their BP during a 2-year follow-up in comparison to patients with normal transaminase levels. Prospectively, stopping heavy alcohol ingestion by a small group of patients decreased 24-hour ambulatory systolic BP by 7.2 mm Hg and diastolic BP by 6.6 mm Hg, while the hypertension prevalence was dropped from 42% to 12%.

Drug-related Causes

Several therapeutic classes of pharmacological agents can cause elevation in the BP values and contribute to resistance to hypertension. The impact of these agents, however, can highly vary among individuals. Given widespread use of, nonnarcotic analgesics, including non-steroidal anti-inflammatory drugs (NSAIDs), aspirin, and acetaminophen, are one of the most common offending agents in terms of worsening BP control. NSAIDs, in particular, are associated with modest but predictable increases in BP.

Medications that can interfere with BP control:

- Non-narcotic analgesics
- Nonsteroidal anti-inflammatory agents
- Selective COX-2 inhibitors
- Sympathomimetic agents
- Alcohol
- Oral contraceptives
- Cyclosporine
- Erythropoietin.

Secondary Causes of Resistant Hypertension

- Obstructive sleep apnea
- Renal parenchymal disease
- Primary hyperaldosteronism
- Renal artery stenosis
- Pheochromocytoma
- Cushing's disease
- Hyperparathyroidism
- Coarctation of aorta.

■ PSEUDORESISTANCE

Poor Blood Pressure Technique

Erroneous measurement of BP can result in the appearance of treatment resistance. Most common mistakes, which include measuring the BP before even allowing the patient to sit quietly and using a cuff that is too small in size, will result in falsely high BP readings. Assessments of office blood pressure measurement technique imply that it is likely a regular clinical drawback.

Poor Adherence

Poor adherence to antihypertensive therapy is a major reason of uncontrolled BP. It is reported that around 40% of newly diagnosed hypertensives discontinue their antihypertensive medicines during the 1st year of treatment. Less than 40% of patients may persist with their prescribed antihypertensive treatment, during 5–10 years of follow-up. The poor adherence is commonly seen at the primary care level. It may be less common among patients who have been seen by specialists.

Lack of BP control is not same as treatment resistance. For an antihypertensive regimen to be failed, it has to have been taken appropriately. This difference is clinically significant as patients with poorly controlled hypertension secondary to lack of adherence need not be subjected to the evaluations and continuous manipulations in treatment regimens that are undertaken for patients with true treatment resistance.

White Coat Effect

White coat effect refers to when clinic BP are persistently elevated while out-of-office values are normal or significantly lower. Studies have indicated that a noteworthy white coat effect is as common in patients with resistant hypertension as in the more general hypertensive population, with a prevalence that ranges from 20% to 30%. Also, as with more general hypertensive patients, patients with resistant hypertension based on a "white coat" phenomenon show less severe target organ damage and also appear to be at less risk to cardiovascular disease as compared with those patients with persistent hypertension during ambulatory BP monitoring.

■ MALIGNANT HYPERTENSION

There are multiple causes of malignant hypertension including the following:

- Medication noncompliance
- Renovascular diseases, such as renal artery stenosis, polyarteritis nodosa, and takayasu arteritis

- Renal parenchymal disease including glomerulonephritis, tubulointerstitial nephritis, systemic sclerosis, hemolytic-uremic syndrome, and systemic lupus erythematosus
- Endocrine dysfunction, such as pheochromocytoma, Cushing disease, primary hyperaldosteronism and renin-secreting tumor
- Coarctation of aorta; drugs or other exposures, including cocaine, phencyclidine, sympathomimetics, erythropoietin and cyclosporine
- Antihypertensive medication withdrawal
- Amphetamines
- Central nervous system disorders, such as head injury, cerebral infarction, and cerebral hemorrhage.

Some of the more common signs or symptoms include:
- Blurry vision
- Headache
- Chest pain
- Irregular heartbeat
- Nosebleed
- Shortness of breath
- Tingling, numbness, burning or prickly skin sensations
- Faintness or dizziness
- Reduced urine output
- Nausea or vomiting
- Altered mental state
- Burst retinal capillaries
- Seizures.

◼ EVALUATION

The evaluation of patients with resistant hypertension should include confirming true treatment resistance and identification of causes contributing to treatment resistance, including secondary causes of hypertension if any; and documentation of target organ damage. Mostly treatment resistance is multifactorial. It is important to assess treatment adherence and use of good BP measurement technique to exclude pseudoresistance.

History

The medical history be obtained in detail and it should document duration and progression of the hypertension; treatment; response to prior medications, including adverse events; current medication use, including herbal and over-the-counter medications; and symptoms of possible secondary causes of hypertension.

Adherence to Treatment

It is important for patients to be asked about how successfully they are taking all of their prescribed doses, including discussion of adverse effects, dosing inconvenience, and out-of-pocket costs, all of which can hamper adherence. Family members can provide more objective estimation about how well a patient is adhering.

Measurement of Blood Pressure

Using a good BP measurement technique is vital for precisely diagnosing resistant hypertension, including having the patient sit quietly for 5 minutes in a chair with his/her back supported before taking the measurement; using a cuff of the correct size with the air bladder encircling at least 80% of the arm (adult large cuff for most patients); and arm supported at heart level during the cuff measurement. A minimum of two readings should be taken at intervals of at least 1 minute. The average of those readings should be taken to correspond to the patient's BP.

Physical Examination

A fundoscopic examination should record the presence and severity of retinopathy. The presence of carotid, abdominal or femoral bruits leads to increased chances of renal artery stenosis. Aortic coarctation or significant aortoiliac disease is suggested by diminished femoral pulses and/or a discrepancy between arm and thigh BPs. Abdominal striae, particularly if pigmented; moon facies; or prominent interscapular fat deposition suggest Cushing's disease.

Ambulatory Blood Pressure Monitoring

Documenting a significant white coat effect needs an unfailing assessment of out-of-office BP values. This is accomplished most objectively with the use of 24-hour ambulatory monitoring. As an alternative, work site measurements by trained health practitioners and/or out-of-office assessments with use of manual or automated BP monitors can be trusted upon. Using good BP technique with validation of the accuracy of readings is essential in the case of self-assessments by patient. Cuffs adequately sized for use with extremely obese patients are usually not available with ambulatory or home automated monitors. Use of wrist monitors may become essential in such cases, but the accuracy of such units can prove inconsistent.

A significant white coat effect should be suspected in patients with resistant hypertension wherein the clinic BP measurements are higher than out-of-office measurements; in patients who repeatedly show signs of overtreatment, mainly orthostatic symptoms; and in patients with chronically high office BP values but target organ damage (LVH, retinopathy, CKD) being absent. In such cases, 24-hour ambulatory BP monitoring is suggested. A mean ambulatory daytime BP of more than 135/85 mm Hg is taken as elevated.[2,3] Out-of-office measurements should be relied on to adjust treatment in case a significant white coat effect is established.

Biochemical Evaluation

Biochemical evaluation of the patient with treatment-resistant hypertension should include a routine metabolic profile (sodium, potassium, glucose, chloride, bicarbonate, blood urea nitrogen and creatinine); urinalysis; and a paired, morning plasma aldosterone and plasma renin or plasma renin activity for screening primary aldosteronism. The aldosterone/renin ratio is an effective screening test for primary aldosteronism, even in the ongoing antihypertensive treatment settings (excluding potassium-sparing diuretics, particularly aldosterone antagonists), having a high negative predictive value. However, a high ratio has a low specificity for primary aldosteronism, probably reflecting the common occurrence of low-renin hypertension in resistant hypertensives. The specificity of the ratio is improvised if a minimum plasma renin activity of 0.5 ng/mL/hour is used in its calculation and/or a plasma aldosterone level ≥15 ng/dL is necessary for the ratio to be considered high. A high ratio (generally 20–30 when plasma aldosterone is reported in ng/dL and plasma renin activity in ng/mL/h) is indicative of primary aldosteronism, but further evaluation is required for confirmation of the diagnosis.

For estimating dietary sodium and potassium intake, calculating creatinine clearance, and measuring aldosterone excretion, a 24-hour urine collected while ingestion of normal diet can be helpful. To do so from the same collection, however, needs that a nonsalt acid (e.g. acetic acid) be used as the preservative for aldosterone. If a 24-hour urine is not used for calculating creatinine clearance, renal function can be estimated by any of a number of validated urine-free formulae. Measurement of 24-hour urinary metanephrines or plasma metanephrines is an efficient screen for patients in whom pheochromocytoma is suspected.

Noninvasive Imaging

It is important to know that imaging for renal artery stenosis should be reserved for patients with an increased level of suspicion. This would include young patients, in particular women, whose presentation suggests the presence of fibromuscular dysplasia and older patients at increased risk of atherosclerotic disease. Depending on the level of training and experience, the preferred imaging modality will differ among institution. For patients with CKD, modalities that do not involve iodinated contrast may be chosen over computed tomography (CT) angiography. Diagnostic renal arteriograms in the absence of suspicious noninvasive imaging are not recommended. Similarly, due to poor specificity, abdominal CT imaging is not recommended for screening adrenal adenomas in the absence of biochemical confirmation of hormonally active tumors (Cushing's syndrome, hyperaldosteronism, and pheochromocytoma).

■ MANAGEMENT

Lifestyle Interventions

- Weight loss
- Dietary salt restriction
- DASH diet and other dietary factors
- Exercise.

Pharmacological Treatment

General Principles

Once all identifiable forms of hypertension, particularly endocrine causes, have been excluded and contributions from the white coat effect and masked uncontrolled hypertension are considered, therapeutic approaches for improved BP control in resistant hypertension can begin. Three mechanistically complementary antihypertensive agents, commonly including a long-acting calcium channel blocker, a blocker of the renin-angiotensin system (ACE inhibitor or ARB), and a diuretic, should already be prescribed and taken by the patient to ensure a proper diagnosis of resistant hypertension.[4]

Specific Therapeutic Regimens

The establishment of the pathogenesis will optimally facilitate the selection of the fourth drug since most cases of resistant hypertension are associated with either volume excess, especially in CKD, or high sympathetic tone. Moreover, it is important to ensure that the most effective antihypertensive agent selected is from certain pharmacological classes while adding a fourth agent (Table 1).

■ CONCLUSION

As a specific subgroup, resistant hypertension has remained understudied. Experimental assessment of patients with resistant hypertension is complicated by the associated high cardiovascular risk that restricts the safe withdrawal of medicines and limits the duration as well as kinds of experimental interventions that can be used to investigate proposed etiologies. The presence of the concomitant disease processes such as diabetes, CKD, atherosclerotic disease, and sleep apnea further limits the studies. Better identification and treatment of patients with resistant hypertension require much additional knowledge and research. While the prevalence and prognosis of resistant hypertension can be projected and assumed, neither is known. Cross-sectional and outcome studies have recognized patient characteristics related to resistant hypertension, but underlying mechanisms of treatment resistance, potential genetic mechanisms in particular, have not been extensively explored. Better guidance to the therapy would demand efficacy assessments of specific multidrug regimens.

TABLE 1: Specific clinical issues associated with treatment resistance.

Issue associated with treatment resistance	Management consideration(s)
Volume control, edema resolution	Thiazide → chlorthalidone → loop diuretic
Heart rate control inadequate	β-blocker, α, β-blocker, verapamil and diltiazem
Renin and aldosterone levels low	Low-salt diet, avoid night-time shift work, amiloride
Renin low, aldosterone normal to high normal	Mineralocorticoid receptor antagonist
Would split dosing of medications improve control?	Evaluate blood pressure pattern according to home and ambulatory blood pressure monitoring
Medication adherence questionable	Initiate indirect or direct methods to detect nonadherence; if nonadherence is documented (partial or complete), discuss frankly, nonjudgmentally with patient and family
Pattern of blood pressure response to medications outside clinician visit times unknown	Identify meal effects on blood pressure, duration of medication effect, relationship of blood pressure to side effects using out-of-office blood pressure monitoring
Sleep disordered breathing; significant anxiety associated with highly variable hypertension	Initiate nondrug strategies concurrently with or separately from antihypertensive drug therapy

■ REFERENCES

1. Hajjar I, Kotchen TA. Trends in prevalence, awareness, treatment, and control of hypertension in the United States, 1988–2000. JAMA. 2003;290:199-206.
2. Lloyd-Jones DM, Evans JC, Larson MG, et al. Differential control of systolic and diastolic blood pressure: factors associated with lack of blood pressure control in the community. Hypertension. 2000;36:594-9.
3. Peralta CA, Hicks LS, Chertow GM, et al. Control of hypertension in adults with chronic kidney disease in the United States. Hypertension. 2005;45:1119-24.
4. The ALLHAT Officers and Coordinators for the ALLHAT Collaborative Research Group. Major outcomes in high-risk hypertensive patients randomized to angiotensin-converting enzyme inhibitor or calcium channel blocker vs diuretic: the Antihypertensive and Lipid-Lowering Treatment to Prevent Heart Attack Trial (ALLHAT). JAMA. 2002;288:2981-97.

Hypertension in Children and Adolescents

Divya Saxena

■ INTRODUCTION

Hypertension (HTN), once thought to be a health condition of adults, is now become a very common health issue of younger population and children, owing to the well-established childhood obesity epidemic. All across the world, the number of healthy children and adolescents being diagnosed with HTN is increasing day-by-day and is now a very well-established entity among children and younger population. High blood pressure (BP) in childhood commonly leads to HTN in adulthood and we all know that HTN is a major long-term condition and a leading cause of premature death among adults throughout the world.

There is evidence that early development of atherosclerosis in children and adolescents is associated with childhood HTN and is a predisposing factor for the early development of coronary artery disease in adults. The reports say that childhood HTN is not associated with cardiovascular disease (CVD) and death.

Despite the high prevalence and potential risks of HTN in children, it often goes unrecognized by the physicians.[1] Normal BP value in children varies according to age, height and sex; therefore there is an urgent need of increasing awareness and education of clinicians about how to diagnose, evaluate and treat the children to combat this increasingly common health problem. More frequent screening of high-risk children and younger population should also be recommended.

■ PREVALENCE

The true incidence of HTN in childhood and adolescent is not known because of the regional difference in the definition of high BP and the BP measurement methodology. However, because of increasing obesity among children, the prevalence of systemic HTN is on increasing trends. Prevalence also varies according to different demographic conditions of even the same country. High BP is consistently greater in boys (15–19%) than in girls (7–12%).

The source of information about the prevalence of HTN in children is mainly from the data of National Health and Nutrition Examination Surveys (NHANES) group.

If we use the recommended three separate measurements methodology in children and adolescents, who have an initial BP measurement of more than or equal to 95th percentile, the prevalence would be somewhere in between 1% and 3%.

Therefore, the actual prevalence of clinical HTN in children and adolescents is 3–5%, but of persistent HTN or previously known as prehypertension (BP from 90th to 94th percentile) is from 2.2% to 3.5% with higher rates among obese or overweight children and adolescents.[2,3]

Prevalence in Other Chronic Conditions

Obesity is the major risk factor for developing HTN in children and adolescents where the prevalence of HTN is 3.8–24.8%. It increases with increasing adiposity and waist circumference. Other than obesity there are various other chronic conditions which are associated with higher rate of high BP in children and adolescents like sleep-disordered breathing (SDB), chronic kidney disease (CKD) and in preterm children.

Sleep-disordered breathing includes condition like primary snoring, sleep fragmentation and obstructive sleep apnea syndrome (OSAS), where the prevalence of high BP ranges from 3.6% to 14% increasing in severity with increasing severity of OSAS.

There is strong evidence in favor of relation between HTN and CKD among children; however, the data regarding HTN leading to CKD in children is lacking, which is more common in adults, whereas in children, certain forms of CKD can lead to HTN. Out of total hypertensive pediatric population 20% may be because of CKD.

There is limited data showing a relation between HTN and preterm birth but low birth weight and preterm birth weight have been identified by few studies as risk factors for HTN and CVD in adults. According to one study, there is a prevalence of 7.3% of HTN among preterm born children though more data are needed to determine the true relation and rate of HTN among these children.[4,5]

■ DEFINITION AND CLASSIFICATION

The American Academy of Pediatrics (AAP)[6] published revised guidelines in 2017 for diagnosing HTN among children and adolescents after about 12 years of the publication of the landmark 2004 Fourth Working Group Report from the National High Blood Pressure Education Program.[7,8] The new guidelines include significant changes to simplify diagnosis and evaluation of HTN in children. If compared with the fourth report these are not only comprehensive but have simpler definitions also, easier to implement in the primary care settings and having stable BP thresholds for adolescents that match the new adult American Heart Association (AHA) and American College of Cardiology (ACC) guidelines. The current definition of high BP, including HTN in children and adolescents, is based on the normative distribution of BP data in healthy children including children from the NHANES and other screening studies.

According to 2017 AAP guidelines, BP levels are to be interpreted on the basis of gender, age, and height because height and gender are important determinants of BP in children. Importantly, however the normative BP tables were created by using data only from normal weight children excluding the BP data from overweight and obese children (i.e. children with BMI ≥85th percentile) that were previously included. As a result, the new BP tables reveal lower thresholds by few mm Hg in comparison to the Fourth Report and are more accurate as truly normative data. In children definitions that categorize BP values were modified by the 2017 AAP guidelines into two age groups. Normal BP for children is still classified less than 90th percentile and HTN is defined at the 95th percentile across three separate visits. The term "prehypertension" has been replaced by the term "elevated blood pressure" as in AHA and ACC guidelines. The pressures between 90th and 95th percentile are described as elevated BP. Staging criteria for stage I and stage II HTN have been revised and for the children more than or equal to 13 years of age, aligned with 2017 AHA and ACC adult HTN guidelines. Additionally in the newer guidelines, there is abandonment of the 99th percentile as a threshold (Table 1).[9-12]

Classification

Flowchart 1 shows modified BP measurement algorithm.

■ NEW NORMATIVE SIMPLIFIED BLOOD PRESSURE TABLE

New normative full BP tables are complicated and lead to under recognition of childhood HTN, so simplified BP table is created based on 90th percentile BP values for children at 5th height percentile. This table is used for initial screening of BP values (Table 2).

■ DIAGNOSIS

It is recommended that persistent HTN in children and adolescents should be diagnosed

TABLE 1: New blood pressure classification for children, adolescents and adults.

HTN classification	Children aged 1–12 years (percentile based)	=13 years (mm Hg based)
Normotensive	<90th percentile	<120/80
Elevated blood pressure	= 90th percentile or = 120/80 mm Hg lower to <95th percentile	<120–129/<80
Stage I hypertension	= 95th percentile to <95th percentile + 12 mm Hg or 130/80 to 139/89 mm Hg (lower)	130–139/80–89
Stage II hypertension	= 95th percentile + 12 mm Hg or = 140/90 mm Hg (lower)	= 140/90

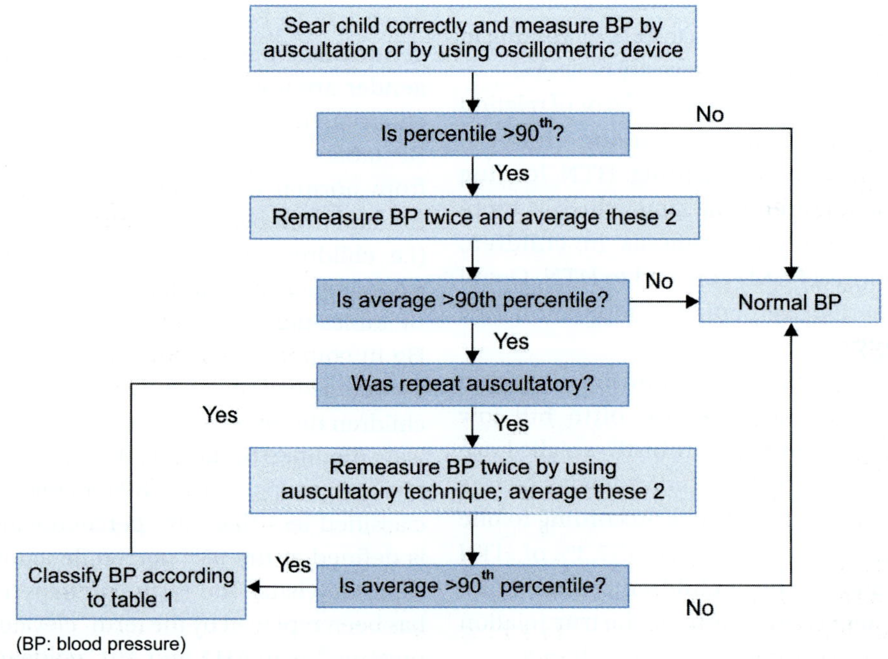

(BP: blood pressure)

Flowchart 1: Modified BP measurement algorithm.

TABLE 2: New normative simplified BP table.

Age (years)	BP (mm Hg)			
	Boys		Girls	
	SBP	DBP	SBP	DBP
1	98	52	98	54
2	100	55	101	58
3	101	58	102	60
4	102	60	103	62
5	103	63	104	64
6	105	66	105	67
7	106	68	106	68
8	107	69	107	69
9	107	70	108	71
10	108	72	109	72
11	110	74	111	74
12	113	75	114	75
13	120	80	120	80

(DBP: diastolic blood pressure; SBP: systolic blood pressure)

on the basis of repeated BP recordings at three separate visits which are greater than 95th percentile for the age, gender and height of the patient or it is more than or equal to 130/80 mm Hg. The age- and height-specific BP percentile may be determined by using calculations for boys or for girls.[11]

SCREENING

These recommendations are based on 2017 AAP recommendation for screening, which are further endorsed by AHA.

- For children without risk factor or conditions associated with HTN, BP is measured beginning at 3–4 years of age during annual health check-ups
- For children more than or equal to 3 years of age with risk factors for HTN, BP measurement is recommended at every healthcare encounter
- Children below 3 years of age with risk factors for HTN should have BP measurements at each health supervision. Children with higher screening BP threshold of systolic or diastolic BP, should be further evaluated.

There are many potential etiologies of isolated elevated BP in children and it may vary considerably on each visit and even during the same visit. So multiple measurements over same time should be obtained before diagnosing HTN.[11]

MEASUREMENT OF BLOOD PRESSURE

The diagnosis of HTN largely depends on accurate measurement of BP because the BP tables are based on auscultatory measurement; therefore, the preferred method of BP measurement is auscultatory. Oscillometric devices are convenient to be used as a screening tool and they minimize operator's error also but they do not provide BP measures, identical to auscultation. Every high BP measurement done by oscillometric device in children is to be confirmed by auscultatory measurement by a standard clinical sphygmomanometer.

Variability in BP measurement of a same subject is due to procedural difference in BP measurements and is observer dependent. Factors responsible for variable BP measurement include cuff size, technique, type of instrument used, number of recordings, etc.[4,5,10,11,13]

Cuff Size and Placement

Use of appropriate cuff size is very important for accurate BP measurement. It is recommended that in every clinical setting, especially in a pediatrician's clinic, cuff of varied sizes should be available, including a standard adult cuff, a large adult cuff and a thigh cuff. When a patient is in between two cuff sizes, the larger of the two cuffs to be used. If smaller cuff is used it may lead to a falsely elevated reading of BP and overestimation of high BP; on the other hand, too wide a cuff may produce lower reading than the actual intra-arterial pressure (Fig. 1).[11,13]

Appropriate cuff size by convention is of a bladder width of at least 40% of the arm circumference at a point midway between the olecranon and the acromion. The cuff length should cover 80–100% of the circumference of arm. The bladder width to length ratio should be at least 1:2.

Points to be Considered while BP Measurements

- The patient should avoid consuming stimulant drugs or food before a BP measurement

- The BP should be measured when a child is sitting quietly for 5 minutes in a chair with his/her back supported and feet resting on the ground. In infants, BP is measured in a supine position
- Blood pressure measurement should be done, when child is relaxed and having normal heart rate, because anxiety can raise heart rates and in turn falsely elevate BP also
- The BP should be measured by auscultatory method by pacing bell of the stethoscope over brachial artery pulse proximal and medial in the cubital fossa and below the bottom edge of the cuff in the right arm, while it is supported at the level of heart. Allowing the arm to hang below the heart will elevate BP levels (Fig. 2)
- The cuff should be of appropriate size and inflated to 20–30 mm Hg above the anticipated systolic BP and then deflated slowly by 2–3 mm Hg per heartbeat (Fig. 3).

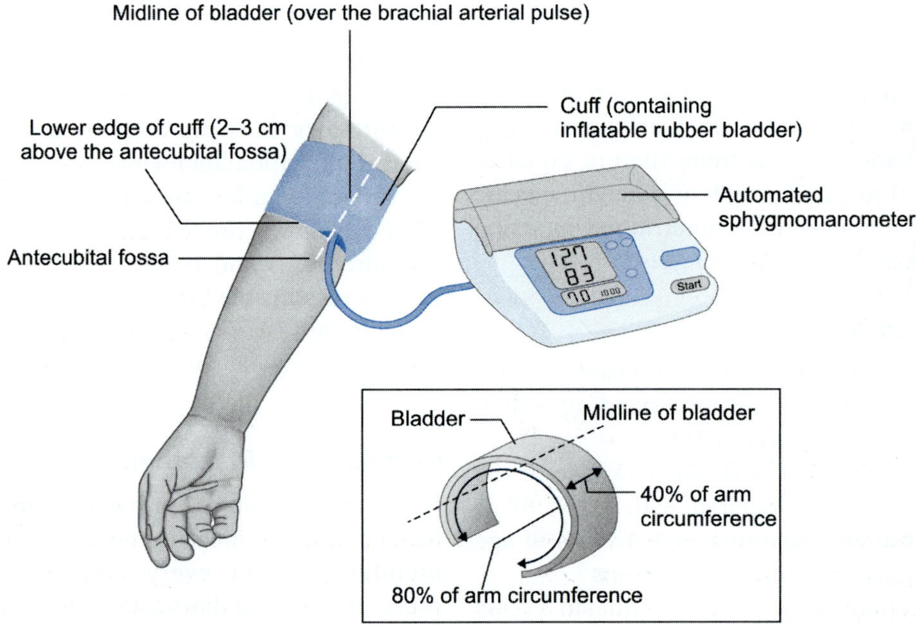

Fig. 1: Cuff size and placement.

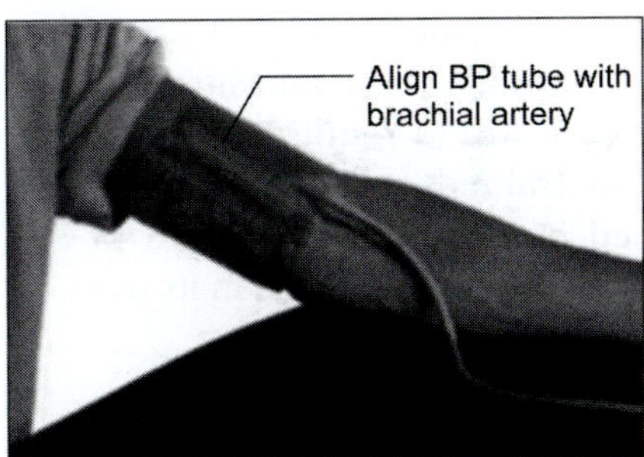

Fig. 2: BP measurement technique.

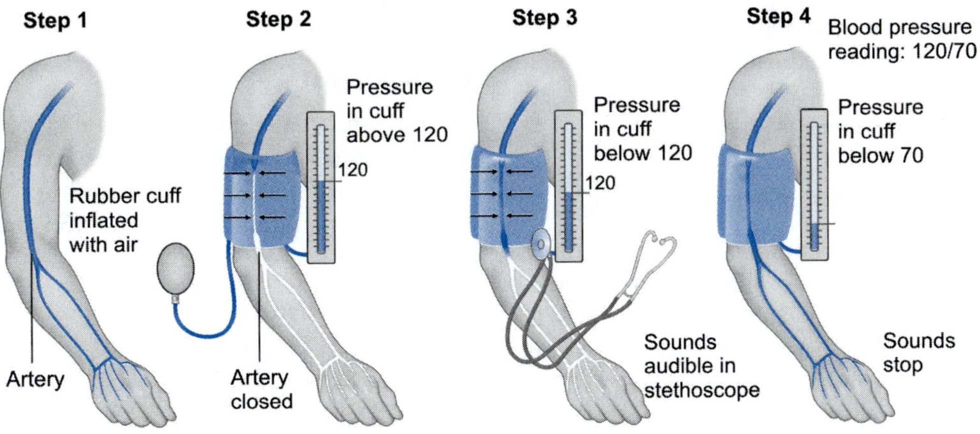

Fig. 3: Stepwise technique of blood pressure measurement.

Ambulatory BP Monitoring

Ambulatory BP monitoring (ABPM) refers to a procedure in which a portable BP device is used to record BP over a specified period, usually 24 hours. It is especially useful in the evaluation of white coat HTN and to evaluate the response to antihypertensive treatment. ABPM should be considered if the clinic measurement is only mildly elevated, or if BP values are normal when measured at home. Conducting ABPM required specific equipment and trained staff, therefore it should be used by experts in the field of pediatric HTN, who are experienced in its use and interpretation.[13]

■ PRIMARY HYPERTENSION

Primary HTN occurs on its own, without an identifiable cause; however, it is now identifiable in children and adolescents. Primary HTN occurs more often in children above 6 years and older adolescents, making up to 85–95% of cases.[10,13,14]

Primary HTN often clusters with other risk factors, including:

- Overweight, obesity
- A family history of high BP
- Type 2 diabetes mellitus
- High cholesterol including low plasma high-density lipoprotein cholesterol and elevated plasma triglycerides
- Too much salt consumption
- Being black or Hispanic
- More common in male gender
- Smoking or exposure to second-hand smoke
- Sedentary lifestyle.

■ SECONDARY HYPERTENSION

Secondary HTN is more common in children than in adults. Younger children with stage II HTN are more likely to have secondary HTN. Renal and renovascular diseases are among the most common secondary causes of HTN in children. Renal disorder accounted (including vascular disorders) for 63–74% of children below 6 years of age according to the recent clinical trials.[10,13,14] Other causes of secondary HTN in children and adolescents include:

- Polycystic kidney disease
- Aortic coarctation

- Adrenal disorders
- Hyperthyroidism
- Pheochromocytoma
- Renal artery stenosis
- Sleep disorders (OSA)
- Certain medication—corticosteroids, oral contraceptive, decongestants, dietary products and recreational drugs
- Environmental exposures—lead, mercury and phthalates
- Neurofibromatosis type-I (NF-1) also known as von Recklinghausen disease, a rare autosomal dominants disorder
- Monogenic forms of HTN.

■ EVALUATION

Once a child is diagnosed as a hypertensive patient, an extensive history and careful physical examination should be done to identify the underlying causes of elevated BP and to detect any end organ damage.[5,13,14]

History

This is the first step while evaluating a child with HTN. A detailed history should be taken.[14]

Perinatal History

Perinatal factors such as maternal HTN, low birth weight, and preterm birth all have been shown to influence BP in childhood and adolescents, so detailed information should be obtained.

Nutritional History

High sodium intake is associated with a 2-fold increase in the incidence of HTN. Consumption of high-fat food, low-fiber diet and sugary beverages are also associated with HTN.

Physical Activity Level

Sedentary lifestyle is a strong predictor of HTN in children and adolescents.

Psychosocial History

Psychosocial history should always be obtained in hypertensive children, because stress, anxiety and depression are associated with early onset of HTN. History of bullying is particularly important in overweight or obese children.

Family History

Family history of HTN in first-and second-degree relatives should be taken carefully.

Physical Examination

A comprehensive physical examination may provide information about the possible causes of HTN and about end organ damage. The child height, weight, elevated BMI and percentile for age should be determined. BP reading should be taken both in upper and lower extremities to rule out coarctation of aorta (Table 3).[14]

Laboratory Evaluation and Imaging Test

Laboratory testing and imaging is to be done in all confirmed cases of HTN to find out the underlying cause of HTN, to detect comorbid condition and to evaluate any end organ damage. Additional testing is required on the basis of individual and family histories, the presence of risk factors and the result of screening tests; children with stage 2 HTN need more extensive evaluation as they may be having secondary HTN.[13,14]

TABLE 3: Etiology of hypertension and suggestive evaluation findings.

Etiology	History findings	Physical examination findings	Possible findings on additional testing
Coarctation of the aorta	• None	• Difference between right and left arm blood pressure • Diminished femoral pulses • Heart murmur • Lower blood pressure in legs than in arms	• Abnormal findings on echocardiography
Cushing syndrome	• Family history of endocrinopathy	• Acne, hirsutism, striae, moon facies, truncal obesity	• Elevated cortisol levels
Drug-induced	• Illicit substance abuse • Amphetamines • Anabolic steroids • Cocaine • Phencyclidine • Caffeine • Diet pills • Ephedra • Performance-enhancing drugs • Oral contraceptives • Steroids sympathomimetics	• Acne, hirsutism, striae (with anabolic steroid use) • Sweating • Tachycardia	• Abnormal findings on urine drug screen

Continued

Continued

Etiology	History findings	Physical examination findings	Possible findings on additional testing
Hyperthyroidism	• Family history of thyroid disorder • Heat intolerance • Rash, sweating, pallor	• Ophthalmopathy • Tachycardia • Thyromegaly • Weight loss	• Suppressed thyroid-stimulating hormone
Mineralocorticoid excess (from congenital adrenal hyperplasia, aldosterone-secreting tumors)	• Family history of endocrinopathy	• Ambiguous genitalia • Muscle weakness	• Elevated plasma aldosterone levels • Hypokalemia • Low plasma renin activity
Obstructive sleep apnea	• Family history of sleep apnea • Snoring or disordered sleep	• Adenotonsillar hypertrophy	• Abnormal findings on polysomnography
Pheochromocy-toma	• Flushing, pallor, palpitations, sweating	• Tachycardia	• Elevated plasma and urine catecholamine levels
Primary hypertension	• Diet high in fat and sodium • Family history of essential hypertension or early cardiovascular disease • Limited physical activity • Patient is in adolescence	• Acanthosis nigricans Obesity	• Hyperlipidemia Impaired glucose tolerance or type 2 diabetes mellitus
Renal artery stenosis	• Prior umbilical artery catheterization	• Abdominal bruit	• Abnormal findings on renovascular imaging
Renal parenchymal disease	• Enuresis • Family history of renal disease • Fatigue • Recurrent urinary tract infections	• Abdominal mass • Edema • Gross hematuria • Growth retardation	• Abnormal blood urea nitrogen or creatinine level • Abnormal findings on urinalysis, urine culture, or renal ultrasonography • Anemia
Rheumatologic disorder	• Family history of autoimmune disease • Fatigue • Joint pain • Rash	• Friction rub • Joint swelling • Malar rash	• Abnormal findings on autoimmune laboratory studies, elevated markers of inflammation

Fasting Laboratory Test

Lipid panel and fasting glucose panel, including fasting insulin levels, should be done in obese or overweight children.

Renin Profiling

Plasma renin level or plasma renin activity is a useful screening test for mineralocorticoid-related diseases.

Hormone

Hormonal levels and 24 hours urine studies should be done to evaluate endocrine HTN.

Retinal Examination

To detect end organ damage, a relationship between HTN and elevated uric acid is suggested by cross-sectional data. It is also associated with other markers of CV risk.

Microalbuminuria

It should be differentiated from proteinuria in CKD, and it is a marker of HTN-related kidney injury and a predictor of CVD in adults.

Imaging

Renal ultrasonography, Doppler renal ultrasonography, CT angiography or MRA with magnetic resonance imaging should be performed when renovascular disease is suspected. Electrocardiography and echocardiography are to be done to detect target organ injury in heart as left ventricular hypertrophy (LVH) or concentric LVH (Table 4).

TABLE 4: Additional testing for children and adolescent with confirmed prehypertension or hypertension etiologies.

Target population	Recommended tests	Purpose
All children with confirmed hypertension	• Blood urea nitrogen and creatinine levels • Complete blood count • Electrolyte levels • Renal ultrasonography • Urinalysis • Urine culture	Rule out underlying renal disease
All children with confirmed hypertension	Fasting glucose level	Rule out diabetes mellitus or hyperlipidemia as comorbid risk factors for cardiovascular disease
Overweight children with prehypertension	Fasting lipid panel	
All children with confirmed hypertension	Echocardiography	Identify target organ damage, including left ventricular hypertrophy and pathologic vascular changes
Children with prehypertension and diabetes or renal disease	Retinal examination	
Children with prehypertension or hypertension and a history suggestive of sleep disorder	Polysomnography	Rule out obstructive sleep apnea
Children with prehypertension or hypertension and a history suggestive of substance use	Drug screen	Rule out underlying substances contributing to or causing elevated blood pressure

HYPERTENSION AND TARGET ORGAN DAMAGE

Hypertension in children and adolescents if left untreated for longer period can cast an impact on many organs and can be linked to future target organ damage. The most prominent clinical evidence of end organ damage in children is LVH along with other intermediate markers of target organ damage like thickening of carotid vessel wall, retinal vascular changes, and patients with severe HTN are also at increased risk of developing hypertensive encephalopathy, seizure, cerebrovascular accidents and congestive heart failure. There is now substantial evidence linking childhood HTN to long-term CV risk and adverse outcomes in adulthood. So every hypertensive child or adolescent should essentially be assessed for any target organ changes.[13]

CONCLUSION

On a population level, HTN in childhood and adolescents is very well-established entity now. It is quite possible that the percentile currently used to define HTN and elevated HTN in childhood underestimate the longitudinal risk. The new AAP guidelines provide an evidence-based approach to the diagnosis, evaluation, and management of abnormal BP values in children and adolescents. Considering the rates of HTN above 3% in asymptomatic children and adolescents, extensive screening programs should be done at school levels also. Increasing obesity linked with HTN in children and adolescents is a rising health concern, that should also be taken seriously. Promoting lifestyle modification by increasing physical activity and well-balanced diet, obesity and thus HTN can be prevented and treated without any additional pharmacological intervention. To attain therapeutic goals, involvement of family and their proper education is necessary. For both clinical and public health benefit, timely identification, examination, and treatment of children with high risk BP is an important step in reducing the excessive future burden of CVD.[9]

REFERENCES

1. Lauer RM, Clarke WR. Childhood risk factors for high adult blood pressure: the Muscatine Study. Pediatrics. 1989;84(4):633-41.
2. Falkner B. Hypertension in children and adolescents: epidemiology and natural History. Pediatr Nephrol. 2010; 25(7):1219-24.
3. Sorof JM, Lai D, Turner J, et al. Overweight, ethnicity, and the prevalence of hypertension in school-aged children. Pediatrics. 2004;113(3 pt 1):475-82.
4. Flynn JT, Kaelber DC, Baker-Smith CM, et al. Clinical practice guideline for screening and management of high blood pressure in children and adolescents. Pediatrics. 2017;140(3): pii:e20171904.
5. Luma GB, Spiotta RT. Hypertension in children and adolescents. Am Fam Physician. 2006;3(9):1558-68.
6. Kaelber DC, Flynn JT. AAP Issues New Pediatric Hypertension Clinical Practice Guideline. AAP Gateway. 2017. [online] Available from http://www.aappublications.org/news/2017/08/21/BloodPressure082117. [Last Accessed January, 2019].
7. Mayo Foundation for Medical Education and Research (MFMER). High Blood Pressure in Children, 1998-2018. [online] Available from https://www.mayoclinic.org/diseases-conditions/high-blood-pressure-in-children/diagnosis-treatment/drc-20373446. [Last Accessed January, 2019].
8. Update on the 1987 Task Force Report on High Blood Pressure in Children and Adolescents: a working group report from the National High Blood Pressure Education Program. National High Blood Pressure Education Program Working Group on Hypertension Control in Children and Adolescents. Pediatrics. 1996;98(4 Pt 1):649-58.
9. Samuels J, Samuel J. New guidelines for hypertension in children and adolescents. J Clin Hypertens (Greenwich). 2018;20(5):837-9.
10. Riley M, Bluhm B. High blood pressure in children and adolescents. Am Fam Physician. 2012;85(7):693-700.
11. Mattoo TK, Stapleton FB, Fulton DR, Kim MS. Definition and Diagnosis of Hypertension in Children and Adolescents. 2018. [online] Available from https://www.uptodate.com/contents/definition-and-diagnosis-of-hypertension-in-children-and-adolescents. [Last Accessed January, 2019].
12. Chobanian AV, Bakris GL, Black HR, et al. The Seventh Report of the Joint National Committee on Prevention, Detection, Evaluation, and Treatment of High Blood Pressure: the JNC 7 report. JAMA. 2003;289(19):2560-72.
13. National High Blood Pressure Education Program Working Group on High Blood Pressure in Children and Adolescents. The fourth report on the diagnosis, evaluation, and treatment of high blood pressure in children and adolescents. Pediatrics. 2004;114(2 Suppl 4th Report):555-76.
14. Flynn JT, Kaelber DC, Baker-Smith CM, et al. Clinical Practice Guideline for Screening and Management of High Blood Pressure in Children and Adolescents. Pediatrics. 2017;140(3):pii:e20171904.

Hypertension in Pregnancy

AN Rai, Mritunjay Kumar Singh

■ INTRODUCTION

Hypertension (HTN) complicates 10–15% of pregnancies worldwide; making it one of the major causes of maternal and perinatal morbidity and mortality worldwide. The distinction between pregnancy-induced hypertension and chronic hypertension is essential for optimal management. With appropriate prenatal care and careful observation of women for signs of pre-eclampsia and then timely delivery to terminate the pregnancy has reduced the number and extent of adverse outcomes, serious maternal—fetal morbidity and mortality. Hypertensive disorder of pregnancy is also associated with negative long term impacts on mother and child.[1]

■ DEFINITION AND CLASSIFICATION OF HYPERTENSIVE DISORDERS IN PREGNANCY

Hypertension in pregnancy is defined as a systolic blood pressure (SBP) more than or equal to 140 mm Hg and/or a diastolic blood pressure (DBP) more than or equal to 90 mm Hg (average of at least 2 measurements taken at least 4 h apart).

- Pregnancy-induced hypertension (>20 weeks of gestation)
  - Gestational HTN[2]
  - Pre-eclampsia:
    - Mild
    - Severe
  - Eclampsia
- Chronic prepregnancy hypertension (<20 weeks of gestation)
- Chronic hypertension with superimposed pre-eclampsia or eclampsia.

■ PREGNANCY-INDUCED HYPERTENSION

Gestational hypertension (GHTN) is characterized by new onset hypertension after 20 weeks of gestation, often near-term, in absence of accompanying proteinuria. Although GHTN usually is benign in nature, but some of these cases may convert into pre-eclampsia or chronic hypertension.

Management of Gestational Hypertension[3]

- Nonsevere hypertension (BP 140–159/90–109 mm Hg) in pregnancy:
  - Start single antihypertensive drug therapy (target DBP <85 mm Hg)

TABLE 1: Drugs used for severe hypertension in pregnancy.

Drug	Dose	Comments
Labetalol	10–20 mg IV, then 20–80 mg every 20–30 min to a maximum dose of 300 mg or Constant infusion 1–2 mg/min IV	Considered a first-line agent Tachycardia is less common and fewer adverse effects Contraindicated in patients with asthma, heart disease, or congestive heart failure
Hydralazine	5 mg IV or IM, then 5–10 mg IV every 20–40 min or Constant infusion 0.5–10 mg/h	Higher or frequent dosage associated with maternal hypotension, headaches and fetal distress—may be more common than other agents
Nifedipine	10–20 mg orally, repeat in 30 min if needed; then 10–20 mg every 2–6 h	May observe reflex tachycardia and headaches

(IV: intravenously; IM: intramuscularly)

- o Maternal, fetal and placental assessment
- o Regular BP monitoring.
- Severe hypertension (BP >160/110 mm Hg) in pregnancy: It is associated with significantly worse maternal and perinatal outcomes, independent of the development of pre-eclampsia and requires urgent pharmacotherapy (Table 1).

Antihypertensive Medications Commonly used in Pregnancy[4]

- *First-line drugs*—oral labetalol, oral methyldopa, long-acting oral nifedipine, or other oral β-blockers (acebutolol, metoprolol, pindolol and propranolol)
- *Second-line drugs*—clonidine, hydralazine and thiazide diuretics
- Angiotensin-converting enzyme (ACE) inhibitors (Grade C) and angiotensin receptor blockers (Grade D) should not be used in pregnant women.

Pre-eclampsia

Pre-eclampsia is the most frequently encountered renal complication of pregnancy. It is characterized by the new onset hypertension (≥140/90 mm Hg after 20 weeks of pregnancy) and proteinuria (>300 mg on 24 h urine collection or +1 on dipstick or protein/creatinine ≥0.3) or in the absence of proteinuria, new onset hypertension with new onset of any one of the following:

- *Thrombocytopenia*—platelet count less than 100,000/μL
- *Renal insufficiency*—serum creatinine above 1.1 mg/dL or doubling of serum creatinine in absence of renal disease
- *Liver dysfunction*—doubling of transaminase level
- Pulmonary edema
- Cerebral or visual symptoms.

Features of Severe Pre-eclampsia

In patients with pre-eclampsia, severe pre-eclampsia can be diagnosed if any of the following criteria is present:

- *Blood pressure*—More than or equal to 160/110 mm Hg on two separate occasions 4 hours apart
- *Thrombocytopenia*—platelet count less than 100,000/μL
- *Renal insufficiency*—serum creatinine above 1.1 mg/dL or doubling of serum creatinine in absence of renal disease or oliguria <500 mL/24 h
- *Liver dysfunction*—doubling of transaminase level or severe right upper quadrant pain or epigastric pain without alternative diagnosis

- Proteinuria above 5 g/24 h
- Pulmonary edema
- Cerebral or visual symptoms
- Serum lactate dehydrogenase above 600 IU/mL.

Pathogenesis

Pre-eclampsia occurs only in presence of the placenta and usually remits when placenta is delivered. The placenta in pre-eclampsia is hypoperfused and ischemic. Pre-eclampsia is characterized by widespread vascular endotheliosis and macroangiopathy in mother induced by circulating factors produced by abnormal placenta. Fetus is immune to the factors shown in Flowchart 1.

Risk Factors for the Development of Pre-eclampsia

- Pre-eclampsia in prior pregnancy
- Family history of pre-eclampsia
- Nulliparity
- Multiple gestation
- Older maternal age
- Molar pregnancy
- Obesity
- Pre-existing hypertension
- Pre-existing chronic kidney disease
- Diabetes mellitus
- Thrombotic vascular disease
- Trisomy 13 fetus
- Fetal hydrops
- High altitude.

Management

- Mild pre-eclampsia:
  - If immature fetus, bed rest mainly in lateral decubitus position
  - Hypertension therapy, if needed
- Severe pre-eclampsia:
  - Admit to labor and delivery area
  - Maternal and fetal evaluation for 24 hours
  - Magnesium sulfate for 24 hours

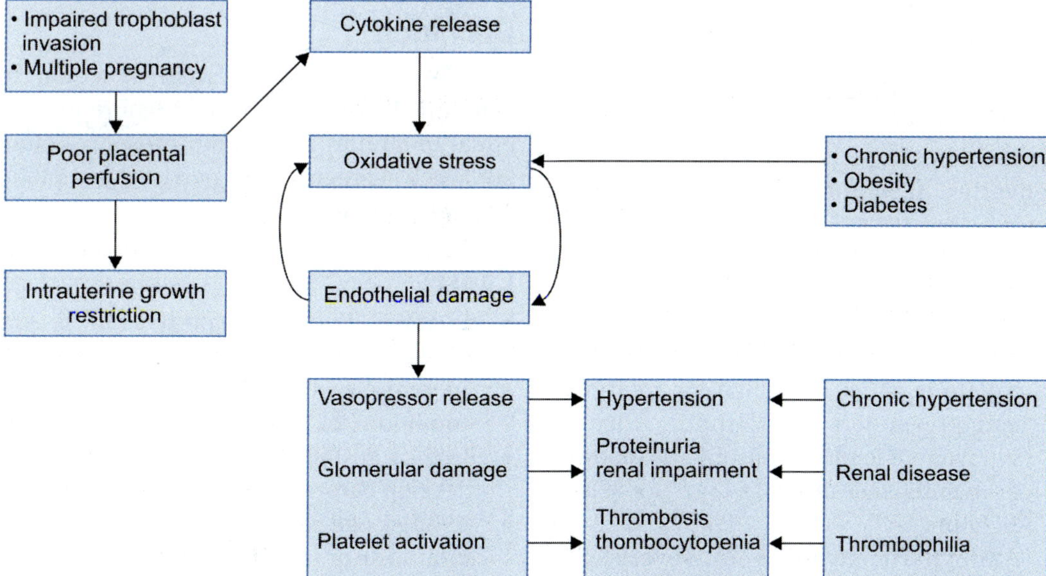

Flowchart 1: Pathogenesis of pre-eclampsia.

- o Antihypertensive if BP more than or equal to 160/110 mm Hg or MAP (mean arterial pressure) more than 125 mm Hg
- o Steroids are indicated in severe intrauterine growth retardation or if gestational age is above 23 weeks.

Prevention of Pre-eclampsia

Low dose aspirin (75–150 mg daily) in high risk persons has shown to reduce the occurrence of pre-eclampsia. Oral calcium supplementation may reduce the likelihood of pre-eclampsia in women whose calcium intake is very low. Vitamin C/E do not protect against pre-eclampsia.

Late Complication of Pre-eclampsia

Several studies have shown that persons with pre-eclampsia have increased risk of cardiovascular disease in later years. And experts suggest yearly evaluation of such persons for blood pressure, lipid profile, blood sugar and body mass index. Healthy lifestyle should also be encouraged in such persons.

Eclampsia

Eclampsia is defined as presence of new onset grand mal seizure in a woman with pre-eclampsia. It occurs in 0.5–4% of deliveries. Eclamptic seizures can occur before labor (25%), during labor (50%) and after delivery (25%).

Management

- *Anticonvulsant therapy*: Magnesium sulfate is agent of choice for treatment and prevention of eclamptic seizures. Intravenous loading dose of 4–6 g, followed by maintenance dose of 1–2 g/h for at least 24 hours.
- Antihypertensives as in severe pre-eclampsia.
- *Definitive treatment*: Delivery following stabilization.

◼ HELLP SYNDROME

The term "HELLP syndrome" is an acronym for the following presentation: Hemolysis, elevated liver enzymes and low platelet count. HELLP syndrome may occur antepartum or postpartum. This syndrome is associated with increased maternal morbidity and mortality; many experts consider this syndrome to be an indication for prompt delivery.

Management

- Initial maternal stabilization followed by delivery is the cornerstone of management
- Platelet transfusion before or after delivery if platelet count is below $20,000/mm^3$ (advised at $<50,000/mm^3$ before cesarean section)
- Before 32 weeks gestation—short course of corticosteroids for fetal lung maturation and improving maternal platelet count may be a viable option.

◼ CHRONIC HYPERTENSION IN PREGNANCY

Definition

Systolic pressure more than or equal to 140 mm Hg, diastolic pressure more than or equal to 90 mm Hg or both presents before 20th week of pregnancy or persists longer than 12 week postpartum.

Causes

- *Primary*: "Essential Hypertension" in 90% of cases
- *Secondary*: Result of other medical condition (i.e. renal disease)
- 15% of gestational HTN cases go on to develop chronic HTN
- 25% risk of developing superimposed pre-eclampsia or eclampsia
- Close monitoring of maternal BP and encouraged to increase the amount of rest.

Prenatal Care for Chronic Hypertensive

- Electrocardiogram should be obtained in women with long-standing hypertension
- *Baseline laboratory tests includes*: Urinalysis, urine culture and serum creatinine, glucose and electrolytes
- Tests to rule out renal diseases, and identify comorbidities such as diabetes mellitus
- Women with proteinuria on a urine dipstick should have a quantitative for urine protein.

Management

- Avoid treatment in women with uncomplicated mild essential HTN as blood pressure may decrease as pregnancy progresses[5]
- May taper or discontinue medicines for women with blood pressure less than 120/80 in 1st trimester
- Reinstitute or initiate therapy for persistent diastolic pressure more than 95 mm Hg, systolic pressure more than 150 mm Hg, or signs of hypertensive end-organ damage
- *Medication of choices*: Oral methyldopa and labetalol.

Highlights

- Occurs in 10–15% of pregnancies
- Diagnosed when BP reads more than 140/90 mm Hg
- Pre-eclampsia means GHTN plus proteinuria
- Protein level above 300 mg/24 h urine sample
- If left untreated, it results in eclampsia (with seizure)
- HELLP syndrome is a complication of pre-eclampsia
- Treatment option includes rest or hospitalization, fetal monitoring, laboratory testing and antihypertensive (methyldopa/hydralazine/labetalol).

■ CONCLUSION

- PIH occurs in 10–15% of pregnancies
- Diagnosed when BP reads more than 140/90 mm Hg
- Pre-eclampsia means GHTN plus proteinuria
- Protein level above 300 mg/24 h urine sample
- If left untreated, it results in eclampsia (with seizure)
- HELLP syndrome is a complication of pre-eclampsia
- Treatment option includes rest or hospitalization, fetal monitoring, laboratories testing and antihypertensive (methyldopa/hydralazine/labetalol).

■ REFERENCES

1. Beckmann CR, Ling FW, Smith RP, Barzansky BM, Herbert WN, Laube DW. Obstetrics and Gynecology, 5th edition. Baltimore, MD: Lippincott Williams & Wilkins; 2006. pp. 188-96.
2. Magloire L, Fuai MF. (2011). Gestational Hypertension. [online] Available from: https://www.uptodate.com/contents/gestational-hypertension. [Last Accessed January, 2019].
3. August P. (2011). Management of Hypertension in Pregnancy and Postpartum Women. [online] Available from: https://www.uptodate.com/contents/management-of-hypertension-in-pregnant-and-postpartum-women. [Last Accessed January, 2019].
4. Bansode BR. (2012). Medicine Update. The Association of Physicians of India. [online] Available from: https://www.apiindia.org. [Last Accessed January, 2019].
5. Butalia S, Audibert F, Côté AM, et al. Hypertension Canada's 2018 Guidelines for the Management of Hypertension in Pregnancy. Can J Cardiol. 2018;34(5):526-31.

Metabolic Syndrome and Hypertension

Anandakumar Amutha, Rajendra Pradeepa, V Mohan

■ INTRODUCTION

Hypertension (HTN) has become a global health issue. Since the disorder remains undiagnosed for a long time, it leads to complications like kidney failure and heart disease. The term metabolic syndrome (MS) is used to refer to a clustering of metabolic risk factors including central obesity, glucose intolerance, hyperinsulinemia, low HDL cholesterol, high triglycerides and HTN. The HTN is also one of the components of MS and is present in more than 80% of patients with MS.[1] The last two decades have seen the emergence of intensified research to investigate ethnic differences in the prevalence of MS and its association with two specific clinical endpoints namely type 2 diabetes mellitus and coronary heart disease (CHD). MS is well recognized as a risk factor for cardiovascular disease (CVD) and cardiovascular mortality.[2] Estimates of MS vary by country, but generally a higher prevalence of MS is seen in non-European groups such as South Asians, Black African-Carribeans, Hispanics and Aboriginals, with significantly lower prevalence in European Whites, Chinese and Japanese.

Hypertension is one of the major components of MS. Recently, the prevalence of HTN has increased and this might be due to the rapid epidemiological transition which occurred over the last 40 years. HTN affects approximately 1 billion individuals worldwide and is an important worldwide public-health challenge. Existing data suggests that the prevalence of HTN has remained stable or has decreased in economically developed countries during the past decade, while it has increased in developing countries.[3] However, the increase in the prevalence rates of HTN needs to be quantified so as to plan for effective prevention strategies which are urgently needed in developing countries like India.

■ BURDEN OF HYPERTENSION

The increase in HTN is expected to disproportionately affect developing nations, with an approximately 89% estimated increase in sub-Saharan Africa from 2000 through 2025 versus a 24% increase in more developed countries. HTN is one of the most common cardiovascular ailments in South Asian countries. The definitions of HTN given by Joint National Committee on Prevention, Detection, Evaluation and Treatment of High Blood Pressure (JNC 7) classification[4] are given here.

Hypertension is defined as systolic blood pressure (BP) level of more than or equal to 140 mm Hg and/or diastolic BP level of more than or equal to 90 mm Hg or being diagnosed as hypertensive by any physician previously. This definition has been modified in JNC 8,[5] where 60 years aged and older individuals have a slightly higher cut off as 150/90 to start pharmacotherapy.

Prehypertension is defined as the area falling between 120 and 139 mm Hg systolic BP and 80–89 mm Hg diastolic BP.

Stage 1 HTN is defined as having a systolic BP 140–159 mm Hg and diastolic BP 90–99 mm Hg.

Stage 2 HTN is defined as having a systolic BP more than or equal to 160 mm Hg and diastolic BP more than or equal to 100 mm Hg.

Prevalence of Hypertension in India

Several studies have reported on the prevalence of HTN from India. As early as 1954, a prevalence of 4% was reported using criteria of more than 160/95 from Kanpur. Later, the prevalence increased during the years 1984–87 to 11% by using JNC V criteria. A higher prevalence of 69% and 55% was recorded among elderly populations aged 60 and above in the urban and rural areas, respectively.[6] Mohan et al. (2001) from urban Chennai, reported 8.4% and 15% prevalence of HTN in adults aged more than 20 years and above in those who belong to the low and middle socio economic group, respectively.[7] A study conducted in the urban areas of Chennai (age group ≥40) reported a higher prevalence of HTN (54%) among low income group and 40% prevalence among high-income group.[8] Misra et al. (2001) reported that in Delhi slums, the prevalence of HTN was 12%.[9]

A region-specific (urban and rural parts of North, East, West and South India) systematic review and meta-analysis reported that about 33% urban and 25% rural Indians are hypertensive. Among them, only 25% rural and 42% urban Indians are aware of their hypertensive status and only 25% rural and 38% of urban Indians are being treated for HTN only. Overall, only one tenth of rural and one fifth of urban Indian hypertensive population have their BP under control.[10]

Gupta et al. (2017) evaluated the trends in HTN prevalence, awareness, treatment and control in an Indian urban population over 25 years.[11] HTN prevalence, awareness, treatment, and control rates are increasing among urban populations in India and better awareness is associated with greater control. A recent study by Shika Singh et al. (2017), in urban Varanasi reported that around one-third of the subjects were hypertensive and half of the study subjects were prehypertensive.[12] Among the study population, the levels of awareness, treatment and control of high BP was very low.

A cross-sectional study conducted in ten Indian states (Screening India's Twin Epidemic (SITE)) showed that among 15,662 subjects, overall 46% had HTN according to JNC 7 report guidelines. Among them, 22.2% were newly diagnosed and 60.1% had prehypertension.[13] In phase I of the Indian Council of Medical Research-India Diabetes (ICMR-INDIAB) study, individuals aged more than or equal to 20 years were surveyed using a stratified multistage sampling design, in three states (Tamil Nadu, Maharashtra and Jharkhand) and one union territory (Chandigarh) of India. BP was measured in all study subjects (n = 14,059). HTN was defined as systolic BP more than or equal to 140 mm Hg, and/or diastolic BP more than or equal to 90 mm Hg and/or use of antihypertensive drugs. Overall age-standardized prevalence of HTN was 26.3% (self-reported: 5.5%; newly detected: 20.8%). Urban residents of Tamil Nadu, Jharkhand, Chandigarh and Maharashtra (31.5, 28.9, 30.7 and 28.1%) had significantly higher prevalence of HTN compared with rural residents (26.2, 21.7, 19.8 and 24.0%, respectively). Figure 1

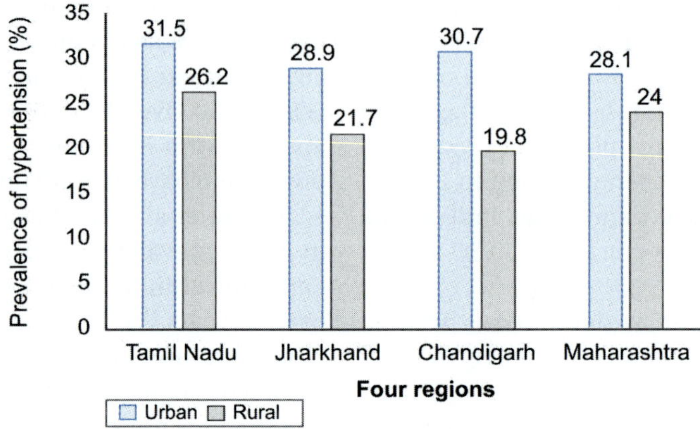

Fig. 1: Prevalence of hypertension in phase 1 of the ICMR-INDIAB (Indian Council of Medical Research-India Diabetes) Study (Bhansali et al. 2015).

shows the prevalence of HTN in phase I of the ICMR-INDIAB study.[14]

Joshi et al. (2012) reported that a positive association (p <0.05) was observed between HTN and age, familial history of cardiovascular disorders, alcohol consumption and diet. In the INDIAB study, Bhansali et al. (2015) reported that age, male gender, urban residence, generalized obesity, diabetes, physical inactivity and alcohol consumption were significantly associated with HTN. Also, salt intake more than or equal to 6.5 g/day showed significantly higher risk for HTN.

■ DEFINITION OF METABOLIC SYNDROME

Unfortunately, there is no internationally agreed definition for MS and hence estimates of MS vary substantially across populations depending on the criteria used. The World Health Organization (WHO) proposed a definition of MS in 1999 and the National Cholesterol Education Program (NCEP) Expert Panel and Adult Treatment Panel III (ATP III) published a working definition in 2001. The International Diabetes Federation (IDF) Consensus group proposed yet another definition in 2005. While most definitions agree on essential components, i.e. glucose intolerance, obesity, HTN and dyslipidemia, they differ in the cut points for criteria of each component of the cluster and the way of combining them to define MS.

Discussions held by IDF and AHA/NHLBI representatives resolved the differences between definitions of metabolic syndrome. In this harmonizing criteria, abdominal obesity need not be a prerequisite for diagnosis but it is just one of five criteria.[15] Presence of any three of five risk factors constitutes a diagnosis of metabolic syndrome. Table 1 presents the criteria for diagnosis of metabolic syndrome using this harmonizing criteria.

Prevalence of Metabolic Syndrome

Several epidemiological studies have confirmed the prevalence of MS in various ethnic groups like Africans, Latin Americans, Chinese, Asian Indians, Australians and Polynesians. The prevalence of the MS varies from 13% in China to 30% in Iran. In a survey in Singapore, the prevalence of the MS varied between the three major ethnic groups— Chinese (15%), Malays (19%) and Indians (20%). All these studies have used either WHO or ATP III criteria for defining the MS.

TABLE 1: Harmonizing criteria for diagnosis of metabolic syndrome (Alberti et al. 2009).[15]

S. No.	Measure*	Categorical cut points
1.	Elevated waist circumference	Population and country specific definitions (>90 cm for males and >80 cm for females for South Asian Indians)
2.	Elevated triglycerides (drug treatment for elevated triglycerides is an alternate indicator)	≥150 mg/dL (1.7 mmol/L)
3.	Reduced HDL-C (drug treatment for reduced HDL-C is an alternate indicator)	<40 mg/dL (1.0 mmol/L) in males <50 mg/dL (1.3 mmol/L) in females
4.	Elevated blood pressure (antihypertensive drug treatment in a patient with a history of hypertension is an alternate indicator)	Systolic BP ≥130 and/or diastolic BP ≥85 mm Hg
5.	Elevated fasting glucose (drug treatment of elevated glucose is an alternate indicator)	≥100 mg/dL

*Any three of five criteria if present, constitutes metabolic syndrome.
(BP: blood pressure; HDL-C: high-density lipoprotein cholesterol)

In the Finn Diane study the overall prevalence of MS was 38% in men and 40% in women according to NCEP diagnostic criteria. A study from Spain reported the prevalence of MS as 31.9%. According to WHO criteria, the prevalence of MS in type 1 diabetes mellitus (T1DM) was found to be 30.7% in Scotland whereas in South India the prevalence of MS in T1DM was 22.2% using harmonizing criteria.[16] The earliest study done by ICMR task force study on prevalence of MS in India reported that the prevalence was 30% in the urban areas of Delhi and 11% in rural Haryana during 1992–94 using ATP III criteria.

Ramachandran et al. in 2003 using a modified ATP III criteria documented a higher prevalence of MS (41%). Deepa et al. in 2002 reported 11.2% prevalence in urban Chennai during 1996–97. Gupta et al. in 2004 reported 25% prevalence using ATP III criteria in Jaipur. Misra et al. carried out a study among the urban slum population in Delhi, reported 30% prevalence of MS. In hypertensive population, the prevalence of MS seems to be very high. In a study of more than 19,000 hypertensive patients attending primary care centers in Spain, MS was present in more than 40% of subjects using the original ATP III definition and it increased to 60% when the IDF criteria were applied.

CONSEQUENCES OF HYPERTENSION AND METABOLIC SYNDROME

By 2020, CVD will become the leading cause of death and disability worldwide. In developing countries, CVD represents up to 75% of deaths from noncommunicable diseases and already accounts for 10% of the developing world's burden of disability. A large cross sectional study from Chennai population reported that nearly 40% of the elderly urban south Indians have MS and it was strongly associated with coronary artery disease.

The Second National Health and Nutrition Examination Survey showed that patients with the MS had a higher risk for cardiovascular death, coronary heart disease and stroke. Furthermore, the higher the number of metabolic abnormalities, the higher the incidence of CVD mortality. More recently, an analysis of data from the Atherosclerosis Risk in Communities study showed that individuals who have the MS without diabetes or CVD still have, poor cardiovascular outcomes.

PREVENTION AND MANAGEMENT OF HYPERTENSION AND METABOLIC SYNDROME

Due to the increased risk of diabetes and CVD in people with the MS, there is an urgent need for strategies to prevent the emerging global epidemic of this condition. Although, there was marked increase in prevalence of HTN over two decades there was little improvement in its management.[17] The primary management goals of the MS are to reduce the risks of CVD and diabetes. Lifestyle modifications, including regular physical activity and even modest weight loss, could reduce the prevalence of the syndrome. Thus, community-wide efforts to change health behaviors are vital to decrease the death and disability resulting from the MS in developing countries.[18]

For management of HTN, WHO had given recommendations as described here.

Primary prevention is to reduce the risk factors which cause the incidence of disease in a population. If the prevention is started earlier, then it will be more effective in the reduction of disease condition. This can be done either by population strategy or in individuals using a high risk strategy. The aim of the population-based strategy is to bring down the average BP in a population which will eventually produce a larger reduction in the incidence of CVDs. This strategy involves a multifactorial approach like nutrition education [Dietary Approaches to Stop Hypertension (DASH) diet], weight reduction, promoting any form of physical activity, behavioral changes, health education, self-care, etc. The high-risk strategy involves the detection of high risk individuals

in families and bringing down their BP and screening them annually to know the status of their condition. By doing this, early intervention could be done to prevent them from developing end stage complications.[19]

Secondary prevention is done once the disease condition has been detected. The affected individuals need to be advised regarding pharmacotherapy, diet and lifestyle management. All individuals should be compliant in taking medications and adhere to follow the specified diet pattern and able to make lifestyle changes.[19]

The main aim of treatment is to reduce the risk of CVD and hence along with appropriate antihypertensive treatment, lifestyle interventions like weight reduction through calorie restricted diet and energy expenditure through physical inactivity should be achieved. To achieve long-term effectiveness, patients should be able to restrict calories of 500–1,000 kcal/day with at least 7–10% weight loss in a year and daily exercise of 30–45 minutes. More intensive exercise programs may have cardiovascular benefits for maintaining body weight. Lifestyle interventions clearly have beneficial effects on BP and lipid profile and also help to reduce the incidence of new-onset diabetes. Moreover, recent data suggest a long-term effect on reduction in cardiovascular morbidity.

Other lifestyle changes related to food selection and diet pattern also have a beneficial effect on certain cardiovascular risk factors and should be encouraged in high risk patients. Lowering salt intake and alcohol consumption has moderate BP-lowering effects, which are enhanced in conjunction with weight loss and increased exercise. A diet rich in fruits, vegetables and low-fat dairy products (DASH diet) substantially lowers BP in comparison with the standard American diet. The Mediterranean diet, which is rich in fruits, vegetables, fish and olive oil, also has a favorable impact on atherogenic dyslipidemia in MS patients. However, pharmacological treatment of BP, dyslipidemia, insulin resistance and obesity will be required in order for most patients to reduce their cardio-metabolic risk.

Mechanism Linking Hypertension and Metabolic Syndrome

Visceral obesity, insulin resistance, oxidative stress, endothelial dysfunction, activated renin–angiotensin system, increased inflammatory mediators and obstructive sleep apnea have been proposed as possible link between MS and HTN. These factors may induce sympathetic overactivity, vasoconstriction, increased intravascular fluid and decreased vasodilatation, leading to development of HTN in those with MS.[20] Flowchart 1 shows the linkage mechanisms between metabolic syndrome and HTN.

Metabolic syndrome in hypertensive patients needs to be treated aggressively including lifestyle changes, treating metabolic risk factors as well in order to reduce cardiovascular risk. Drugs like ACE inhibitor and angiotensin receptor blocker should be given preference as they have protective effect on newly diagnosed diabetes.[21] A patient centric approach for the HTN and MS includes modification of unhealthy lifestyle that aggravates the underlying pathology. The treatment includes sodium and calorie restriction, alcohol and smoking cessation, weight reduction and increased physical activity and use of medication wherever indicated.

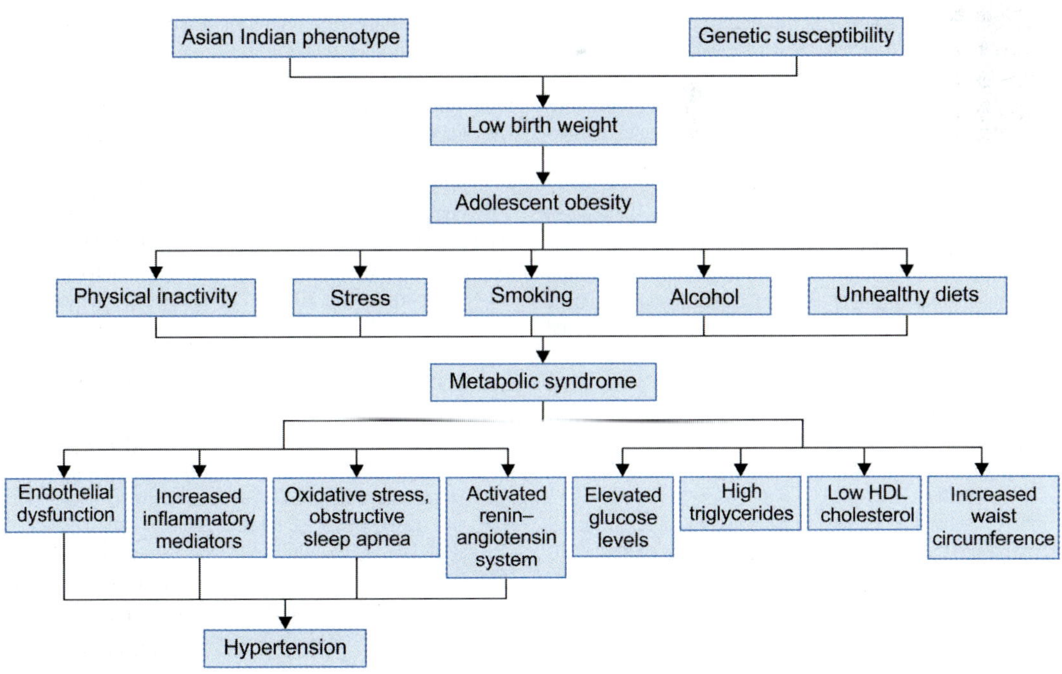

Flowchart 1: Mechanism linking metabolic syndrome and hypertension in Asian Indians.

■ CONCLUSION

Prevention of metabolic syndrome and hypertension are the need of the hour as they pose increased risk for diabetes and CVD. Strategies like lifestyle modification, including regular physical activity, weight loss and healthy eating behaviors could help reduce the prevalence of MS. Since Asian Indians have a stronger genetic predisposition to diabetes and CVD, community wide efforts are necessary to reduce the morbidity and mortality resulting from MS and hypertension.

■ REFERENCES

1. Duvnjak L, Bulum T, Metelko Ž. Hypertension and the metabolic syndrome. Diabetologia Croatica. 2008;37(4): 83-9.
2. Isomaa B, Almgren P, Tuomi T, et al. Cardiovascular morbidity and mortality associated with the metabolic syndrome. Diabetes Care. 2001;24(4):683-9.
3. Kearney PM, Whelton M, Reynolds K, et al. Worldwide prevalence of hypertension: a systematic review. J Hypertens. 2004;22(1):11-9.
4. Chobanian AV, Bakris GL, Black HR, et al. The Seventh Report of the Joint National Committee on Prevention, Detection, Evaluation, and Treatment of High Blood Pressure: the JNC 7 report. JAMA. 2003;289(19):2560-72.
5. Page MR. The JNC 8 hypertension guidelines: an in-depth guide. Am J Manag Care. 2014;20(Spec No. 1):E8.
6. Hypertension Study Group. Prevalence, Awareness, treatment and control of hypertension among the elderly in Bangladesh and India: a multicentric study. Bull World Health Organ. 2001;79(6):490-500.
7. Mohan V, Shanthirani S, Deepa R, et al. Chennai Urban Population Study (CUPS No. 4). Intra-urban differences in the prevalence of the metabolic syndrome in southern India—the Chennai Urban Population Study (CUPS No. 4). Diabet Med. 2001;18(4):280-7.
8. Ramachandran A, Snehalatha C, Vijay V, et al. Impact of poverty on the prevalence of diabetes and its complications in urban southern India. Diabet Med. 2002;19(2):130-5.
9. Misra A, Pandey RM, Devi JR, et al. High prevalence of diabetes, obesity and dyslipidemia in urban slum population in northern India. Int J Obes Relat Metab Disord. 2001;25(11):1722-9.
10. Anchala R, Kannuri NK, Pant H, et al. Hypertension in India: a systematic review and meta-analysis of prevalence, awareness, and control of hypertension. J Hypertens. 2014;32(6):1170-7.
11. Gupta R, Gupta VP, Prakash H, et al. 25-Year trends in hypertension prevalence, awareness, treatment, and control in an Indian urban population: Jaipur Heart Watch. Indian Heart J. 2017;70(6):1-6.
12. Singh S, Shankar R, Singh GP. Prevalence and associated risk factors of hypertension: a cross-sectional study in urban Varanasi. Int J Hypertens. 2017;2017:5491838.
13. Joshi SR, Saboo B, Vadivale M, et al. SITE Investigators. Prevalence of diagnosed and undiagnosed diabetes and hypertension in India—results from the Screening India's Twin Epidemic (SITE) study. Diabetes Technol Ther. 2012;14(1):8-15.
14. Bhansali A, Dhandania VK, Deepa M, et al. Prevalence of and risk factors for hypertension in urban and rural India: the ICMR-INDIAB study. J Hum Hypertens. 2015;29(3):204-9.
15. Alberti KG, Eckel RH, Grundy SM, et al. Harmonizing the metabolic syndrome: a joint interim statement of the International Diabetes Federation Task Force on Epidemiology and Prevention; National Heart, Lung, and Blood Institute; American Heart Association; World Heart Federation; International Atherosclerosis Society; and International Association for the Study of Obesity.
16. Billow A, Anjana RM, Ngai M, et al. Prevalence and clinical profile of metabolic syndrome among type 1 diabetes mellitus patients in southern India. J Diabetes Complications. 2015;29(5):659-64.
17. Roy A, Praveen PA, Amarchand R, et al. Changes in hypertension prevalence, awareness, treatment and control rates over 20 years in National Capital Region of India: results from a repeat cross-sectional study. BMJ Open. 2017;7(7):e015639.
18. Mohan V, Deepa M. The metabolic syndrome in developing countries. Diabetes Voice. 2006;51:15-7.
19. Muruganathan A. Dean's Oration. Hypertension in India: the way forward. Hypertension. 2017;1:293-8.
20. Yanai H, Tomono Y, Ito K, et al. The underlying mechanisms for development of hypertension in the metabolic syndrome. Nutr J. 2008;7:10.
21. Ratto E, Leoncini G, Viazzi F, et al. Metabolic syndrome and cardiovascular risk in primary hypertension. J Am Soc Nephrol. 2006;17(4 Suppl 2):S120-2.

White Coat Hypertension and Masked Hypertension

Sasidharan PK, Arathi N

INTRODUCTION

Hypertension is a well-known risk factor for cardiovascular diseases since long. In the 1940s, it was shown that blood pressure (BP) measured at home by family member could be as much as 30 mm Hg lower than readings taken by physicians at their office.[1] The concept of casual and basal blood pressure (BBP) was introduced in the 1940s, in which it was shown that when people were allowed to relax for 90 minutes the BP might be 20–30 mm Hg lower than when first recorded. In this study, the casual blood pressure (CBP) was defined as the initial BP taken without any rest and the BBP was the minimum value obtained after a prolonged period of rest. It was found in this study that the BBP was a better predictor of cardiovascular risk.[2] For clinical practice, hypertension has always been defined by an arbitrary threshold, based on the casual measurements above which an individual is identified as being hypertensive, and below which they are classified as normotensive. A major implication of this is that anyone who tends to exhibit an exaggerated increase of pressure during the clinic measurement will be labeled as hypertensive.[3]

The terms white coat hypertension and masked hypertension refers to the variability of a patients' BP measurements between the physician's office and the patients' home environment. A patient with white coat hypertension has high BP levels in the physician's office and normal BP in their typical environment. Masked hypertension on the other hand is the situation where the BP is normal when measured at the physician's office, but is higher at the home environment. It is also termed as "Isolated home hypertension", "Isolated ambulatory hypertension", "Reverse white coat hypertension" and "White coat normotension".[4] White coat hypertension can lead to unnecessary drug prescription, but overall causes less harm to patients than sustained hypertension.[5] But several observations suggest that masked hypertension is not an innocent phenomenon, but has almost the similar risks for cardiovascular events as sustained hypertension.

WHITE COAT HYPERTENSION

White coat hypertension was first discovered by Riva Rocci in 1896, who described this phenomenon as an increase in BP experienced only during a physician's visit. This was not quantitatively researched until 1983, when the term "White Coat Syndrome" was first described in 1983 by Manacia et al, on the basis of continuous intra-arterial BP recordings, that the heart rate and the systolic as well as the diastolic blood pressure (DBP) rose when a doctor entered the patient's room.[6,7] White coat hypertension is a condition in which patients have high BP levels when they are measured at the physician's office, but normal BP levels during their daily lives and while in their home environment.[8,9]

These entities are now being recognized more with the availability of noninvasive method for continuous BP monitoring. For years, conventional clinic measurements alone were used for defining BP status. But it was found that a single clinic BP alone was not predictor of the cardiovascular outcomes. The papers on ambulatory BP measurements were first introduced by Sokolov et al. in 1960 and it was found to be a better predictor of cardiovascular outcomes as compared to CBP.[10,11]

White Coat Effect Versus White Coat Hypertension

Some authors use the terms white coat effect and white coat hypertension interchangeably.[5] The more distinctive term "Isolated Office Hypertension" has been suggested in order to minimize confusion with white coat effect.[8] The World Health Organization proposed the term "Isolated Clinic Hypertension" to describe those patients who have hypertension in the office, but normal ambulatory BP.[12] If one accepts isolated office hypertension as classical white coat hypertension, there will still be the need of a term to describe all other patients with a transient disparity between the office BP and ambulatory BP. White coat hypertension or isolated office hypertension is diagnosed when office BP is more than or equal to 140/90 mm Hg on at least three occasions, while the average day time or 24-hour BP is less than 135/85 mm Hg. Self-measurement of BP has been proposed

as a useful alternative to ambulatory blood pressure monitoring (ABPM) to measure the average day time BP.[8] On the other hand, the Eighth Joint National Committee in the United States maintains that hypertension should be treated pharmacologically in those individuals older than 60 years who have a BP measurement of 150/90 mm Hg or higher and those younger than 60 years with a BP of 140/90 mm Hg or higher.[13] White coat effect on the other hand, is defined as a "transient" elevation in the office BP measurement induced by an alerting response to a doctor or nurse.[5,8] It usually averages about 20/10 mm Hg with the maximal rise taking place 1–4 minutes after the doctor/nurses arrival, but can last up to 10–15 minutes only.[5] White coat effect, therefore, can occur in both normotensive and hypertensive individuals and is not substantially influenced by reassurance and familiarization with the technique of BP measurement.[5] The white coat effect can result in diagnosing a person as having essential hypertension when their daily blood pressures are within normal limits. These misdiagnosed patients are typically described as having white coat hypertension, which it is truly not.[14] A person with a high office BP and a large white coat effect may also show elevated average day time or 24-hour BP and thus have hypertension with white coat effect. "White coat hypertension" is a form of "white coat effect" with more sustained elevation of BP. The failure to adequately diagnose white coat hypertension with standardized measurements has led to inappropriate prescription and overuse of antihypertensive medications for individuals who are not persistently hypertensive.[15]

When to Suspect White Coat Hypertension?

None of the hypertension guidelines elaborate on how a practicing physician may suspect white coat hypertension. At the bed side the possibility of a white coat hypertension should be kept in mind in the clinical context of repeated office pressures in the hypertensive range for many years without any evidence of left ventricular hypertrophy, retinal changes or albuminuria. All these strongly indicate that the BP is not sustained.[16] Furthermore, in white coat hypertension, despite increasing the medication, generally little change is elicited in the office in the systolic and diastolic pressures. In true recalcitrant hypertension, the medication usually affects some lowering of BP though not to an acceptable level.[16] Also, office measurements of systolic pressure are known to quickly settle to reduced values on repeated estimation, whereas white coat systolic pressures tend to vary up and down by large amount on repeated measurements.[17] It should also be suspected in female sex, nonsmokers, recent onset hypertension, obesity, elderly, and when only one or two of BP measurements are made before diagnosis in the office environment.[17,18]

A "slow breathing test", causing a fall in BP after 1 minute of recording high BP, was supposed to indicate white coat hypertension. A rise in pressure determined by an unknown and unintroduced physician (The white coat test) or response to public speaking to an audience of strangers, also confirm the white coat diagnosis. None of these have become standards.[19,20]

Importance of Identifying White Coat Hypertension

This aspect is very important since the future management of the entity is dependent on its identification. Several studies have shown that people with raised office BP, but normal average BP on an ABPM, have risk of major cardiovascular events which is comparable to that of clinically normotensive subjects and the risks are less than those with sustained high BP.[21,22] But white coat hypertension has

been even shown to have greater prevalence of target organ damage and metabolic abnormalities than normotensive subjects.[23] Therefore, antihypertensive drug treatment should be instituted in patients with white coat hypertension when there is evidence of target organ damage or a high cardiovascular risk.[5,8] Therefore, identification of white coat hypertension should be followed by a search for metabolic risk factors and organ damage. Lifestyle intervention, close monitoring and regular assessment of risk factors are recommended for individuals with uncomplicated white coat hypertension not requiring pharmacological treatment.[5,8]

White coat effect does not predict future target organ damage or cardiovascular morbidity or mortality in most of the studies, but the contrary has been observed in two studies.[24-28] White coat effect and white coat hypertension affects 15–30% of presumable hypertensive individuals.[29] Some consider this as prehypertensive phase requiring more intense follow-up.[14,30-33]

Physiological Mechanism of White Coat Effect

A few authors believe that the white coat phenomenon is a common, periodic, neuro-endocrine reflex conditioned by anticipation of getting a high BP reading and the fear of what this measurement may indicate concerning future illness. It does not change with time or with prolonged association with the physician, particularly with advancing years, it may be even superimposed on essential hypertension.[16] The use of microneurography, which measures the sympathetic nerve traffic of skin and muscle, has shown that there is profound activation of skin nerves and associated inhibition of muscle nerve traffic, which were demonstrated in participants when physicians either took BP or physicians were present during these measurements.

This is similar to a defense reaction that has been demonstrated in animals when they are exposed to emotional stressors. These emotional factors like anxiety or stress may be responsible for the microneurographic response and the origin of white coat hypertension.[34,35] Patients with white coat hypertension have been shown to be more prone to higher levels of anxiety compared with both normotensive individuals.[36] However, research has also shown that patients who are prone to white coat hypertension do not hyper react to all emotional stimulus, but only to those associated with the physician's office or the physician.[37] Research by Ogedegbe et al. have suggested that those who experience white coat hypertension may have been classically conditioned to have high anxiety at physician's office as a result of negative or painful experiences with the medical office or the physician.[36] The patient's perception of their BP level has also been demonstrated to contribute to the situational anxious response. Labeling a patient as hypertensive solely based on office readings can have a negative effect on their BP levels, thus increasing the risk of demonstrating white coat hypertension in future office visits.[38] White coat hypertension based on ambulatory measurements was demonstrated most clearly in those participants who saw themselves as hypertensive during their office visit, regardless of whether their perceptions were medically correct or not.[38]

Diagnosis of White Coat Hypertension

Diagnosis of white coat hypertension requires preferentially, the use of ABPM. However, since the lack of clinical features is a characteristic of white coat hypertension, this factor restricts the use of ABPM as a diagnostic tool.[39,40] On the basis of obvious treatment implications, it is important for physicians to distinguish patients whose BP obtained in the clinic accurately reflect the actual BPs. In the recent years, 24-hour ambulatory monitoring of BP has become increasingly valuable in diagnosis of white coat effect and there is some indication that ambulatory methods of BP monitoring are more closely related to the outcome and target organ pathology than BP measurements made in the clinic.[41,42] Ambulatory monitoring may be used to confirm the diagnosis of white coat hypertension within 3 months after first recording and then every 6 months, to provide continued monitoring of these patients, as there is a risk of developing true hypertension.[41] In the office setting, measuring the patient's BP in a quiet room with an automatic device may reduce the magnitude of difference between office and out of office BP measurements.[42,43] Findings have demonstrated that a significant proportion of patients diagnosed as having resistant hypertension were truly experiencing the white coat effect. So it has been recommended that patients who start to have mild or moderately high BP measurements should not be treated with medication unless there is target organ damage and their BP remains high after 3–6 visits.[43-45]

Ambulatory Blood Pressure Measurement

Almost all adults have higher systolic blood pressure (SBP) when taken by ABPM or by the patients themselves.[46] It has been observed that the average multiple office BP recordings are as much as 10/5 mm Hg higher than the ambulatory BP readings. The difference is usually small and lies within the usual daily variation and does not warrant a change in the management.[46] It is only when the pressure difference is significant and the ABPM configuration is characteristic that a diagnosis of white coat hypertension is warranted. The degree of pressure elevation in susceptible patients is also physician dependent, some physicians causing a higher degree of white coat effect than others.[16] With the advent of the ABPM, the appreciation and understanding of hypertension as a whole and white coat hypertension in particular, has drastically improved.[16] The 24-hour BP can be divided into the following segments for the ease of understanding:[16]

- From the time of attachment of the monitor till the first 3–4 hours
- The rest of the morning hours, through the afternoon, and evening until bedtime
- During sleep
- Upon awakening and until the recorder is removed.

Each segment has a unique pattern defining its white coat character. In the first minutes of the recording, the SBP and DBP reaches the highest of the values in the entire 24 hours. During the next 2–3 hours, the pressure falls more slowly to the lowest day time value.[29] In this segment of the ABPM, the pulse pressure tends to be wider, as the SBP rises disproportionately than the diastolic. This has been used as an indicator of the white coat effect.[27-49] During the rest of the daytime period, the ABPM recording plateaus with minor variations alone. During the night time, there is a normal circadian fall in the BP, which also occurs in approximately half of the hypertensive population as well.[50] The BP falls 10–20% lower than the mean daytime BP. If the fall is <10%, it is called as nondippers or blunted dip. The patients with essential hypertension are known to lose the circadian night time dip and has been linked to increased cardiovascular risk.[51-55] The final segment, during the time of awakening and the subsequent couple of hours, is characterized by a rise in BP until the recording device is removed.

The White Coat Character of ABPM

First segment: During the first segment of the ABPM, the initial increase in the BP when the device is connected, is universal. The initial rise followed by fall produces the bimodal pattern of BP tracing, suggestive of white coat effect, so is the widening of the pulse pressure.[47-49] An initial sympathetic surge causes the initial surge followed by an endocrine surge, which causes the slow dissipation.[50]

Second segment: The second segment may show three variations:

1. The first response is the normal response to exercise. There will be a rise in the SBP and less elevation of DBP. Following the exercise, the pressure falls back rapidly to the previous plateau levels
2. The second response occurs when the patient experiences a white coat response to various triggers. The white coat effect raises the SBP more than the DBP and a widening of the pulse pressure. This has been recognized as a marker of this condition.[51,52] The white coat phenomenon is essentially systolic. There may be a modest increase in the DBP, but there have been no reports of isolated or pure diastolic white coat hypertension. The triggers that have been identified as precipitating white coat events include, the arrival at the doctor's office, entering into the examination room, arrival of the physician to the patient's bedside, undergoing the physical examination and the actual recording of the BP. Each of the aforementioned stages of a doctor's visit provoked a white coat effect. Anticipation of visit provoked some BP elevation but the arrival at doctor's office produced a full-blown white coat episode. While waiting for the doctor, this peak tends to resolve to some extent. Admission to the consultation room caused another pressure rise and manually taking the BP by the cuff and manometer produced another peak, which is the highest.[6,52] Anxiety elevates BP but does not appear to be the trigger for the white coat episodes.[54]

This has been proven in a study where no significant difference in BP could be noted up on subjecting to anxiety in white coat persons when compared to nonwhite coats.[55,56] Mental stress has been considered as a trigger for the white coat episode in one study, but has been disproved in other studies.[45,57] The mechanism of these triggers is thought to be due to a conditioned reflex that, once established, persisted for years, visit after visit[58]

3. The third variation seen is when the patient actually has an essential hypertension and is complicated by the white coat effect. In this instance, the pressure rises through the afternoon and the evening and reaches abnormally high levels.

The third segment: The nocturnal dip in white coat hypertension has not generally been elucidated. This physiological night time dip in pressure occurs in approximately half of the hypertensive adult population.[59] It occurs in approximately the same proportion in treated hypertensives with white coat effect. When this happens in treated individuals, the dip may be significantly lowered by medications, but tends to be without symptoms or complications.

The final segment: In a series, the awakening and subsequent couple of hours, provoked white coat episodes. But this did not peak as much as when the device is connected.[16]

Self-monitoring of Blood Pressure

It has been shown in some studies that self-monitoring of BP may be superior in evaluating the effects of antihypertensive therapy.[60] In the recent years, there has been availability of recorders, including automated machines, which enable the patient to measure the blood pressure at places outside the physician's office. In a study, which compared the BP taken at physician's office with that of 24-hour ambulatory BP and self-monitored BP at home by the patient, it was found that home BP were consistently lower than the clinic BP measurements. It was also observed that the home BP is a simple and convenient method of out of office BP and it correlated closely with the 24-hour ambulatory BP recordings and hence, can be used as a substitute for resource limited settings, where ambulatory BP monitors may be scarcely available. The inherent limitations of home BP measurements is that it reflects only basal or near BBPs. It is therefore possible that an individual's BP might be normal while the subject is relaxed at home, but high when the subject is under stress. Considering the large number of hypertensive population, it is difficult or impossible to subject every hypertensive to home monitoring or ABPM. Therefore, the true clinical indications for home monitoring of BP are—(1) Suspicion of white coat hypertension, (2) Identification of white coat effect in hypertensives, and (3) Identification of true and false resistant hypertension. There is some evidence to suggest that white coat hypertension is associated with an increased risk of developing sustained hypertension.[61] Therefore, it can be considered as a prerunner of systemic hypertension.

Management

The mainstay of treatment of white coat hypertension is not pharmacological. Since white coat hypertension is a form of ill-sustained hypertension, the risk factors are the same as that of sustained hypertension. Hence, the management includes, weight reduction, regular exercise, following a balanced diet, smoking cessation, control of diabetes and stress management, etc; pharmacological treatment should be withheld.[62] White coat hypertension may also be addressed through the development of therapeutic relationship between the physician and the patient. Effective communication and relation building can reduce the patient's anxiety about their illness. Empathy and trust to the patient are also important to reduce white coat hypertension. This will reduce patient anxiety as well as improve treatment adherence.[63]

■ MASKED HYPERTENSION

The combination of office BP measurements with the help of either ambulatory BP or home BP, allows clinician to identify at least four patterns of BP status.[3] These include:

- Those normotensives by both methods (True normotensives)
- Hypertensive on clinic measurements and normotensive by home BP (white coat hypertensives)
- Normotensive by clinic measurement and hypertensive by home BP (Masked hypertension), and
- Hypertensive by both methods (Sustained hypertension).

For hypertension by home BP, the term masked hypertension was introduced, since it is not detected by routine methods.[64] The difference between masked hypertension and white coat hypertension is that masked hypertension has the same risk for future cardiovascular events as sustained hypertension may have. The high cardiovascular risk and a failure to be diagnosed by conventional methods, makes it worth to get more insight into this phenomenon and its consequences, so that adequate measures can be taken.[65-68] It has been shown that masked hypertension is independently associated with increased aortic stiffness, renal injury, and end organ damage such as left ventricular hypertrophy, increased pulse wave velocity and carotid intima media thickness.[69,70] Masked hypertension also represents a group of patients who are either not receiving treatment or receiving inadequate treatment. For treated patients, this condition should be termed as masked uncontrolled hypertension.[71]

Risk Factors, Causes and Sub types of Masked Hypertension

There are two major groups of factors that might lead to masked hypertension—(1) Factors that selectively raise the ambulatory BP and hence the clinic BP could be relatively low, and (2) There could be a second group of factors that affect both the sets of measurements.[67,72]

The factors that selectively increase the ambulatory BPs include the following:

- *Smoking*: Smokers tend to have higher day time ambulatory BPs when compared to the clinic BPs.[73] There is a tendency for smokers to be more masked hypertensives than nonsmokers.[74] Smoking also has a predictive effect on masked hypertension[75]
- *Alcohol*: The pressor effect of alcohol also contributes to masked hypertension. The association has been nonsignificant though[76]
- *Physical activity*: Studies have shown that subjects who were not physically active during the day had high day time BPs.[77] The elevation of BP in masked hypertensives appears to be more marked during day than at night[75]
- *Stress*: Exposure to stress and unmanaged stress during the day time hours is an important factor contributing to masked hypertension.

Factors that may have an effect on both the office and the ambulatory BP—It has been found that those who have a higher home BP than the office BP were older, more likely to be males, had a history of diabetes, stroke or coronary artery disease.[65,78-80] Shortened sleep time, often starting in adolescents and obstructive sleep apnea have been associated with masked hypertension.[81-83]

Subtypes of Masked Hypertension

The subtypes of masked hypertension might have a prognostic and therapeutic implication in the long run.[84] Such a classification was introduced by Yano and Bakris.[85] These include:

- *Morning hypertension*: This is the most common subtype of masked hypertension. There is a physiological rise in BP in early morning with fall in the late morning and early afternoon. If the office BP is taken late in the morning, this may cause a masked hypertension
- *Day time hypertension*: It is caused by lifestyle factors like stress, cigarette smoking and physical activity.[37,86-88] The predominant day time hypertension is also seen during smoking, heavy drinking and poor exercise tolerance[85]
- *Nocturnal hypertension*: Nondippers may cause masked hypertension. This pattern is seen in obese, those with high salt intake, sleep apnea, chronic kidney disease (CKD), and those with autonomic dysfunction. This increase in morning surge is associated with increase in mortality.[89]

The prevalence of masked hypertension varies considerably depending on population characteristics.[90] Masked hypertension has been identified in more than one-third of untreated African Americans and more than 40% of low-income South Africans.[91-93] In a Japanese study, the incidence of masked hypertension was 11% after a follow-up period of 8 years.[94] Depending on the various study population settings, the definition of masked hypertension and technique of BP measurement, the prevalence ranged between 8–38%.[84] A meta-analysis showed a prevalence of 16.8% based on 28 studies.[94] In a Brazilian study on type 2 diabetes mellitus presenting with prehypertension, 30% had masked untreated hypertension.[95] An Indian study has shown that nearly 60% of treated patients with CKD had masked uncontrolled hypertension.[96]

Diagnosis

Unlike patients with white coat hypertension, who are easy to identify given their elevated BP at office, the objective of making diagnosis of masked hypertension is to identify patients who have persistently elevated out of office BP and thus are not receiving treatment or are treated inadequately.[97] The gold standard for identifying patients with masked hypertension is ambulatory BP measurement. But studies have, however, suggested that self-monitoring of BP correctly classifies most cases of masked hypertension.[97] A meta-analysis has shown that there was no significant difference in the detection of masked hypertension by home monitoring of BP and ABPM.[5] In a study in 1993, where home and clinic BPs were measured in a group of healthy young subjects, 10% were hypertensive at home and were overweight, had high insulin levels, low high density lipoproteins, suggesting their high risk. The increased availability of self-monitoring of BP devices makes it relatively easier to identify patients with masked hypertension. One of the problems with home monitoring and diagnosis of masked hypertension is that BP tends to be higher in the morning than in the evening and there is no consensus as to at what time of the day the BP has to be measured. It has been suggested that masked hypertension may be a precursor of true hypertension. One study had demonstrated persistence and reproducibility of masked hypertension in 40% children over a 3-year period. In the HARVEST study, over a 6-year follow-up, the masked hypertensives were twice as likely to develop sustained hypertension as the normotensives.[98]

Prognostic Significance and Clinical Implications

It was shown that patients with masked hypertension had higher left ventricular mass and more carotid atherosclerosis than true normotensives. In this regard, they were comparable to true hypertensives.[12] This finding suggests that they may be at increased risk of cardiovascular morbidity. There have been many other studies that were published after this pioneer study which also showed the same findings.[99-103] There are also studies proving the association of masked hypertension with high levels of C reactive protein and diminished endothelial function.[103] Metabolic risk factors were more frequent in masked hypertension than in patients with uncontrolled hypertension.[104] There was higher serum glucose level and urinary albumin to creatinine ratio in masked hypertensives than in normotensives.[105]

The clinical implication is that masked hypertension is a phenomenon worth further investigation. The clue to the presence of a masked hypertension is a patient presenting with target organ damage, with an apparently normal office BP. The practical point is that out of office BP monitoring should be encouraged for those who are at high risk of a masked hypertension. These include smokers, alcoholics, obese people, diabetics, those under job stress, prehypertensives, etc. The phenomenon should also be suspected in those who had a raised office BP measurement at some time, family history of hypertension in both the parents, multiple risks for cardiovascular disease and diabetic patients. They should be followed up periodically. In a country like India proper clinical evaluation regarding diet and lifestyle habits could predict the chances of having masked hypertension and the focus should be on modifying these, rather than documenting masked hypertension.

Masked Hypertension in Treated Individuals

Masked hypertension is of importance in treated patients because, it gives a false impression that the BP is adequately controlled. It has been shown that the prevalence of masked hypertension is higher in treated individuals. A morning office recording of a normal BP in the office may coincide with the peak levels of medication, whereas the trough levels later in the day may be associated with hypertensive range of BP. It has been shown that drug treatment converts an overt hypertension into a masked uncontrolled hypertension rather than to a normotension.[106] It has also been noted that those with a higher pretreatment SBP, had a disproportionate reduction in the SBP at the office than ABPM, known as the Wilders principle, which says pretreatment BP is a determinant of antihypertensive response.[107] Increased prevalence of masked uncontrolled hypertension may be due to noncompliance to medication, except on the day of office visit. The significance of masked uncontrolled hypertension is normalizing the office BP, ignoring the out of office BP increases the number of individuals with masked uncontrolled hypertension.[108] The logical explanation to this is that some patients with sustained hypertension were converted into masked hypertension and some with masked hypertension were converted into sustained normotensives. Thus with drug treatment, which may render a patient normotensive or masked hypertensive, the cardiometabolic risk was higher when compared to an untreated hypertensive. Antihypertensive just initiates a transition from sustained hypertension to masked hypertension to sustained normotension. Also, the cardiometabolic risk of a treated patient who is normotensive, is still higher than a normal individual with the same BP.[108]

Treatment and Prevention of Masked Hypertension

It is established that treatment of hypertension leads to reduction in cardiovascular morbidity and mortality. This reduction is not related to any specific antihypertensive agent.[109] As mentioned above, the treatment of patients with masked hypertension should yield similar results as that of sustained hypertension in terms of cardiovascular morbidity and mortality. But lack of such evidence does not obviate the need to treat this group of people, since the relationship between BP and cardiovascular risk is continuous. Thus, treatment should not be withheld from this group. The high prevalence of masked uncontrolled hypertension among treated individuals is due to suboptimal dosage of antihypertensive prescribed by the physician and failure to select long-acting antihypertensive medications. The optimal treatment of masked hypertension requires the use of combination of drug therapy along without of office BP measurement in achieving sustained normotension.[110]

In a Spanish study, which followed up treated hypertensive patients for 4 years for cardiovascular events, showed that night time SBP is the single most important predictor of cardiovascular risk rather than day time BP.[52] Using an updated data from Spanish registry, it was found that the clinical characteristics of masked uncontrolled hypertensive patients were male sex, elderly, obese, diabetes and longer duration of hypertension. All these increased the risk of future cardiovascular disease.[111,112] This study, therefore, favored the use of both day time and night time ABPM especially in high risk patients. An algorithm was proposed for treating patients with masked hypertension.[113] All patients with high normal BP at the office, may undergo home monitoring of BP or ambulatory BP measurement. If they are found to have masked hypertension,

a 24-hour ABPM may be repeated within 2 months to confirm the diagnosis. Once masked hypertension is confirmed, patients may undergo comprehensive cardiovascular risk assessment and they should be treated with antihypertensive medications, similar to patients with sustained hypertension.

■ CONCLUSION

The above write up is to give a concept of labile hypertension and the factors which cause them. Hypertension epidemic itself is due to the changed lifestyle of our people resulting from globalization, urbanization, consumerism, improper education, self-centeredness, and the resultant loss of human values and the overall influence of USA on our lifestyle. It is difficult for a practitioner in India to make routine ABPM or do mandatory home monitoring in the current scenario due to the large volume of patients and poor resources. This is especially so for our society since the priorities should be different. India still lacks basic facilities like safe drinking water, good waste management, clean surroundings and good sanitation. People still do not have access to balanced diet and they are not even aware of good lifestyle practices nor are they empowered for it. Let us advocate each patient about the general measures on preventing hypertension and modifying their diet and lifestyle. Instead of looking for masked hypertension and white coat hypertension in each individual patient, let us study their diet and lifestyle and give appropriate advice on modifying them including tips on stress management. But let us be aware of the concepts described above and identify those who could be having these phenomena by studying their clinical features and aberrations in lifestyle. Use ABPM and home BP monitoring only for research purposes for the time being, till we achieve the living standards of the developed world with very few patients and enough resources.

■ REFERENCES

1. Ayman P, Goldshine AD. Blood pressure determinations by patients with essential hypertension. The difference between clinic and home readings before treatment. Am J Med Sci. 1940:200;465-74.

2. Alam GM, Smirk FH. Casual and basal blood pressures in British and Egyptian men. Br Heart J. 1943;5(3):152-5.

3. Pickering TG, Eguchi K, Kario K. Masked Hypertension: A review. Hypertens Res. 2007;30(6):479-88.

4. Pickering TG, Davidson K, Gerin W, et al. Masked Hypertension. Hypertension. 2002;40(6):795-6.

5. Celis H, Fagard RH. White coat hypertension: A clinical review. Eur J Intern Med. 2004;15(6):348-57.

6. Mancia G, Bertinieri G, Grassi G, et al. Effects of blood pressure measures by the doctor on the patients blood pressure and heart rate. Lancet. 1983;2(8352):695-8.

7. Sipahioglu NT Sipahioglu F. Closer look at white-coat hypertension. World J Methodol. 2014;4(3):144-50.

8. Mancia G, De Backer G, Dominiczak A, et al. 2007 Guidelines for the management of arterial hypertension: The Task Force for the Management of Arterial Hypertension of the European Society of Hypertension (ESH) and of the European Society of Cardiology (ESC). J Hypertens. 2007;25(6):1105-87.

9. Pickering TG, James GD, Boddie C, et al. How common is white coat hypertension? JAMA. 1988;259(2):225-8.

10. Sokolov M, Werdegar D, Kain HK, et al. Relationship between level of blood pressure measured casually and by portable recorders and severity of complications in essential hypertension. Circulation. 1966;34(2):279-98.

11. Perloff D, Sokolow M, Cowan R. The prognostic value of ambulatory blood pressure. JAMA. 1983;249(20):2792-8.

12. Guidelines subcommittee: 1993 Guidelines for the management of mild hypertension: Memorandum from a World Health Organization/International society of Hypertension meeting. J Hypertension. 1993;11:905-18.

13. James PA, Oparil S, Carter BL, et al. 2014 evidence based guidelines for the management of high blood pressure in adults: report from the panel members appointed to the Eighth Joint National Committee (JNC 8). JAMA. 2014;311(5):507-20.

14. Verdecchia P, Schillaci G, Borgioni C, et al. Identification of subjects with white coat hypertension and persistently normal ambulatory blood pressure. Blood Press Monit. 1996;1(3):217-22.

15. Dolan E, Stanton A, Atkins N, et al. Determinants of white coat hypertension. Blood Press Monit. 2004;9(6):307-9.

16. Bloomfield DA, Park A, et al. Decoding white coat hypertension. World J Clin Cases. 2017;5(3):82-92.

17. Khan TV, Shakir-Shatnawi Khan S, Akhondi A, et al. White coat hypertension: Relevance to clinical and emergency medical service personnel. Med Gen Med. 2007;9(1):52.

18. Ramli AS, Halmey N, Teng CL, et al. White coat effect and white coat hypertension: One and the same? Malays Fam Physician. 2008;3(3):158-61.

19. Thalenberg JM, Póvoa RM, Bombig MT, et al. Slow breathing test increases the suspicion of white coat hypertension in the office. Arq Bras Cardiol. 2008;91(4):243-9.

20. Saladini F, Benetti E, Malipiero G, et al. Does home blood pressure allow for a better assessment of white coat effect than ambulatory blood pressure? J Hypertens. 2012;30(11):2118-24.

21. Verdecchia P, Palatini P, Schillaci G, et al. Independent predictors of isolated clinic hypertension. J Hypertens. 2001;19(6):1015-20.

22. Owens P, Atkins N, O'Brien E, et al. Diagnosis of white coat hypertension by ambulatory blood pressure monitoring. Hypertension. 1999;34(2):267-72.

23. Mancia G, Facchetti R, Bombelli M, et al. Long term risk of mortality associated with selective and combined elevation in office, home and ambulatory blood pressure. Hypertension. 2006;47(5):846-53.

24. Parati G, Mancia G. White coat effect: semantics, assessment and pathophysiological implications. J Hypertens. 2003;21(3):481-6.

25. Lantelme P, Milon H, Vernet M,et al. Difference between office and ambulatory blood pressure or real white coat effect: Does it matter in terms of prognosis? J Hypertens. 2000;18(4):383-9.

26. Verdecchia P, Schillaci G, Borgioni C, et al. Prognostic significance of white coat effect. Hypertension. 1997;29(6):1218-24.

27. Munakata M, Saito Y, Nunokawa T, et al. Clinical significance of blood pressure triggered by a doctor's visit in patients with essential hypertension. Hypertens Res. 2002;25(3):343-9

28. Mulè G, Nardi E, Cottone S, et al. Relationship between ambulatory white coat effect and left ventricular mass in arterial hypertension. Am J Hyperten. 2003;16(6):498-501.

29. O'Brien E, Beevers G, Lip GY. ABC of hypertension: Blood pressure measurement. BMJ. 2001;322:1110-4.

30. Pierdomenico SD, Mezzetti A, Lapenna D, et al. White coat hypertension in patients with newly diagnosed hypertension: Evaluation of prevalence by ambulatory blood monitoring and impact on cost of health care. Eur Heart J. 1995;16(5):692-7.

31. Bidlingmeyer I, Burnier M, Bidlingmeyer M, et al. Isolated office hypertension: A prehypertensive state? J Hypertens. 1996;14(3):327-32.

32. Muscholl MW, Hense HW, Bröckel U, et al. Changes in left ventricular structure and function in patients with white coat hypertension: Cross sectional survey. BMJ. 1998;317(7158):565-70.

33. Gustavsen PH, Høegholm A, Bang LE, et al. White coat hypertension is a cardiovascular risk factor: A 10 year follow up study. J Hum Hypertens. 2003;17(12):811-7.

34. Mancia G, Bombelli M, Seravalle G, et al. Diagnosis and management of patients with white-coat and masked hypertension. Nat Rev Cardiol. 2011;8(12):686-93.

35. Grassi G, Turri C, Vailati S, et al. Muscle and skin sympathetic nerve traffic during the white coat effect. Circulation. 1999;100(3):222-5.

36. Ogedegbe G, Pickering TG, Clemow L, et al. The misdiagnosis of Hypertension: the role of patient anxiety. Arch Int Med. 2008;168(22):2459-65.

37. Parati G, Pomidossi G, Casadei R, et al. Comparison of the cardiovascular effects of different laboratory stressors and their relationship with blood pressure variability. J Hypertens. 1988;6(6):481-8.

38. Gerin W, Marion RM, Friedman R, et al. How should we measure blood pressure in the doctor's office? Blood Press Monit. 2001;6(5):257-62.

39. Spruill TM, Pickering TG, Schwartz JE, et al. The impact of perceived hypertension status on anxiety and the white coat effect. Ann Behav Med. 2007;34(1):1-9.

40. Parati G, Stergiou GS. Self measured and ambulatory blood pressure in assessing the white coat phenomenon. J Hypertens. 2003;21(4):677-82.

41. O'Brien E. Is the case for ABPM as a routine investigation in clinical practice overwhelming? Hypertension. 2007;50(2):284-6.

42. Verdecchia P, Clement D, Fagard R, et al. Task force III: Target organ damage, morbidity and mortality. Blood Press Monit.1999;4(6):303-17.

43. Clement DL, De Buyzere ML, De Bacquer DA, et al. Prognostic value of ambulatory blood pressure recordings in patients with treated hypertension. N Eng J Med. 2003;348(24):2407-15.

44. Grossman E. Ambulatory blood pressure monitoring in the diagnosis and management of hypertension. Diabetes care. 2013;36(Suppl 2):S307-11.

45. Pickering TG, Hall JE, Appel LJ, et al. Recommendations for blood pressure measurement in humans and experimental animals: Part 1: Blood pressure measurement in humans: A statement for professionals from the subcommittee of professional and public education of the American Heart Association Council on High Blood Pressure Research. Circulation. 2005;111(5):697-716.

46. Meyers MG, Valdivieso MA. Use of automated blood pressure recording device, the Bp TRU to reduce the white coat effect in routine practice. Am J Hypertens. 2003;16(6):494-7.

47. Muxfeldt ES, Bloch KV, Nogueira Ada R, et al. True resistant hypertension: Is it possible to be recognized in the office? Am J Hypertens. 2005;18(12 Pt 1):1534-40.

48. Cohen DL, Townsend RR, et al. How significant is white coat hypertension? J Clin Hypertens (Greenwich). 2010;12(8):625-6.

49. Rasmussen SL, Torp-Pedersen C, Borch-Johnsen K, et al. Normal values for ambulatory blood pressure and differences between casual blood pressure and ambulatory blood pressure: Results from a Danish population survey. J Hypertens. 1998;16(10):1415-24.

50. Yoon HJ, Ahn Y, Kim KH, et al. Can pulse pressure predict the white coat effect in treated hypertensive patients? Clin Exp Hypertens. 2012;34(8):555-60.

51. Hermida RC, Ayala DE, Calvo C, et al. Pulse pressure differences between normotensive and white coat hypertensive subjects. Am J Hypertens. 2003;16(S1):50A.

52. Verdecchia P, Schillaci G, Borgioni C, et al. Ambulatory blood pressure: a potent predictor of total cardiovascular risk in hypertension. Hypertension. 1998;32(6):983-8.

53. De la Sierra A, Redon J, Banegas JR, et al. Prevalence and factors associated with circadian blood pressure patterns in hypertensive patients. Hypertension. 2009;53(3):466-72.

54. Koroboki E, Manios E, Psaltopoulou T, et al. Circadian variation of blood pressure and heart rate in normotensives, white coat, masked, treated and untreated hypertensives. Hellenic J Cardiol. 2010;53(6):432-8.

55. O'Brien E, Sheridan J, O'Malley K. Dippers and non dippers. Lancet. 1988;2(8607):397.

56. Giorgini P, Striuli R, Petrarca M, et al. Long term blood pressure changes induced by the 2009 L'Aquila earthquake: Assessment by 24 hour ambulatory monitoring. Hypertens Res. 2013;36(9):795-8.

57. Nakao M, Shimosawa T, Nomura S, et al. Mental arithmetic is a useful diagnostic evaluation in white coat hypertension. Am J Hypertens. 1998;11(1 Pt 1):41-5.

58. Siegel WC, Blumenthal JA, Divine GW. Physiological, psychological and behavioral factors and white coat hypertension. Hypertension.1990;16:140-6.

59. Lantelme P, Milon H, Gharib C, et al. White coat effect and reactivity to stress: cardiovascular and autonomic nervous system responses. Hypertension. 1998;31(4):1021-9.

60. Cottier C, Julius S, Gajendragadkar SV, et al. Usefulness of home BP determination in treating borderline hypertension. JAMA. 1982;248(5):555-8.

61. Martin CA, McGrath BP. White coat hypertension. Clin Exp Pharmacol Physiol. 2014;41(1):22-9.

62. Chrysant SG. Treatment of white coat hypertension. Curr Hypertens Rep. 2000;2(4):412-7.

63. Cobos B, Haskard-Zolnierek K, Howard K. White coat hypertension: improving the patient-health care practitioner relationship. Psychol Res Behav Manag. 2015;8:133-41.

64. Pickering TG, Davidson K, Gerin W, et al. Masked Hypertension. Hypertension. 2002;40(6):795-6.

65. Sega R, Trocino G, Lanzarotti A, et al. Alterations of cardiac structure in patients with isolated office, ambulatory or

home hypertension. Day from the general population. PAMELA study. Circulation. 2001;104(12):1385-92.

66. Fagard RH, Cornelissen VA. Incidence of cardiovascular events in white coat, masked and sustained hypertension versus true normotension: a meta analysis. J Hypertens. 2007;25(11):2193-8.

67. Bobrie G, Clerson P, Ménard J, et al. Masked hypertension: A systematic review. J Hypertens. 2008;26(9):1715-25.

68. Verberk WJ, Kessels AG, de Leeuw PW. Prevalence, causes and consequences of masked hypertension: A meta-analysis. Am J Hypertens. 2008;21(9):969-75.

69. Tientcheu D, Ayers C, Das SR, et al. Target organ complications and cardiovascular events associated with masked hypertension and white-coat hypertension: Analysis from the Dallas heart study. J Am Coll Cardiol. 2015;66(20):2159-69.

70. Hänninen MR, Niiranen TJ, Puukka PJ, et al. Target organ damage and masked hypertension in general population. The Finn Home study. J Hypertens. 2013;31(6):1136-43.

71. Nabil N, Dzubur A, Durak A, et al. Blood pressure control in hypertensive patients, cardiovascular profile and the prevalence of masked uncontrolled hypertension. Med Arch. 2016;70(4):274-9.

72. Pickering TG, Shimbo D, Haas D, et al. Ambulatory Blood pressure monitoring. N Engl J Med. 2006;354(22):2368-74.

73. Ogedegbe G. Causal mechanisms of masked hypertension: Socio-psychological aspects. Blood Press Monit. 2010; 15(2):90-2.

74. Mann SJ, James GD, Wang RS, et al. Elevation of ambulatory blood pressure in hypertensive smokers. A case-control study. JAMA. 1991:265(17):2226-8.

75. Liu JE, Roman MJ, Pini R, et al. Cardiac and arterial target organ damage in adults with elevated ambulatory and normal office blood pressure. Ann Intern Med. 1999;131(8):564-72.

76. Wing LM, Brown MA, Beilin LJ, et al. 'Reverse white coat hypertension' in older hypertensives (JSH 2004). J Hypertens. 2002;20(4):639-44.

77. Japanese Society of Hypertension. Japanese Society of Hypertension guidelines for the management of hypertension. Hypertens Res. 2006;29(Suppl):S1-105.

78. Kario K, Pickering TG, Matsuo T, et al. Stroke prognosis and abnormal nocturnal blood pressure falls in older hypertensives. Hypertension. 2001;38(4): 852-7.

79. Selenta C, Hogan BE, Linden W, et al. How often do office blood pressure measurement fails to identify true hypertension? An exploration of white-coat normotension. Arch Fam Med. 2000;9(6):533-40.

80. Ohkubo T, Kikuya M, Metoki H, et al. Prognosis of masked hypertension detected by 24 hour ambulatory blood pressure monitoring, 10 year follow up from the Ohasama Study. J Am Coll Cardiol. 2005;46(3):508-15.

81. Mastui Y, Eguchi K, Ishikawa J, et al. Sub clinical arterial damage in untreated masked hypertensive subjects detected by home blood pressure measurement. Am J Hypertens. 2007;20(4):385-91.

82. Mezick EJ, Hall M, Matthews KA. Sleep duration and ambulatory blood pressure in black and white adolescents. Hypertension. 2012;59(3):747-52.

83. Li F, Huang H, Song L, et al. Effects of obstructive sleep apnea hypopnea syndrome on blood pressure and c-reactive protein in male hypertension patients. J Clin Med Res. 2016;8(3):220-4.

84. Gupta A, Gupta P. Masked hypertension: current scenario. Medicine Update. 2012;2.

85. Yano Y, Bakris GL. Recognition and management of masked hypertension: a review and novel approach. J Am Soc Hypertens. 2013;7(3):244-52.

86. Ungar A, Pepe G, Monami M, et al. Isolated ambulatory hypertension is common in out patients referred to a hypertension centre. J Hum Hypertens. 2004;18(12):897-903.

87. Yamasue K, Hayashi T, Ohshige K, et al. Masked Hypertension in elderly managerial employees and retirees. Clin Exp Hypertens. 2008;30(3):203-11.

88. Cavelaars M, Tulen JH, van Bemmel JH, et al. Determinants of ambulatory blood pressure response to physical activity. J hypertens. 2002;20(10):2009-15.

89. Israel S, Israel A, Ben-Dov IZ, et al. The morning blood pressure surge and all cause mortality in patients referred for ambulatory blood pressure monitoring. Am J Hypertens. 2011;24(7):796-801.

90. Franklin SS, O'Brien E, Staessen JA, et al. Masked Hypertension. Understanding its complexity. European Heart J. 2017;38(15):1112-8.

91. Sterne JA, Egger M, Smith GD. Systematic reviews in health care: Investigating and dealing with publication and other biases in meta-analysis. BMJ. 2001;323(7304): 101-5.

92. Eager M, Davey Smith G, Schneider M, et al. Bias in meta-analysis detected by simple, graphical test. BMJ. 1997;315(7109):629-34.

93. Duval S, Tweedie R. Trim and fill: A simple funnel plot based method of testing and adjusting for publication bias in meta-analysis. Biometrics. 2000;56(2):455-63.

94. Ugajin T, Hozawa A, Ohkubo T, et al. White coat hypertension as a risk factor for the development of home hypertension: The ohasama study. Arch Intern Med. 2005;165(13):1541-6.

95. Leitão CB, Canani LH, Kramer CK, et al. Masked hypertension, urinary albumin excretion rate and echocardiographic parameters in putatively normotensive type 2 diabetic patients. Diabetes care. 2007;30(5):1255-60.

96. Drawz PE, Alper AB, Anderson AH, et al. Masked hypertension and elevated night time blood pressure in

CKD. Prevalence and association with organ damage. Clin J Am Soc Nephrol. 2016;11(4):642-52.

97. Pickering TG, Miller NH, Ogedegbe G, et al. Call to action on use and reimbursement for home blood pressure monitoring: executive summary: a joint scientific statement from the American Heart Association Society Of Hypertension and Preventive Cardiovascular Nurses Association. Hypertension. 2008;52(1):1-9.

98. Shahab ST, Gudbrandsson T, Jamerson K, et al. Isolated home hypertension in Tecumseh, Michigan. Croat Med J. 1993;34:325-31.

99. Palatini P, Winnicki M, Santonastaso M, et al. Prevalence and clinical significance of isolated ambulatory hypertension in young subjects screened for stage 1 hypertension. Hypertension. 2004;44(2):170-4.

100. Kotsis V, Stabouli S, Toumanidis S, et al. Target organ damage in "white coat hypertension" and "masked hypertension". Am J Hypertens. 2008;21(4):393-9.

101. Manios E, Michas F, Tsivgoulis G, et al. Impact of pre hypertension on carotid artery intima media thickening: actual or masked? Atherosclerosis. 2011;214(1):215-9.

102. Hoshide S, Ishikawa J, Eguchi K, et al. Masked nocturnal hypertension and target organ damage in hypertensives with well controlled self measures home blood pressure. Hypertens Res. 2007;30(2):143-9.

103. Veerabhadrappa P, Diaz KM, Feairheller DL, et al. Endothelial-dependent flow-mediated dilation in African Americans with masked hypertension. Am J Hypertens. 2011;24(10):1102-7.

104. Yoon HJ, Ahn Y, Park JB, et al. Are metabolic risk factors and target organ damage more frequent in masked hypertension than in white coat hypertension? Clin Exp Hypertens. 2010;32(7):480-5.

105. Ishikawa J, Hoshide S, Eguchi K, et al. Masked Hypertension defined by ambulatory blood pressure monitoring is associated with an increased serum glucose level and urinary albumin-creatinine ratio. J Clin Hypertens (Greenwich). 2010;12(8):578-87.

106. Pareek AK, Messerli FH, Chandurkar NB, et al. Efficacy of low-dose chlorthalidone and hydrochlorothiazide as assessed by 24-h ambulatory blood pressure monitoring. J Am Coll Cardiol. 2016;67(4):379-89.

107. Schmieder RE, Schmidt ST, Riemer T, et al. Disproportional increase in office blood pressure compared with 24-hour ambulatory blood pressure with antihypertensive treatment: Dependency on pretreatment blood pressure levels. Hypertension. 2014;64:1067-72.

108. Franklin SS, Thijs L, Li Y, et al. Masked Hypertension in diabetes mellitus: Treatment implications for clinical practice. Hypertension. 2013;61(5):964-71.

109. Lenfant C, Chobanian AV, Jones DW, et al. Seventh report of the Joint National committee on the prevention, detection, evaluation and treatment of high blood pressure (JNC 7): resetting the hypertension sails. Hypertension. 2003;41(6):1178-9.

110. Lewington S, Clarke R, Qizilbash N, et al. Age-specific relevance of usual blood pressure to vascular mortality; A meta-analysis of individual data for one million adults in 61 prospective studies. Lancet. 2002;360(9349):1903-13.

111. Wald DS, Law M, Morris JK, et al. Combination therapy vs monotherapy in reducing blood pressure, meta-analysis on 11,000 participants from 42 trials. Am J Med. 2009;122(3):290-300.

112. Banegas JR, Ruilope LM, de la Sierra A, et al. High prevalence of masked uncontrolled hypertension in people treated with hypertension. Eur Heart J. 2014;35(46):3304-12.

113. Ogedegbe G, Agyemang C, Ravenell JE, et al. Masked hypertension: evidence of the need to treat. Curr Hypertens Rep. 2010;12(5):349-55.

Perioperative Hypertension

Dev B Pahlajani

INTRODUCTION

Hypertension is a global healthcare challenge and it is responsible for cardiac failure, coronary atherosclerotic vascular disease (CAVD), kidney failure, stroke, ocular complications, and intracranial bleed. It is estimated that more than 1 billion individuals worldwide suffer from hypertension. Several studies from India have shown prevalence rate ranging from 40% to 70% in the adults above the age of 60 years, age at which many of them are likely to undergo major or minor cardiac or noncardiac surgery. As many as 25% of patients who undergo major noncardiac surgery and 80% of those undergoing cardiac surgery suffer from perioperative hypertension.

Perioperative hypertension by definition would include preoperative hypertension detected while undergoing preoperative checkup, or during surgery or in the postoperative period.

RISK OF SURGERY

There is a direct relationship between risk of surgery and severity of hypertension. Thus, it is essential to understand the risk of surgical procedure and management of hypertension in these patients.

It is the most common risk factor for perioperative cardiovascular complications and emergencies. While pre-existing hypertension could be responsible for aggravation, emergencies could arise because of de novo hypertension during surgery. Such an aggravated situation could lead to precipitation of acute myocardial infarction (AMI), acute coronary syndrome, stroke, intracranial bleed or acute left ventricular failure as well as acute renal injury. It is prudent to ensure maintenance of the optimum level of blood pressure, which could keep the patient in cardiovascular and cerebrovascular stability. In systemic review and meta-analysis of 30 observational studies, preoperative hypertension was associated with 35% increase in cardiovascular complications which included dysrhythmias, myocardial ischemia or AMI, neurological complications, and renal failure in patients with diastolic blood pressure more than or equal to 110 mm Hg immediately before surgery.[1] While diastolic blood pressure is a certain risk factor for such serious complications, the data of systolic blood pressure is lacking. Isolated hypertension in patients who undergo endarterectomy and coronary artery bypass graft surgery (CABG) is associated with greater risk of cardiovascular morbidity.[2]

Increased pulse pressure has been reported to be an independent risk factor for postoperative neurological complications and cardiac failure.[3] Postoperative hypertension occurs in 5–25% patients and is particularly infrequently observed in post-CABG patients. It could occur in over next 1–3 days following surgery.

Intraoperative hypertension could be defined as systolic blood pressure more than 20% of preoperative blood pressure and diastolic blood pressure more than 110 mm Hg or mean arterial pressure of more than 105 mm Hg and could appear within 20 minutes after induction of anesthesia.

Some of the life-threatening emergencies that can arise from intraoperative hypertension include:

- Aortic dissection
- Left ventricular failure with pulmonary edema
- AMI
- Non-ST elevation MI
- Eclampsia
- Acute renal failure
- Hypertensive encephalopathy
- Precipitation of stroke
- Intracranial bleed.

Acute elevation of blood pressure more than 20% in intraoperative period could be considered as hypertensive emergency. Sudden increase in diastolic and systolic blood pressure above 180 and 120 mm Hg in the past was defined as malignant hypertension. However, currently blood pressure guidelines replace this term with hypertensive emergency or crisis.

PATHOPHYSIOLOGY OF HYPERTENSIVE CRISIS

Hypertensive crisis could result from discontinuation of antihypertensive medications and autonomic hyperactivity, collagen disease, some of the stimulants used inadvertently during surgery, kidney failure, eclampsia, and renal hypertension.

A pathophysiology such as hypertensive crisis is related to humoral vasoconstrictors like catecholamine secretion, which increase systemic vascular resistance. This leads to injury to the endothelium, which further increases the blood pressure with deposition of platelets and fibrin. Platelet and fibrin deposition leads to further release of vasoconstrictive substances precipitating renal failure, hypertensive encephalopathy, and acute coronary syndrome. Factors which lead to severe hypertension during surgery include sympathetic aggravation as a result of pain and stress of surgery and some specific types of surgical procedures like carotid endarterectomy and intra-abdominal, and intrathoracic peripheral vascular surgery. Several other causes of hypertension have been identified viz.

- Intraoperative drugs, which included inadvertently administered vasopressor drugs by anesthetist or surgeon
- Hypervolemia due to overzealous infusion of fluids
- Light anesthesia and surgical stimulation
- Some of the equipment-related events like ventilator problem, hyperventilation, and stuck valve
- Awareness under general anesthesia.

PREOPERATIVE EVALUATION OF HYPERTENSION

It is important to rule out white coat hypertension by taking at least three readings on different occasions in sitting and standing position. If needed, ambulatory blood pressure monitoring may be performed.

- Detailed examination of the cardiovascular system by history taking, physical examination, electrocardiogram (ECG), and two-dimensional echo to ensure that the patient is free from associated acute coronary syndrome, left ventricular failure, pre-existing coronary artery disease, and to ensure that the patient is in a good hemodynamic condition
- Assess kidney function

- Neurological status for any current or pre-existing history of transient ischemic attacks or stroke
- Diabetes
- Presence of multiple coexisting risk factors which are commonly associated with hypertension and could increase the risk of surgery.

Precautions

- It may be prudent to differ elective major surgery in patients with systolic blood pressure of greater than 180 mm Hg or diastolic blood pressure of 110 mm Hg or more
- *Beta-blockers*: Patients who are on chronic treatment with β-blockers for hypertension and/or underlying ischemic heart disease should be continued on β-blockers. Their abrupt withdrawals could lead to precipitation of acute coronary syndrome or hypertensive crisis and inadvertent tachycardia
- In β-blocker naïve patients, β-blockers should not be started in the preoperative period particularly on the day or two of planned or emergency surgery
- Medical treatment should be continued until the day of surgery in patients with hypertension
- In patients with hypertension who undergo major surgery, it is advisable to discontinue angiotensin converting enzyme (ACE) inhibitors or angiotensin receptor blockers (ARBs) perioperatively. Some of the earlier reports have indicated increased adverse outcomes in patients who have continued ACE inhibitors or ARBs prior to or during major surgery. Such adverse outcomes are probably related to contraction of intravascular volume as well as blunting of the compensatory activation of renin–angiotensin–aldosterone system. Both these mechanisms will lead to prolonged hypotension and adverse outcomes. The data on the potential risk and benefit of ACE inhibitors in the perioperative condition are limited. However, there is some evidence to suggest that stopping ACE inhibitors or ARB, 24 hours before noncardiac surgery had lesser risk of primary composite end point of all cause death or myocardial ischemia[4,5]

- Special attention needs to be paid to diuretics that can lead to hypovolemia and electrolyte imbalance. Hypokalemia could lead to lethal arrhythmias
- Clonidine poses a specific problem due to abrupt preoperative discontinuation and may lead to sudden surge of blood pressure and potentially serious life-threatening complications like acute coronary syndrome or intracranial bleed or acute kidney injury.

▪ INTRAOPERATIVE MANAGEMENT AND CARE BY ANESTHETIST

- Intubation should be rapid and smooth without parasympathetic stimulation, which could cause bradycardia and hypotension
- Balanced anesthesia to avoid extensive sympathetic flow
- Watch for arrhythmias and signs of ischemia on ECG monitoring
- Direct laryngoscopy to be kept to the minimum
- In severe hypertension with end-organ involvement to monitor blood pressure through radial artery cannulation
- Avoid hypotension and maintain patient in fluid and electrolyte balance.

▪ DRUG MANAGEMENT OF HYPERTENSION DURING OR AFTER SURGERY

Drugs that are commonly used to treat intra-operative and postoperative hypertension are broadly classified as:
- *Beta blockers*: Labetalol and esmolol

- *Calcium channel blockers*: Nicardipine and clevidipine
- *Angiotensin-converting enzyme inhibitor*: Enalaprilat
- *Vasodilators*: Fenoldopam, hydralazine, nitroglycerine, and nitroprusside.

Their dose, duration, and route depend on the severity of the hypertension and involvement of the end organ

While β-blockers like esmolol and vasodilator nitroglycerine would be preferred for cardiovascular complications, for neurological complications drugs like nicardipine, fenoldopam, clevidipine, and labetalol would be the preferred choice. For acute severe hypertension when blood pressure needs to be controlled rapidly, nitroprusside would be a better choice.

Drugs for Control of Hypertension

- *Labetalol:* It is a selective α1- and non-selective β-adrenergic receptive blocker. It is safe and is one of the ideal drug for intraoperative and postoperative hypertension particularly in cardiovascular and neurological complications and hypertension during pregnancy. It decreases peripheral vascular resistance without significantly lowering cardiac output. Some of the contraindications include patients with sinus bradycardia, heart block, cardiac failure, and bronchial asthma. It should be administered in the continuous infusion after giving loading dose of 20 mg, which could be increased to 60 mg. It is administered at the infusion rate of 1–2 mg/min after the initial loading dose. Its action starts within 2–5 minutes lasting for about 4 hours.
- *Esmolol*: It is a rapidly acting β-blocker administered intravenously at a loading dose of 500–1000 µg/kg/min. The maintenance of infusion should be kept at 50 µg/kg/min, which can be increased to 400 µg/kg/min. However, its duration is short, lasting for 10–20 minutes and

therefore the maintenance after the desired blood pressure has been achieved can be carried further with oral drugs

- *Nicardipine*: This second-generation dihydropyridine calcium channel blocker is a short-acting drug. It is recommended for patients with ischemic stroke with diastolic blood pressure of more than 120 mm Hg or systolic blood pressure of 220 mm Hg. The drug can be administrated at 5 mg/h. However, one should not increase it to more than 15 mg/h. Once the target blood pressure has been achieved, the dose should be reduced progressively or patient can be put on oral antihypertensive drugs. One can switch to oral nicardipine 20 mg capsule thrice a day or it should be administered as nicardipine 50 mg ER tablets in the dose of 100 mg/day.
- *Clevidipine*: This is third-generation dihydropyridine calcium channel blocker. It is ultrashort acting and it is a powerful vasodilator and increases coronary blood flow and increases the stroke volume. It maintains renal blood flow. It is administered at an infusion rate of 1–2 mg/h with increasing dose depending on blood pressure. Most patients are treated up to 16 mg/h. Its half-life is short for 2 minutes with duration of action for 10 minutes. Clevidipine has been shown to reduce the blood pressure effectively in the postoperative hypertension. Systemic review and meta-analysis including four studies reported clevidipine to be more effective than other hypertensive drugs in the management of perioperative hypertension without adverse events
- In the ECLIPSE (Evaluation of CLevidipine In the Perioperative Treatment of Hypertension Assessing Safety Events) trial was compared with nitroglycerine and nitroprusside for control of hypertension. It was found to be more effective than nitroglycerine and sodium nitroprusside

in maintaining blood pressure within prespecified range though there was no difference in MI, stroke, or renal dysfunction between three drugs[6]

- *Fenoldopam*: It is a peripheral vasodilator and acts as the peripheral dopamine 1 receptor agonist. It promotes natriuresis and diuresis by causing renal artery vasodilation and activation of dopamine receptors in renal tubules. However, it can cause tachycardia and increase intraocular and intracranial pressure. Cases have been reported with rebound hypertension. The drug can be administered by infusion of 0.1 μg/kg/min increasing up to maximum of 1.5 μg/kg/min. Its onset is rapid, with duration of 30–60 minutes

- *Hydralazine*: It is an age-old drug, which has been used orally as a vasodilator for hypertension and apart from its oral use, it is effective intravenously in acute emergencies. It is administered in the dose of of 10–20 mg bolus and followed by continuous infusion of 1.5–5 μg/kg/min. Its half-life is about 4 hours. Hydralazine is best to be avoided in pregnant woman and patients with dissecting aneurysms

- *Nitroglycerine*: It is a commonly used vasodilator particularly in patients who get into left ventricular failure either during or after surgery due to hypertension. It is administered intravenously. It is an arterial and venous dilator. The dose should be started at an infusion rate of 5 μg/min can be increased up to 50 μg/min. Its action is short lasting

- *Nitroprusside*: It is ultrashort acting drug with action starting within few seconds. It is arterial and venodilator and is used in very severe cases. The initial infusion rate is 0.25–0.3 μg/kg/min to achieve the target blood pressure. Due to its sudden hypotension it could lead to decreased cerebral perfusion and therefore avoided in encephalopathy and cerebrovascular

accidents. It is accumulated in body and its prolonged administration could result in cyanide accumulation.

◼ RECENT GUIDELINES

American Heart Association or American College of Cardiology (ACC or AHA) guidelines writing committee recommended to control the blood pressure to the levels of less than 130/80 mm Hg before undertaking major elective procedure in either inpatient or outpatient setting. For patients unable to take oral medications, the committee recommends it is advisable to use intravenous medication.[7]

Those with diastolic blood pressure of more than 110 mm Hg should preferably be postponed until the blood pressure is brought down at the optimum level.

Careful watch should be kept during induction of anesthesia for surgery since it can result in 20–30 mm Hg rise in blood pressure with tachycardia and this is true of patients who have untreated hypertension prior to surgery.

Inhibition of sympathetic nervous system and blunting of baroreceptor control with anesthesia could lead to intraoperative hypertension. Patients with severe hypertension of more than 210 mm Hg systolic and 105 mm Hg diastolic would get exaggerated response during induction.

Should one differ the surgery if preoperative hypertension is detected in an individual?

Data from some of the earlier studies in 1970s indicated that uncontrolled hypertension resulted in cardiovascular instability and posed risk for precipitation of cardiovascular events. That is why it used to be recommended practice that surgery needed to be postponed, if blood pressure was not under control preoperatively. However, hypertension guidelines have undergone several changes over the years. Data from 70s and 80s was based on inadequate number of patients, with earlier anesthetic agents and not so sophisticated monitoring systems. With availability of effective medications, which can promptly control hypertensive crisis and safer anesthesia such old guidelines are no more valid. In patients in stage I and II hypertension, one could go ahead and perform surgery since mild-to-moderate preoperative hypertension is not a major risk for complications. No doubt there is a linear relationship between the extent of hypertension and cardiovascular risk, this association tends to disappear when adjustment is made of accompanying risk factors such as cardiac failure and previous MI. As a matter of fact ACC/AHA guidelines on perioperative evaluation and care for noncardiac surgery do not identify hypertension as a risk factor that should lead to differing or cancelling surgery. European Society of Cardiology/European Society of Anesthesia guidelines have similar recommendations. However, it is important not to disregard the importance of preoperative hypertension since hypertension is associated with multiple comorbidities particularly unrecognized and undiagnosed coronary artery disease. This could become manifest during surgery, particularly anesthesia. European guidelines recommend delaying surgery in patients, who are found to have blood pressure reading greater than 180 mm Hg systolic or 110 mm Hg diastolic.[8] However, one has to strike balance between the immediate need of surgery versus risk of hypertension.

◾ CONCLUSION

- Significant number of elderly patients have preoperative hypertension
- Preopertive normotensive patients could develop intraoperative hypertension
- Hypertension is frequently observed following CABG
- Patients who have pre- or intraoperative hypertension could continue to remain hypertensive in postoperative period

- Perioperative hypertension carries a risk of precipitating AMI, acute coronary syndrome, intracranial hemorrhage, acute renal failure and aortic dissection
- There are excellent drugs to control perioperative hypertension and hypertensive crisis
- It is not necessary to postpone surgery if the patient needs it unless there are other compelling comorbidities like renal failure, acute coronary syndrome, AMI, cardiac failure or stroke.

◾ REFERENCES

1. Howell SJ, Sear JW, Foex P. Hypertension, hypertensive heart disease and perioperative cardiac risk. Br J Anaesth. 2004;92:570-83.
2. Aronson S, Boisvert D, Lapp W. Isolated systolic hypertension is associated with adverse outcomes from coronary artery bypass grafting surgery. Anaesth Analog. 2002;94:1079-84.
3. Fontes ML, Aronson S, Mathew JP, et al. Pulse pressure and risk of adverse outcome in coronary bypass surgery. Anesth Analg. 2008; 107:1122-29.
4. Schirmer U, Schürmann W. Preoperative administration of angiotensin-converting enzyme inhibitors. Anaesthesist. 2007;56:557-61.
5. Brabant SM, Bertrand M, Eyraud D, et al. The hemodynamic effects of anesthetic induction in vascular surgical patients chronically treated with angiotensin II receptor antagonists. Anesth Analg. 1999;89:1388-92.
6. Aronson S, Dyke CM, Stierer KA, et al. The ECLIPSE trials: comparative studies of clevidipine to nitroglycerin, sodium nitroprusside, and nicardipine for acute hypertension treatment in cardiac surgery patients. Anesth Analg. 2008;107(4):1110-21.
7. Whelton PK, Carey RM, Aronow WS, et al. 2017 ACC/AHA/AAPA/ABC/ACPM/AGS/APhA/ASH/ASPC/NMA/PCNA Guideline for the Prevention, Detection, Evaluation, and Management of High Blood Pressure in Adults. A Report of the American College of Cardiology/American Heart Association Task Force on Clinical Practice Guidelines. Hypertension. 2018;71(6):1269-324.
8. Williams B, Mancia G, Spiering W, et al. 2018 ESC/ESH Guidelines for the management of arterial hypertension. Eur Heart J. 2018;39(33):3021-104.

Hypertension in Elderly

Jyotirmoy Pal, Uddalak Chakraborty, Tanuka Mandal, Tarun Kumar Paria, Purbasha Biswas

■ INTRODUCTION

Hypertension is a very important public health problem all over the world. It follows iceberg pattern where unknown number of cases far exceeds known cases. Hypertension is a threat to life at all ages and in both sexes. Prevalence of hypertension is increasing alarmingly in developing countries and is now one of the leading causes of morbidity and mortality among the elderly. Prevalence of hypertension in India in the last three decades has increased manifold, approximately by about 30 times among urban residents whereas about 10 times among rural residents. Average life span all over the globe has been increasing. In the year of 1961, Indian elderly were 5.63%, numbering around 24.7 million whereas in 2001, it has risen to 7.4% (76.6 million). By considering current demographic trend, it is projected that in middle of this century geriatric population will go up to 324 million, i.e. four times of the current aged population. Increase in hypertension prevalence in elderly is due to changes in arterial structure and function accompanying aging process. Subjects with uncontrolled or poorly controlled hypertension are known to have higher risk of developing coronary artery disease (CAD), congestive heart failure (HF), cerebrovascular disease and stroke. The elderly population in India is second largest in the world. According to 2011 Census, 8.1% are of the age 60 years and above.

■ PHYSIOLOGICAL CHANGES IN OLD AGE

- Decreased vascular compliance
- Decreased baroreceptor sensitivity
- Increased salt-sensitivity of blood pressure (BP)
- Increased total and central adiposity
- Neurohumoral changes in aging.

Consequences of decreased vascular compliance are relative increase in systolic pressure, increase in pulse pressure [systolic blood pressure–diastolic blood pressure (SBP–DBP)], decreased DBP and lower intravascular volume. Decreased baroreceptor sensitivity results in increased BP variability, impaired BP homeostasis with early morning BP surge, postural (orthostatic) hypotension, postprandial hypotension and orthostatic hypertension. Two-thirds of older hypertensives are sodium sensitive. This is because decreased glomerular filtration rate (GFR), increased proximal tubular reabsorption, and decreased production of natriuretic factors. Neurohumoral changes are

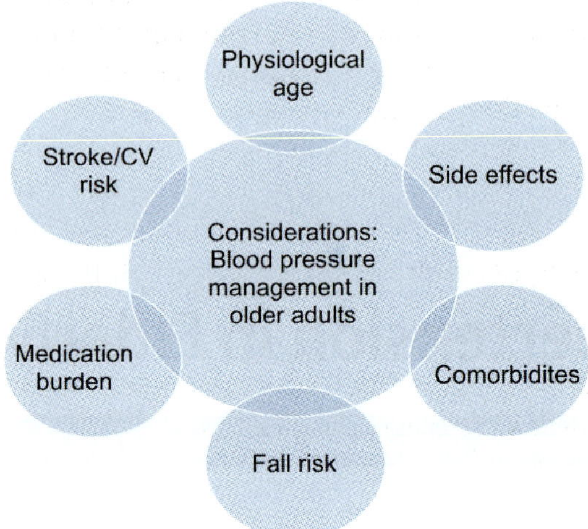

Fig. 1: Blood pressure management in older patients.

in form of decreased beta-receptor sensitivity, increased norepinephrine, increased renin activity and increased aldosterone activity (Fig. 1).

BLOOD PRESSURE MEASUREMENT

For measuring BP, patient should have taken rest for 5 minutes and he/she should not have taken caffeine or tobacco in last 30 minutes. Patient should be made to sit with support behind his/her back and legs should remain uncrossed with arm at heart level. The use of android sphygmomanometer is nowadays recommended by World Health Organization (WHO).

Radial artery should be palpated during initial cuff inflation, which helps in determining the level of SBP and rules out presence of auscultatory gap, which if not done, can underestimate SBP or overestimate DBP. Auscultatory gap is commonly seen in elderly, female sex, increased arterial stiffness and atherosclerosis.

If the pulseless radial or brachial artery can be palpated after occlusion by the cuff, pseudohypertension should be suspected. Lack of understanding of this entity can falsely over-diagnose hypertension and injudicious use of antihypertensive drugs.

Bell of the stethoscope should be lightly applied over the brachial artery for auscultation because Korotkoff sounds are low pitched. BP measurements are recorded to the nearest 2 mm Hg. Three measurements should be done and average of the last two measurements should be taken as the value for that visit. Three visits with six measurements should be taken to diagnose systemic hypertension.

White coat hypertension is more commonly seen in elderly, Home monitoring and ambulatory blood pressure monitoring (ABPM) have got advantage in this population. ABPM (24 h) can detect dipper, nondipper, and early morning surge pattern, which is associated with severe CV events.

CLINICAL ISSUES

- White coat hypertension
- Labile hypertension
- Pseudohypertension
- Postural hypotension
- Secondary hypertension
- Resistant hypertension
- Polypharmacy and drug interaction
- Nonadherence.

Measuring only office BP may give erroneous result in BP due to white coat hypertension. For that purpose, 24 hours ABPM should be considered. There is fluctuation in BP from day-to-day, hour-to-hour due to arterial stiffness, and decreased Windkessel effect of aorta. Higher prevalence of atherosclerosis gives rise to a substantial portion of patients with pseudohypertension. Loss of autonomic tones, baroreceptor sensitivity gives rise to postural hypotension and postprandial hypotension. After a high-carbohydrate meal, supine BP declines and heart rate increases without an increase in plasma norepinephrine levels.

Secondary hypertension should be suspected, if there is sudden surge of SBP and DBP, particularly DBP, occurrence of malignant hypertension and presence of resistant hypertension. Common secondary causes of hypertension are chronic kidney disease, renovascular hypertension, obstructive sleep apnea and hypothyroidism. Resistant hypertension is seen due to arterial stiffness, higher baseline BP, comorbidities, increase salt intake, sedentary lifestyle, nicotine, alcohol intake, poor compliance, volume overload and nonsteroidal anti-inflammatory drug (NSAID) use.

▪ EVALUATION

Fasting blood sugar (FBS), postprandial blood sugar (PPBS), lipid profile, complete blood count, urinalysis with microscopic examination and electrocardiogram are reasonable for an initial evaluation.

▪ TREATMENT ISSUES IN ELDERLY

- Antihypertensive drugs are strongly advocated in elderly, though most data are on patients with age less than 80 years
- Hypertension in the Very Elderly Trial (HYVET) demonstrated clear benefits if antihypertensive therapy is used above age more than 80 years of age

Goals to be Achieved

- Below 80 years target BP 140/80 mm Hg is desirable, but above 80 years, SBP 140–45 mm Hg is desirable
- In elderly BP lowering below 130/70 mm Hg not desirable due to increased incidence of orthostatic fall.

As per Eighth Joint National Committee (JNC 8)

"In the general population aged 60 years or older, initiate pharmacologic treatment to lower BP at SBP of 150 mm Hg or higher or DBP of 90 mm Hg or higher and treat to a goal SBP lower than 150 mm Hg and goal DBP lower than 90 mm Hg.
(Recommendation: grade A)

In the general population aged 60 years or older, if pharmacologic treatment for high BP results in lower achieved SBP (e.g., <140 mm Hg) and treatment is not associated with adverse effects on health or quality of life, treatment does not need to be adjusted.
(Recommendation: grade E)

Treatment Issues

Nonpharmacological Treatment

Lifestyle changes particularly weight loss, avoidance of sedentary lifestyle and reduced sodium intake are beneficial in controlling BP in elderly hypertensive. However, these changes have to be in moderation, as they should not compromise with the quality of life in the elderly as ischemic heart disease (IHD), cardiac failure, renal failure, peripheral vascular disease and orthopedic problems are also coexistent in this population.

Pharmacological Treatment

What guidelines say?
As per American Heart Association (AHA) 2011,

"The initial antihypertensive drug should be started at the lowest dose and gradually increased depending on the BP response to the maximum tolerated dose. If the antihypertensive response to the initial drug is inadequate after reaching full dose (not necessarily maximum recommended dose), a second drug from another class should be added, provided the initial drug is tolerated. If the person is having no therapeutic response or significant adverse effects, a drug from another class should be substituted. If a diuretic is not the initial drug, it is usually indicated as the second drug. If the antihypertensive response is inadequate after reaching the full dose of two classes of drugs, a third drug from another class should be added. When the BP is 20/10 mm Hg above goal, drug therapy should generally be initiated with two antihypertensive drugs, one of which should be a thiazide diuretic; however, in the elderly, treatment must be individualized."

AHA 2017 new recommendations: Treatment of hypertension is recommended for noninstitutionalized ambulatory community-dwelling adults (≥65 years of age), with an average SBP more than or equal to 130 mm Hg with SBP treatment goal of less than 130 mm Hg. For older adults (≥65 years of age) with hypertension and a high burden of comorbidity and/or limited life expectancy, clinical judgment, patient preference, and a team-based approach to assess risk or benefit are reasonable for decisions regarding intensity of BP lowering and choice of antihypertensive drugs. BP lowering is reasonable to prevent cognitive decline and dementia (Table 1).

TABLE 1: Recommendations for treatment of hypertension in older persons.

COR	LOE	Recommendations for treatment of hypertension in older persons
I	A	Treatment of hypertension with a SBP treatment goal of less than 130 mm Hg is recommended for noninstitutionalized ambulatory community-dwelling adults (≥65 years of age) with an average SBP of 130 mm Hg or higher
IIa	C-EO	For older adults (≥65 years of age) with hypertension and a high burden of comorbidity and limited life expectancy, clinical judgment, patient preference, and a team-based approach to assess risk/benefit is reasonable for decisions regarding intensity of BP lowering and choice of antihypertensive drugs

(BP: blood pressure; SBP: systolic blood pressure)

As per JNC 8,

"In the general nonblack population, including those with diabetes, initial antihypertensive treatment should include a thiazide-type diuretic, calcium channel blocker (CCB), angiotensin-converting enzyme (ACE) inhibitor, or angiotensin receptor blocker (ARB).

Moderate Recommendation—Grade B

In the general black population, including those with diabetes, initial antihypertensive treatment should include a thiazide-type diuretic or CCB.

For general Black population: Moderate Recommendation—Grade B

For Black patients with diabetes: Weak Recommendation—Grade C"

As per Indian Hypertension Guidelines-III,

Elderly hypertensives should be started with CCB or diuretic.

JNC 8 Appointed Panel Members Blood Pressure Guideline Older Adult Recommendation

"In the general population aged 60 years or older, initiate pharmacologic treatment to lower BP at SBP of 150 mm Hg or higher or DBP of 90 mm Hg or higher and treat to a goal SBP lower than 150 mm Hg and goal DBP lower than 90 mm Hg" (Fig. 2).

(Strong Recommendation—Grade A)

"In the general population aged 60 years or older, if pharmacologic treatment for high BP results in lower achieved SBP (e.g., <140 mm Hg) and treatment is not associated with adverse effects on health or quality of life, treatment does not need to be adjusted."

(Expert Opinion—Grade E)

It came as a surprise to the hypertension community when the JNC 8 defined a higher BP target for people above the age of 60 years. Of course, the decision to recommend a target of 150/90 mm Hg was well justified by the committee and based on the existing literature, applying a

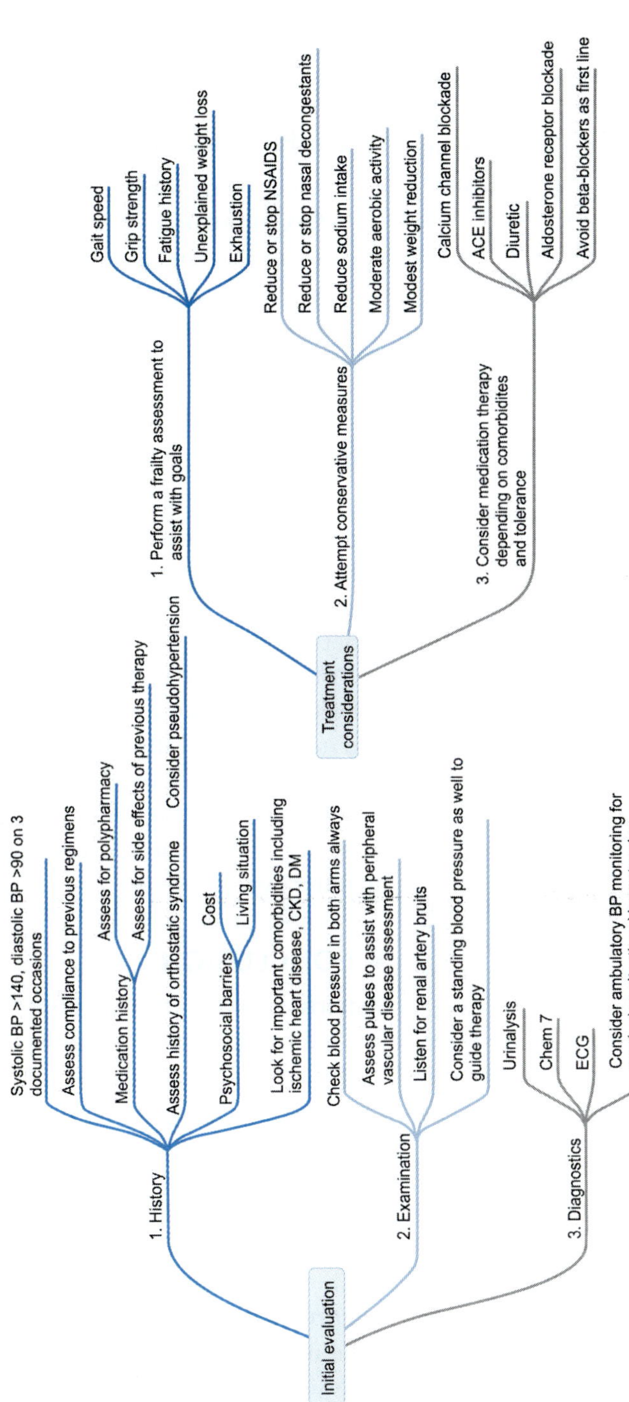

(ECG: electrocardiogram; CKD: chronic kidney disease; DM: diabetes mellitus; NSAIDS: nonsteroidal anti-inflammatory drugs; Chem 7: sodium, potassium, creatinine; ACE: angiotensin-converting enzyme)

Fig. 2: A proposed scheme to identify and individualized important aspects in the care of patients over 60 years of age with hypertension.

new and rigorous pipeline to examine the existing evidence, in keeping with Institute of Medicine recommendations. However, the 150/90 mm Hg target in the elderly was still a decision against the general "the lower the better" trend. And it was not accepted by all committee members; opponents of this target published a "minority report" outlining their views and interpretation of the evidence in more detail compared with the statements in the JNC 8 report.

Summary of All Guidelines

- Start with small dose
- Increase gradually with monitoring
- Add next drug if not controlled
- Observe side effects and drug interaction, noncompliance
- Choice of drug according to concomitant diseases and other drugs
- Ordinarily CCBs and diuretics are first-line of choice.

■ INDIVIDUAL CLASS OF DRUGS

Diuretics

Decrease blood volume, decrease peripheral resistance and so BP. They are very effective in elderly with stiff peripheral artery. But at the same time causes increase of age-related physiological changes and further depletion of blood volume, increases postural hypotension. Electrolyte imbalance causing more arrhythmia. Impaired glucose tolerance, hyperuricemia, hypokalemia and hypomagnesemia. But thiazide diuretics maintain bone mineral density (BMD) and increase blood calcium level. Loop diuretics decrease blood calcium level.

Calcium Channel Blocker

It is effective in elder population because of increased vascular stiffness, decreased vascular compliance and diastolic dysfunction. Adverse effects are postural hypotension, ankle edema and headache. These are effective in preventing dementia.

ACE Inhibitor and ARBs

- Reduce peripheral resistance without reflex stimulation of HR and contractility
- Indications are hypertension with HF/diabetes mellitus (DM)/nephropathy/postacute myocardial infarction (AMI)/angina and also effective in preventing dementia.

Beta-blocker

They are not used as first choice but used when hypertension associated with arrhythmias, post-AMI, HF, hyperthyroidism, essential tremor, anxiety neurosis and preoperative hypertension.

Adherence is most important issue in elderly hypertension. Frequent nonadherence and noncontrol of BP occur due to dementia, low socioeconomic condition, isolation, cost, side effects, treating complications, and all these issues are to be addressed while dealing an older hypertensive.

■ CONCLUSION

Hypertension has been an important cause of morbidity and mortality in elderly population. Multifactorial contributors coupled with physiological changes due to aging make hypertension in the elderly a tad bit different from hypertension in younger adults. Early detection and prompt treatment of geriatric hypertension has been beneficial to prevent morbidity and mortality. A careful and rational treatment approach considering age of the patient may avoid drug related complications in the elderly.

■ REFERENCES

1. Puspanjali S, TP Sherin Raj. Demography of aging in India. Indian J Gerontol. 2005;19:327-42.

2. Franlin SS, Jacobs MJ, Wong ND, et al. Predominance of isolated systolic hypertension among middle age and elderly US hypertensives analysis based on National Health and Nutrition Examination Survey (NHANES) III. Hypertension. 2001;37:869-74.

3. Franklin SS, Khan SA, Wong ND, et al. Is pulse pressure more important than systolic blood pressure in predicting coronary heart disease event. Circulation. 1999;100:354-60.

4. Dalal PM. Hypertension. In: Jhala (Ed). A report on community survey for casual hypertension in old Bombay. Bombay: Sir HN Hospital Research Society; 1980.

5. Reaven GM. Insulin resistance, hyper-insulinemia and hyper-triglyceridemia in the etiology clinical course of hypertension. Am J Med. 1991;90:7S-12S.

6. Mohan JC. Prevalence, awareness, treatment and control and risk factors of hypertension in India and its neighborhood: Newer data and older perspective. Indian Heart J. 2006;58:7-9.

7. Anderson GH, Blackman N, Streeten DH. The effect of age on prevalence of secondary forms of hypertension in 4429 consecutively referred patients. J Hyperns. 1994;12:609-15.

8. Chobanian AV, Bakris GL, Black HL. Seventh report of the Joint National Committee on Prevention, Detection, Evaluation, and Treatment of High Blood Pressure. Hypertension. 2003;42:1206-52.

9. National High Blood Pressure Education Program Working Group. Report on Hypertension in the elderly. Hypertension. 1994;23:275-85.

10. Psaty BM, Lumley T, Furberg CD, et al. Health outcomes associated with various anti-hypertensive therapies used as first line agents: a network meta-analysis. JAMA. 2003;289:2534-44.

11. ALLHAT Officers and Coordinators for the ALLHAT Collaborative Research Group. The Antihypertensive and Lipid-Lowering Treatment to Prevent Heart Attack Trial. Major outcomes in high risk hypertensive patients randomized to angiotensin converting enzyme inhibitor or calcium channel blocker vs diuretic. The Antihypertensive and Lipid-Lowering Treatment to prevent Heart Attack Trial (ALLHAT). JAMA. 2002;288:2981-97.

12. Staessen JA, Fagard R, Thijs L, et al. Randomised double blind comparison of placebo and active treatment for older patients with isolated systolic hypertension. The Systolic Hypertension in Europe (Syst-Eur) Trial Investigators. Lancet. 1997;350:757-64.

13. SHEP Cooperative Research Group. Prevention of stroke by antihypertensive drug treatment in older persons with isolated systolic hypertension. JAMA. 1996;265:3255-64.

14. Schiffrin EL. Effects of antihypertensive drugs on vascular remodeling: do they predict outcome in response to antihypertensive therapy? Curr Opin Nephrol Hypertens. 2001;10:617-24.

15. Yusuf S, Sleight P, Progue J. Effects of angiotensin converter inhibitor, ramipril, on cardiovascular events in high-risk patients. The outcomes Prevention Evaluation Study Investigators. N Engl J Med. 2000;342:145-53.

16. Linholm LH, Ibsen H, Dahlof B, et al. Cardiovascular morbidity and mortality in patients with diabetes in the losartan intervention for Endpoint reduction in hypertension study (LIFE): a randomized trial against atenolol. Lancet. 2002;359:1004-10.

17. Dahlof B, Lindholm LH, Hansson L, et al. Morbidity and mortality in the Swedish Trail in Old patients with hypertension. Lancet. 1991;338:315-9.

18. Frishman WH, Landau A, Cretkovic A. Combination drug therapy with calcium-channel blockers in the treatment of systemic hypertension. J Clin Pharmacol. 1993;33:752-5.

19. Madhukumar S, Gaikwad V, Sudeepa D. An Epidemiological study of Hypertension and its risk factors in Rural Population of Bangalore Rural District. Al Ameen J Med Sci. 2012;5(3):264-70.

20. Pradeepa R, Mohan V. Hypertension and pre hypertension in developing countries. Indian J Med Res. 2008;128:688-90.

21. Hafez G, Bagchi K, Mahaini R. Caring for the elderly: A report on the status of care for the elderly in the Eastern Mediterranean Region. East Mediterr Health J. 2000;6(4):636-43.

22. Aronow WS, Fleg JL, Pepine CJ, et al. ACCF/AHA 2011 Expert Consensus Document on Hypertension in the Elderly. A Report of the American College of Cardiology Foundation Task Force on Clinical Expert Consensus Documents. J Am Coll Cardiol. 2011;57(20):2037-114.

23. World health organization. World Health Day. [online] Available from: https://www.who.int/campaigns/world-health-day [Last accessed February, 2019].

24. Ministry of Home Affairs. SRS Statistical Report 2011: SRS Statistical Report Tables. Available at: http://www.censusindia.gov.in/vital_statistics/SRS_Report/12SRS%20Statistical%20Report%20Table%20-%2020111.pdf [Last accessed February, 2019].

25. Currie, Gemma, Delles, Christian. Blood pressure targets in the elderly. J Hypertension. 2018;36(2):234-6.

26. Available from: https://cdn.ymaws.com/www.thenpa.org/resource/resmgr/annual_conference/2018_annual_conference/2018_speaker_handouts/J1844_Chronic_Care_Managemen.pdf

Blood Pressure Variability and Target Organ Damage

NR Rau, Shivashankara

■ INTRODUCTION

Hypertension is the most common significant single contributor to the global burden of disease and mortality which accounts for more than 12.8% of all deaths annually. The prevalence of high blood pressure (BP) globally is expected to increase over the next decade. The most common treatable risk factors of hypertension are stroke, coronary artery disease, heart failure, chronic kidney disease, and aortic and peripheral arterial disease, accounting for about 50% of the risk.[1] BP fluctuates in response to various changes in sleep patterns, physical and mental activities and responds to autonomic, humoral, mechanical, myogenic and environmental stimuli. Marked spontaneous oscillations over short and long-term periods are a characteristic of BP. Owing to this, there may be radical differences in office blood pressure monitoring (OBPM) or home blood pressure monitoring (HBPM) as compared to his/her average day and night time BP, which results in a challenge in diagnosing and prescribing treatments to patients.

Although BP regulation aims at reducing the incidence of target-organ damage, prevention of cardiovascular disease (CVD) and premature death in hypertensive patients; the current antihypertensive therapy does not ameliorate all hazards associated with hypertension. While they cause a meaningful change, i.e. reduction by approximately one-third; the results are suboptimal at best.[2] Usual BP, the general right underlying BP level, is widely regarded as the primary determinant of vascular risk associated with BP and benefits from antihypertensive therapy. Although the diagnosis of high BP appears to be straightforward, misdiagnosis is not rare in clinical practice, and there are still several unresolved issues regarding optimal BP classification after many years of research. Guidelines for the American Heart Association[3] on measurement of BP states that current clinical readings are generally agreed as a surrogate marker for the true BP of a patient and are considered to be the essential component of BP in determining its adverse effects. For instance, the phenomena of isolated office hypertension (i.e. high BP at the doctor's office despite normal BP out of office) and masked hypertension (i.e. normal BP in the doctor's office and high BP out of office) lead to frequent over- and underdiagnosis of BP-associated cardiovascular (CV) risk.[4]

Over the past few decades, there has been mounting evidence to the effect that in addition to the absolute BP values, high blood pressure variability (BPV) is associated with the development, progression, and severity of cardiac, renal and vascular damage along with increased risk of CV mortality.[5-7] Indeed, when the subject at high CV risk is compared with those at low risk, higher BPV values appear to have a more significant prognostic value.[8]

Also, there is a prevalent assumption among physicians treating hypertension that as long as the diastolic pressure is adequate for maintaining coronary perfusion, the lower the BP, the better. There is a poor understanding of the component of BP causing said vascular events. Mean BP (average of multiple readings of either systolic or diastolic BP) is essential, but other factors, such as variability (variation in BP with time) or instability of BP (transient BP fluctuations) may also play a role in most vascular events. However, according to the current paradigm, an effective pharmacological regime provides a continuous, indiscriminate reduction of BP over 24 hours. The results of the study Ambulatory Blood Pressure Monitoring for Cardiovascular Event Prediction challenge conventional understanding and have the potential to affect significant changes in hypertension management.[9]

CIRCADIAN RHYTHM AND BLOOD PRESSURE VARIATION IN STANDARD AND HIGH BLOOD PRESSURE PATIENTS

Sleep usually involves calmness and detachment from the outside environment, resulting in a reduction of BP at night in general. This decline does not occur under conditions of total deprivation of sleep. Ultimately, Millar-Craig et al.[10] used continuous intra-arterial monitoring to establish the circadian rhythm of BP. In people with normal BP or uncomplicated hypertension, BP declines to the lowest levels during night sleep (night dip), rises abruptly with morning awakening (morning surge), and reaches near peak or peak values during the first hours of diurnal activity. In usual dippers, the average sleep-time BP is lower than the day-time average by 10–20%. Intrinsic factors (*neurohumoral regulation*) and extrinsic factors (physical activity, sleep deprivation or quality, and dietary sodium) influence the timing and amplitude of the natural rhythm of BP. Also, the natural rhythm of BP can also be affected by behavioral factors (mental activity and emotional status) and lifestyle factors (alcohol drinking and smoking).[11] Sleep disturbances, including sleep restriction, sleep apnea, insomnia and shift work, have also been found to induce CV system stress and play a role in CV disorder development.

The normal circadian BP rhythm is preserved when hypertension first develops. Later, as target organ damage jeopardizes systemic BP regulation, the circadian rhythm is distorted, with a tendency to increase variability and excessive morning BP surge. Finally, BP can increase sleep time to produce a nondipper pattern.[10] In nondipper or riser patterns, diabetes, poststroke, congestive heart failure, sleep apnea syndrome, orthostatic hypotension or medicated hypertension are often associated with conditions. Otherwise, a morning BP surge pattern is associated with smoking, alcohol consumption, over 60 years of age, cold weather, increased arterial stiffness, impaired baroreflex or orthostatic hypertension.[12]

Blood Pressure Variability

While average clinical BP values remain the gold standard for hypertension diagnosis and therapy, recent research in hypertensive subjects has proven both pathological and prognostic in the evaluation and quantification of BPV, in addition to normal BP values. For example, substantial evidence shows that increased BPV is associated independently with a higher risk of target-organ damage, CV events and mortality. As a result, controlling BPV can contribute to optimal CV protection in hypertensive patients in addition to reducing absolute BP levels. Variations in BP over time can be defined as a BP variable in simplistic terms. These fluctuations in BP are created through a complex combination of multiple CV control mechanisms or during the change from every day to environmental situations.[13]

The extent of these variations differs from person to person and is high in patients with diminished mechanisms of CV control.[14] Typical examples of these routine fluctuations are increased BP following physical activity or psychological stress and decreased levels of BP during relaxation or sleep.[13] Studies of high CV risk populations showed high BPV values as reliable predictors of CV mortality and morbidity in individual subjects, even to a greater extent than average BP values. BPV can be classified into five different types, depending on the time measurements evaluated—very short, short, mid-term, long-term and very long-term.[15] Concise term BPV can be defined as variability beat to beat, while variability over 24 hours is referred to as short-term BPV.

Variability daily is identified as mid-term BPV. In BP measurements that are less than or greater than 5 years is long-term and very long-term BPV visits-to-visit variabilities. There is a healthy relationship between levels of BPV and BP; higher levels of BP, higher levels of BPV. In practice, different indices were used to measure different types of BPV; they are extensively reviewed by Parati et al.[15] BPV is usually expressed as a standard 24-hour mean BP deviation [standard deviation (SD)].[16] To measure all five different types of BPV, the SD and coefficient of variation are used. These two indices are particularly crucial for the long-term measurement of BPV. Alternative indices for measuring short-term BPV are proposed or in practice.

The variability of beat to beat can be estimated from the frequency domain spectral analysis.[15] Recently, average real variability for short-term BPV has been proposed.[17] It calculates the average of the absolute differences over 24 hours between consecutive BP measurements. It reflects the short-term within-subject variability as it focuses on the sequence of BP readings.[15] It is known that various intrinsic and extrinsic factors influence various types of BPV. Wei Li et al. demonstrated that BPV is influenced by various demographic, clinical and biochemical factors in a population-based study of adult Chinese subjects with different ethnicities.[18] The authors also found that an average night-time systolic BP, an average daytime diastolic BP, triglycerides, fasting blood glucose and apolipoprotein A were associated with BPV significantly and independently.

Very Short-term BPV

Very short-term BPV refers to beat-to-beat fluctuations in BP due to the interplay of different CV control systems, such as the baroreceptor reflex, the renin-angiotensin system, the myogenic vascular response and the release of endothelial nitric oxide, as well as changes in behavioral and emotional mechanisms.[19-21] Usually, noninvasive finger cuffs that track finger BP levels continuously through infrared photoplethysmography are evaluated in a laboratory via intra-arterial recording or under ambulatory conditions.[19,22] Standard deviations of BP values or BP fluctuations from spectral analyzes at different frequency bands are often used as the main indicators for very short-term BPV assessment.[19]

Although its practical usefulness and reliability are questionable, concise-term BPV has been used as a tool to diagnose and treat patients with CVD, as well as to study the mechanism of action of antihypertensive drugs.[19,21,23] The detection of changes in beat-to-beat BPV can also help to select antihypertensive drugs rationally.[20] Hypertensive patients with labile blood pressure, e.g. may have increased sympathetic modulation of vascular tone and may, therefore, respond well to sympathetic antihypertensive drugs.[21]

Short-term-Blood Pressure Variability

Studies that recorded intra-arterial BPV over a day were the first to attempt to relate short-term BPV to increased CV mortality and target organ damage.[5,24] Ambulatory blood pressure monitoring (ABPM) is the most common 24-hour method for analyzing BPV behavior. This method can determine if the loss of the expected circadian BP rhythm is associated with CV morbidity and mortality in hypertensive patient subpopulations,[25,26] as well as in the general population.[27,28] In this sense, the kidney is especially susceptible to variations in pressure, as are vascular territories (macro and microcirculation), and ABPM detects myocardium.[27,29]

There is no universal consensus as to which of these parameters better reflect the increased risk of CV and the need for further mathematical subanalysis of 24-hour BP recording to determine a parameter for predicting CV events.[30] In several studies, both absolute elevated night-time BP and nondipping profile were addressed. Several studies have shown that elevated night-time BP is more effective in predicting morbidity of CV compared to the mean values of awake or 24-hour BP.[25,29,31-33] In addition, the detection of a blunted nocturnal decline in dipped BP, or even an increase in inverted dipper BP values, was found to be associated with a higher prevalence of vascular damage, increased risk of CV and death.[34,35] Morning blood pressure surge (MBPS) was associated with target organ damage, including left ventricular hypertrophy (LVH), albuminuria,

increased intima-media carotid thickness, arterial stiffness, reduced reserve coronary flow and silent cerebrovascular disease.[36,37]

Discrepancies, however, were found in clinical trials that identified MBPS as a risk factor for CV disease. Some,[35,38] but not all studies,[39,40] found a positive association between MBPS regardless of the 24-hour BP levels with CV outcomes in both hypertensive and the general community. Despite these various studies, the threshold at which an MBPS becomes pathological remains unclear and can account for the heterogeneity of the clinical studies results.[36] Therefore, new MBPS measures have been investigated that may more effectively predict CV risk. However, there is still no consensus on the real prognostic significance of MBPS and also whether MBPS targeting is more beneficial than clinic BP targeting.[41] Despite this, in today's clinical practice, BP appears to be an important target of antihypertensive treatment for hypertension management.[36]

Mid-term, Long-term and Very Long-term Blood Pressure Variability

Long-term BPV refers to changes in BP daily, visit-to-visit and season-to-season.[7,22] Relatively unclear are the factors that contribute to long-term BPV. Long-term BPV may result from poor control of BP in treated patients, such as inadequate physician treatment, poor patient adherence or inappropriate methods of BP measurement.[7,22] It can also be influenced by individual behavioral changes as well as environmental factors, such as outdoor temperatures and differences between different seasons during the daylight hours.[22,42] For example, BPV was found to be higher in winter than in summer, possibly because of increased sodium retention and vascular resistance due to increased sympathetic activity.[42]

Some studies have also suggested that increased arterial stiffness contributes to long-term BPV pathogenesis. Day-to-day BPV can be evaluated by ABPM over 48 hours or by HBPM data collected over several days, weeks or months, whereas visit-to-visit BPV is usually evaluated by ABPM or OBPM, usually spaced by visits over weeks, months and years.[7,22] However, the reliability of using OBPM to evaluate long-term BPV has been questioned as it does not consider the normal activities of the patient and requires frequent BP measurement visits to the physician.[7,22]

A recent cross-sectional single-center study showed significant differences between single OBPM and following BP measurement methods.[43] Sometimes in-office measurements are also inaccurate, mainly due to the effect of white coat, inadequate or uncalibrated devices, and suboptimal measuring techniques (e.g. incorrect cuff size, no rest before measurement).[44,45] While a large number of recommendations have been published on correct OBPM techniques; these guidelines are not generally translated into primary care practice.[45,46] There is strong evidence that increased long-term BPV is associated with increased risk of stroke, CV events and death, including all-cause mortality.[47,48] It may, therefore, be clinically important to measure long-term BPV, as it can provide useful insights into the long-term control of the patient's BP and the effectiveness of the current antihypertensive therapy.[7]

Tools to Measure Blood Pressure Variability

Different tools allow BPV measurement. One of them is 24-hour ABPM that helps to determine the BPV accurately. In principle, ABPM enables BP to be recorded 24 hours (or even longer) and evaluates various parameters such as mean BP, variations between daytime and night-time, pressure loads, the area under the curve and variability of pulse pressure.

Also, a 24-hour ABPM measurement enables short-term BPV to be evaluated between measurement intervals not longer than 15 minutes.[49] These different evaluations facilitated by ABPM are valuable for clinical hypertension management as they increase the accuracy of the diagnosis and prediction of CV risk.[50] Absolute indications for ABPM include the identification of white coat or masked hypertension and abnormal BP patterns lasting 24 hours and evaluation of the effectiveness of antihypertensive treatment.[51] Some of ABPM's limitations include night-time discomfort, occasional failure to detect accurate artifact measurements, limited device availability and high cost. In addition to these repeated measurements, HBPM or OBPM can be acquired with a well-calibrated automated BP monitoring device. BPV can be determined from these values by calculating the SD or variation coefficient.

■ BLOOD PRESSURE VARIABILITY AND CARDIAC HYPERTROPHY

Early available data suggest that mean BP values obtained through 24-hour BP monitoring predict the presence of LVH more effectively than a single measurement of BP.[26] Increase in 24-hour BPV assessment[52] or daytime[25] recorded with ABPM was associated with a higher degree of hypertensive CV complications, such as left ventricular (LV) systolic dysfunction.[53] Most of the studies examining the association between BPV and LVH examined short-term variability.[53-55] In a general population, the night-time BP nondipper pattern and the exaggerated MBPS evaluated with ABPM are associated with increased LV mass and CV morbidity[56] and with a CV remodeling in hypertensive patients.[57] A recent meta-analysis of the correlation between short-term BPV and LV mass indexes, however, suggests a weak positive correlation between BPV and

LV mass[58,59] while another study showed that higher visit-to-visit BPV predicts CV events in hypertensive LVH patients.[60]

In addition, several problems have been detected in the evaluation of the CV impact of short-term and long-term BPV, including limited reproducibility of BPV, the lack of standard reference values, and limitations of conventional devices for ABPM.[61] Considering the limitations of the evaluation of the clinical relevance of BPV, preclinical studies have clearly contributed to the actual knowledge of the role of BPV in CVD. The sinoaortic denervated (SAD) rat represents an excellent experimental model to investigate the consequences of BPV on target organs because SAD increases fluctuation in BP without affecting mean values. Specifically, the ablation of carotid and aortic baroreceptor afferents in SAD rats induces a chronic increase in short-term BPV with normal average BP level.[62]

■ BLOOD PRESSURE VARIABILITY AND CHRONIC KIDNEY DISEASE

End-stage renal disease individuals are characterized by marked variations in BP and changes in the circadian rhythm of BP. However, no short-term human BPV study has found influence in determining the development or progression of renal dysfunction on the prognostic role of BPV on mean BP levels. Few studies have shown that an increase in short-term BPV can be positively correlated with impaired renal function evaluated with microalbuminuria or glomerular filtration rate estimates.[7,63] However, longitudinal studies have found that night-time BP nondipper or inverted dipper patterns evaluated over 24-hour ABPM are independent predictors of poor kidney prognosis, as evaluated by many kidney function markers.[64,65] HBPM was found to have a predictive value for renal

function impairment[66,67] but the same results were not found in all studies. Visit-to-visit BPV may be important in predicting the risk of nephropathy and chronic kidney disease development and progression.[68,69]

■ BLOOD PRESSURE VARIABILITY CEREBROVASCULAR DYSFUNCTION AND BRAIN DAMAGE

Hypertension is the most critical risk factor for atherosclerotic carotid lesion and cerebral small vessel disease that contribute to stroke and cognitive decline in the elderly.[70] Therefore, detecting the early involvement of these vascular territories may have the potential to prevent future brain damage before clinical manifestations occur.[71] Increased short- and long-term BPV was suggested as an independent risk factor for stroke in elderly patients with high BP.[72] Cerebral infarction was associated with a disturbed nocturnal decline in BP, whereas a substantial morning pressure rise and a sizeable nocturnal decline in BP were both associated with cerebral hemorrhage.[36]

In the case of cognitive dysfunction, BPV is associated with low scores in cognitive testing in the elderly[73] and was claimed as a predictor of cognitive decline in subjects of common age.[74] Also, the long-term BPV in young subjects was associated with worse psychomotor speed and verbal memory in 25 years of follow-up, regardless of BP levels.[75] The combination of short-term BPV and early carotid artery damage was detected over a decade ago and is also confirmed in recent studies.[76,77] Nondipping pattern and exaggerated MBPS were associated with increased carotid intima-media thickness values and high blood inflammatory marker levels in older adults with high CV risk[38,78] and middle-aged hypertensive subjects. Also, daily BPV is not only associated with carotid artery atherosclerosis, but also with arterial rigidity and endothelial function in normotensive and mild-moderate individuals with hypertension.[79,80] As the link between the pathophysiological mechanisms of stroke and cognitive impairment, it appears that cerebral small vessel disease (CSVD) may be linked to silent cerebral injury. Short-term variability has recently been associated with the presence of subclinical CSVD in subjects of hypertension, regardless of BP and other clinical covariates.[81]

■ BLOOD PRESSURE VARIABILITY AS A TARGET FOR ANTIHYPERTENSIVE TREATMENT: SHORT AND LONG-TERM STUDIES

In clinical practice, BPV's independent role in predicting organ damage and CV morbidity remains controversial. Despite this, numerous publications have analyzed in recent years whether antihypertensive drugs affect BPV reduction, regardless of BP values. Besides, few studies discussed the link between decreasing BPV with pharmacological treatment and improving target organ damage and consequently reducing CV events.

Most of the data come from post-hoc analysis of clinical trials and databases using various classes of antihypertensive drugs and separate clusters of target organ damage and CV outcomes. The studies also used various phenotypes of BPV. Some assessed the effect of antihypertensive medicines on ABPM's short-term BPV, while others used HBPM's long-term BPV, visit-to-visit or longer intervals such as between seasons.

Recently, a systematic review was carried out to assess the differences in effectiveness in stroke prevention between classes of antihypertensive drugs. Compared to other drugs, inter-individual variation in SBP was significantly reduced by calcium channel blockers (CCB) and nonloop diuretic drugs and increased by angiotensin-converting enzyme (ACE) inhibitors, angiotensin blockers (ARB) and β-adrenergic blockers (βB).[82] A post-hoc analysis of two major clinical trials compared the variability of both in-visit and ABPM between amlodipine and atenolol-based treatment groups and the variability within BPV between placebo and atenolol and diuretic-based treatment groups. As a result, amlodipine decreased the risk of BPV over time, while atenolol had opposite effects.[83]

An ABMP database meta-analysis showed that subjects treated with telmisartan or amlodipine had a higher smoothness index than others treated with losartan, valsartan or Ramipril.[84] The same ABPM database was further evaluated, and the smoothness index and treatment-on-variability index inferred BPV. Compared to various monotherapies, telmisartan/amlodipine combination was associated with a smoother 24-hour BP reduction profile as well as significantly lower and smoother BP levels over 24-hour.[85]

A randomized, double-blind, placebo-controlled study with four parallel therapy arms (placebo, candesartan, indapamide and amlodipine) analyzed ABPM data for short-term BPV. In summary, treatment with amlodipine and indapamide was associated with a significant reduction in BPV.[86] It investigated the effect of two combinations of antihypertensive drugs [(olmesartan/CCB) and (olmesartan/diuretic)] on home blood pressure variability (HBPV) and arterial stiffness. The study showed that in addition to home BP reduction, the combination of ARB/CCB improved HBPV.

Also, the reduction in HBPV was partly attributable to this combination's reduction in arterial stiffness.[87] A randomized, open-label, blinded-endpoint trial studied the time-dependent valsartan/hydrochlorothiazide combination therapy efficacy of ABPM-measured BPV administration. The results showed that the proportion of subjects with properly controlled outpatient BP after combination therapy was significantly higher during bedtime than when they were awakened.[88]

Patients treated with atenolol and lacidipine were compared to intraindividual visit-to-visit variations of both clinical and 24-hour mean BP of clinic BP. In conclusion, there is no significant difference between βB and CCB treatment in the visit-to-visit BPV.[89] Short-term BPV indices were studied in a cohort of patients treated either alone or in combination with CCB, diuretics, ACE inhibitors, ARBs or βB. Patients treated with CCB and diuretics alone or combinations had lower BPV compared to other classes of medicines.[90] Antihypertensive drug class effect on the daily variability of HBP following an investigation into a recent minor cerebrovascular event. In patients treated with CCB/diuretics, variability in SBP was reduced compared with both ACE inhibitors and ARBs.[91]

In patients with LVH randomized to losartan-and atenolol-based treatment, the association of visit-to-visit BPV with target organ damage and CV outcomes has been recently analyzed. As a result, higher variability of BP in treatment, regardless of mean BP, was associated with later events of stroke and composite CV, but not with myocardial infarction or target organ damage.[63] However, in a post-hoc study of elderly patients, the association between visit-to-visit BP variability and cognitive impairment was not associated with BP-mediated reduction medication.[92]

A study compared the variability of visit-to-visit BP between old and old subjects and between two combinations of treatments, i.e. ARB/CCB and ARB/diuretic. In the ARB/CCB group, the long-term variability was lower than in the other group, particularly in the very old and isolated patients with systolic hypertension.[93] A prospective, randomized trial analyzed visit-to-visit and seasonal BP variations in elderly patients receiving ARB/CCB or ARB/diuretics combination. In the ARB/CCB group, visit-to-visit BPV was substantially lower than in the ARB/diuretic group. About seasonal variability, no significant differences were found between groups.[94]

For their effects on HBPV, another study compared a combination of a CCB/ACE inhibitors with the corresponding monotherapies and placebo. The study demonstrated that CCB/ACE inhibitors reduces HBPV more effectively than other treatments.[95] Recently, the effects on intra-individual visit-to-visit BPV of three CCB-based treatments (CCB/ARB, CCB/βB, CCB/diuretic) have been studied, confirming previous observations. There was no difference between groups in the maximum BPs. In the CCB/diuretic group, however, BPV was lower than in the CCB/βB group. At each visit, daily at home, and by ABPM, simultaneous evaluation of the efficacy of a fixed-dose combination of perindopril/amlodipine in the doctor's office was assessed in another study. A significant reduction in BP levels and a beneficial effect on the improvement of BPV detected on different parameters related to BPV could be demonstrated.[96]

Together, this data suggests that CCB may be more effective in reducing BPV and specific CV outcomes than other antihypertensive drugs alone or in combination as a monotherapy or in addition to diuretics.

■ CONCLUSION

To summarize, the concept of BPV though has been evaluated for several decades; its clinical implication is still far from clear. Despite the availability of clinical evidence showing that BPV could cause damage to the target organ, in routine clinical practice, it did not achieve desired significance. Reasons for this could be the lack of high-quality tests evaluating a direct relationship between the reduction of BPV and reduction of CV risk and the difficulty of measuring BPV in a busy ambulatory setting. In patients with hypertension, diabetes mellitus and chronic kidney disease, both short and long-term BPVs are independently associated with target organ damage and CV events. Some antihypertensive medicines, either as monotherapy or in combination, reduce short-and long-term BPV effectively.

Nevertheless, available data suggest that CCB are more capable of attenuating long-term BPV and effective BPV management of hypertension compared to other therapeutic classes, rather than merely controlling average BP levels. This concept can then be regarded as clinically meaningful. It is reasonable to include BPV in the hypertension management diagnostic armamentarium.

■ REFERENCES

1. Lawes CM, Vander Hoorn S, Rodgers A. Global burden of blood-pressure related disease, 2001. Lancet. 2008; 371(9623):1513-8.
2. Gradman AH. Sleep-time blood pressure: a validated therapeutic target. J Am Coll Cardiol. 2011;58(11):1174-5.
3. Pickering TG, Hall JE, Appel LJ, et al. Recommendations for blood pressure measurement in humans and experimental animals: part 1: blood pressure measurement in humans: a statement for professionals from the Subcommittee of Professional and Public Education of the American Heart Association Council on High Blood Pressure Research. Circulation. 2005;111(5):697-716.
4. Papadogiannis DE, Protogerou AD. Blood pressure variability: a confounder and a cardiovascular risk factor. Hypertens Res. 2011;34:162-3.
5. Parati G, Pomidossi G, Albini F, et al. Relationship of 24-hour blood pressure mean and variability to severity of target-organ damage in hypertension. J Hypertens. 1987; 5(1):93-8.
6. Hansen TW, Thijs L, Li Y, et al. Prognostic value of reading-to-reading blood pressure variability over 24 hours in 8938 subjects from 11 populations. Hypertension. 2010;55(4):1049-57.
7. Parati G, Ochoa JE, Bilo G. Blood pressure variability, cardiovascular risk, and risk for renal disease progression. Curr Hypertens Rep. 2012;14(5):421-31.
8. Dolan E, O'Brien E. Is it daily, monthly, or yearly blood pressure variability that enhances cardiovascular risk? Curr Cardiol Rep. 2015;17(11):93.
9. Hermida RC, Ayala DE, Mojon A, et al. Decreasing sleep-time blood pressure determined by ambulatory monitoring reduces cardiovascular risk. J Am Coll Cardiol. 2011;58:1165-73.
10. Millar-Craig MW, Bishop CN, Raftery EB. Circadian variation of blood-pressure. Lancet. 1978;1(8068):795-7.
11. Peixoto AJ, White WB. Circadian blood pressure: clinical implications based on the pathophysiology of its variability. Kidney Int. 2007;71(9):855-60.
12. Kario K, White WB. Early morning hypertension: what does it contribute to overall cardiovascular risk assessment? J Am Soc Hypertens. 2008;2(6):397-402.
13. Parati G. Blood pressure variability, target organ damage and antihypertensive treatment. J Hypertens. 2003;21(10):1827-30.
14. Mancia G, Parati G, Di Rienzo M, et al. BP variability. In: Zanchetti A, Mancia G (Eds). Handbook of hypertension: Pathophysiology of hypertension. Amsterdam: Elsevier Science BV; 1997. pp. 117-69.
15. Parati G, Ochoa JE, Lombardi C, et al. Blood pressure variability: assessment, predictive value, and potential as a therapeutic target. Curr Hypertens Rep. 2015;17(4): 537.
16. Su DF, Miao CY. Blood pressure variability and organ damage. Clin Exp PharmacolPhysiol. 2001;28(9):709-15.
17. Mena L, Pintos S, Queipo NV, et al. A reliable index for the prognostic significance of blood pressure variability. J Hypertens. 2005;23(3):505-11.
18. Li W, Yu Y, Liang D, Jia EZ. Factors Associated with Blood Pressure Variability Based on Ambulatory Blood Pressure Monitoring in Subjects with Hypertension in China. Kidney and Blood Pressure Res. 2017;42(2):267-75.
19. Parati G, Ochoa JE, Lombardi C, et al. Assessment and management of blood-pressure variability. Nat Rev Cardiol. 2013;10(3):143-55.
20. Höcht C. Blood pressure variability: prognostic value and therapeutic implications. ISRN Hypertens. 2013:398485.
21. Stauss HM. Identification of blood pressure control mechanisms by power spectral analysis. Clin Exp Pharmacol Physiol. 2007;34(4):362-8.
22. Chenniappan M. Blood pressure variability: assessment, prognostic significance and management. J Assoc Physicians India. 2015;63(5):47-53.
23. Souza HC, Martins-Pinge MC, da Silva VJ, et al. Heart rate and arterial pressure variability in the experimental reno-vascular hypertension model in rats. Auton Neurosci. 2008;139(1):38-45.
24. Grassi G, Bombelli M, Brambilla G, et al. Total cardiovascular risk, blood pressure variability and adrenergic overdrive in hypertension: evidence, mechanisms and clinical implications. Curr Hypertens Rep. 2012;14(4):333-8.
25. Palatini P, Penzo M, Racioppa A, et al. Clinical relevance of night time blood pressure and of daytime blood pressure variability. Arch Intern Med. 1992;152(9):1855-60.

26. Mancia G, Zanchetti A, Agabiti-Rosei E, et al. Ambulatory blood pressure is superior to clinic blood pressure in predicting treatment-induced regression of left ventricular hypertrophy. SAMPLE Study Group. Study on Ambulatory Monitoring of Blood Pressure and Lisinopril Evaluation. Circulation. 1997;95(6):1464-70.

27. Madden JM, O'Flynn AM, Dolan E, et al. Short-term blood pressure variability over 24 h and target organ damage in middle-aged men and women. J Hum Hypertens. 2015;29(12):719-25.

28. Madden JM, O'Flynn AM, Fitzgerald AP, et al. Correlation between short-term blood pressure variability and left-ventricular mass index: a meta-analysis. Hypertens Res. 2016;39(3):171-7.

29. Sega R, Facchetti R, Bombelli M, et al. Prognostic value of ambulatory and home blood pressures compared with office blood pressure in the general population: follow-up results from the Pressioni Arteriose Monitorate e Loro Associazioni (PAMELA) study. Circulation. 2005;111(14):1777-83.

30. O'Brien E, Parati G, Stergiou G. Ambulatory blood pressure measurement: what is the international consensus? Hypertension. 2013;62(6):988-94.

31. Fagard RH, Van Den Broeke C, De Cort P. Prognostic significance of blood pressure measured in the office, at home and during ambulatory monitoring in older patients in general practice. J Hum Hypertens. 2005;19(10):801-7.

32. Staessen JA, Thijs L, Fagard R, et al. Predicting cardiovascular risk using conventional vs ambulatory blood pressure in older patients with systolic hypertension. Systolic Hypertension in Europe Trial Investigators. JAMA. 1999;282(6):539-46.

33. Clement DL, De Buyzere ML, De Bacquer DA, et al. Prognostic value of ambulatory blood-pressure recordings in patients with treated hypertension. N Engl J Med. 2003;348(24):2407-15.

34. Hansen TW, Li Y, Boggia J, et al. Predictive role of the night time blood pressure. Hypertension. 2011;57(1):3-10.

35. Metoki H, Ohkubo T, Kikuya M, et al. Prognostic significance for stroke of a morning pressor surge and a nocturnal blood pressure decline: the Ohasama study. Hypertension. 2006;47(2):149-54.

36. Kario K. Prognosis in relation to blood pressure variability: pro side of the argument. Hypertension. 2015;65(6):1163-9.

37. Turak O, Afsar B, Ozcan F, et al. Relationship between elevated morning blood pressure surge, uric acid, and cardiovascular outcomes in hypertensive patients. J Clin Hypertens (Greenwich). 2014;16(7):530-5.

38. Li Y, Thijs L, Hansen TW, et al. Prognostic value of the morning blood pressure surge in 5645 subjects from 8 populations. Hypertension. 2010;55(4):1040-8.

39. Verdecchia P, Angeli F, Mazzotta G, et al. Day-night dip and early-morning surge in blood pressure in hypertension: prognostic implications. Hypertension. 2012;60(1):34-42.

40. Bombelli M, Fodri D, Toso E, et al. Relationship among morning blood pressure surge, 24-hour blood pressure variability, and cardiovascular outcomes in a white population. Hypertension. 2014;64(5):943-50.

41. Asayama K, Wei FF, Liu YP, et al. Does blood pressure variability contribute to risk stratification? Methodological issues and a review of outcome studies based on home blood pressure. Hypertens Res. 2015;38(2):97-101.

42. Floras JS. Blood pressure variability: a novel and important risk factor. Can J Cardiol. 2013;29(5):557-63.

43. Burkard T, Mayr M, Winterhalder C, et al. Reliability of single office blood pressure measurements. BMJ Heart. 2018;104(14):1173-9.

44. Sheppard JP, Martin U, Gill P, et al. Prospective Register of Patients Undergoing Repeated Office and Ambulatory Blood Pressure Monitoring (PROOF-ABPM): protocol for an observational cohort study. BMJ Open. 2016;6(10):e012607.

45. Sebo P, Pechere-Bertschi A, Herrmann FR, et al. Blood pressure measurements are unreliable to diagnose hypertension in primary care. J Hypertens. 2014;32(3): 509-17.

46. Levy J, Gerber LM, Wu X, et al. Non adherence to recommended guidelines for blood pressure measurement. J Clin Hypertens (Greenwich). 2016;18(11):1157-61.

47. Kikuya M, Ohkubo T, Metoki H, et al. Day-by-day variability of blood pressure and heart rate at home as a novel predictor of prognosis: the Ohasama study. Hypertension. 2008;52(6):1045-50.

48. Muntner P, Shimbo D, Tonelli M, et al. The relationship between visit-to-visit variability in systolic blood pressure and all-cause mortality in the general population: findings from NHANES III, 1988 to 1994. Hypertension. 2011;57(2):160-6.

49. Nobre F, Mion Junior D. Ambulatory Blood Pressure Monitoring: Five Decades of more light and Less Shadows. Arq Bras Cardiol. 2016;106(6):528-37.

50. Turner JR, Viera AJ, Shimbo D. Ambulatory blood pressure monitoring in clinical practice: a review. Am J Med. 2015;128(1):14-20.

51. O'Brien E, Parati G, Stergiou G. Ambulatory blood pressure measurement. Hypertension. 2013;62:988-94.

52. Frattola A, Parati G, Cuspidi C, et al. Prognostic value of 24-hour blood pressure variability. J Hypertens. 1993;11(10): 1133-7.

53. Tatasciore A, Zimarino M, Tommasi R, et al. Increased short-term blood pressure variability is associated with early left ventricular systolic dysfunction in newly diagnosed untreated hypertensive patients. J Hypertens. 2013;31(8):1653-61.

54. Ryu J, Cha RH, Kim DK, et al. The clinical association of the blood pressure variability with the target organ damage in hypertensive patients with chronic kidney disease. J Korean Med Sci. 2014;29(7):957-64.

55. Gomez Angelats E, Sierra C, Coca A, et al. Lack of association between blood pressure variability and left ventricular hypertrophy in essential hypertension. Med Clin (Barc). 2004;123(19):731-4.

56. Kaneda R, Kario K, Hoshide S, et al. Morning blood pressure hyper-reactivity is an independent predictor for hypertensive cardiac hypertrophy in a community-dwelling population. Am J Hypertens. 2005;18(12 Pt 1):1528-33.

57. Yano Y, Hoshide S, Inokuchi T, et al. Association between morning blood pressure surge and cardiovascular remodelling in treated elderly hypertensive subjects. Am J Hypertens. 2009;22(11):1177-82.

58. Juhanoja EP, Niiranen TJ, Johansson JK, et al. Agreement between ambulatory, home, and office blood pressure variability. J Hypertens. 2016;34(1):61-7.

59. Madden JM, O'Flynn AM, Fitzgerald AP, et al. Correlation between short-term blood pressure variability and left-ventricular mass index: a meta-analysis. Hypertens Res. 2016;39(3):171-7.

60. Vishram JK, Dahlof B, Devereux RB, et al. Blood pressure variability predicts cardiovascular events independently of traditional cardiovascular risk factors and target organ damage: a LIFE sub study. J Hypertens. 2015;33(12):2422-30.

61. Parati G, Bilo G, Valentini M. Blood pressure variability: methodological aspects, pathophysiological and clinical implications. In: Mancia G, Grassi G, Kjeldsen SE (Eds). Manual of Hypertension of the European Society of Hypertension,. London: Inform a Healthcare. 2008. pp. 61-71.

62. Parati G, Lantelme P. Blood pressure variability, target organ damage and cardiovascular events. J Hypertens. 2002;20(9):1725-9.

63. Manios E, Tsagalis G, Tsivgoulis G, et al. Time rate of blood pressure variation is associated with impaired renal function in hypertensive patient's. J Hypertens. 2009;27(11):2244-8.

64. Felicio JS, de Souza AC, Kohlmann N, et al. Nocturnal blood pressure fall as predictor of diabetic nephropathy in hypertensive patients with type 2 diabetes. Cardiovasc Diabetol. 2010;9:36.

65. Tsioufis C, Andrikou I, Thomopoulos C, et al. Comparative prognostic role of night time blood pressure and non-dipping profile on renal outcomes. Am J Nephrol. 2011;33(3):277-88.

66. Matsui Y, Ishikawa J, Eguchi K, et al. Maximum value of home blood pressure: a novel indicator of target organ damage in hypertension. Hypertension. 2011;57(6):1087-93.

67. Tamura K, Azushima K, Umemura S. Day-by-day home measured blood pressure variability: another important factor in hypertension with diabetic nephropathy? Hypertens Res. 2011;34(12):1249-50.

68. Kawai T, Ohishi M, Kamide K, et al. The impact of visit-to-visit variability in blood pressure on renal function. Hypertens Res. 2012;35(2):239-43.

69. Tsioufis C, Andrikou I, Thomopoulos C, et al. Comparative prognostic role of night time blood pressure and non-dipping profile on renal outcomes. Am J Nephrol. 2011;33(3):277-88.

70. James PA, Oparil S, Carter BL, et al. 2014 evidence-based guideline for the management of high blood pressure in adults: report from the panel members appointed to the Eighth Joint National Committee (JNC 8). JAMA. 2014;311(5):507-20.

71. Filomena J, Riba-Llena I, Vinyoles E, et al. Short-term blood pressure variability relates to the presence of subclinical brain small vessel disease in primary hypertension. Hypertension. 2015;66(3):634-40.

72. Hashimoto T, Kikuya M, Ohkubo T, et al. Home blood pressure level, blood pressure variability, smoking, and stroke risk in Japanese men: the Ohasama study. Am J Hypertens. 2012;25(8):883-91.

73. Brickman AM, Reitz C, Luchsinger JA, et al. Long-term blood pressure fluctuation and cerebrovascular disease in an elderly cohort. ArchNeurol. 2010;67(5):564-9.

74. Bohm M, Schumacher H, Leong D, et al. Systolic blood pressure variation and mean heart rate is associated with cognitive dysfunction in patients with high cardiovascular risk. Hypertension. 2015;65(3):651-61.

75. Yano Y, Ning H, Allen N, et al. Long term blood pressure variability throughout young adulthood and cognitive function in midlife: the Coronary Artery Risk Development in Young Adults (CARDIA) study. Hypertension. 2014;64(5):983-8.

76. Zakopoulos NA, Tsivgoulis G, Barlas G, et al. Time rate of blood pressure variation is associated with increased common carotid artery intima-media thickness. Hypertension. 2005;45(4):505-12.

77. Chen Y, Xiong H, Wu D, et al. Relationship of short-term blood pressure variability with carotid intima-media thickness in hypertensive patients. Biomed Eng Online. 2015;14:71.

78. Nagai M, Hoshide S, Ishikawa J, et al. Visit-to visit blood pressure variations: new independent determinants for carotid artery measures in the elderly a thigh risk of cardiovascular disease. J Am Soc Hypertens. 2011;5(3):184-92.

79. Song H, Wei F, Liu Z, et al. Visit-to-visit variability in systolic blood pressure: correlated with the changes of arterial stiffness and myocardial perfusion in on-treated hypertensive patients. Clin Exp Hypertens. 2015;37(1):63-9.

80. Liu Z, Zhao Y, Lu F, et al. Day-by-day variability in self-measured blood pressure at home: effects on carotid artery atherosclerosis, brachial flow-mediated dilation, and endothelin1 in normotensive and mild-moderate hypertensive individuals. Blood Press Monit. 2013;18(6):316-25.

81. Nagai M, Kario K. Visit-to-visit blood pressure variability, silent cerebral injury, and risk of stroke. Am J Hypertens. 2013;26(12):1369-76.

82. Webb AJ, Fischer U, Mehta Z, et al. Effects of antihypertensive-drug class on inter individual variation in blood pressure and risk of stroke: a systematic review and meta-analysis. Lancet. 2010;375(9718):906-15.

83. Rothwell PM, Howard SC, Dolan E, et al. Effects of beta blockers and calcium-channel blockers on within-individual variability in blood pressure and risk of stroke. Lancet Neurol. 2010;9(5):469-80.

84. Parati G, Schumacher H, Bilo G, et al. Evaluating 24-h antihypertensive efficacy by the smoothness index: a meta-analysis of an ambulatory blood pressure monitoring database. J Hypertens. 2010;28(11):2177-83.

85. Parati G, Dolan E, Ley L, et al. Impact of antihypertensive combination and mono treatments on blood pressure variability: assessment by old and new indices. Data from a large ambulatory blood pressure monitoring database. J Hypertens. 2014;32(6):1326-33.

86. Zhang Y, Agnoletti D, Safar ME, et al. Effect of antihypertensive agents on blood pressure variability: the Natrilix SR versus candesartan and amlodipine in the reduction of systolic blood pressure in hypertensive patients (X-CELLENT) study. Hypertension. 2011;58(2):155-60.

87. Matsui Y, O'Rourke MF, Hoshide S, et al. Combined effect of angiotensin II receptor blocker and either a calcium channel blocker or diuretic on day-by-day variability of home blood pressure: the Japan Combined Treatment With Olmesartan and a Calcium-Channel Blocker Versus Olmesartan and Diuretics Randomized Efficacy Study. Hypertension. 2012;59(6):1132-8.

88. Hermida RC, Ayala DE, Mojon A, et al. Chronotherapy with valsartan/hydrochlorothiazide combination in essential hypertension: improved sleep-time blood pressure control with bedtime dosing. Chronobiol Int. 2011;28(7):601-10.

89. Mancia G, Facchetti R, Parati G, et al. Visit-to-visit blood pressure variability in the European Lacidipine Study on Atherosclerosis: methodological aspects and effects of anti-hypertensive treatment. J Hypertens. 2012;30(6): 1241-51.

90. Levi-Marpillat N, Macquin-Mavier I, Tropeano AI, et al. Antihypertensive drug classes have different effects on short-term blood pressure variability in essential hypertension. Hypertens Res. 2014;37(6):585-90.

91. Webb AJ, Wilson M, Lovett N, et al. Response of day-to-day home blood pressure variability by antihypertensive drug class after transient ischemic attack or non-disabling stroke. Stroke. 2014;45(10):2967-73.

92. Wijsman LW, deCraen AJ, Muller M, et al. Blood pressure lowering medication, visit-to-visit blood pressure variability, and cognitive function in old age. Am J Hypertens. 2016;29(3):311-8.

93. Rakugi H, Ogihara T, Saruta T, et al. Preferable effects of olmesartan/calcium channel blocker to olmesartan/diuretic on blood pressure variability in very elderly hypertension: COLM study sub analysis. J Hypertens. 2015;33(10):2165-72.

94. Sato N, Saijo Y, Sasagawa Y, et al. Visit-to-visit variability and seasonal variation in blood pressure: Combination of Antihypertensive Therapy in the Elderly, Multicentre Investigation (CAMUI) Trial sub analysis. Clin Exp Hypertens. 2015;37(5):411-9.

95. Mancia G, Omboni S, Chazova I, et al. Effects of the lercanidipine-enalapril combination vs. the corresponding monotherapies on home blood pressure in hypertension: evidence from a large database. J Hypertens. 2016;34(1): 139-48.

96. Karpov YA, Gorbunov VM, Deev AD. Effectiveness of fixed-dose perindopril/amlodipine on clinic, ambulatory and self-monitored blood pressure and blood pressure variability: an open-label, non-comparative study in the general practice. High Blood Press Cardiovasc Prev. 2015;22(4):417-25

Secondary Hypertension

Management of Hypertension in Chronic Kidney Disease

Sankar D Navaneethan

■ INTRODUCTION

Hypertension is the leading cardiovascular risk factor worldwide and a significant contributor to kidney disease progression independent of diabetes and other renal risk factors. Among patients with chronic kidney disease (CKD), hypertension is extremely common (with prevalence over 80%) and contributes to the progression of CKD and development of end-stage kidney disease (ESKD).[1] Further, resistant hypertension defined as blood pressure (BP) more than 140/90 mm Hg despite being on more than or equal to 3 BP lowering medications is 2–3 times more common among those with kidney disease. Pathophysiology of CKD associated hypertension is multifactorial with different mechanisms contributing to hypertension. Irrespective of this, BP lowering significantly reduces cardiovascular and renal risk in those with different comorbidities including among those with CKD. In this chapter, we will focus on various issues relating to the management of hypertension in those with pre-existing CKD (who are not on dialysis)—(A) BP targets recommended for CKD population; (B) role of various agents used to lower BP in CKD and specific considerations in CKD; and (C) a systematic approach to managing these high-risk patients.

■ GUIDELINE RECOMMENDATIONS FOR BLOOD PRESSURE TARGETS IN KIDNEY DISEASE

Several guidelines have recommended BP targets for those with CKD based on available clinical trial evidence (Table 1). The Kidney Disease: Improving Global Outcomes (KDIGO) 2012 clinical practice guideline recommends systolic blood pressure (SBP) of ≤140 mm Hg and diastolic blood pressure (DBP) of ≤90 mm Hg in nonalbuminuric CKD patients, and ≤130/80 mm Hg in those with albuminuria.[2] The American College of Physicians published clinical guidelines for pharmacologic treatment of hypertension in adults of age ≥60 years with SBP ≥150 mm Hg. It recommended a goal SBP <150 mm Hg to reduce the risk of death.[3] For individuals within this age group with high cardiovascular risk, clinicians should consider initiating or intensifying treatment to achieve a target SBP <140 mm Hg to reduce the risk of stroke or cardiac events. While it stated that individuals with CKD and (estimated) glomerular filtration rate (eGFR) <45 mL/min/1.73 m^2

TABLE 1: Major randomized trials of blood pressure targets and all-cause mortality and end-stage renal disease outcomes, in nondialysis-dependent chronic kidney disease.

Author and year	Targeted blood pressure (mm Hg)	Achieved blood pressure (mm Hg)	Incident ESRD	All-cause mortality
Klahr et al. 1994	MAP ≤92 vs. MAP ≤107	126/77 vs. 134/81	No difference	No difference
Wright et al. 2002	MAP ≤92 vs. 102–107	128/78 vs. 141/85	% risk reduction: 6 (95% CI–29 to +31)	1.6% vs. 1.9% (not statistically significant)
Ruggenenti et al. 2005	DBP <90 vs. SBP/DBP <130/80	130/80 vs. 134/82	No difference (p = 0.99)	–
Wright et al. 2015 and Cheung et al. 2017	SBP <120 vs. <140	CKD subgroup: 123/67 vs. 137/74	CKD subgroup: HR 0.57 (95% CI 0.19–1.54)	CKD subgroup: HR 0.72 (95% CI 0.53–0.99)

(ESRD: end-stage renal disease; CKD: chronic kidney disease; HR: hazard ratio; CI: confidence interval ; DBP: diastolic blood pressure; MAP: mean arterial pressure; SBP: systolic blood pressure)

generally have increased cardiovascular risk, specific recommendations were not issued for those with CKD. Systolic Blood Pressure Intervention Trial (SPRINT) trial was terminated early in the year 2015 based on an interim analysis showing that group with SBP <120 mm Hg had a 25% lower risk of cardiovascular disease and 27% lower risk of all-cause mortality than the group assigned to an SBP <120 mm Hg.[4] Subsequently, the American College of Cardiology/American Heart Association (ACC/AHA) 2017 Hypertension Guidelines recommended antihypertensive treatment to a BP goal of <130/80 mm Hg in patients with CKD.[5] The ACC/AHA guidelines chose an SBP target of <130 mm Hg rather than <120 mm Hg (the intensive goal in SPRINT) due to the concerns about applying the results from SPRINT to a broader population. Specifically, BP was measured in the SPRINT trial using multiple automated BP measurements which on average is expected to be lower than routine clinic measurements. The 2018 European Society of Hypertension/European Society of Cardiology guidelines recommend an SBP target of 130–139 mm Hg and DBP of 70–79 mm Hg for patients with CKD.[6]

■ CONCERNS OF INTENSIVE BP LOWERING IN CHRONIC KIDNEY DISEASE

Intensive BP reduction is also associated with adverse outcomes. For instance, SPRINT trial reported increased risks of adverse events such as acute kidney injury (AKI), electrolyte disturbances such as hypokalemia, hyponatremia and hypotension. Intensive BP lowering did not lead to higher risk of orthostatic hypotension or injurious falls in the SPRINT trial, but other studies have raised concerns about these unintended consequences. More importantly, BP is generally measured using strict protocol in clinical trials which does not occur in routine clinical settings. Therefore, we must consider tradeoffs when making decisions with individual patients. Pill burden along with more frequent physician visits and BP checks, and side effects including AKI (which may have long-term impacts) are among the downsides of intense BP control which patients should be aware of. Clinicians should provide the best available information on risks, benefits, and uncertainties to patients so that they can make informed decisions.[7]

■ MANAGEMENT OF HYPERTENSION IN KIDNEY DISEASE

Lifestyle Modification or Sodium Restriction

A substantial body of evidence provides support to the notion that lifestyle modification which includes regular exercise and dietary modifications can have substantial effects on BP. These therapies can facilitate reducing pill burden (by reducing number of medications) in highly motivated individuals who achieve and sustain lifestyle changes.[8] Sodium restriction should be considered as an important component of all medication regimens for managing hypertension in kidney disease. Several studies confirmed the likely antihypertensive effects of a low-sodium diet, and some argue that a low-sodium diet might be even more effective than treatment with valsartan when added to patients already taking lisinopril. In a double-blind, randomized controlled trial that included patients with stage 3–4 CKD, a low-sodium diet resulted in significantly decreased ambulatory blood pressure (~10 mm Hg), albuminuria and extracellular volume.[9] Current guideline recommendations for CKD patients range from <2.3 g/day by the National Kidney Foundation—KDOQI guidelines to <1.5 g/day by the United States Department of Health.

Medications

Renin–Angiotensin–Aldosterone Blockers

Renin–angiotensin–aldosterone blockers which include angiotensin-converting enzyme inhibitors (ACEIs) and angiotensin II receptor blockers (ARBs) have emerged as the mainstays for managing hypertension in CKD. Both KDIGO and the recently published AHA/ACC guidelines endorse these agents as the first line therapy for those with CKD stage 3 or higher or those patients with albuminuria of at least 300 mg/day. In a meta-analysis of studies enrolling patients with albuminuria and at least one other cardiovascular risk factor, we showed that both ACEI and ARB reduced the risk of progression of kidney disease compared with placebo by 20–30%. Further, compared with placebo, both ACEI and ARB decreased the odds of cardiovascular events [odds ratio 0.82 (95% CI, 0.71–0.92) for ACEI and 0.76 (95% CI, 0.62–0.89) for ARB, respectively].[10] Similar findings have been reported by other studies and meta-analyzes demonstrating renal and cardiovascular benefits of these agents among those with CKD and albuminuria. Evidence supporting combination therapy with ACEI and ARB is limited. Notably, several trials such as the Ongoing Telmisartan Alone and in Combination with Ramipril Global Endpoint Trial (ONTARGET) and the Veterans Affairs Nephropathy in Diabetes Trial in patients with diabetic nephropathy demonstrated a higher risk of hyperkalemia and acute kidney injury when ACEI and ARB were used in combination.[11] Therefore, ACEI/ARB combination therapy cannot be justified in those with CKD. Role of aldosterone antagonists in those with kidney disease has been discussed under the diuretics section.

Calcium Channel Blockers

Calcium channel blockers include the dihydropyridine calcium channel blockers which are more specific for vascular smooth muscle, causing arterial vasodilation with fewer effects on cardiac muscle. On the other hand, nondihydropyridine calcium channel blockers such as verapamil and diltiazem are not routinely used in the management of hypertension due to their potential for drug interactions and other side effects such as heart block and bradycardia. Dihydropyridine calcium channel blockers have not been examined in the CKD population extensively. However, their antihypertensive potential has been demonstrated as they have been used as an active comparator in trials testing ACEI and ARB in CKD. Peripheral edema is the most common side effect that limits the widespread use of these agents; however, often CKD patients are on diuretics which might address this vexing issue. Where do they fit in BP management in CKD? In CKD with uncontrolled hypertension, dihydropyridine calcium channel blockers are an appropriate choice for who are already on an ACEI or ARB and a diuretic. These agents could also be considered as a second agent in those who are not volume overloaded and do not require a diuretic.

Thiazide Diuretics

Thiazides diuretics have been widely used as BP-lowering agents for more than five decades and block the Na-Cl cotransporter in the distal convoluted tubule of the nephron. Two widely used agents in this group are hydrochlorothiazide (HCTZ) which has a half-life of 15 hours and chlorthalidone with a half-life of up to 60 hours. Studies have demonstrated that thiazides reduce cardiovascular outcomes, including stroke, heart failure, coronary events and death in the general population but trials examining these agents in those with CKD are limited. Their efficacy remains intact in those with eGFR more than 30 mL/min/1.73 m^2, and clinical practice guidelines recommend switching from thiazides to loop diuretics when GFR falls less than 30 mL/min/1.73 m^2. It is important to note that hydrochlorothiazide 25 mg reduced mean blood pressure by about 7 mm Hg in patients with stage 4–5 CKD and another trial showed chlorthalidone was effective in lowering blood pressure in patients with advanced CKD.[12] Therefore, their role in advanced CKD cannot be excluded, and ongoing trials would provide us with some additional data. Clinicians should consider the fact that higher thiazide doses are necessary to achieve a therapeutic effect in those with kidney disease. This is because these agents act on the luminal side of the tubular epithelium. In CKD, with the reduction in tubular mass, a lesser amount of drug is secreted into the tubular lumen thereby arguing for the higher dose. Side effects such as electrolytes abnormalities, including hypokalemia, hyponatremia and hyperuricemia, are well-known and should be monitored closely while on these agents.

Loop Diuretics

Loop diuretics, another widely used diuretics in the CKD population, act by inhibiting the Na-K-2Cl cotransporter in the apical membrane of kidney tubular epithelial cells located in the thick ascending limb of the loop of Henle. One downside with this class is that they are short-acting and hence not considered a traditional antihypertensive agent except for managing volume overload which in turn helps reduce blood pressure. Often, higher doses of loop diuretics are needed to achieve a therapeutic effect in CKD. In those with severe or refractory volume overload (such as those with advanced CKD and congestive heart failure), a combination of a loop and thiazide diuretics provide additional antihypertensive and volume reduction benefit. Adverse events noted are similar to thiazides which include volume depletion and AKI, electrolyte abnormalities, including hypokalemia suggesting the need for close monitoring of laboratory data during its use.

■ MINERALOCORTICOID RECEPTOR BLOCKERS

Mineralocorticoid receptor blockers (MRBs) or aldosterone antagonists competitively inhibit aldosterone binding to the mineralocorticoid receptor resulting in reduced sodium reabsorption at the expense of reduced potassium excretion. Both spironolactone and eplerenone have a well-established role in those with heart failure. In CKD, aldosterone antagonists reduced proteinuria and blood pressure in those with mild-to-moderate CKD and who were treated with ACEI or ARB, but increase the risk of hyperkalemia and gynecomastia.[13] Clinical trials have not documented whether adding aldosterone antagonists to ACEI or ARB would reduce the risk of major cardiovascular events or ESKD in those with CKD. It is important to note that PATHWAY-2 trial demonstrated that in those with resistant hypertension who were on three drugs, spironolactone was the most effective add-on drug (compared to doxazosin or placebo).[14] As with ACEI and ARBs, hyperkalemia is the major limiting side effect, precluding the widespread use of MRBs. Do these agents fit our treatment approach in CKD? They are an appropriate choice for CKD patients with resistant hypertension and/or hypokalemia as long as serum potassium is being monitored.

Beta-blockers

Beta-blockers such as carvedilol and nebivolol have vasodilating effects, and in fact the reduction in systemic vascular resistance might mediate the antihypertensive effect.[15] Role of beta-blockers is well-established in those with heart failure with reduced ejection fraction and after acute myocardial infarction. They are not widely recommended to be used as monotherapy for hypertension control in the general population and those with CKD. Increased sympathetic activity is known to be a contributor to hypertension in CKD and thereby might have a role in hypertension control in this population. Bradycardia is the most common concern, and these agents are cleared by hepatic metabolism. However, atenolol has only limited hepatic clearance, and drug levels are dependent on kidney elimination posing risk for bradycardia in those with AKI.

Direct Vasodilators and Centrally Acting Alpha-Agonists

These agents are often reserved for those with resistant hypertension. In fact, recently released AHA guidelines on resistant hypertension noted that no large trials have tested their efficacy and hence should be used with caution.[16] Current available direct vasodilators include hydralazine and minoxidil. Hydralazine is rapidly metabolized by the liver to inactive metabolites, whereas minoxidil is also primarily hepatically metabolized and may be dosed only once daily in CKD. Side effects of minoxidil include hirsutism which often is dose-dependent. The centrally acting α-agonists clonidine and guanfacine act by stimulating alpha 2-receptors in the brainstem and eventually reducing sympathetic outflow. Both medications frequently cause dry mouth, sedation and bradycardia, and exhibit rebound hypertension upon abrupt cessation. Further, more than 50% of the drug gets excreted in the urine and thus requires close monitoring for side effects in those with CKD.

Prescribing Algorithm

In the setting of nondialysis-dependent CKD and in the absence of specific indications for other drugs, ACEI or ARB is the appropriate first-line therapy for hypertension (especially in those with albuminuria) and are endorsed by the clinical practice guidelines. Second-line treatment could include diuretics as CKD patients often have volume overload. If volume overload is not a concern, calcium channel blocker is a good second-line agent. Otherwise, calcium channel blockers are appropriate as a third agent in CKD. MRBs are an appropriate choice if the BP remains uncontrolled while on ACEI or ARB, diuretic and a calcium channel blocker. If BP remains uncontrolled while on a triple-drug regimen, secondary causes should be ruled out (based on the clinical scenario) as recommended by

TABLE 2: Recommended agents for management of hypertension in nondialysis-dependent chronic kidney disease.

Recommended prescription order	Antihypertensive class	Side effects	Guideline recommendation
First	ACEI or ARB	Acute kidney injury hyperkalemia	Yes
Second	Diuretic	Electrolyte abnormalities	Yes
Third	Calcium channel blockers	Peripheral edema	Yes
Fourth	MRA and beta-blockers	Hyperkalemia, gynecomastia	No
Reserved for resistant hypertension	Vasodilators and alpha-agonists	Hirsutism, hypotension, dry mouth, edema	No

(ACEI: angiotensin-converting enzyme inhibitor; ARB: angiotensin II receptor blocker; MRA: mineralocorticoid receptor antagonist)

the AHA's scientific statement on resistant hypertension.[15] Other agents that could be considered as the fourth-line of agents are discussed in Table 2.

CONCLUSION

Appropriate management of hypertension in CKD reduces both cardiovascular and kidney adverse outcomes. In addition to the well-established use of an ACEI or ARB, lifestyle modification including dietary salt restriction and appropriate use of diuretic therapy make up the mainstay of hypertension treatment in patients with CKD. Based on clinical trial evidence, a BP target of 130/80 mm Hg is recommended by several guidelines across the globe for those with CKD.

REFERENCES

1. Webster AC, Nagler EV, Morton RL, et al. Chronic kidney disease. Lancet. 2017;389(10075):1238-52.
2. Kidney International. (2012). KDIGO Clinical Practice Guideline for the management of blood pressure in chronic kidney disease. Vol 2, Issue 5. pp. 1-85. [online] Available from http://www.kdigo.org/clinical_practice_guidelines/pdf/KDIGO_BP_GL.pdf [Last Accessed January 2019].
3. Qaseem A, Wilt TJ, Rich R, et al. Pharmacologic treatment of hypertension in adults aged 60 years or older to higher versus lower blood pressure targets: a clinical practice guideline from the American College of Physicians and the American Academy of Family Physicians. Ann Intern Med. 2017;166(6):430-7.
4. Wright JT Jr, Williamson JD, Whelton PK, et al. A randomized trial of intensive versus standard blood-pressure control. N Engl J Med. 2015; 373(22):2103-16.
5. Whelton PK, Carey RM, Aronow WS, et al. 2017 ACC/AHA/AAPA/ABC/ACPM/AGS/APhA/ASH/ASPC/NMA/PCNA Guideline for the Prevention, Detection, Evaluation, and Management of High Blood Pressure in Adults: Executive Summary: A Report of the American College of Cardiology/American Heart Association Task Force on Clinical Practice Guidelines. Hypertension. 2018;71(6):1269-1324.
6. Williams B, Mancia G, Spiering W, et al. 2018 Practice guidelines for the management of arterial hypertension of the European Society of Hypertension (ESH) and the European Society of Cardiology (ESC). Blood Press. 2018;27(6):314-40.
7. Walther CP, Chandra A, Navaneethan SD. Blood pressure parameters and morbid and mortal outcomes in nondialysis-dependent chronic kidney disease. Curr Opin Nephrol Hypertens. 2018;27(1):16-22.
8. Appel LJ, Champagne CM, Harsha DW, et al. Effects of comprehensive lifestyle modification on blood pressure control: main results of the PREMIER clinical trial. JAMA. 2003;289(16):2083-93.
9. Saran R, Padilla RL, Gillespie BW, et al. A randomized crossover trial of dietary sodium restriction in stage 3-4 CKD. Clin J Am Soc Nephrol. 2017;12(3):399-407.
10. Maione A, Navaneethan SD, Graziano G, et al. Angiotensin-converting enzyme inhibitors, angiotensin receptor blockers and combined therapy in patients with micro- and macroalbuminuria and other cardiovascular risk factors: a systematic review of randomized controlled trials. Nephrol Dial Transplant. 2011;26(9):2827-47.

11. Mann JF, Schmieder RE, McQueen M, et al. Renal outcomes with telmisartan, ramipril, or both, in people at high vascular risk (the ONTARGET study): a multicenter, randomized, double-blind, controlled trial. Lancet. 2008;372(9638):547-53.

12. Karadsheh F, Weir MR. Thiazide and thiazide-like diuretics: an opportunity to reduce blood pressure in patients with advanced kidney disease. Curr Hypertens Rep. 2012;14(5): 416-20.

13. Navaneethan SD, Nigwekar SU, Sehgal AR, et al. Aldosterone antagonists for preventing the progression of chronic kidney disease: a systematic review and meta-analysis. Clin J Am Soc Nephrol. 2009;4(3):542-51.

14. Williams B, MacDonald TM, Morant S, et al. Spironolactone versus placebo, bisoprolol, and doxazosin to determine the optimal treatment for drug-resistant hypertension (PATHWAY-2): a randomized, double-blind, crossover trial. Lancet. 2015;386(10008):2059-68.

15. Sinha AD, Agarwal R. Clinical pharmacology of antihypertensive therapy for the treatment of hypertension in chronic kidney disease. Clin J Am Soc Nephrol. 2018. pii: CJN.04330418.

16. Carey RM, Calhoun DA, Bakris GL, et al. Resistant hypertension: Detection, evaluation, and management: a scientific statement from the American Heart Association. Hypertension. 2018;72(5):e53-90.

Hypertension in Patients with Renal Parenchymal Disease, Chronic Renal Failure, and Chronic Dialysis

Narinder P Singh, Anish K Gupta, Gurleen Kaur

■ INTRODUCTION

Among noncommunicable diseases (NCDs) arena, chronic kidney disease (CKD) is a key determinant of adverse health outcomes and is associated with an eight to 10-fold increase in cardiovascular mortality. The global account of CKD is considerable and has risen dramatically over the past 20 years. Global Burden of Disease (GBD) 2016 report documented that CKD had rapidly moved up the ranks of causes of global deaths and positioned 11th on the list. Morbidity and mortality due to CKD have increased, more prominent driver by population growth and aging. Diabetes followed by hypertension was the leading drivers of CKD globally. The estimated global crude prevalence of CKD was 147.6 million in 1990 which increased to 275.9 million cases in 2016. Diabetes and hypertension contributed 50.6% and 23.3%, respectively, of the increased CKD disability-adjusted life years (DALYs). India at present has the world's largest population of diabetics, and obesity has long been recognized as an emerging epidemic. The CURES cohort suggested that every fifth person in India is hypertensive. Treatment of hypertension is imperative and it must be acknowledged that these increases in acute kidney injury (AKI), CKD and/or end-stage renal disease (ESRD), happening worldwide, have occurred despite the universal application of strategies of renoprotection over the last two decades, more especially the widespread use of angiotensin-converting enzyme (ACE) inhibitors or angiotensin II receptor blocker (ARBs). A stepwise approach in combination of lifestyle changes and pharmacological therapy should be used to achieve blood pressure target in patients with kidney disease. In this review we will discuss management of hypertension in kidney disease.

■ PATHOGENESIS OF HYPERTENSION IN CHRONIC KIDNEY DISEASE

The relationship between hypertension and kidney disease is complex and multifactorial (Box 1). Pathogenesis of hypertension in CKD is characterized by retention of sodium and water leading to increases in plasma volume and results in increase of cardiac output. The hypertension is continued by imbalance in the vasoactive system including activation of vasoconstriction systems (renin angiotensin aldosterone, sympathetic system, RAAS) and decreased production of vasodilatory agents such as NO and prostaglandins. Secondary

> **Box 1: Factor implicated in the pathogenesis of hypertension in chronic kidney disease.**
>
> - Impaired sodium excretion—expansion of ECF volume—volume overload (volume-dependent)
> - Activation of RAS—direct vasoconstriction and sympathetic activation
> - Electrolyte disturbances
> - Sympathetic activation—direct vasoconstriction stimulation of renin release
> - SHPT (by raising the intracellular calcium concentration leading to vasoconstriction)
> - Imbalance in prostaglandins or kinins—vasoconstriction
> - Endothelin—direct vasoconstriction renal injury
> - Impaired vasodilatation secondary to reduced endothelial nitric oxide synthesis
> - Structural changes of the arteries
> - Sleep apnea, obesity and metabolic syndrome
> - Drugs: Erythropoiesis-stimulating agents, NSAIDs, oral contraceptives, sympathomimetic agents, steroids-mineralocorticoids and glucocorticoids, cyclosporine, tacrolimus, vascular endothelial growth factor inhibitors, illicit drugs and herbal supplements
> - Increase in central pulse pressure and isolated systolic hypertension secondary to increased vascular wall stiffening and absence of normal nocturnal decline in blood pressure
>
> (CKD: chronic kidney disease; ECF: extracellular fluid; NSAID: nonsteroidal anti-inflammatory drugs)

hyperparathyroidism with increase in intra-cellular calcium leads to vasoconstriction and causes hypertension.

Blood Pressure Variability in Chronic Kidney Disease

In healthy individuals normally blood pressure (BP) follows a circadian pattern and BP has a tendency to be the highest during the morning and gradually declining from late evening onwards and lowest in the night and shoots up just after waking in the morning. A fall of more than 10% in systolic and diastolic BP in the night, compared to daytime readings, is normal and termed as "dippers". Patients with a nocturnal fall less than 10% are defined as nondippers pattern that can be a useful marker of hypertension severity. Among CKD patients and those on maintenance hemodialysis the prevalence of nondippers is 74–82%. The phenomenon of nondipping pattern have been associated with greater risk of cardiovascular complications in CKD population. Extracellular volume expansion, uremic neuropathy and restless leg syndrome are associated with nondipping pattern in patients with CKD.

Managing Hypertension in Chronic Kidney Disease

Nonpharmacologic (lifestyle changes) and pharmacologic treatment are both necessary to achieve the target BP. A combination of nonpharmacological lifestyle change and pharmacological therapy are the key strategies to achieve target BP in patients with CKD. Ambulatory blood pressure monitoring (ABPM) was the gold standard for detecting of hypertension. High blood pressure (HBP) was no more far behind to ABPM in terms of detecting white coat and masked hypertension (HTN). Individualize BP targets and pharmacotherapy should be based on the age, presence of comorbidities and end-organ damage (cardiovascular disease and retinopathy), CKD progression and treatment resistance. Recommendation of various guidelines on BP target and intervention are demonstrated in Table 1.

Nonpharmacological Management

Lifestyle modification offers the potential to lower BP in a simple, inexpensive and

TABLE 1: Various guidelines on management of hypertension in nondialysis-dependent CKD patients.

	Ualb (Uprot) mg/24 h	BP Threshold	BP Target	Intervention
KDIGO 2012				
CKD patients without/with diabetes (DM-/DM+)				
	<30	>140/90 mm Hg	≤140/90 mm Hg	Agent: no recommendation
	≥30	>130/80 mm Hg	≤130/80 mm Hg	Agent: ACE inhibitor or ARB
Kidney transplants				
	Any	>130/80 mm Hg	≤130/80 mm Hg	Agent: time after transplantation, use of calcineurin inhibitors
Children				
	Any	≤50th percentile	>90th percentile	Agent: ACE inhibitor or ARB
Elderly				
	• Tailor, age, comorbidities, other therapies • Gradual escalation • Close attention to adverse events—electrolyte disorders, acute deterioration in kidney function, orthostatic hypotension and drug side effects			
Lifestyle and pharmacological treatments				
	Individualize of targets and agents according to age, CVD, comorbidities, risk of CKD progression, retinopathy (DM) and tolerance of treatment, inquire about postural dizziness, check for postural hypotension regularly			
Lifestyle modification				
	-	--	BMI 20–25 kg/m^2	Achieve/maintain healthy weight
	-	-	<90 mmol/day (<2 g/day) of sodium	Lower salt intake
	-	-	≥30, 5x/week	Exercise program
	-	-	≤2 drinks/day (male); ≤1 drink/ day (female)	Limit alcohol intake
CHEP	CKD without albuminuria		<140/90 mm Hg (nondiabetic CKD) <130/80 mm Hg (diabetes)	
	CKD with albuminuria		<140/90 mm Hg (nondiabetic CKD) <130/80 mm Hg (diabetes)	

Continued

Continued

	Ualb (Uprot) mg/24 h	BP Threshold	BP Target	Intervention
JNC 8	CKD without albuminuria		<140/90 mm Hg	
	CKD with albuminuria		<140/90 mm Hg	
SH and ASH	CKD without albuminuria		<140/90 mm Hg	
	CKD with albuminuria		<140/90 mm Hg	
NICE	CKD without albuminuria		<140/90 mm Hg (nondiabetic CKD) <130/80 mm Hg (diabetes)	
	CKD with albuminuria		<130/80 mm Hg	
ESC and ESH	CKD without albuminuria		<140 mm Hg SBP	
	CKD with albuminuria		<130 mm Hg SBP	
ACC/AHA 2017[2]	CKD	≥130/80 mm Hg	<130/80 mm Hg	
	CKD after renal transplantation	≥130/80 mm Hg	<130/80 mm Hg	

(ACE: angiotensin-converting enzyme; ARB: angiotensin II receptor blocker; BP: blood pressure; CKD: chronic kidney disease; CVD: cardiovascular disease; KDIGO: kidney disease: improving global outcomes; DM: diabetes mellitus; CHEP: Canadian Hypertension Education Program; ESH/ESC: European Societies of Hypertension and Cardiology; NICE: National Institute for Health and Clinical Excellence; JNC 8: Eighth Joint National Committee (USA); AHA: American Hypertension Association; ACC: American College of Cardiology; SBP: systolic blood pressure)

effective fashion while also improving a range of other outcomes such as changes in lipid levels resulting from diet and exercise and liver function through moderation of alcohol intake. KDIGO 2012 guidelines recommends maintaining a healthy weight (BMI 20–25 kg/m^2), lowering salt intake to <90 mmol (<2 g) per day of sodium (corresponding to 5 g of sodium chloride), an exercise program compatible with cardiovascular health and tolerance, aiming for at least 30 minutes 5 times per week exercise and limiting alcohol intake to no more than one standard drink per day for women and no more than two standard drinks per day for men.[1] Restrict dietary protein to ≤1.4 g/kg/day for CKD stages 1–2 or 0.6–0.8 g/kg/day for CKD stages 3–4.

Pharmacological Management

Progression of CKD depends on nonmodifiable risk factors such as CKD types (diabetic nephropathy, glomerulonephritides, polycystic kidneys disease, nephrons mass and presence of CVD) and factors that can be modified with medical management include proteinuria, hypertension, obesity, high protein intake, anemia, dyslipidemia, smoking, hyperuricemia and hypoproteinemia.[3] As per

KDIGO guideline goal BP target in patients with CKD should be <140/90 mm Hg and in CKD patients with/without diabetes and/or albuminuria (>30 mg/24 h), goal BP target should be <130/80 mm Hg. If target BP is achieved, the patient should be recommended for lifestyle modifications to manage risk factors and regularly monitor BP. ACE inhibitor or ARB or a calcium channel blocker should be started if BP is above the target. Obtain SCr and K levels 7–10 days after initiation of an ACE inhibitor or ARB and/or with changes in anti-RAAS therapy. Increase in SCr 30% above baseline within 3 months of initiating anti-RAAS therapy may be acceptable. Close monitoring is required as it increases risk of hyperkalemia (if K^+>6 mmol/L stop ACE inhibitor/ARBs). If during follow-up visits, BP is not at the desired target, compliance to medication and lifestyle modifications should be reinforced and the dose of the ACE inhibitor or ARB should be optimized. Coadministration of calcium channel blocker (CCB), diuretic, α-blocker, or β-blocker is also acceptable (Table 2). NSAIDs, COX-2 antagonists, or potassium sparing diuretics can develop hyperkalemia if these drugs are used in combination with ACE inhibitors or ARBs. Inquire about postural dizziness and periodic check for postural hypotension. Despite concurrent use of three anti-hypertensive agents at optimal doses, at least one of which is a diuretic (defined as resistant hypertension), if BP is not achieved at target levels, then further intervention is required. Patients whose BP is controlled on four antihypertensive medications are also considered to have resistant hypertension (controlled resistant hypertension). There is need to address several factors that contribute to the pathogenesis of resistant hypertension (Flowchart 1).

Managing Hypertension in Dialysis Population

Patients who are just initiating dialysis are volume overloaded leads to an elevation in blood pressure. Volume overload is often an overlooked factor in managing hypertension. Erythropoietin-induced hypertension and untreated sleep apnea are other important causes. Pathogenesis of hypertension in hemodialysis patients include sympathetic overactivity, activation of the RAAS, arteriosclerosis, changes in endothelium-derived vasoactive peptides, increases in intracellular calcium, and decreases in renalase. Blood pressure should be monitored every 30–60 minutes during a dialysis session and more frequently in unstable patients. Compared with predialysis and postdialysis BP measurements, diagnosis of hypertension is better made by using home BP recordings

TABLE 2: Recommended antihypertensive agents for patients with CKD and HTN.

Classification of patients	First line	Second line	Third line	Fourth line
Diabetic CKD with or without HTN	ACE inhibitor or ARB	Thiazide or loop diuretics	ND-CCB (may also be considered 2nd line)	Aldosterone antagonist
Nondiabetic CKD + HTN + proteinuria	ACE inhibitor or ARB	Thiazide or loop diuretics	ND-CCB (may also be considered 2nd line)	Aldosterone antagonist
Nondiabetic CKD + HTN but without proteinuria (<200 mg/g)	No agents preferred; consider a diuretic	ACE inhibitor or ARB or CCB	Aldosterone antagonist	NA

(ACE: angiotensin-converting enzyme; ARB: angiotensin II receptor blocker; CKD: chronic kidney disease; CCB: calcium channel blocker; HTN: hypertension; ND-CCB: nondihydropyridine calcium channel blockers; NA: not available)

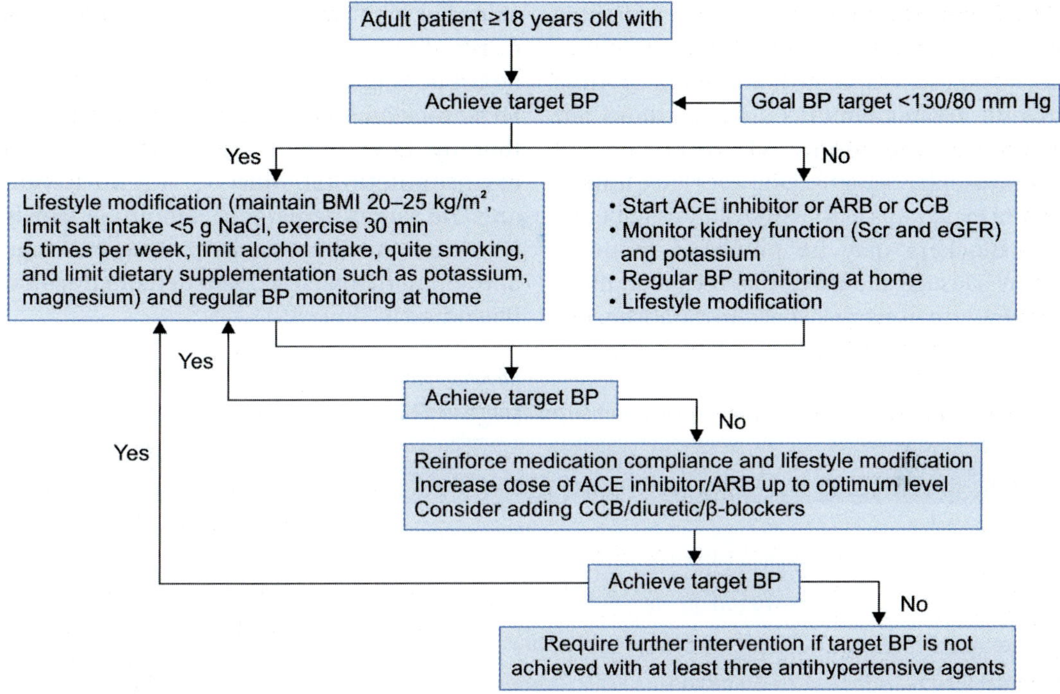

(ACE: angiotensin-converting enzyme; ARB: angiotensin II receptor blocker; CCB: calcium channel blockers; eGFR: estimated glomerular filtration rate; Scr: serum creatinine; BP: blood pressure; BMI: body mass index; NaCl: sodium chloride)

Flowchart 1: Management of hypertension in chronic kidney disease.

or interdialytic ambulatory BP recordings.[4] Clinical decisions in managing interdialytic BP should be based on systolic blood pressure (SBP) and diastolic blood pressure (DBP), but not on mean arterial BP. Reducing the target dry weight can control the high blood pressure and should be adjusted before antihypertensive agents are added. Dry weight can be defined as the lowest tolerated postdialysis weight at which there are minimal signs or symptoms of either hypovolemia or hypervolemia. Achievement of "dry weight" using a combination of clinical assessment of edema, fluid in lungs, jugular venous pressure (JVP) and serous cavities, blood pressure, chest X-ray and echocardiography. This should be achieved over 3–6 weeks in young adults and 12–14 weeks in older individuals and those with vascular pathologies.

Bioimpedance, relative plasma volume (RPV) monitoring, and plasma natriuretic peptides are more accurate methods for assessing dry weight. Periodic clinical assessment should be done to reassess dry weight. Lowering dialysate Na based on predialysis plasma Na level may reduce interdialytic weight gain and thirst. Management of increased fluid accumulation should be to achieve a low sodium intake, increased UF, and/or increased dialysis treatments. Treatment recommendations should be use of long duration sessions with low ultrafiltration rate and practice nocturnal hemodialysis. Delivery of dialysis of at least 4 hours duration three times a week may facilitate volume and hypertension control. Start antihypertensive medications if the blood pressure remains elevated despite the attainment of "dry weight". Use of antihypertensive agent is preferably during the evening with a once per day dosing schedule. ACE inhibitors or ARBs provide greater benefits such as more left ventricular hypertrophy (LVH) regression and cardiovascular benefits. Diuretics have little to no role in patients with ESRD dialysis patients. Beta-blockers may be preferred to other agents. Dosage should not be escalated more frequently than every 4 weeks. In the absence of side effects, the dose of each antihypertensive agent should be increased to a high dose before adding another antihypertensive agent. Hypertension is common with erythropoietin therapy. Low initial doses of subcutaneous erythropoietin should be administered, and the target hematocrit should be slowly achieved. Antihypertensive drugs, dosage and supplement in CKD and hemodialysis are illustrated in Table 3.

TABLE 3: Antihypertensive drugs, dosage and supplement in CKD and hemodialysis.

Drugs	Usual dose	GFR <10 mL/min	Removal with hemodialysis	Supplement for dialysis
Diuretic				
Acetazolamide	250 mg q6–8 h	Avoid	Unknown	N/A
Amiloride	5–10 mg qd	Avoid	N/A	N/A
Furosemide	40–80 mg bid	100%	None	None
Hydrochlorothiazide	25–50 mg qd	Avoid	None	N/A
Indapamide	2.5 mg qd	Avoid	None	N/A
Metolazone	5–10 mg qd	100%	None	None
Spironolactone	50–100 mg qd/bid	Avoid	N/A	N/A
Torsemide	5–10 mg bid	100%	Avoid	None
Beta-blockers				
Acebutolol	400–600 mg qd/bid	30–50%	30%	150 mg
Atenolol	50–100 mg qd	25–50%	50%	25–50 mg
Bisoprolol	2.5–20 mg qd	100%	None	None
Carvedilol	25 mg bid	50%	None	None
Esmolol	50–150 µg/kg/min IV	100%	None	None
Labetalol	200–600 mg bid	100%	None	None
Metoprolol	50–100 mg	100%	None	50%
Propranolol	80–160 mg bid	100%	None	None
Sotalol	160 mg qd	15–30%	50%	50 mg
Timolol	10–20 mg bid	100%	None	None
CCB				
Amlodipine	2.5–10 mg qd	100%	None	None
Diltiazem	180–360 mg	100%	None	None
Felodipine	5–10 mg qd	100%	None	None

Continued

Continued

Drugs	Usual dose	GFR <10 mL/min	Removal with hemodialysis	Supplement for dialysis
Nifedipine XL	30–90 mg qd	100%	None	None
Verapamil CD	180–360 mg qd	100%	None	None
ACE				
Benazepril	5–40 mg qd	50–75%	Negligible	5–10 mg
Captopril	12.5–50 mg tid	50%	50%	12.5–25 mg
Enalapril	2.5–10 mg q12h	50%	50%	2.5–5 mg
Fosinopril	10 mg qd	75%	None	None
Lisinopril	2.5–10 mg qd	25–50%	50%	2.5–5 mg
Perindopril	2–8 mg/day	25–50%	50%	2 mg
Ramipril	5–10 mg qd	25–50%	20%	2.5 mg
ARB				
Candesartan	8–35 mg/day	100%	None	None
Irbesartan	75–300 mg/day	100%	None	None
Losartan	50–100 mg qd	100%	None	None
Olmesartan	10–40 mg/day	100%	None	None
Telmisartan	40–80 mg/day	100%	None	None
DIR				
Aliskiren	150–300 mg qd	Unknown	Unknown	Unknown
Central α-agonist				
Clonidine	0.1–0.3 mg bid/tid	100%	5%	None
Guanethidine	10–100 mg qd	50% (avoid)	None	None
Methyldopa	250–500 mg bid/tid	q12–24h	60%	250–500 mg
Reserpine	0.05–0.25 mg qd	Avoid	None	None
α$_2$-blockers				
Doxazosin	1–16 mg qd	100%	None	None
Prazosin	1–15 mg bid	100%	None	None
Terazosin	1–20 mg qd	100%	None	None
Vasodilator				
Diazoxide	150–300 mg bolus	100%	None	None
Hydralazine	25–50 mg tid/qid	q8–16h	25–40%	None
Minoxidil	5–30 mg bid	100%	None	None
Nitroprusside	0.25–0.8 mg/kg/min IV	100%	None	None

(ACE: angiotensin-converting enzyme; ARB: angiotensin II receptor blocker; CKD: chronic kidney disease; CCB: calcium channel blockers; DIR: direct inhibitors of renin)

Managing Paradoxical Hypertension

Paradoxical hypertension appears at the end of dialysis when water removal is completed. The causes of paradoxical hypertension include ultrafiltration, hypovolemia, pre-existing hypertension, hypercalcemia, improvement of hypoxia and antihypertensives that are removed during dialysis, e.g. ACE inhibitors. Management includes nifedipine 10 mg, with quick response or captopril 10 mg predialysis, isotonic normal saline NaCl, or correction of hypovolemia.

Managing Hypertension in Kidney Transplant Patient

Choice of antihypertensive agent in kidney transplant patient is based on some parameters such as level of urine albumin, hemodynamic stability, altered graft perfusion immediately after transplantation, drug-drug interaction (with immunosuppressive agents or other drugs), comorbid conditions and impact on graft function and all-cause mortality. Initially after transplantation, CCB (dihydropyridine) is preferred over ACE inhibitors/ARB. In patients with proteinuria with mild graft dysfunction, ARB is the preferred drug. Loop diuretics can be used as add-on therapy.

■ CONCLUSION

Hypertension is both a cause and consequence of CKD. The CURES cohort suggested that every fifth person in India is hypertensive. Considering the high prevalence of CKD risk factors it has long been presumed that CKD represents a major public health problem in India, at least in urban cities.

In patients with CKD, hypertension is a common comorbid condition that increases the risk of progression of CKD and the risk of cardiovascular complications. Reduction of BP to less than 130/80 mm Hg, slowing the progression of kidney disease and reducing cardiovascular disease (CVD) risk are goals of antihypertensive therapy. However, this BP goal is not attained by the majority of CKD patients. Stringent control of hypertension using a RAAS inhibitor-based treatment regimen is an evidence-based approach to slow the progression of CKD and reduce CVD risk. Most CKD patients require multiple antihypertensive drugs to reduce BP to target level. Clinical evidence indicates that initial fixed-dose RAAS inhibitor-based combination therapy is more effective and more efficient than stepped-care therapy or sequential monotherapy for lowering BP to target levels and reduces the risk of adverse events.

■ REFERENCES

1. Andrassy KM. Comments on 'KDIGO 2012 Clinical Practice Guideline for the Evaluation and Management of Chronic Kidney Disease'. Kidney Int. 2013;84(3):622-3.
2. Whelton PK, Carey RM, Aronow WS, et al. 2017 ACC/AHA/AAPA/ABC/ACPM/AGS/AphA/ASH/ASPC/NMA/PCNA guideline for the prevention, detection, evaluation, and management of high blood pressure in adults. Executive summary: A report of the American College of Cardiology/American Heart Association Task Force on Clinical Practice Guidelines. Hypertension. 2018;71(6):1269-324.
3. Abraham G, Arun KN, Gopalakrishnan N, et al. Management of hypertension in chronic kidney disease: consensus statement by an expert panel of Indian nephrologists. J Assoc Physicians India. 2017;65(Suppl 2):6-22.
4. Singh NP, Mathukiya S, Aggarwal N, et al. Correlation between home, clinic, and ambulatory blood pressure monitoring among CKD patients. J Am Soc Nephrol 2018;29 (Kidney Week Edition):1063.

Primary Hyperaldosteronism and Other Mineralocorticoid Hypertension

Minal Mohit

■ INTRODUCTION

Adrenal glands are made of two parts—(1) cortex and (2) medulla. The cortex is further three layered—(1) zona glomerulosa, (2) zona fasciculata, and (3) zona reticularis. Zona glomerulosa is mainly responsible for aldosterone (mineralocorticoid) synthesis, zona fasciculata for glucocorticoid synthesis and zona reticularis for androgen synthesis. Medulla is the central core secreting mainly catecholamines. Zona glomerulosa functions under regulation of renin–angiotensin system, zona fasciculata functions under adreno-corticotropic hormone (ACTH) influence (Flowchart 1).

■ PRIMARY ALDOSTERONISM

Primary hyperaldosteronism, also known as Conn's Syndrome was first described in 1955 by Jerome W Conn.[1]

Definition

As per ESCPG (Endocrine Society Clinical Practice Guideline) in 2008,[2] it is defined as a group of disorders in which aldosterone production is inappropriately high, relatively autonomous, and independent of the renin–angiotensin system and in which aldosterone secretion is not suppressed by sodium loading. Hypokalemia, which was formerly included in the definition, is now no more considered a rule (Flowchart 2).

Causes of Primary Aldosteronism

Besides the aldosterone-producing adenoma (APA) as originally described by Conn, there are six subtypes of primary aldosteronism (PA). Idiopathic hyperaldosteronism (IHA) is the most common form of PA, it is characterized by bilateral adrenal hyperplasia (Table 1).

Pathobiology of Primary Aldosteronism

The three major pathologic disorders asso-ciated with PA are—(1) adenoma, (2) hyper-plasia and (3) carcinoma.

Adrenocortical Adenoma

It occurs somewhat more frequently in the left than in the right adrenal. Adenomas usually measure less than 2 cm in diameter and have a golden yellow color.

Idiopathic Hyperaldosteronism

It is the most common subtype (63%). IHA has less florid clinical and biochemical manifestations compared with APA.

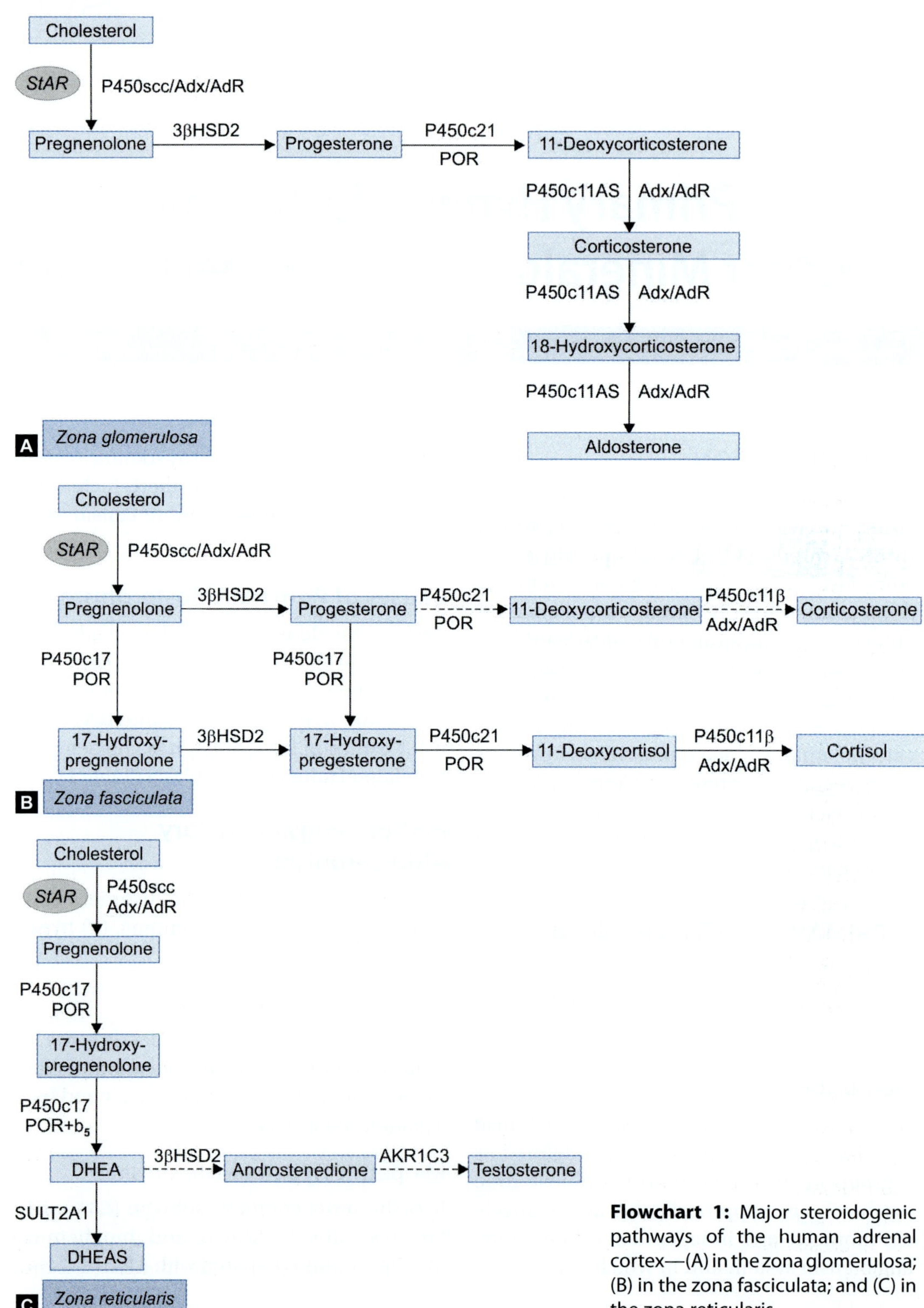

Flowchart 1: Major steroidogenic pathways of the human adrenal cortex—(A) in the zona glomerulosa; (B) in the zona fasciculata; and (C) in the zona reticularis.

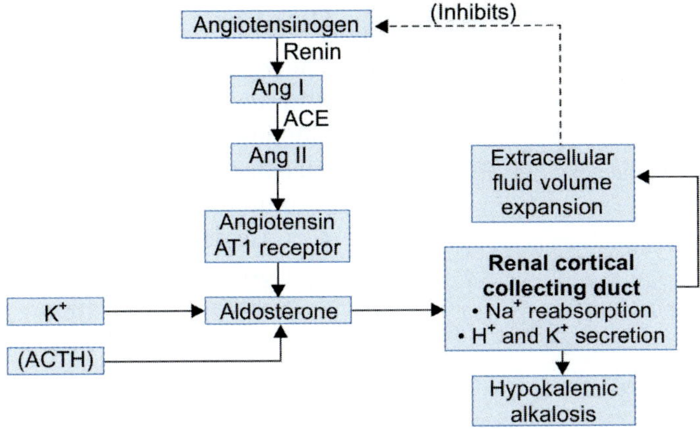

(ACE: angiotensin-converting enzyme; ACTH: adrenocorticotropic hormone; Ang: angiotensin)

Flowchart 2: Renin–angiotensin–aldosterone system in primary aldosteronism.

TABLE 1: Forms of primary aldosteronism and their prevalence rates.

Disorder	Prevalence, (%)
Bilateral idiopathic adrenal hyperplasia	63
Aldosterone-producing adenoma	33
Primary (unilateral) adrenal hyperplasia	<1
Aldosterone-producing adrenocortical carcinoma	<1
Ectopic (nonadrenal) aldosterone-producing adenomas	Rare
Familial hyperaldosteronism (FH)	
• Type I (FH I)—glucocorticoid-remediable hyperaldosteronism	0.5
• Type II (FH II)—adrenocorticotropic hormone (ACTH)-independent familial hyperaldosteronism	3–4

Adrenal Carcinoma

It is a rare cause of PA. Histologically carcinomas are difficult to distinguish from adenomas, but are almost invariably larger than 3 cm in diameter and include areas of necrosis, calcification, and pleomorphic nuclei.[3]

Prevalence of Primary Aldosteronism

The prevalence of PA varies from 5% to 13% of all patients with hypertension.

Clinical Manifestations of Primary Aldosteronism

Most patients are asymptomatic. Hypertension may be the only finding. Hypokalemia may be discovered on routine work-up for hypertension. Symptoms of hypokalemia may be present at times such as muscle weakness, very rarely muscle paralysis, or more commonly, polyuria, polydipsia, nocturia (secondary to nephrogenic diabetes insipidus), paresthesia and rarely tetany.[4] Malignant hypertension may be present at times; on the other extreme, normotensive hyperaldosteronism has been reported[5] (Box 1).

In PA, the normal circadian pattern of BP with nocturnal dipping is preserved with decreased variability.[5]

Aldosterone has a role in tissue damage (inflammation, fibrosis and remodeling) (Flowchart 3). Patients with PA have greater target organ damage as compared to age and blood pressure (BP) matched essential

Box 1: Clinical manifestations of primary aldosteronism.

- Hypertension due to extracellular fluid volume expansion and sympathetic activation
- Hypokalemia, hypomagnesemia and metabolic alkalosis
- Cardiac arrhythmias
- Renal dysfunction
- Nephrogenic diabetes insipidus
- Muscle weakness
- Paresthesias and tetany
- Flaccid paralysis

hypertensive patients. Also prevalence of metabolic (insulin resistance) syndrome is increased in PA compared to essential hypertension[6] (Box 2).

Epidemiology of Primary Aldosteronism

The disease affects all ages, including children. At any age, adenomas are more common in females, IHA affects both males and females equally. In children, growth failure may be the presenting feature.

Diagnosis of Primary Aldosteronism

The Endocrine Society Published Clinical Practice Guidelines on the detection, diagnosis and treatment of PA in 2008 with specific diagnostic work-up.[2] Sequential steps recommended for work up include:
- Case detection (screening)
- Confirmation of the diagnosis
- Subtype classification.

Screening

Clinical criteria and methods of screening for PA are summarized in flowchart 4.

All patients to be screened include:
- Patients with hypertension and hypokalemia (spontaneous or diuretic induced)
- Young patients with hypertension
- Patients with early onset of cerebrovascular attack (age <50 years)
- Patients with positive family history of early stroke in a first-degree relative
- Patients with hypertension and adrenal incidentalomas
- *Resistant hypertension*: BP that remains above goal despite concurrent use of three antihypertensive agents of different classes, or that requires a minimum of four agents to achieve therapeutic goal

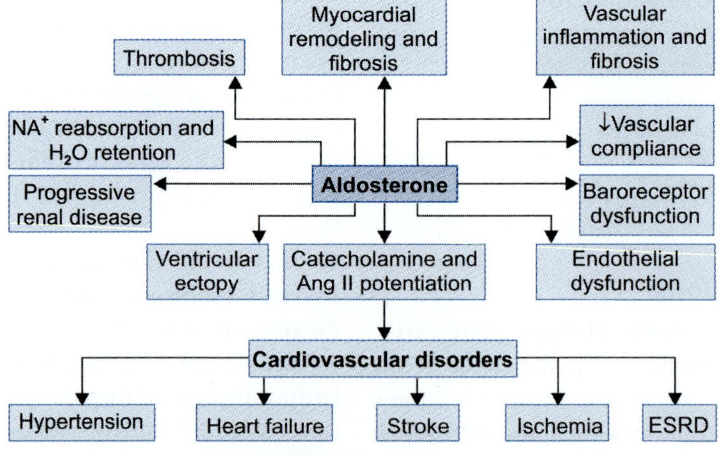

(Ang: angiotensin; ESRD: end-stage renal disease)

Flowchart 3: Ill-effects of aldosterone on tissues leading to cardiovascular damage.

Box 2: Cardiovascular disease in primary aldosteronism.

- Increase in the relative risk of:
  - Stroke (4.2 ×)
  - Myocardial infarction (6.5×)
  - Atrial fibrillation (12.1×)
- Increased left ventricular hypertrophy and diastolic dysfunction
- Increased stiffness of large arteries
- Widespread tissue fibrosis
- Increased remodeling of resistance vessels

- Secondary hypertension is being considered for other reasons.

Assessment of the Renin–angiotensin–aldosterone Axis

- *Plasma and urinary aldosterone:* Raised plasma aldosterone in a normokalemic patient is the fundamental abnormality. If serum potassium is less than 3 mmol/L, potassium supplementation should be administered and normokalemia established before aldosterone is measured. Alternatively, 24-hour urinary aldosterone excretion rate can be assessed. Conditions where 24-hour urinary aldosterone excretion rate may be normal in PA include significant hypokalemia, renal failure, incomplete collection of urine and variability in rates of hepatic metabolism of aldosterone. Unlike plasma aldosterone, the urinary aldosterone excretion rate decreases with age[7-10]
- A variant with isolated 11-deoxycorticosterone (DOC) excess has periodic aldosterone hypersecretion
- *Plasma renin activity (PRA):* In PA, PRA is usually low or undetectable
- *Aldosterone–renin ratio:* Hiramatsu et al. introduced the aldosterone–renin ratio in 1981.[11] It is recognized across the globe as the most reliable means of screening for PA. Values more than 30 when plasma aldosterone concentration (PAC) is

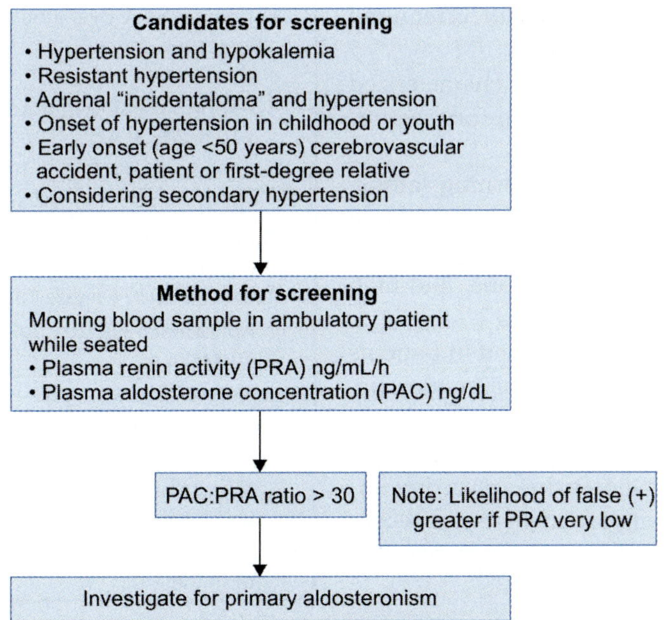

Flowchart 4: Algorithm for case detection in primary aldosteronism.

Box 3: Drugs to be changed during the test.

- If results not diagnostic, and if hypertension (HT) can be controlled with other meds, withdraw meds that may affect the aldosterone/renin ratio for at least 2 weeks:
    - Beta-adrenergic blockers, central α2- agonists and nonsteroidal anti-inflammatory drugs
    - Angiotensin-converting enzyme inhibitors, angiotensin receptor blockers, renin inhibitors and dihydropyridine calcium channel antagonists
    - Potassium-wasting diuretics
- If necessary to maintain HT control:
    - Hydralazine (with verapamil slow-release, to avoid reflex tachycardia)
    - Prazosin, doxazosin and terazosin
    - α-methyldopa

expressed in ng/dL and PRA as ng/mL/h (conventional units) or equivalent to 750 when PAC is reported as pmol/L (SI units) and PRA in conventional units; or equivalent to 60 when both are in SI units; are considered positive. To interpret this ratio without potential error, a minimum PAC value more than 15 ng/dL is required (Box 3)

- Secondary aldosteronism is characterized by elevated plasma aldosterone values together with a normal ratio
- *Prerequisites of the test*: morning sample for PAC and PRA, normokalemia, liberal dietary sodium intake, and discontinuation of spironolactone, eplerenone, and high dose amiloride for 5–6 weeks
- False positive results are seen in patients on β-receptor blockers, renal impairment, and old age
- False negative results are seen in patients on diuretics, angiotensin-converting enzyme (ACE) inhibitor, angiotensin receptor blockers (ARBs) and dihydropyridine calcium-channel blockers.

Establishment of the Diagnosis of Primary Aldosteronism

There are four aldosterone suppression tests to confirm or exclude the diagnosis.[2] Three of them are salt loading tests that can be conducted by increasing dietary sodium, infusing saline or administering exogenous mineralocorticoid or through combination of these approaches. The fourth test depends on inhibition of aldosterone secretion by an ACE inhibitor (Box 4).

Box 4: Four confirmation tests for the diagnosis of primary aldosteronism with normal and abnormal values.

- Oral sodium loading test: Increase dietary Na^+ intake to 300 mmol/day × 3 days; verify by 24-h urine Na^+ excretion; slow-release KCl to maintain normokalemia
    - Abnormal: Urinary aldosterone excretion >12 mg/24 h
    - Normal: Urinary aldosterone secretion ≤12 mg/24 h
- Intravenous saline suppression test: 2 L normal saline IV over 4 hours; measure plasma aldosterone concentration (PAC) at baseline and at 4 hours
    - Abnormal: PAC ≥15 ng/dL (baseline) and ≥10 ng/dL at 4 h
    - Indeterminate: PAC 5–10 ng/dL at 4 h
    - Normal: PAC <5 ng/dL at 4 h
- Fludrocortisone suppression test: 4 days high Na^+ diet + slow-release NaCl 30 mEq TID + fludrocortisone acetate 100 µg q6h
    - Abnormal: PAC >6 ng/dL on day 4 (upright, 10 AM)
    - Normal: PAC ≤6 ng/dL
- Captopril challenge test: Captopril 25–50 mg orally in seated patient
    - Abnormal: Absence of suppression of PAC by 30% from baseline
    - Normal: Suppression of PAC by 30% from baseline

Dexamethasone suppression test is used to differentiate glucocorticoid-remediable aldosteronism (GRA) from other causes of PA.

Primary Aldosteronism Subtype Classification

Adrenal Venous Sampling

In order to differentiate unilateral disease due to APA from bilateral disease due to hyperplasia, adrenal venous sampling is considered the "gold standard".[2] On the side of the tumor, aldosterone:cortisol ratios measured in the blood collected from the adrenal veins are significantly higher than those found in the inferior vena cava (IVC), whereas on the contralateral side, aldosterone secretion is suppressed (Box 5).

Adrenal Scintigraphy

I^{131}-labeled or 6-β-$[^{75}Se]$ selenomethyl- nor-cholesterol can be used to image the adrenals and to distinguish between APA and IHA.

Computed Tomography and Magnetic Resonance Imaging

Neither computed tomography (CT) nor magnetic resonance imaging (MRI) is accurate in distinguishing between APA and IHA.[35] A negative imaging test does not exclude a surgically curable form of PA.

Box 5: Interpretation of the results of adrenal venous sampling for subtype classification in primary aldosteronism.

- Calculate aldosterone: Cortisol ratios for IVC and each adrenal vein = "cortisol-corrected aldosterone ratios" (CCARs)
- AV cortisol should be ≈10-fold higher than IVC value, if the catheter is positioned correctly
- Unilateral disease: CCAR >4 (high to low side)
- Bilateral disease: CCAR <3 (high to low side)
- Indeterminate: CCAR 3–4

(AV: adrenal vein; IVC: inferior vena cava)

Treatment of Primary Aldosteronism

In case of PA due to APA or unilateral hyperplasia, surgery is recommended, whereas, medical management with aldosterone antagonists is offered to patients with bilateral disease (Flowchart 5).

Surgical Treatment

In a patient with APA, the recommended approaches are:

- Unilateral laparoscopic adrenalectomy via transperitoneal anterior approach is the standard approach[2]
- *Enucleation:*[12] This might result in sub-optimal correction as multiple satellite nodules and/or hyperplastic tissue surround the extirpated adenoma that

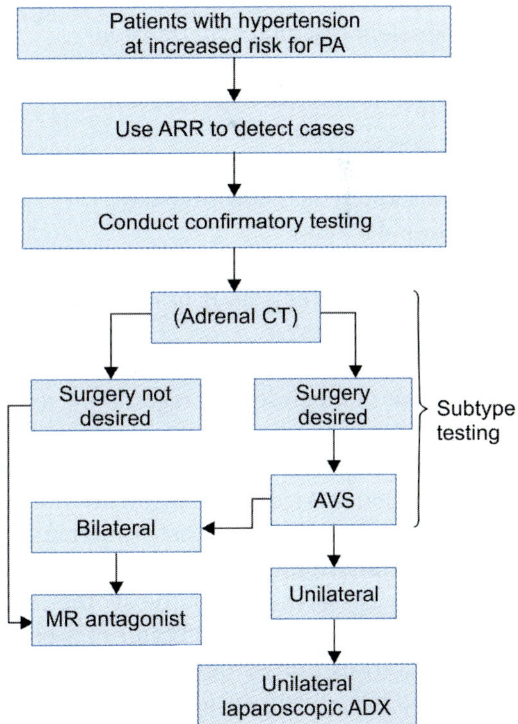

(ARR: aldosterone renin ratio; ADX: adrenalectomy; AVS: adrenal vein sampling; PA: primary aldosteronism)

Flowchart 5: Algorithm for establishing and treating primary aldosteronism.

might contribute to hypersecretion of aldosterone.

Preoperative preparation includes treatment with low dose spironolactone (12.5–50 mg daily). This gives smoother perioperative course with better control of BP and plasma potassium levels.

Postoperatively, BP usually decreases progressively over a period of weeks to months. Factors associated with resolution of hypertension postoperatively include:[13]

- Having one or no first-degree relatives with hypertension
- Preoperative use of two or fewer antihypertensive agents
- Duration of hypertension less than 5 years
- *Higher preoperative PAC:* PRA ratio
- Higher urinary aldosterone secretion
- Preoperative response to spironolactone
- Coexistent essential hypertension
- Older age
- Longer duration of hypertension.

Medical Treatment

- Low sodium diet (<80 mEq/day)
- Spironolactone
- *Eplerenone (50 mg twice daily)*: Drug of choice in men as it is not androgen antagonist
- Amiloride (2.5–20 mg daily), an aldosterone independent antagonist of renal tubule sodium transport.

Despite improvement in electrolyte status, the BP response is suboptimal and additional drugs are required such as calcium channel blockers (nifedipine) and ACE inhibitors (enalapril). Drugs that block the synthesis of aldosterone, trilostane an inhibitor of 3-beta-hydroxysteroid-dehydrogenase (3βHSD), have also been used to lower BP in PA.[14] The adrenolytic drug, mitotane is of value in aldosterone secreting carcinoma. Future might have aldosterone synthase inhibitors. In GRA, exogenous glucocorticoid is highly effective.

Aldosterone-producing Adrenal Carcinoma

It is a rare condition with a prevalence of 3–5% of all aldosterone-producing tumors. The prognosis is poor, with a median survival rate of 14 months and a 5-year survival rate of 24%. The diagnosis is suspected when:

- The adrenal tumor is greater than 3 cm in diameter
- The presence of calcification
- Biochemistry showing secretion of cortisol or androgen or both in addition to aldosterone
- Uptake of labeled cholesterol adrenal scanning agent, which also localizes the metastases.

Treatment

Adrenalectomy is done once the diagnosis is made, but that is only palliative. Mitotane has shown some benefits.[15]

Glucocorticoid-remediable Aldosteronism

It is autosomal dominant in inheritance. Hypertension in children or young adults is the most common feature of the syndrome. Patients often have resistant hypertension and hypokalemia. GRA results from expression of aldosterone synthase in the zona fasciculata. ACTH is the dominant control mechanism of aldosterone secretion in GRA.

Mineralocorticoids Other than Aldosterone

17-α-hydroxylase Deficiency

It is rare autosomal recessive disorder and the disease affects both adrenal and gonadal glands. The genetic mutations result in 17α-hydroxylase/17, 20-lyase deficiency. Consequent defects in cortisol synthesis and compensatory secretion of ACTH stimulate the synthesis of 11 DOC and corticosterone B by the zona fasciculata. High concentrations of DOC lead to hypertension, hypokalemia and suppression of the renin–angiotensin–aldosterone axis. In the gonads, the condition leads to pseudohermaphroditism in males and primary amenorrhea in females.[16]

Treatment

Glucocorticoids and sex steroids replacement.

11β-hydroxylase Deficiency

It is a rare cause of mineralocorticoid hypertension, autosomal recessive condition. It is accompanied by hyperandrogenism and contributes to 8–16% of cases of congenital adrenal hyperplasia.[17] Clinically, this disorder presents with variable degree of virilization and hypertension. The diagnosis is established by high basal or ACTH stimulated levels of 11-deoxycortisol. PRA is usually elevated in 21-hydroxylase deficiency and suppressed in 11β-hydroxylase deficiency.

Treatment

Glucocorticoid replacement to reduce ACTH secretion, thereby reducing the stimulus for excess DOC and adrenal androgen production. If the hypertension does not respond to glucocorticoid alone, then mineralocorticoid receptor antagonists or calcium channel blockers can be used.

Deoxycorticosterone Excess States

The DOC overproduction causing mineralocorticoid excess may be primary (caused by adrenal adenomas, malignancy, or hyperplasia) or secondary, depending on the amount of excess ACTH secretion. In patients with primary hyperdeoxycorticosteronism hypertension and hypokalemia are accompanied by suppressed urinary and plasma aldosterone levels.[18]

Treatment

Mineralocorticoid receptor blockade therapy before unilateral adrenalectomy.

Corticosterone Excess States

Corticosterone-producing adrenal tumors are extremely rare and usually are carcinomas. Hypertension and hypokalemia with elevated plasma corticosterone but suppressed aldosterone and renin levels.

Congenital Apparent Mineralocorticoid Excess Syndrome

The syndrome of congenital apparent mineralocorticoid excess is due to deficiency of 11βHSD2. The persistence of cortisol resulting from deficiency in 11βHSD leads to marked elevation in mineralocorticoid activity (Flowchart 6). Clinically, the patients present during childhood, with symptoms of hypertension, muscle weakness, impaired growth, and polyuria with polydipsia (secondary to nephrogenic DI). Lab abnormalities include hypokalemia, metabolic alkalosis, suppressed PRA and aldosterone, hypercalciuria and evidence of renal insufficiency.[19]

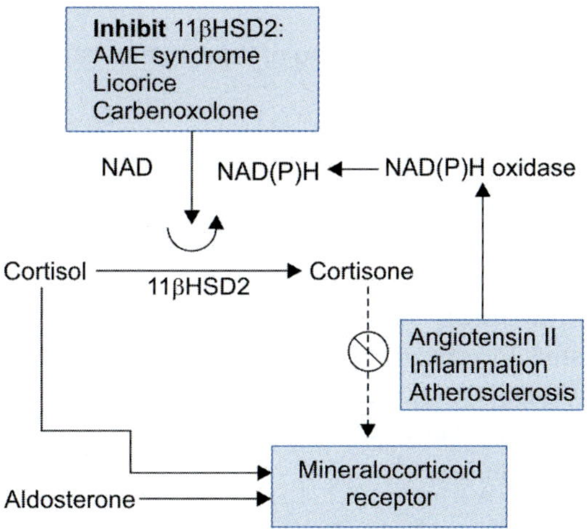

(AME: apparent mineralocorticoid excess; HSD: hydroxysteroid dehydrogenase)

Flowchart 6: Role of 11βHSD2 in metabolizing cortisol (which activates the mineralocorticoid receptor) and to cortisone (which does not).

Diagnosis

Twenty-four hour urinary free cortisol—urine free cortisone ratio. A normal ratio ranges from 0.3 to 0.5, but in 11βHSD2 deficiency, the ratio varies from 5 to 18. Genetic testing is performed to confirm the diagnosis.

Differential Diagnosis

Mineralocorticoid excess with low aldosterone secretion

- 17α-hydroxylase deficiency
- 11β-hydroxylase deficiency
- Liddle's syndrome
- 11-deoxycorticosterone-producing tumors
- Ectopic ACTH secretion
- Liquorice or carbenoxolone ingestion.

Treatment

- Dexamethasone
- Amiloride or triamterene
- Spironolactone
- Thiazide diuretic
- Renal transplantation.

Acquired Apparent Mineralocorticoid Excess Syndrome

This is due to ingestion of liquorice or carbenoxolone.

Liquorice

Ingestion of liquorice and carbenoxolone results in hypertension and hypokalemia accompanied by low plasma aldosterone and renin levels. Liquorice contains a steroid, glycyrrhetinic acid, which inhibits 11βHSD2.[20] Consumption of liquorice 50 g a day for 2 weeks or longer is enough to cause to hypertension.[21]

Carbenoxolone

Carbenoxolone is a hemisuccinate derivative of glycyrrhetinic acid. It was developed originally as an antiulcer drug but was found to cause sodium retention, hypertension, hypokalemia and suppression of the renin–angiotensin–aldosterone system. Carbenoxolone also inhibits 11βHSD2 activity. Carbenoxolone also inhibits its reductase forms (11βHSD1). This is responsible for the clinical differences between liquorice and carbenoxolone ingestion.

Ectopic ACTH Syndrome

Hypertension, hypokalemia and metabolic alkalosis can be found in patients with ectopic ACTH syndrome. The symptoms are less common in patients with pituitary dependent or ACTH–independent Cushing's syndrome. One proposed hypothesis is that cortisol secretion is so high in ectopic ACTH syndrome that it exceeds the metabolic capacity of 11βHSD2.

Glucocorticoid Resistance States

Glucocorticoid resistance causes increased total and free plasma cortisol levels and also increased urinary cortisol values. This leads to hypertension and signs of androgen excess, but the classical signs of cortisol excess as in Cushing's are not seen. ACTH levels are also increased, causing high adrenal androgen, corticosterone, and DOC secretion. Low dose dexamethasone suppression is absent, and despite of glucocorticoid resistance, signs of adrenal insufficiency are not seen.

Treatment

Dexamethasone up to 3 mg daily.

Primary (Essential) Hypertension

Of all the cases labeled as essential hypertension, approximately 25% of patients have low-renin hypertension. This group of patients achieves greater BP reduction with mineralocorticoid antagonism than with other antihypertensive drugs.[22]

Exogenous Mineralocorticoid States

Exogenous steroids are administered for long term to patients with Addison's disease or patients who have undergone bilateral adrenalectomy. Large doses of aldosterone, DOC, 9α-fludrocortisone, 9α-fluoropredni-solone or hydrocortisone can result in initial sodium retention, hypokalemia, and decreased PRA and aldosterone secretion. High salt intake in this period leads to hypertension. After a while, mineralocorticoid escape phenomenon happens and the initial symptoms are resolved, normalizing sodium retention and restoring hypokalemia.

Activating Mutations of the Mineralocorticoid Receptor

A gain of function mutation in the mineralo-corticoid receptor causes early onset hyper-tension that is exacerbated in pregnancy.

Disorders of the Renal Tubular Epithelium that Mimic Primary Mineralocorticoid Excess

Liddle's Syndrome

In Liddle's syndrome, activity of epithelial sodium channel is enhanced as the result of varying mutations in a short segment of the cytoplasmic tail of the β or γ subunits.

Patients with Liddle's syndrome present in youth, with excess sodium retention, hypertension and varying degree of hypo-kalemia. It is an autosomal dominant condi-tion. It does not respond to spironolactone therapy. It lacks hyperandrogenism and has normal urinary cortisol:cortisone ratio.

Treatment

Potassium sparing diuretics such as amiloride or triamterene, which directly close apical membrane sodium channel in principal cells.

■ CONCLUSION

Hypertension is a common presentation in our daily outpatient department (OPD). To treat it and dismiss every case as essential hypertension is not the right approach. To keep an eye open for mineralocorticoid hypertension is essential. It is indeed challenging to diagnose hyperaldosteronism, but it is definitely helpful in treating our patients. Hypertension, which has been long standing, along with hypokalemia can be treated either by surgical intervention or by medical management, preventing long-term sequelae. Genetic variants of PA can be diagnosed prenatally and the baby can be prevented from many complications, both cerebrovascular and cardiovascular.

■ REFERENCES

1. Conn JW. Primary aldosteronism: a new clinical syndrome. J Lab Clin Med. 1955;45:6-17.
2. Funder JW, Carey RM, Fardella C, et al. Case detection, diagnosis, and treatment of patients with primary aldosteronism: an Endocrine Society. Clinical Practice Guideline. J Clin Endocrinol Metab. 2018;93:3266-81.
3. Neville AM, OM,ill MJ. Histopathology of the human adrenal cortex. Clin Endocrinol Metab. 1985;14:791-820.
4. Ferriss JB, Brown JJ, Fraser R, et al. Primary hyper-aldosteronism. Clin Endocrinol Metab. 1981;10:419-52.
5. Imai Y, Abe K, Munakata M, et al. Circadian blood pressure variations under different pathophysiological conditions. J Hypertens Suppl. 1990;8:S125-32.
6. Funder JW. The role of aldosterone and mineralocorticoid receptors in cardiovascular disease. Am J Cardiovasc Drugs. 2007;7:151-7.
7. Milliez P, Girerd X, Plouin PF, et al. Evidence for increased rate of cardiovascular events in patients with primary aldosteronism. J Am Coll Cardiol. 2005;45:1243-8.
8. Young WF Jr: Primary aldosteronism: renaissance of a syndrome. Clin Endocrinol. 2007;66:607-18.
9. Cain JP, Tuck ML, Williams GH, et al. The regulation of aldosterone secretion in primary aldosteronism. Am J Med. 1972;53:627-37.
10. Edwards C, Landon J. Corticosteroids. In: Lorraine JA Bell EJ (Eds). Hormone Assays and Their Clinical Application. New York: Churchill Livingstone; 1976. pp. 519-79.
11. Hiramatsu K, Yamada T, Yukimura Y, et al. A screening test to identify aldosterone-producing adenoma by measuring plasma renin activity. Results in hypertensive patients. Arch Intern Med. 1981;141:1589-93.
12. Nakada T, Kubota Y, Sasagawa I, et al. Therapeutic outcome of primary aldosteronism: adrenalectomy versus enucleation of aldosterone-producing adenoma. J Urol. 1995;153:1775-80.

13. Sawaka AM, Young WF Jr, Thompson GB, et al. Primary aldosteronism: factors associated with normalization of blood pressure after surgery. Ann Intern Med. 2001;135:258-61.

14. Winterberg B, Vetter W, Groth H, et al. Primary aldosteronism: treatment with trilostane. Cardiology. 1985;72(Suppl 1): 117-21.

15. Tenschert W, Maurer R, Vetter H, et al. Primary aldosteronism by carcinoma of the adrenal cortex. Klin Wochenschr. 1987;65:428-32.

16. Yanase T, Simpson ER, Waterman MR. 17 alpha-hydroxylase/17,20-lyase deficiency: from clinical investigation to molecular definition. Endocr Rev. 1991;12:91-108.

17. Zachmann M, Tassinari D, Prader A. Clinical and biochemical variability of congenital adrenal hyperplasia due to 11 beta-hydroxylase deficiency. A study of 25 patients. J Clin Endocrinol Metab. 1983;56:222-9.

18. Biglieri EG, Irony I, Kater CE. Identification and implications of new types of mineralocorticoid hypertension. J Steroid Biochem. 1989;32:199-204.

19. Palermo M, Shackleton CH, Mantero F. Urinary free cortisone and the assessment of 11 beta-hydroxysteroid dehydrogenase activity in man. Clin Endocrinol (Oxf). 1996;45:605-11.

20. MacKenzie MA, Hoefnagels WH, Jansen RW, et al. The influence of glycyrrhetinic acid on plasma cortisol and cortisone in healthy young volunteers. J Clin Endocrinol Metab. 1990;70:1637-43.

21. Sigurjonsdottir HA, Franzson L, Manhem K, et al. Liquorice-induced rise in blood pressure: a linear dose-response relationship. J Hum Hypertens. 2001;15:549-52.

22. Buhler FR, Bolli P, Kiowski W, et al. Renin profiling to select antihypertensive baseline drugs. Renin inhibitors for high-renin and calcium entry blockers for low-renin patients. Am J Med. 1984;77:36-42

Catecholamines, Hypertension, and Pheochromocytoma—Genomic Insights

Kalyani Sridharan, Riddhi Das Gupta, Nihal Thomas

■ INTRODUCTION

Pheochromocytomas and paragangliomas (PPGLs) are neuroendocrine tumors that overproduce catecholamines. They are a rare but an important and treatable cause of hypertension. Recent advances have broadened the genetic landscape of PPGLs and this could make personalized biochemical and genetic testing possible in this disease.

■ CATECHOLAMINE BIOSYNTHESIS

Catecholamine biosynthesis starts with conversion of tyrosine to dihydroxyphenylalanine (DOPA) by the enzyme tyrosine hydroxylase (TH) which is the rate-limiting step in the pathway. This enzyme is present in the sympathetic nerves and adrenal and extra-adrenal chromaffin cells explaining the catecholamine production at these tissue sites. The expression of this enzyme is decreased in biochemically silent tumors. The DOPA is further decarboxylated by aromatic L-amino acid decarboxylase to dopamine (DA). In dopaminergic neurons the DA thus formed is released. However, in noradrenergic neurons, the DA enters the storage vesicles where the membrane-bound enzyme dopamine β-hydroxylase converts dopamine to norepinephrine (NE). In the adrenal medullary chromaffin cells the NE is further converted to epinephrine (EP) due to the presence of the enzyme phenylethanolamine N-methyl transferase (PNMT) and is stored in the chromaffin granules.

■ CATECHOLAMINE METABOLISM

Unique about the metabolism of catecholamines is the fact that it happens in the same cells where it is produced. There are two distinct enzyme pathways of catecholamine metabolism. One involves O-methylation of the catecholamines and the other involves deamination. The former pathway is mediated by catecholamine-O-methyl transferase (COMT) and occurs predominantly in the adrenal and extra-adrenal chromaffin tissue. The end products of this pathway are 3-methoxytyramine (3MT), normetanephrine (NMN) and metanephrine (MN) produced, respectively from DA, NE and EP. The latter pathway involves the enzyme monoamine oxidase (MAO) and occurs predominantly at the sympathetic nerve endings and results in the production of 3,4-dihydroxyphenylglycol (DHPG). O-methylation of DHPG produces 3-methoxy 4-hydroxyphenylglycol (MHPG). Hepatic extraction and metabolism of DHPG and MHPG result in the production of vanillylmandelic acid (VMA).

Due to the relatively constant production of MNs from the catecholamines leaking from the storage granules independent of catecholamine release, plasma or urinary MNs rather than catecholamines are the biochemical tests of choice in diagnosis of PPGLs.

HYPERTENSION IN PPGLS

Eighty to ninety percent of patients with PPGLs present with hypertension of which half will have sustained hypertension.[1] Around 5–15% will be normotensive. This latter group includes patients with low or absent catecholamine production. The clinical phenotypes of hypertension in PPGLs depend on the biochemical phenotype of the catecholamine produced, the pattern of secretion and the content of catecholamines. Sustained hypertension is frequent in NE secreting PPGL due to continuous and constitutive secretory pattern in these tumors.[2] Children more often present with sustained hypertension than paroxysmal hypertension.[3] Paroxysmal hypertension is more common in PPGLs secreting EP as this tumor phenotype is more differentiated and follows a regulated secretory pattern which limits continuous and unregulated catecholamine secretion.[2] Also, it is responsive to stimuli causing sudden catecholamine release leading to paroxysms.

BIOCHEMICAL PHENOTYPES IN PPGLS

The biochemical phenotype of PPGLs depends upon the pattern of expression of enzymes in the catecholamine biosynthetic cascade within the tumor. Tumor arising from extra-adrenal sites that lack dopamine hydroxylase and PNMT predominantly secrete dopamine while those with a slightly better differentiation profile lacking only PNMT secrete NE. Adrenal pheochromocytomas predominantly secrete EP due to the expression of PNMT which is induced by glucocorticoids from the surrounding adrenal cortical cells.[4] In most cases the categorization of PPGLs as adrenergic vs. noradrenergic is made from the level of increase in the plasma MN and NMN. Adrenergic PPGLs have an increase in MN above the upper cut-off and a tumor-derived increase in MN of more than 5% of the combined increase in MN and NMN;[5] noradrenergic PPGLs have an increase in plasma NMN with either a lack of increase in MN or an increase in MN of less than 5% that of combined MN and NMN.[6] Predominantly, dopamine secreting PPGLs have a solitary increase in plasma 3MT indicating a poorer tumor differentiation and an increased risk of malignancy and are frequently associated with succinate dehydrogenase B (SDHB) and SDHD mutations. Biochemically silent PPGLs can be difficult to diagnose due to the absence of secretion of catecholamines or its metabolites. In these cases chromogranin A may be used as a neuroendocrine tumor-marker.[7]

GENETIC PHENOTYPE OF PPGLS AND ITS BIOCHEMICAL AND CLINICAL CORRELATION

Historically, it was believed that 10% of PPGLs harbored germline mutations. However, with advances in gene sequencing methods currently between 30% and 40% of PPGLs are known to harbor germline mutations in over 15 susceptibility genes.[6] A substantial proportion of sporadic tumors have been shown to harbor somatic mutations. Hereditary PPGLs most frequently involve five genes leading to syndromic presentation: Von Hippel-Lindau (VHL) syndrome, multiple Endocrine Neoplasia 2 (MEN2), familial paragangliomas due to mutations in the genes encoding subunits of succinate dehydrogenase (SDH)—SDHB and SDHD, and neurofibromatosis 1 (*NF1*). Other genes that are less frequently involved include *SDHC*,

SDHA, SDHAF2, TMEM127, MAX, fumarate hydratase (FH), malate dehydrogenase (*MDH2*), isocitrate dehydrogenase (IDH) and *HIF2A.*

In view of the high rate of inherited mutations in PPGLs genetic testing should be considered in all cases of PPGLs and is particularly recommended in those with a family history, a syndromic presentation, young age at onset, bilateral adrenal PPGLs or metastatic or multifocal disease.

The genetic landscape of PPGLs will be detailed by means of a series of case vignettes.

CASE 1

An 18-year-old woman presented with severe hypertension for the past 3 months. There was no history to suggest renal disease. There was no history of weakness of limbs, no weight gain or cushingoid features. On evaluation she was found to have elevated urinary NMNs (24 h urine NM—5,700 µg; upper lab limit—600 µg/24 h). Computed tomography (CT) of the abdomen (Fig. 1) revealed bilateral adrenal masses of sizes 7 × 6.3 cm and 2 × 1.5 cm and a nodule in the tail of pancreas. Mutational analysis for *VHL* gene was positive (NM_000551.3:c.463+3A>G) (Fig. 2). She underwent right adrenalectomy, left cortical sparing adrenalectomy and distal pancreatectomy. Postoperative period was uneventful and she remained normotensive on follow-up.

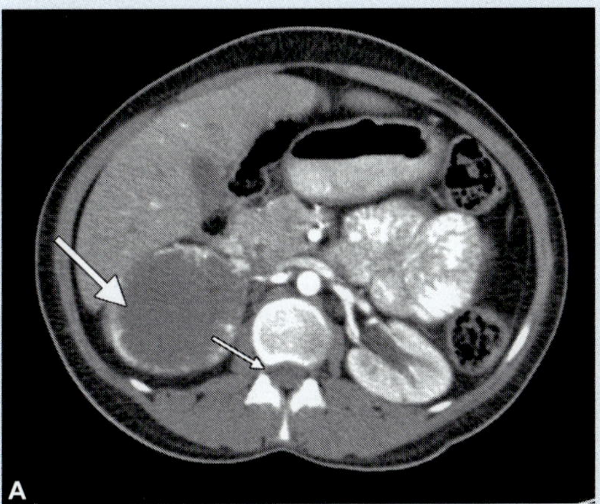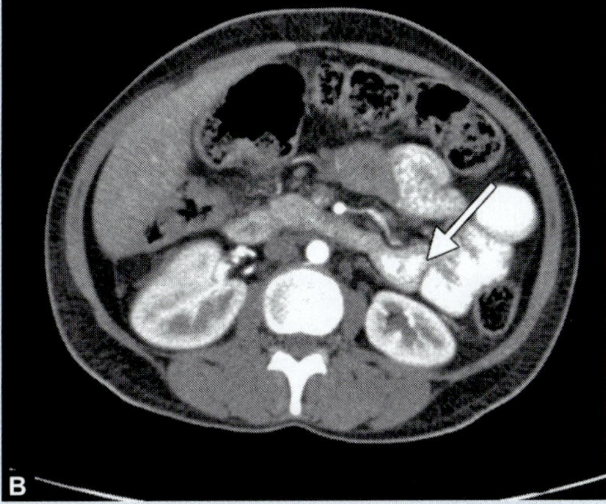

Figs. 1A and B: Computed tomography of the abdomen showing bilateral adrenal masses in the patient as depicted by the arrows.

Mutations in the *VHL* gene is one of the most common mutations identified in PPGLs. The PPGL in *VHL* has a penetrance of 7–20%.[8] These tumors have a noradrenergic biochemical phenotype, and are located in the adrenals though they can also occur in extra-adrenal locations. Around 50% of the tumors are bilateral. Malignancy is less common. Most of the mutations are missense mutations.[9] Large deletions are uncommon in *VHL* with PPGLs and even when present, they tend to associate with unilateral rather than bilateral PPGLs.[10] The *VHL* gene on chromosome 3p encodes a VHL tumor suppressor protein which binds to hypoxia inducible factor (HIF) α subunit and promotes its degradation. VHL mutations, therefore, result in stabilization of HIF α which then translocates to the nucleus and upregulates genes involved in angiogenesis and cell proliferation which would otherwise be upregulated only during hypoxia.[11] The PPGLs due to VHL mutations, like SDHx mutations, lack PNMT expression and therefore do not produce EP irrespective of their adrenal or extra-adrenal location. The suggested optimal time for screening for PPGL in VHL is at 5 years of age considering the early age at onset of these tumors.[12] Due to the increased frequency of multifocal and recurrent PPGLs, long-term follow-up is necessary in these patients.

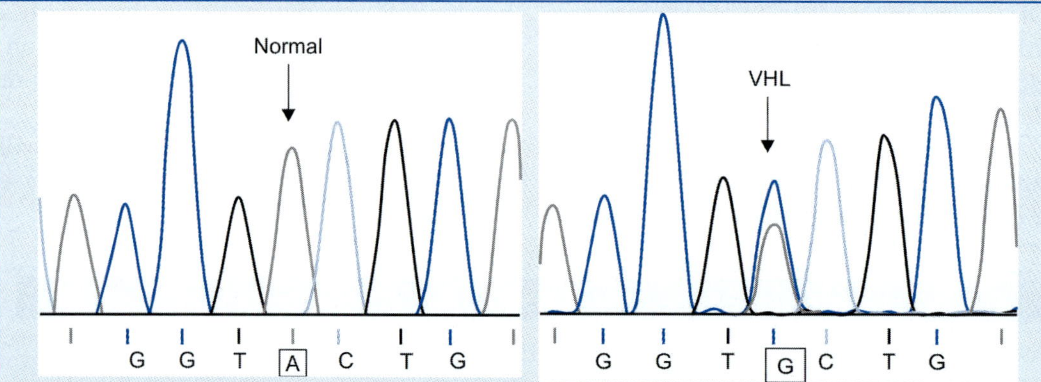

Fig. 2: Depiction of a normal *VHL* gene on the left and a point mutation in the gene on the right.
Source: Molecular lab; Department of Molecular Pathology, CMC, Vellore.

CASE 2

A 35-year-old male presented with history of hypertension, diabetes mellitus and progressive weight loss of 3 months duration. Physical examination was normal. On evaluation his routine biochemistry, renal function tests, cardiac imaging and thyroid functions were normal. The urinary NMN was elevated (6,682 µg/24 h; upper limit of normal—600 µg/24 h) while urinary MN was normal (192 µg/24 h; upper limit of normal—350 µg/24 h). CT of the abdomen revealed a 6.5 × 4.6 × 3.4 cm retroperitoneal mass (Fig. 3A) and bone metastasis (arrow in Fig. 3B). Bone scan showed multiple metastasis (Fig. 4A). Biopsy of the mass was paraganglioma. In view of presentation with malignant abdominal paraganglioma with metastasis genetic testing for *SDHB* gene was done which was positive (Fig. 4B). Patient received palliative chemotherapy.

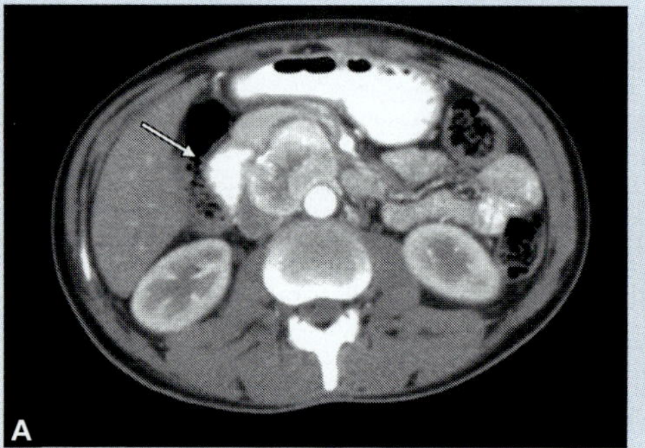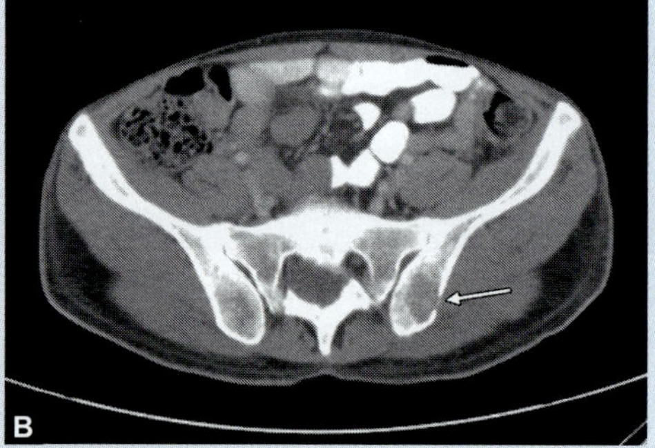

Figs. 3A and B: (A) Computed tomography of the abdomen depicting a retroperitoneal tumor on the left and; (B) Bone metastasis on the right (arrows).

Familial paraganglioma syndromes are due to mutations in the various subunits of SDH—SDHB, SDBD, SDHC, SDHA and its accessory factor SDHAF2. SDH along with its subunits forms the complex II of the mitochondrial respiratory electron transport chain. It converts succinate to fumarate and mediates the transfer of electrons from Kreb cycle to oxidative phosphorylation. Mutations in SDH result in mitochondrial dysfunction and decreased cellular energy production.[13] It also results in accumulation of succinate. This inhibits prolyl hydroxylases which mediate HIF degradation.[14] So the net result of SDH mutation is stabilization of HIF and a pseudohypoxic phenotype. Accumulation of succinate also results in DNA hypermethylation of genes involved in catecholamine biosynthetic pathway thereby causing an immature cellular phenotype that is nonsecretory or dopamine secreting.[15]

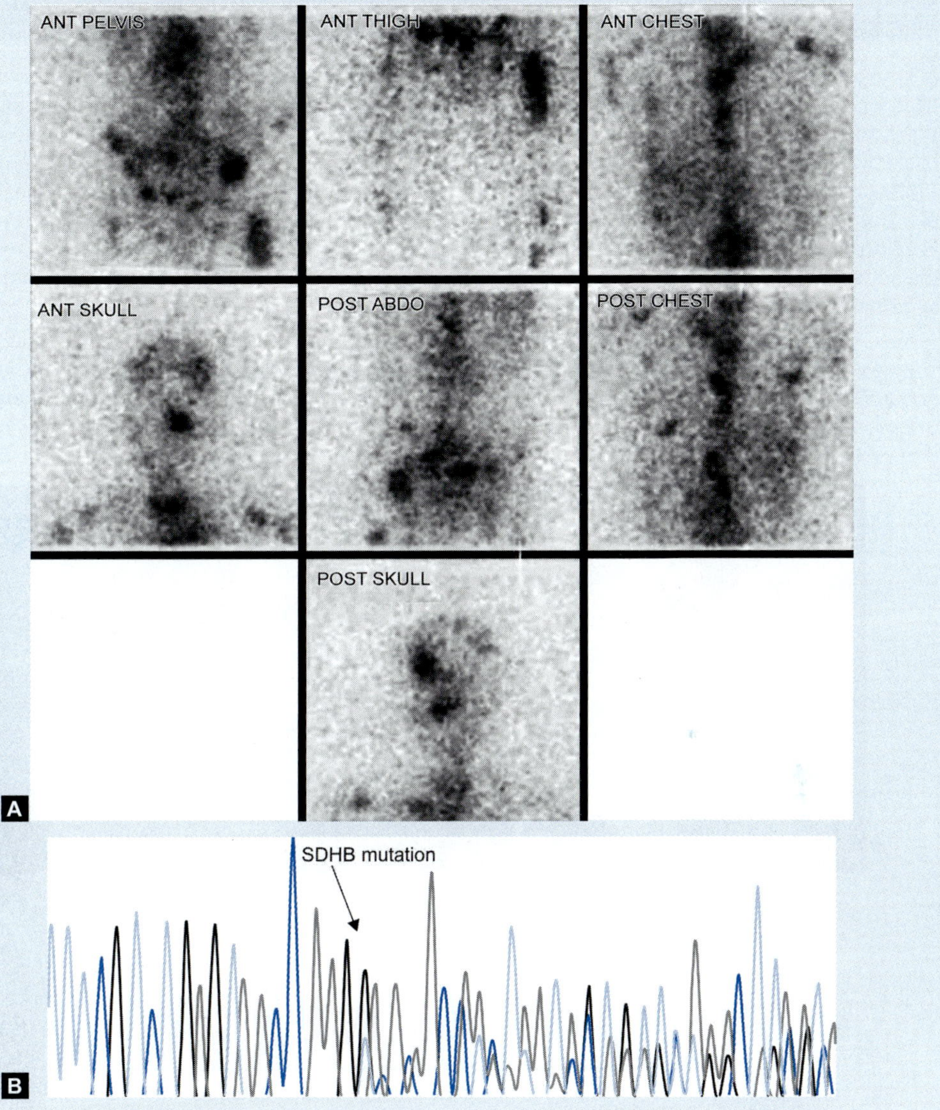

Figs. 4A and B: (A) Bone scan depicting multiple metastasis; (B) Succinate dehydrogenase B (SDHB) mutation in the patient.
Source: (A) Bone scan - Department of Nuclear Medicine, CMC, Vellore; (B) Molecular lab, Department of Molecular Pathology; CMC, Vellore.

Succinate dehydrogenase B mutations typically result in abdominal and thoracic PPGLs and less commonly head and neck PPGLs or adrenal pheochromocytomas. Unlike SDHD mutations, the penetrance is not high[16] but the mutation carries a high risk of malignancy and metastases.[17] Due to the poorly differentiated tumor phenotype in VHL and SDHx mutations, ^{18}F-flurodeoxyglucose positron emission tomography (PET) is superior as compared to ^{123}MIBG (metaiodobenzylguanidine) or ^{18}F-flurodopamine PET.[18]

Tumor tissue immunohistochemistry (IHC) for SDHB has been shown to guide genetic analysis and significantly cut down the costs.[19] Negative IHC for SDHB indicates presence of SDH subunit mutation.[20]

In carriers with SDHB and SDHD mutations it is recommended that surveillance starts at 5–7 years of age and includes annual measurement of NMN and 3MT.[6]

CASE 3

A 31-year-old gentleman reported in a case series earlier,[21] presented with a 4-month history of episodic headache, palpitations and sweating along with difficult-to-control hypertension. Family history was significant for a history of bilateral carotid body tumors in two younger siblings. On examination he had bilateral nonpulsatile neck swelling which had been progressing slowly over the past 5 years. His urinary NMN was elevated (3,540 μg/24 h; upper normal limit—600 μg/24 h) while urinary MN was normal. Imaging of the abdomen revealed right adrenal mass and two abdominal paragangliomas while magnetic resonance imaging (MRI) of the neck revealed bilateral carotid body tumors (Figs. 5A and B). He underwent resection of the abdominal lesions and later excision of the bilateral carotid body tumors. Genetic testing of the patient and his siblings was positive for SDHD mutation (Fig. 5C).

Succinate dehydrogenase D mutations are the most common cause of head and neck paragangliomas.[22] They less commonly cause abdominal paragangliomas and adrenal pheochromocytomas. The penetrance of SDHD mutation is high (75%),[23] unlike SDHB. *SDHD* gene is maternally imprinted and therefore, the disease shows a paternal transmission with most carriers of maternally inherited mutations remaining disease free.

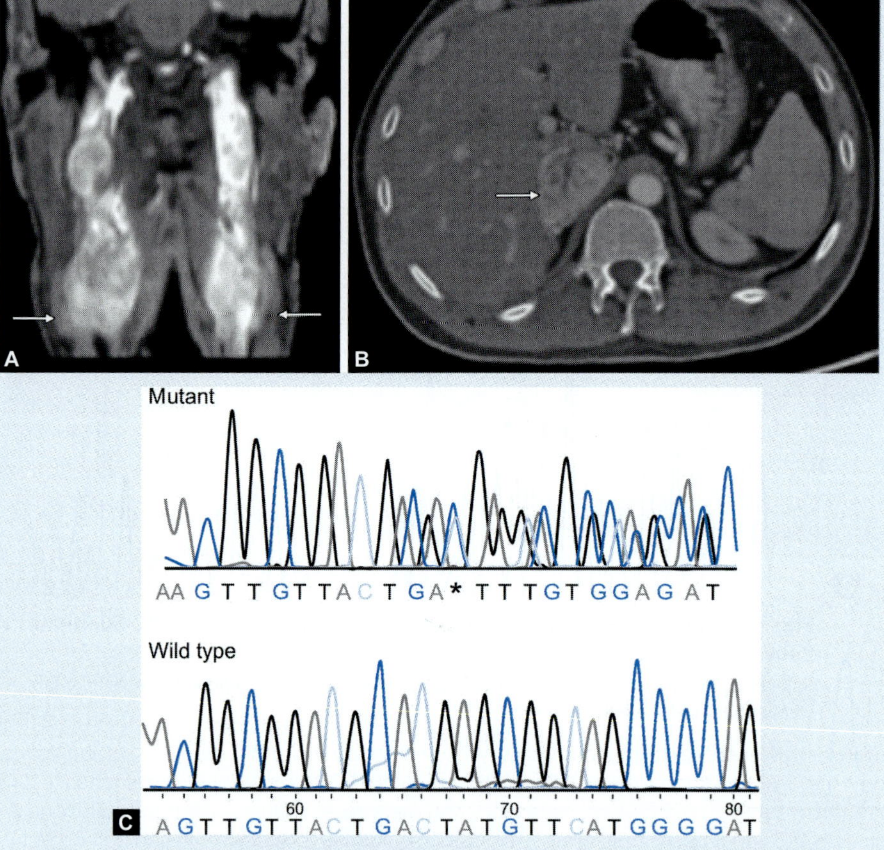

Figs. 5A to C: (A) Magnetic resonance imaging of head and neck showing bilateral carotid body tumors (arrows); (B) MRI of abdomen showing right adrenal mass (arrow); (C) Succinate dehydrogenase D (SDHD) mutation in the patient.

Source: (C) Molecular lab, Department of Molecular Pathology; CMC, Vellore.

CASE 4

A 44-year-old gentleman presented with a history of uncontrolled hypertension of 2 years duration and recent onset of diabetes mellitus. On evaluation he was found to have elevated 24 hours urinary VMA on two occasions (16 mg and 12 mg/24 h; normal <7 mg/24 h). Routine biochemistry also suggested parathyroid hormone (PTH)-dependent hypercalcemia (serum calcium—11 mg/dL, serum phosphate—3.5 mg/dL and serum PTH—131 pg/mL). CT imaging of the abdomen revealed bilateral adrenal masses. MIBG scan revealed uptake in both adrenal glands (Fig. 6A). Ultrasonography of the neck showed a right parathyroid adenoma (Fig. 6B). He underwent bilateral adrenalectomy and excision of the right parathyroid adenoma along with right hemithyroidectomy as thyroid appeared bulky on the right side. Biopsy was reported as parathyroid adenoma and medullary thyroid carcinoma. It was followed up with a total thyroidectomy. Genetic testing was positive for RET (rearranged in transfection) mutation at codon 634 (Fig. 7).

Multiple endocrine neoplasia 2 is due to mutations in the RET proto-oncogene located on chromosome 10. Mutation of RET results in dysregulated kinase signaling RAS/RAF/MAPK and PI3K/AKT/mTOR.[24] Activation of these pathways results in cell proliferation and tumorigenesis. These tumors lack HIF2α expression unlike SDHx mutations and therefore have a differentiated phenotype and increased PNMT expression leading to adrenergic phenotype. PPGLs in MEN2A have a penetrance of around 50% and occur in third to fourth decade of life. The PPGLs are almost always in adrenals and are frequently bilateral and very rarely malignant. Screening for PPGLs is recommended beginning from childhood.

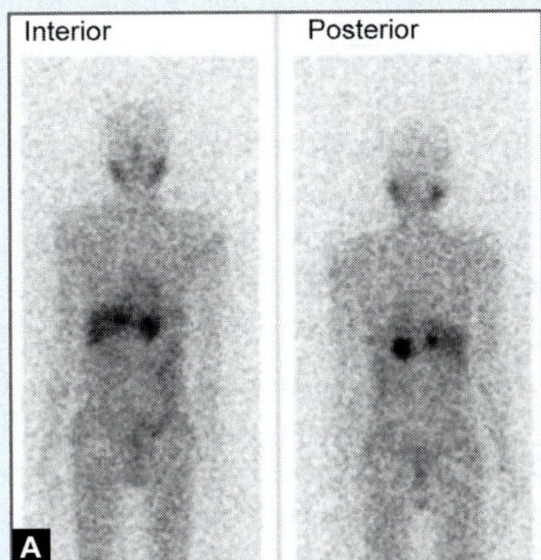

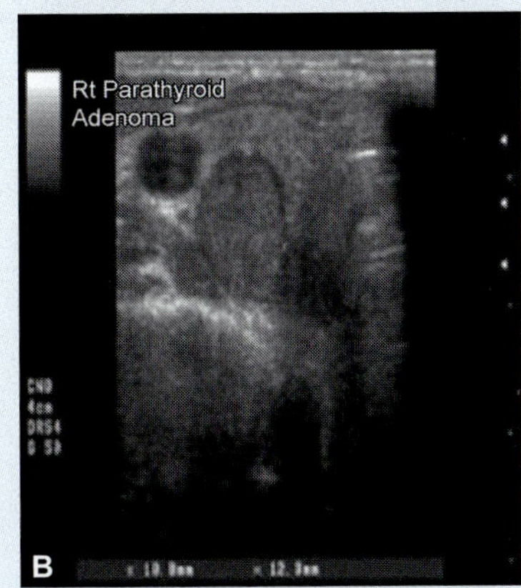

Figs. 6A and B: (A) MIBG (metaiodobenzylguanidine) scan with bilateral adrenal uptake; (B) Right parathyroid adenoma.

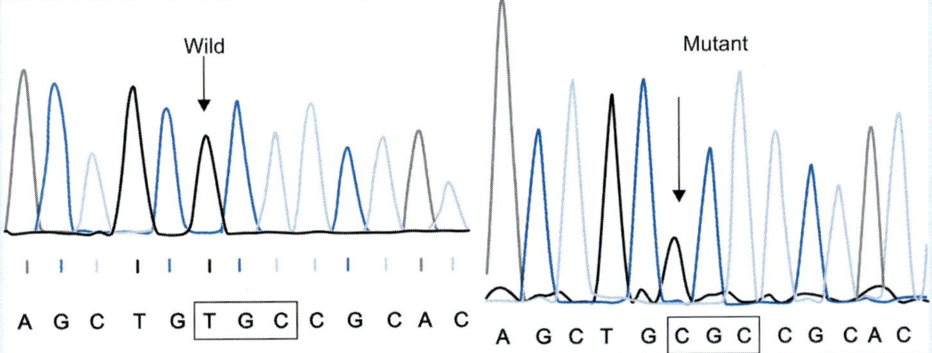

Fig. 7: *RET* gene with wild type allele on the left and mutant on the right.
Source: Molecular lab, Department of Molecular Pathology; CMC, Vellore.

■ OTHER MUTATIONS

Neurofibromatosis 1 can have PPGLs mostly confined to adrenals, frequently bilateral and adrenergic. Penetrance is low (<5%). The incidence is 0.1–5.7% in patients with NF-1 in general and 50% in those with NF-1 and hypertension.[25]

Other less commonly involved genes include SDHC mutations which predominantly result in head and neck PPGLs. More recently mutations in SDHA and SDHAF2 have also been identified with familial paragangliomas.

TMEM127 is a putative tumor suppressor gene which acts as a negative regulator of mTOR. The PPGLs associated with *TMEM127* are adrenergic and adrenal in location and less commonly associated with malignancy.[26] The age at presentation of PPGLs is slightly older in *TMEM127*.

MAX plays an important role in MYC/MAX/MXD1 signaling.[26] The PPGLs associated with MAX mutations are mostly adrenal and bilateral. However, risk of malignancy is high and the biochemical phenotype though predominantly adrenergic, is often mixed.[6] It is believed to show paternal transmission.

More recently identified mutations in FH, ICD and prolyl hydroxylases (PDH) result in PPGLs with a noradrenergic phenotype.

■ GENE CLUSTERS IN PPGLS

The PPGL susceptibility genes can be divided into two clusters—cluster 1 includes pseudohypoxic phenotype while cluster 2 genes are those involved in kinase signaling.[27] Cluster 1 is again subdivided into 1a which includes the SDHx, FH, ICD and MDH2 mutations while 1b includes VHL, HIF2α and PDH mutations.[27] Tumors of the cluster 1 genes are vascular and show overexpression of vascular endothelial growth factor (VEGF). Cluster 2 genes include *RET, NF1, TMEM127,* and *MAX.* Cluster 1 mutations have an immature phenotype, are extra-adrenal or adrenal in location, and are predominantly noradrenergic. Cluster 2 mutations have a mature phenotype, are adrenergic, and are located in the adrenals.

■ GENOTYPE–PHENOTYPE CORRELATION AND IMPLICATIONS FOR GENETIC TESTING

As described earlier, the genotype–phenotype correlation affecting the biochemical and clinical presentation can be used to guide genetic testing. In patients with syndromic or familial presentation, targeted genetic testing of the specific mutation is recommended. In apparently sporadic disease next generation sequencing (NGS) panel would be cost effective. According to a study at a tertiary referral center in India 32.7% of patients with PPGLs harbored germline mutations and 15.3% had mutations in *VHL* gene[28] which was the most common mutation. Similar rates were obtained from another tertiary care center where 32% of PPGLs had germline mutations and 12% had VHL mutations.[29] In the former study, VHL mutation was also the most common mutation in apparently sporadic unilateral pheochromocytoma. Carefully chosen targeted gene testing based on data on genotype–phenotype correlation can identify the mutation in the majority of the patients. Despite the high throughput nature of NGS, data has to be interpreted cautiously taking into consideration clinical and biochemical phenotype, as a variant of undetermined significance picked up on NGS need not necessarily be pathological.

■ CONCLUSION

Pheochromocytomas and paragangliomas are a rare but treatable cause of secondary hypertension. Newer gene sequencing methods have widened the genetic landscape of PPGLs. Several studies have tried to define the genotype and phenotype correlation of PPGLs. This knowledge would help in genetic testing and clinical decision making in patients with PPGLs.

■ REFERENCES

1. Zelinka T, Eisenhofer G, Pacak K. Pheochromocytoma as a catecholamine producing tumor: implications for clinical practice. Stress. 2007;10(2):195-203.

2. Zuber SM, Kantorovich V, Pacak K. Hypertension in Pheochromocytoma: Characteristics and Treatment. Endocrinol Metab Clin North Am. 2011;40(2):295-311.

3. Barontini M, Levin G, Sanso G. Characteristics of pheochromocytoma in a 4- to 20-year-old population. Ann N Y Acad Sci. 2006;1073:30-7.

4. Eisenhofer G, Rundquist B, Aneman A, et al. Regional release and removal of catecholamines and extraneuronal metabolism to metanephrines. J Clin Endocrinol Metab. 1995;80(10):3009-17.

5. Eisenhofer G, Timmers HJ, Lenders JW, et al. Age at diagnosis of pheochromocytoma differs according to catecholamine phenotype and tumor location. J Clin Endocrinol Metab. 2011;96(2):375-84.

6. Eisenhofer G, Klink B, Richter S, et al. Metabologenomics of phaeochromocytoma and paraganglioma: An integrated approach for personalised biochemical and genetic testing. Clin Biochem Rev. 2017;38(2):69-100.

7. Kimura N, Miura W, Noshiro T, et al. Plasma chromogranin A in pheochromocytoma, primary hyperparathyroidism and pituitary adenoma in comparison with catecholamine, parathyroid hormone and pituitary hormones. Endocr J. 1997;44(2):319-27.

8. Woodward ER, Maher ER. Von Hippel-Lindau disease and endocrine tumour susceptibility. Endocr Relat Cancer. 2006;13(2):415-25.

9. Ong KR, Woodward ER, Killick P, et al. Genotype-phenotype correlations in von Hippel-Lindau disease. Hum Mutat. 2007;28(2):143-9.

10. Lomte N, Kumar S, Sarathi V, et al. Genotype phenotype correlation in Asian Indian von Hippel-Lindau (vHL) syndrome patients with pheochromocytoma/paraganglioma. Fam Cancer. 2018;17(3):441-9.

11. Robinson CM, Ohh M. The multifaceted von Hippel-Lindau tumour suppressor protein. FEBS Lett. 2014;588(16):2704-11.

12. Binderup ML, Bisgaard ML, Harbud V, et al.; Danish vHL Coordination Group. Von Hippel-Lindau disease (vHL). National clinical guideline for diagnosis and surveillance in Denmark. 3rd edition. Dan Med J. 2013;60(12):B4763.

13. Pacak K. Pheochromocytoma: a catecholamine and oxidative stress disorder. Endocr Regul. 2011;45(2):65-90.

14. Favier J, Amar L, Gimenez-Roqueplo AP. Paraganglioma and phaeochromocytoma: from genetics to personalized medicine. Nat Rev Endocrinol. 2015;11(2):101-11.

15. Cascón A, Comino-Méndez I, Currás-Freixes M, et al. Whole-exome sequencing identifies MDH2 as a new familial paraganglioma gene. J Natl Cancer Inst. 2015; 107(5). pii: djv053.

16. Heesterman BL, Bayley JP, Tops CM, et al. High prevalence of occult paragangliomas in asymptomatic carriers of SDHD and SDHB gene mutations. Eur J Hum Genet. 2013;21(4):469-70.

17. Amar L, Bertherat J, Baudin E, et al. Genetic testing in pheochromocytoma or functional paraganglioma. J Clin Oncol. 2005;23(34):8812-8.

18. Timmers HJ, Chen CC, Carrasquillo JA, et al. Comparison of 18F-fluoro-L-DOPA, 18F-fluoro-deoxyglucose, and 18F-fluorodopamine PET and 123I-MIBG scintigraphy in the localization of pheochromocytoma and paraganglioma. J Clin Endocrinol Metab. 2009;94(12):4757-67.

19. Papathomas TG, Oudijk L, Persu A, et al. SDHB/SDHA immunohistochemistry in pheochromocytomas and para-gangliomas: a multicenter interobserver variation analysis using virtual microscopy: a Multinational Study of the European Network for the Study of Adrenal Tumors (ENS@T). Mod Pathol. 2015;28(6):807-21.

20. Pai R, Manipadam MT, Singh P, et al. Usefulness of Succinate dehydrogenase B (SDHB) immunohistochemistry in guiding mutational screening among patients with pheochromocytoma-paraganglioma syndromes. APMIS. 2014;122(11):1130-5.

21. Kapoor N, Pai R, Ebenazer A, et al. Familial carotid body tumors in patients with SDHD mutations: a case series. Endocr Pract. 2012;18(5):e106-10.

22. Baysal BE, Willett-Brozick JE, Lawrence EC, et al. Prevalence of SDHB, SDHC, and SDHD germline mutations in clinic patients with head and neck paragangliomas. J Med Genet. 2002;39(3):178-83.

23. Benn DE, Gimenez-Roqueplo AP, Reilly JR, et al. Clinical presentation and penetrance of pheochromocytoma/paraganglioma syndromes. J Clin Endocrinol Metab. 2006;91(3):827-36.

24. Dahia PL. Pheochromocytoma and paraganglioma pathogenesis: learning from genetic heterogeneity. Nat Rev Cancer. 2014;14(2):108-19.

25. Gruber LM, Erickson D, Babovic-Vuksanovic D, et al. Pheochromocytoma and paraganglioma in patients with neurofibromatosis type 1. Clin Endocrinol (Oxf). 2017;86(1): 141-9.

26. Vicha A, Musil Z, Pacak K. Genetics of pheochromocytoma and paraganglioma syndromes: new advances and future treatment options. Curr Opin Endocrinol Diabetes Obes. 2013;20(3):186-91.

27. Mercado-Asis LB, Wolf KI, Jochmanova I, et al. Pheochromocytoma: A genetic and diagnostic update. Endocr Pract. 2018;24(1):78-90.

28. Pandit R, Khadilkar K, Sarathi V, et al. Germline mutations and genotype-phenotype correlation in Asian Indian patients with pheochromocytoma and paraganglioma. Eur J Endocrinol. 2016;175(4):311-23.

29. Pai R, Ebenazer A, Paul MJ, et al. Mutations seen among patients with pheochromocytoma and paraganglioma at a referral center from India. Horm Metab Res. 2015;47(2):133-7.

Coarctation of Aorta

Suresh T Yavagal

■ INTRODUCTION

In India about 84 million adult population is suffering from hypertension (HTN). 90% of them have essential HTN. Prevalence increases from 15% in young adults to more than 60% in adults aged 65 years and above. Incidence of secondary HTN is 5–10% of all hypertensives. Incidence of coarctation of aorta (CoA) is 0.2%. In the study reported by Kota et al.[1] out of 12,650 children below 18 years of age 1.06% had HTN. 93% had secondary HTN. Most common cause was intrinsic renal disease. But in infants CoA was most common cause of HTN (40%).

Coarctation of aorta is a congenital abnormality of the heart producing obstruction to blood flow through the aorta. It consists of constricted aortic segment comprising localized medial thickening with some infolding of the media and superimposed neointimal tissue. It may be a shelf-like structure or a membranous curtain-like structure with an eccentric or a central opening. Most commonly it is located at the junction of the ductus arteriosus with the aortic arch just distal to the origin of left subclavian artery. Rarely the coarcted segment is present in the lower thoracic or abdominal aorta. Coarctation can occur in isolation, in association with bicuspid aortic valve, or with major cardiac malformations.[2] CoA accounts for 5–8% of children born with congenital heart disease.[3] The majority of coarctations are newly diagnosed in childhood—less than 25% are recognized beyond 10 years of age.[4] Significant coarctation requires the presence of proximal HTN along with echocardiographic or angiographic evidence of CoA with gradient greater than 20 mm Hg across the coarctation.

■ CLINICAL FEATURES

Majority of adult patients are asymptomatic. Patient may present with the history of headache, giddiness, epistaxis, lower limb fatigue, or claudication pain on exertion. Clinical examination will show HTN in upper limbs and reduced pressure in lower limbs (Fig. 1). Systolic blood pressure difference must be at least 10 mm Hg. Radiofemoral pulse delay is present. Pulse will be high volume in upper limbs and reduced or absent in lower limbs. Abdominal aortic pulsation is feeble or absent. Apical impulse will be heaving type suggesting left ventricular hypertrophy. Auscultation will reveal a systolic murmur in the interscapular region. There may be a widespread crescendo-

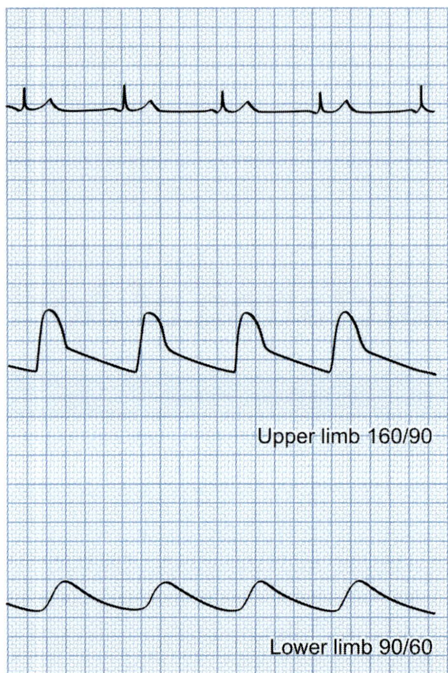

Fig. 1: Hypertension in upper limbs and reduced pressure in lower limbs.

decrescendo systolic murmur throughout the chest due to intercostal collateral arteries. Fundoscopic examination will show "Cork Screw" tortuosity of retinal arteries.

INVESTIGATIONS

Electrocardiogram shows left ventricular hypertrophy. X-Ray chest will show LV contour of the apex. Figure of three configuration over proximal descending aorta is due to prestenotic and poststenotic dilatation. Bilateral or unilateral rib notching is seen in II to IX ribs in 50% of cases. It appears as an erosion of the under surface of posterior rib generally at its outer third. Echocardiogram will show a posterior shelf with expanded isthmus and transverse aortic arch. There will be high velocity jet with diastolic persistence through the coarctation site. There will be slow upstroke in abdominal aortic velocity. MRI will provide detailed information of the coarctation. Cardiac catheterization and angiocardiogram is reserved for interventional procedure.

TREATMENT

Antihypertensive drugs are needed for HTN. Treatment of coarctation includes either surgery or balloon dilatation and stenting. Surgical repair is to relieve in the obstruction. But recoarctation occurs in 10% and there is aneurysm formation at the site in 2–27%. After treating coarctation antihypertensive drugs are either not required or required in lower dose. Until recently surgical repair was the gold standard for native coarctation. Today transcatheter-based dilatation and stent implantation has emerged as viable therapeutic option for native and recurrent coarctation as it is less invasive and demonstrates lower complication rate and long-term outcome (Figs. 2 and 3).

HYPERTENSION IN COARCTATION OF AORTA

Upper limb HTN of varying degrees occurs in CoA. There are three theories for the genesis of HTN—mechanical, neural and renal.

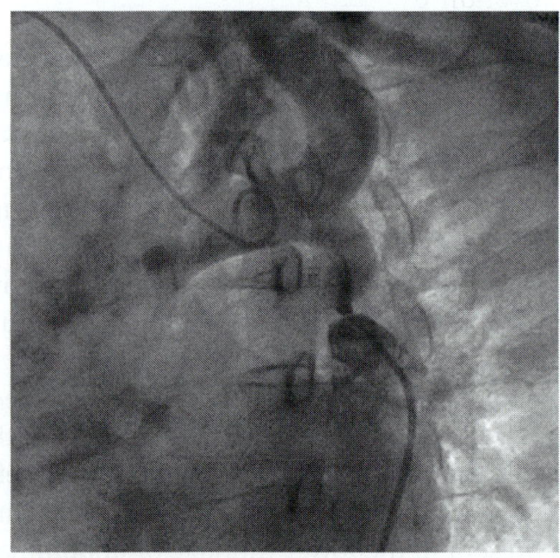

Fig. 2: Coarctation of aorta.

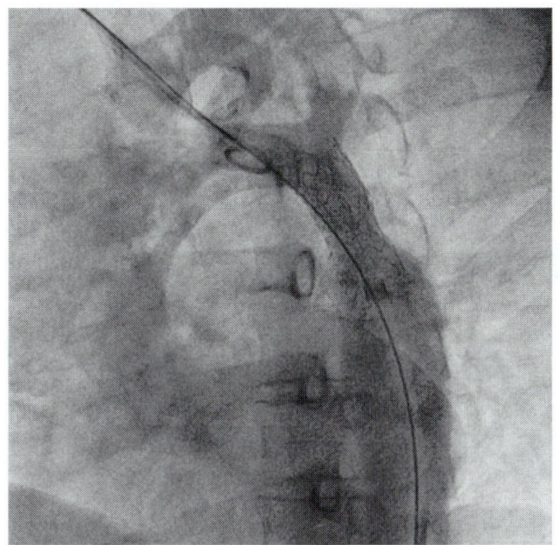

Fig. 3: After balloon angioplasty and stenting.

Mechanical theory proposes that resistance to circulation at the zone of coarctation leads to disproportionate upper limb HTN. Neural theory focuses on the distensibility of precoarct segment of aorta. Elevated driving pressure in the proximal aorta during early infancy will reset the baroreceptors to a higher basal rate which leads to HTN. Renal mechanism states that renal arteries originating from the lower pressure postcoarct of aorta will lead to reduced renal blood flow with subsequent activation of renin angiotensin aldosterone system. HTN may persist or appear later after a successful surgery or intervention because changes in vascular reactivity, arterial wall compliance, and abnormal baroreceptors reflex function persist even after the obstruction is corrected. Although HTN is common in CoA the incidence of hypertensive retinopathy or papilledema is rare. Incidence of toxemia of pregnancy is also less in CoA.[5]

RESISTANT HYPERTENSION

If one comes across multidrug-resistant HTN in adulthood one must look for CoA as it may be a causative factor; Balloon dilatation and stenting the coarcted segment help in controlling the blood pressure.[6]

CONCLUSION

Coarctation of aorta is one of the causes of secondary HTN. It is the most common cause for secondary HTN in infants. In all adults with resistant HTN CoA should be looked for. Balloon angioplasty and stenting is the current treatment of choice with excellent results.

REFERENCES

1. Kota SK, Kota SK, Meher LK, et al. Clinical analysis of hypertension in children: an urban Indian study. Saudi J Kidney Dis Transpl. 2013;24(4):844-52.
2. Doshi AR, Rao PS. Coarctation of Aorta-management options and decision making. Pediat Therapeut. 2012;S5: 006.
3. Van Praagh R, Vlad P. Dextrocardia, mesocardia, and levocardia: the segmental approach to diagnosis in congenital heart disease. In: Keith JD, Rowe RD, Vlad P (Eds). Heart Disease in Infancy and Childhood, 3rd edition. New York: Macmillan Publishers Limited; 1978. pp. 638-95.
4. Moss AJ, Adams FH. In: Emmanouildes GC, Allen HD, Riemenschneider TA, Gutgesell HP (Eds). Heart Disease in Infants, Children and Adolescents, 4th edition. Baltimore: Williams & Wilkins; 1989.
5. Satpathy M, Mishra BR (Eds). Clinical Diagnosis of Congenital Heart Disease. New Delhi: Jaypee Brothers Medical Publishers; 2008. p. 392.
6. Meller SM, Fahey JT, Setaro JF, et al. Multi-drug-resistant hypertension caused by severe aortic coarctation presenting in late adulthood. J Clin Hypertens (Greenwich). 2015;17(4):313-6.

Hypertension due to Central Nervous System Dysfunction

K Mugundhan

■ INTRODUCTION

Hypertension causes central nervous system (CNS) damages in many ways and it affects both small vessels and large vessels in cerebral circulation. It is an important risk factor for both ischemic and hemorrhagic stroke. An acute elevation of blood pressure (BP) can present with features of hypertensive encephalopathy (headache, seizure, and altered sensorium) and chronic hypertension can present as vascular dementia. Like hypertension causes CNS damages, reversal also can occur, i.e. CNS disease also causes severe paroxysmal hypertension. Hypertension causing CNS problems is well recognized and understood but paroxysmal hypertension which occurs secondary to CNS disorders is poorly understood and exact mechanism is not clear. Paroxysmal hypertension occurs in many neurological disorders like stroke, brainstem lesions, epilepsy, carotid endarterectomy, electroconvulsive therapy, neuroleptic malignant/serotonin syndrome, general anesthesia, spinal cord disease, and scorpion envenomation. This paroxysmal hypertension occurs as a result of abnormal overactivity of sympathetic nervous system or underactivity of parasympathetic nervous system from CNS insults (Table 1).

TABLE 1: Secondary hypertension—CNS disorders.

Stroke	Brainstem diseases	Carotid endarterectomy
Epilepsy	Electroconvulsive therapy	General anesthesia
Myelopathy	Scorpion envenomation	Neuroleptic malignant syndrome

■ CENTRAL NEURAL PATHWAY

Baroreceptors are present in carotid sinus and aorta which sensitize systemic arterial pressure and blood volume. It plays an important role in BP homeostasis and acts as afferent receptor in the central neural BP pathway. It sends information about BP and volume to vasomotor centers in medulla through glossopharyngeal nerve and vagus nerve. Nucleus tractus solitarius in the brainstem receives information about systemic arterial pressure first and then it sends impulses to other vasomotor centers in the brain depending on the response it desires. The important sympathetic vasomotor centers in brainstem are rostral ventrolateral medulla, rostral ventromedial medulla, raphe nucleus, midbrain, and hypothalamus paraventricular nucleus. Parasympathetic center in the brainstem are dorsal nucleus of vagus and nucleus ambiguous (Figs. 1A and B).

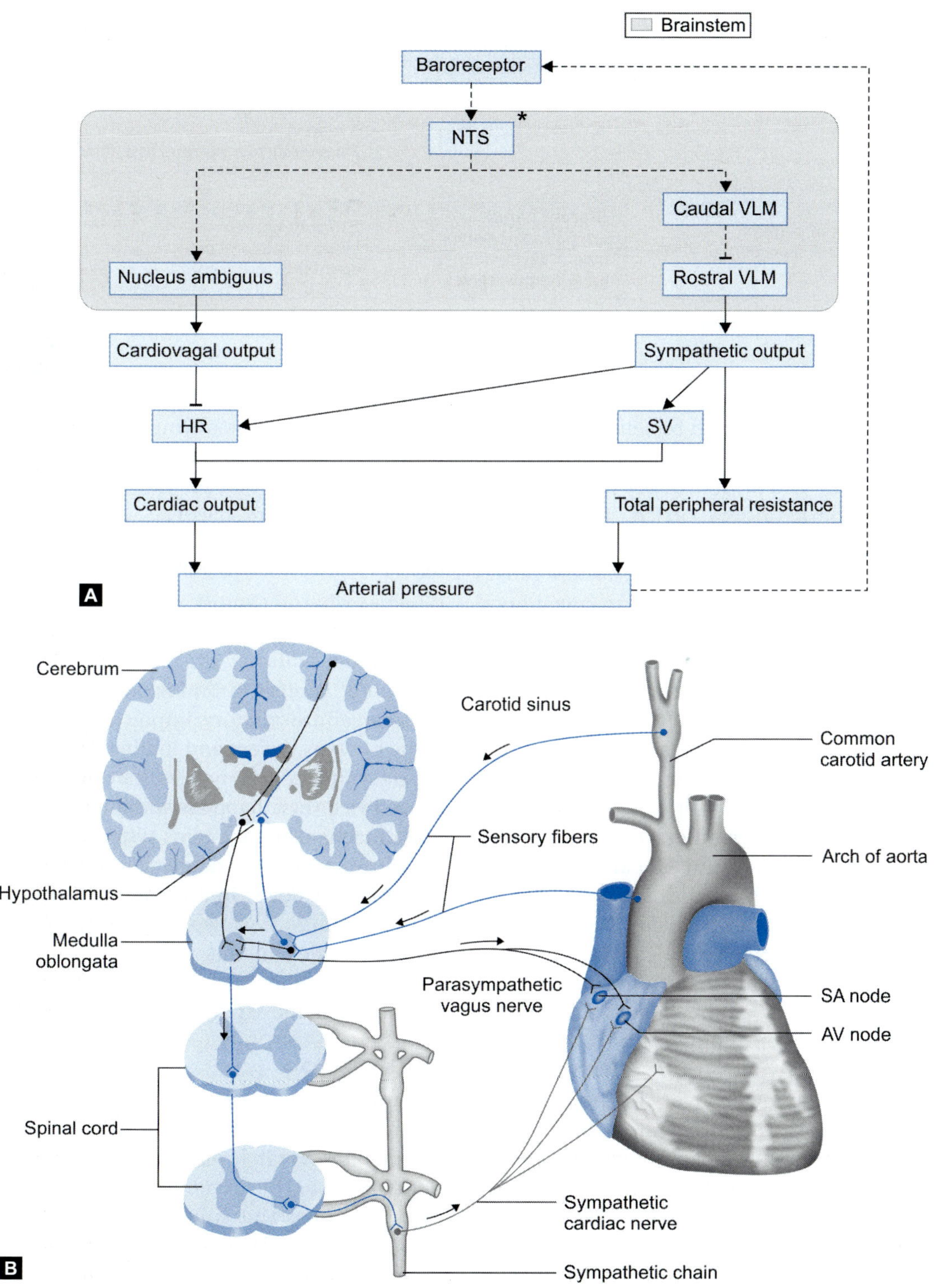

Figs. 1A and B: (A) Depicts baroreflex feedback pathway in flowchart; (B) Depicts organs, blood vessels, nerves, and neural centers involved in baroreflex pathway.

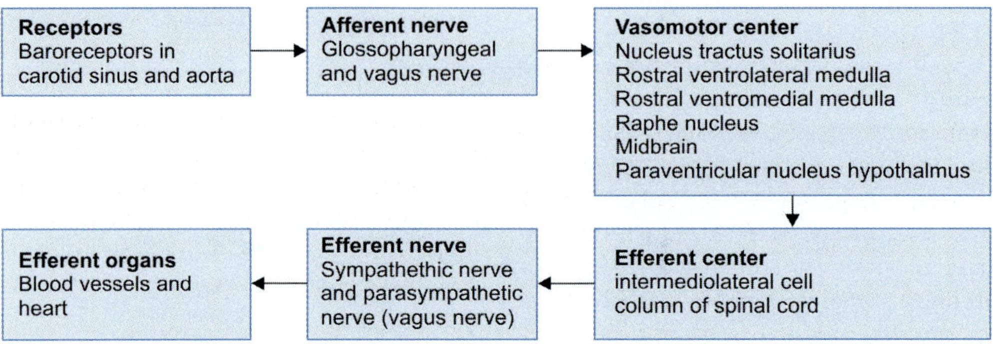

Flowchart 1: Baroreflex—Feedback control.

Vasomotor center controls sympathetic fibers in the spinal cord by sending signals to the intermediolateral cell column of the spinal cord from where first order preganglionic sympathetic fibers arise and supply blood vessels, heart, and other structures. Sympathetic nerve fibers activation causes vasoconstriction, increase in peripheral resistance, heart rate, cardiac output, and BP.[1] Vasomotor center also has control over parasympathetic nervous system by sending signals to dorsal motor nucleus and nucleus ambiguous of vagus nerve which supplies heart. Resting heart rate is predominantly under parasympathetic control. Parasympathetic nerve fibers activation leads to bradycardia, reduces cardiac output, and decreases systemic arterial pressure. Other mechanism by which CNS influences BP includes release of hormones like vasopressin from posterior pituitary and adrenocorticotropic hormone from anterior pituitary. Both contribute to sodium-dependent hypertension. Hypothalamus exerts its control over BP through its connections with brain stem and limbic system. Among the hypothalamus nucleus, paraventricular nucleus and dorsomedial part of hypothalamus are involved in BP control. Dorsomedial hypothalamus mainly involves in stress-induced hypertension and paraventricular nucleus involves with body homeostasis.[2] Even though posterior hypothalamus regulates sympathetic nervous system, it has less role in BP compared to paraventricular nucleus and dorsomedial hypothalamus (Flowchart 1).

Baroreflex—Feedback Control

Whenever baroreceptors in carotid sinus or aorta sensitize low systemic arterial pressure and blood volume, it sends impulse to vasomotor centers in brainstem. Vasomotor centers send excitatory impulse to sympathetic nervous system and inhibitory impulse to parasympathetic nervous system to increase BP and vice versa happens with high BP. This reflex mechanism maintains systemic arterial pressure at normal range (Flowchart 1).[3] However, any defect in this pathway can lead to reflex failure and hypotension or hypertension. Defect in this pathway at various levels is identified as a cause of secondary hypertension due to CNS dysfunction.

Pathogenesis

Disorders which affect this CNS pathway of BP control can cause paroxysmal hypertension. Lesion at several levels of central neural pathway, i.e. baroreceptors, brainstem, hypothalamus, and spinal cord can cause severe paroxysmal hypertension. How various lesions in CNS pathway causes hypertension will be discussed below.

Stroke

It is a well-known fact that high BP occurs following massive infarct in cerebral hemisphere. This high BP protects brain from cerebral ischemia. The probable explanation of paroxysmal hypertension in stroke is due to cerebral edema which affects paraventricular nucleus of hypothalamus and interrupts baroreceptor reflex pathway leading to excess sympathetic activation and high BP. Similarly in lateral medullary syndrome due to infarction of nucleus tractus solitarius and interruption of baroreceptor reflex pathway high BP occurs.[4] When plasma catecholamines were measured in stroke patients with high BP, they were elevated threefold times of upper limit of normal value transiently for 3–4 weeks following stroke. Cushing reflex is characterized by bradycardia, hypertension, and irregular breathing. Here secondary hypertension occurs due to raised intracranial hypertension from cerebral edema.

Brain Lesions

Tumors of fourth ventricle and basilar artery aneurysm have been seen in association with high BP.[5,6] Mass lesions in brainstem irritate or compress vasomotor centers which leads to abnormal firing of sympathetic neurons and elevate BP. Hypertension is also noted in vascular loops compressing medulla and in this patient hypertension is reversed by surgical decompression.

Carotid Endarterectomy

Carotid endarterectomy which is now widely done for carotid stenosis also associated with paroxysmal hypertension. Cases have been reported that in postoperative period some of the patients who underwent carotid endarterectomy developed severe hypertension resembling pheochromocytoma and were treated with alpha-blockers.[7,8] The most probable explanation for this scenario is the damage of afferent pathway of baroreflex circuit (baroreceptors in carotid sinus and afferent fibers) caused by surgery. When these patients were followed up BP normalized in 4–6 weeks. Similarly bilateral lymph node neck dissection for cancer damages afferent fibers of baroreflex pathway and associated with paroxysmal hypertension.

Spinal Cord Disease

Quadriplegic patients with cervical cord disease were noted to have paroxysmal sweating, paleness, and high BP whenever bladder is obstructed or catheter is kinked and this BP normalizes with release of obstruction. Stretching of bladder sends impulses to intermediolateral cell column of spinal cord and causes reflex activation of autonomic nervous system (ANS). Normally higher center modulates this reflex activation of ANS. Loss of this modulation in cervical spinal cord injury due to cut down of impulse from vasomotor center to intermediolateral cell column leads to abnormal ANS activation with bladder distension and results in paroxysmal hypertension.

Epilepsy and Electroconvulsive Therapy

Sometimes seizures are associated with high BP. Seizures which originate in thalamus, hypothalamus, or temporal lobe can present with paroxysmal hypertension. Seizure activates limbic and insular structures which has control over ANS. In these patients plasma catecholamines, norepinephrine, prolactin, and adrenocorticotrophic hormone are elevated transiently following seizures. Some patients after electroconvulsive therapy develop severe hypertension in the range of 250/150 mm Hg and it is similar to hypertension that occurs following epilepsy.

Neuroleptic Malignant Syndrome and Serotonin Syndrome

Both these syndromes are caused by antipsychiatric medications. And these syndromes are suspected when psychiatric patients present to emergency department with altered sensorium, hyperthermia, rigidity, and sympathetic overactivity. Sympathetic overactivity results in diaphoresis, tachycardia, and hypertension. D2 receptor blockade in hypothalamus, nigrostriatal, and mesolimbic causes symptoms of neuroleptic malignant syndrome and hypothalamus D2 receptor blockade is responsible for sympathetic mediated hypertension. In serotonin syndrome excess serotonin acts on midline raphe nuclei in brainstem which is one of the vasomotor centers in brainstem and contributes to paroxysmal hypertension.

Toxins

Scorpion envenomation causes morbidity and mortality by ANS overactivity. BP above 200 mm Hg systolic and acute pulmonary edema are well-known complications of scorpion envenomation.[9] Neurotoxins released by scorpion bite act on voltage-dependent sodium channel and keep sodium channel in open position leading to prolong, repetitive firings in somatic, sympathetic, and parasympathetic neurons both in central and periphery.

Diagnosis

In the above discussed conditions, diagnosis of secondary hypertension is made by understanding the pathophysiology of disease. But we need to exclude other factors that contribute hypertension before attributing hypertension due to CNS dysfunction. For example, pheochromocytoma can present with CNS symptoms, stroke, and high BP. If hypertension is attributed to stroke, pheochromocytoma may be missed. It should be suspected in any stroke patient presenting at young age whose BP is resistant to routine antihypertensives and alpha-blocker is needed to control hypertension. Plasma free metanephrine, catecholamines, 24 hours urinary catecholamines, and metanephrine are measured in patient with suspected pheochromocytoma, and they are elevated several times above reference value when it is present. Nuclear imaging using metaiodobenzylguanidine is done to locate the pheochromocytoma. Coarctation of aorta, renal artery stenosis, thyroid disorder, and Conn's adenoma are other causes of secondary hypertension that should be evaluated before attributing hypertension to CNS dysfunction. Echocardiogram, ultrasonogram abdomen, renal artery Doppler, thyroid function test, renal function test, arterial-blood gas test, urine routine, and plasma aldosterone renin ratio are done to rule out secondary causes.

Management

Treatment of secondary hypertension due to CNS dysfunction depends on the medical conditions in which it occurs. Antihypertensive drugs are used as rescue to control paroxysmal hypertension till underlying CNS disease is treated. Treatment of underlying CNS diseases is essential as it reverses the mechanism which causes paroxysmal hypertension.

Stroke

As already discussed high BP occurs following ischemic stroke but lowering of BP worsens cerebral ischemia. The American Heart Association guidelines recommend lowering of BP if BP is above 220/130 mm Hg in patient who is not a candidate for thrombolysis. BP should be lowered to 185/110 mm Hg for patient who is a candidate for thrombolysis and maintain below 180/105 mm Hg after thrombolysis.[10] Short-acting and rapidly reversal drugs are used to avoid hypotension. Most commonly used drugs are labetalol, nicardipine, and enalaprilat

> **Box 1: Antihypertensives in stroke**
>
> - Labetalol—10 mg over 2 min, repeat every 10–20 min until desired BP is achieved, maximum dosage per day is 300 mg
> - Nicardipine—5 mg/h infusion, increase 2.5 mg/h every 15 min until desired BP is achieved, maximum dose is 15 mg/h

> **Box 2: Scorpion envenomation antidote**
>
> - Antidote for scorpion envenomation is alpha-blocker prazosin that blocks toxin mediated sympathetic drive

(Box 1). Hypertension associated with hemorrhagic stroke can cause rebleed and worsening of neurological deficit. Guidelines recommend BP should be reduced to less than 180/90 mm Hg in hemorrhagic stroke and whether BP can be reduced to 140/90 mm Hg is still controversial.

Spinal Cord Disease and Scorpion Envenomation

Paroxysmal hypertension occurring in quadriplegic patients due to spinal cord disease is treated by combining beta-blockers with alpha-blockers (doxazosin, terazosin, or prazosin). Bladder distension should be avoided with proper catheter drainage. Transcutaneous electrical nerve stimulation can be used as an alternative therapy in some cases to control BP in spinal cord disease. Alpha blocker is an effective antidote for scorpion envenomation (Box 2).

Electroconvulsive Therapy and Epilepsy

Anesthetists use ganglionic blockade to manage severe hypertension during electroconvulsive therapy as it is more effective than labetalol plus nicardipine combination. Intravenous bolus of 15 mg trimethaphan camsylate is used as ganglionic blockade[11] to treat hypertension associated with electroconvulsive therapy. Paroxysmal hypertension associated with diencephalic epilepsy is best treated with noncompetitive alpha-blockers phenoxybenzamine, as it cannot be displaced by norepinephrine released from excessive sympathetic drive.

CONCLUSION

Severe hypertension is a recognized complication of CNS dysfunction and BP monitoring is essential in above discussed clinical situations. Appropriate drugs should be chosen based on clinical scenario and timely administration is needed to prevent organ damage. Other causes of hypertension should be evaluated whenever high BP is not responding to antihypertensives even after underlying CNS disease improves.

REFERENCES

1. Guyenet PG. The sympathetic control of blood pressure. Nat Rev Neurosci. 2006;7(5):335-46.
2. Hilton SM. Hypothalamic regulation of the cardiovascular system. Br Med Bull. 1966;22(3):243-8.
3. Cowley AW Jr, Liard JF, Guyton AC. Role of the baroreceptor reflex in daily control of arterial blood pressure and other variables in dogs. Circ Res. 1973;32(5):564-76.
4. Hachinski V. Hypertension in acute ischemic strokes. Arch Neurol. 1985;42(10):1002.
5. Reis DJ, Doba N. Hypertension as a localizing sign of mass lesions of brainstem. N Engl J Med. 1972;287(26):1355-6.
6. Emanuele MA, Dorsch TR, Scarff TB, et al. Basilar artery aneurysm simulating pheochromocytoma. Neurology. 1981;31(12):1560-1.
7. Streifer JY, Israel D, Melamed E. The hyperperfusion syndrome: an under-recognized complication of carotid endarterectomy. Isr Med Assoc J. 2004;6(1):54-6.
8. De Toma G, Nicolanti V, Plocco M, et al. Baroreflex failure syndrome after bilateral excision of carotid body tumors: an underestimated problem. J Vasc Surg. 2000;31(4):806-10.
9. Gueron M, Ilia R, Sofer S. The cardiovascular system after scorpion envenomation. A review. J Toxicol Clin Toxicol. 1992;30(2):245-58.
10. Jauch EC, Saver JL, Adams HP Jr, et al. Guidelines for the early management of patients with acute ischemic stroke: a guideline for healthcare professionals from the American Heart Association/American Stroke Association. Stroke. 2013;44(3):870-947.
11. Petrides G, Maneksha F, Zervas I, et al. Trimethaphan (Arfonad) control of hypertension and tachycardia during electroconvulsive therapy: a double-blind study. J Clin Anesth. 1996;8(2):104-9.

Sleep Apnea and Hypertension

Vasili Pradeep, Alladi Mohan

"Sleep that knits up the raveled sleave of care,
The death of each day's life, sore labor's bath,
Balm of hurt minds, great nature's second course,
Chief nourisher in life's feast."

William Shakespeare
Macbeth, Act 2 Scene 2

■ INTRODUCTION

Nearly one-third of a human's life is spent sleeping. Earlier sleep was considered to be a passive and homogeneous state. Presently, sleep is understood to consist of cyclic periods of complex and changing brain activity, behavior and physiology.[1-6] Sleep disturbances, particularly obstructive sleep apnea (OSA) is considered as the most common secondary cause of hypertension associated with resistant hypertension.[2] The relationship between OSA and hypertension has been a point of interest for decades, with untreated OSA being associated with an increased risk for developing new-onset hypertension.[6]

■ EPIDEMIOLOGY

Hypertension is a major public health problem globally including in India.[7] Prevalence of hypertension in India has been estimated to be 29.8% [95% confidence interval (CI) 26.7–33.0)]. It has been estimated that, nearly 33% urban and 25% rural subjects in India are hypertensive.[8] Published epidemiological data from India suggest that the prevalence of OSA and OSA syndrome (OSAS) in community-based studies ranged from 3.5% to 13.7% and 1.7% to 3.6%, respectively.[9-11]

■ SLEEP AND CIRCADIAN HEMODYNAMIC RHYTHMS

Blood pressure and heart rate undergo a series of changes during different stages of sleep and these changes are principally neurogenic in origin. In non-rapid eye movement (NREM) sleep, central sympathetic outflow decreases and cardiac vagal tone increases resulting in decreased heart rate and blood pressure, which manifests as dipping pattern of blood pressure.[12] During rapid eye movement (REM) sleep, a surge in sympathetic outflow results in increased heart rate and blood pressure.[13]

■ TERMINOLOGY OF SLEEP DISORDERED BREATHING

OSA is defined as occurrence of an average five or more episodes of obstructive respiratory events per hour of sleep with either sleep related symptoms or comorbidities or more than or equal to 15 such episodes without any sleep-related symptoms or comorbidities. OSAS is defined as OSA associated with daytime symptoms, most often excessive sleepiness.[3-5] Apnea is defined as cessation of inspiratory airflow for at least 10 seconds or more. It can be either central or obstructive depending upon the cause. Central sleep apnea is characterized by decreased or complete withdrawal of respiratory drive in pontomedullary junction to the muscles of respiration.[14] OSA occurs due to complete or partial collapse of pharynx during sleep. It can be further classified as mild (5–15), moderate (15–30) and severe (>30) based on apnea-hypopnea index (AHI), which is a measure of frequency of apneas and hypopneas detected during each hour of sleep using polysomnography.[15]

■ PATHOPHYSIOLOGIC LINK BETWEEN OSA AND HYPERTENSION

As described in the evidence-based Indian initiative on obstructive sleep apnea (INOSA) guidelines,[16] OSA is an independent risk factor for systemic hypertension. An increased prevalence of hypertension has been observed in patients with OSA. Increase in one additional apneic event per hour of sleep has been observed to enhance the odds of developing hypertension by about 1. Further, the odds of developing hypertension increases by 13% with 10% decline in nocturnal oxygen saturation. It has also been observed that OSA is an important but often undetected cause in patients with resistant hypertension.

Prevalence of OSA in patients with primary hypertension has been found to be more than 30% and moderate-to-severe OSA can be detected in two-thirds of the patients with drug-resistant hypertension.[17] Owing to multifactorial etiology of both OSA and hypertension, various interlinked factors are considered to play an important role in their pathophysiology.

Age and Obesity

Age and obesity are two important confounding variables in understanding the pathophysiological link between OSA and hypertension. It has been observed that patients with OSA have an increased risk of cardiovascular complications like atrial fibrillation and hypertension, which are more evident at a younger age. Treating the OSA patients with continuous positive airway pressure (CPAP) resulted in decreased incidence of atrial fibrillation.[18] While OSA patients are frequently found to be obese, OSA has also been documented in nonobese individuals.

Autonomic Nervous System Changes

Due to repetitive cycles of hypoxemia and hypercapnia secondary to episodic OSA, reflex sympathetic and parasympathetic activation occurs. These autonomic derangements results in increased catecholamine levels, which persist during daytime, ultimately contributing to hypertension. Effective CPAP therapy has been observed to result in decreased urinary catecholamine levels especially in patients with severe OSA.[19]

Inflammatory and Cytokine-mediated Effects

OSA promotes oxidative stress, which leads to systemic inflammation and cardiovascular morbidity. Patients with OSA are found to have elevated levels of several biomarkers of systemic inflammation. However, further data are required to establish whether these biomarkers indicate a worse prognosis and whether therapeutic interventions directed at these markers could alter the pathogenesis.[20]

Renin–angiotensin–aldosterone System

A significant correlation has been observed between plasma aldosterone concentration and OSA severity in patients with resistant hypertension indicating the involvement of renin–angiotensin–aldosterone system in the pathogenesis of this condition. Evidence also suggests that increased dietary salt intake leads to increased severity of resistant hypertension in patients with moderate to severe OSA.[21]

Nocturnal Fluid Redistribution

Disturbances in fluid volume regulation are involved in the pathogenesis of both hypertension and OSA. In patients with OSA, nocturnal fluid shift rostrally due to postural change leads to narrowing of already compromised upper airway diameter predisposing them to further increased episodes of OSA and consequently leading to nondipping pattern of nocturnal blood pressure.[21]

Sleep Insufficiency

OSA leads to impaired sleep quality. Sleep deprivation cause a sufficient increase in sympathetic activity, arterial stiffening and venous endothelial dysfunction, which further leads to hypertension and other cardiovascular complications.[22]

Organ System Involvement

Central Nervous System

As a result of chronic intermittent hypoxia, areas of brain that regulate sympathetic outflow are predominantly affected leading to hypertension in patients with OSA. *Delta-FosB* gene expression has been observed to be increased in median preoptic nucleus, organum vasculosum of the lamina terminalis, nucleus of the solitary tract, subfornical organ and rostral ventrolateral medulla due to chronic intermittent hypoxia. These suggest a direct effect of OSA in cerebral vasculature resulting in complications like hypertension and stroke.[23]

Respiratory System

Repeated episodes of hypoxemia and hypercapnia in patients with OSA lead to pulmonary vascular remodeling resulting in hypoxic pulmonary vasoconstriction. Over a period of time, pulmonary venous hypertension ensues. Both hypoxic pulmonary vasoconstriction and pulmonary venous hypertension along with abnormal production of inflammatory mediators results in vascular cell proliferation and aberrant vascular remodeling results in pulmonary arterial hypertension.[24]

Cardiovascular System

The mechanisms underlying cardiovascular complications in OSA include sympathetic activation, changes in intrathoracic pressure, sleep disturbances, oxidative stress and vascular inflammation from nocturnal hypoxia and reoxygenation cycles, among others.[25] Sympathetic activation is thought to be the most common mechanism leading to tachy-arrhythmias, especially atrial fibrillation, in patients with OSA. Other mechanisms, which account for cardiovascular complications in OSA include coagulation factors, endothelial damage, platelet activation and an increase in inflammatory mediators. As a consequence of these mechanisms, there will be increased blood pressure, pulmonary hypertension, arrhythmias and congestive heart failure.[26,27]

Endocrine System

In people with metabolic syndrome, which is a cluster of coexisting metabolic diseases namely hyperglycemia, hypertension, hyper-uricemia and obesity, presence of OSA is categorized in syndrome Z. It constitutes a collection of interrelated metabolic disorders that increases the chance of developing heart disease, stroke and diabetes mellitus. CPAP decreases postprandial dyslipidemia after 2 months of therapy. More complex mechanisms are involved in patients with diabetes mellitus and OSA with hypertension signifying multifactorial involvement of these metabolic disorders.[28]

Kidneys

Renal sympathetic denervation in patients with OSA and resistant hypertension has been found to be an effective therapy for reducing severity of resistant hypertension, glucose intolerance and OSA. However, further studies are needed in this regard before considering it as a therapy for patients with OSA and hypertension.[29]

◼ EFFECT OF OSA TREATMENT ON HYPERTENSION

Lifestyle modification and dietary practices such as weight reduction, moderate exercise, and decreasing dietary salt intake have been shown to reduce the incidence of resistant hypertension in patients with OSA.[21,30] Effective management of OSA results in decreased morbidity and mortality (Fig. 1). CPAP therapy in patients with OSA

has been found to reduce the occurrence of resistant hypertension and facilitates significant reduction in blood pressure in those with resistant hypertension. Further studies are needed in this regard before considering CPAP therapy as a preventive measure for hypertension in patients with OSA. Oral appliances are considered as a better alternative in patients with mild-to-moderate OSA, who cannot tolerate CPAP therapy. However, CPAP yielded better polysomnography outcomes than oral appliances, especially in reducing AHI.[31] Even though significant weight reduction occurs with bariatric surgery, there is no significant reduction in AHI in patients.[32]

◼ CONCLUSION

Available evidence suggests OSA as an important modifiable and preventable cause of hypertension. Timely diagnosis of OSA and institution of CPAP therapy with good compliance is considered to be potentially beneficial in patients with hypertension.

◼ REFERENCES

1. Konecny T, Kara T, Somers VK. Obstructive sleep apnea and hypertension: an update. Hypertension. 2014;63:203-9.
2. Pedrosa RP, Drager LF, Gonzaga CC, et al. Obstructive sleep apnea: the most common secondary cause of hypertension associated with resistant hypertension. Hypertension. 2011;58:811-7.
3. Iber C, Ancoli-Israel S, Chesson A, Quan SF; for the American Academy of Sleep Medicine. The AASM manual for the scoring of sleep and associated events—rules, terminology and technical specifications, 1st edition. Westchester: American Academy of Sleep Medicine; 2007.
4. Berry RB, Budhiraja R, Gottlieb DJ, et al; American Academy of Sleep Medicine. Rules for scoring respiratory events in sleep: update of the 2007 AASM Manual for the Scoring of Sleep and Associated Events. Deliberations of the Sleep Apnea Definitions Task Force of the American Academy of Sleep Medicine. J Clin Sleep Med. 2012;8:597-619.
5. Jafari B, Mohsenin V. Polysomnography. Clin Chest Med. 2010;31:287-97.
6. Marin JM, Agusti A, Villar I, et al. Association between treated and untreated obstructive sleep apnea and risk of hypertension. JAMA. 2012;307:2169-76.

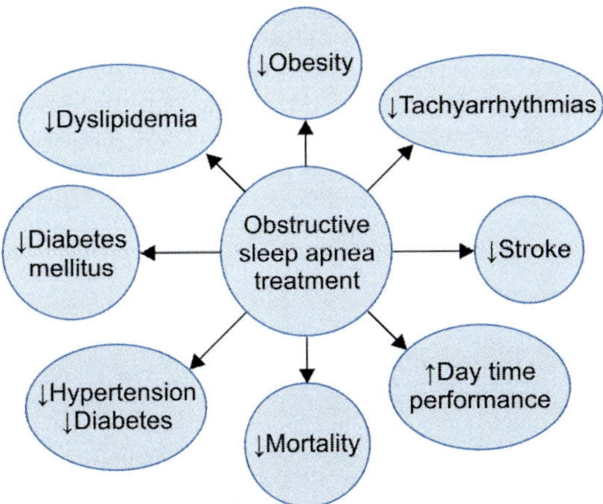

Fig. 1: Beneficial effects of treatment of obstructive sleep apnea.

7. Mackay J, Mensah G. Atlas of heart disease and stroke. Geneva: World Health Organization; 2004.

8. Anchala R, Kannuri NK, Pant H, et al. Hypertension in India: a systematic review and meta-analysis of prevalence, awareness, and control of hypertension. J Hypertens. 2014;32:1170-7.

9. Sharma SK, Ahluwalia G. Epidemiology of adult obstructive sleep apnea syndrome in India. Indian J Med Res. 2010;131:171-5.

10. Udwadia ZF, Doshi AV, Lonkar SG, et al. Prevalence of sleep disordered breathing and sleep apnea in middle-aged urban Indian men. Am Respir Crit Care Med. 2004;169: 168-73.

11. Sharma SK, Kumpawat S, Banga A, et al. Prevalence and risk factors of obstructive sleep apnea syndrome in a population of Delhi, India. Chest. 2006;130:149-56.

12. Floras JS. Hypertension and Sleep Apnea. Can J Cardiol. 2015;31:889-97.

13. Somers VK, Dyken ME, Mark AL, et al. Sympathetic-nerve activity during sleep in normal subjects. N Engl J Med. 1993;328:303-7.

14. Javaheri S, Dempsey JA. Central sleep apnea. Compr Physiol. 2013;3:141-63.

15. Fleetham J, Ayas N, Bradley D, et al. Canadian Thoracic Society guidelines: diagnosis and treatment of sleep disordered breathing in adults. Can Respir J. 2006;13:387-92.

16. Sharma SK, Katoch VM, Mohan A, et al; Indian Initiative on Obstructive Sleep Apnoea (INOSA) Guidelines Working Group. Consensus & evidence-based INOSA Guidelines 2014 (first edition). Indian J Med Res. 2014;140:451-68.

17. Franklin KA, Lindberg E. Obstructive sleep apnea is a common disorder in the population-a review on the epidemiology of sleep apnea. J Thorac Dis. 2015;7:1311-22.

18. Lavergne F, Morin L, Armitstead J, et al. Atrial fibrillation and sleep-disordered breathing. J Thorac Dis. 2015;7:575-84.

19. Pinto P, Bárbara C, Montserrat JM, et al. Effects of CPAP on nitrate and norepinephrine levels in severe and mild-moderate sleep apnea. BMC Pulm Med. 2013;13:13.

20. Testelmans D, Tamisier R, Barone-Rochette G, et al. Profile of circulating cytokines: impact of OSA, obesity and acute cardiovascular events. Cytokine. 2013;62:210-6.

21. Pimenta E, Stowasser M, Gordon RD, et al. Increased dietary sodium is related to severity of obstructive sleep apnea in patients with resistant hypertension and hyperaldosteronism. Chest. 2013;143:978-83.

22. Dettoni JL, Consolim-Colombo FM, Drager LF, et al. Cardiovascular effects of partial sleep deprivation in healthy volunteers. J Appl Physiol. 2012;113:232-6.

23. Knight WD, Little JT, Carreno FR, et al. Chronic intermittent hypoxia increases blood pressure and expression of FosB/DeltaFosB in central autonomic regions. Am J Physiol Regul Integr Comp Physiol. 2011;301:R131-9.

24. Kholdani C, Fares WH, Mohsenin V. Pulmonary hypertension in obstructive sleep a pnea: is it clinically significant? A critical analysis of the association and pathophysiology. Pulm Circ. 2015;5:220-7.

25. Javaheri S, Barbe F, Campos-Rodriguez F, et al. Sleep Apnea: Types, Mechanisms, and Clinical Cardiovascular Consequences. J Am Coll Cardiol. 2017;69:841-58.

26. Jean-Louis G, Zizi F, Clark LT, et al. Obstructive sleep apnea and cardiovascular disease: role of the metabolic syndrome and its components. J Clin Sleep Med. 2008;4:261-72.

27. Drager LF, McEvoy RD, Barbe F, et al. Sleep Apnea and Cardiovascular Disease: Lessons From Recent Trials and Need for Team Science. Circulation. 2017;136:1840-50.

28. Phillips CL, Yee BJ, Marshall NS, et al. Continuous positive airway pressure reduces postprandial lipidemia in obstructive sleep apnea: a randomized, placebo-controlled crossover trial. Am J Respir Crit Care Med. 2011;184(3):355-61.

29. Witkowski A, Prejbisz A, Florczak E, et al. Effects of renal sympathetic denervation on blood pressure, sleep apnea course, and glycemic control in patients with resistant hypertension and sleep apnea. Hypertension. 2011;58:559-65.

30. Furlan SF, Braz CV, Lorenzi-Filho G, et al. Management of Hypertension in Obstructive Sleep Apnea. Curr Cardiol Rep. 2015;17:108.

31. Li W, Xiao L, Hu J. The comparison of CPAP and oral appliances in treatment of patients with OSA: a systematic review and meta-analysis. Respir Care. 2013;58:1184-95.

32. Dixon JB, Schachter LM, O'Brien PE, et al. Surgical vs conventional therapy for weight loss treatment of obstructive sleep apnea: a randomized controlled trial. JAMA. 2012;308:1142-9.

Therapeutic Aspects: Pharmacologic and Nonpharmacologic Interventions

Nonpharmacological Interventions in Hypertension and their Impact

KK Pareek, Saket Goyal

"The doctor of the future will give no medicine, but will interest his patients in the care of the human frame, in diet, and in the cause and prevention of disease"
—**Thomas Edison**

INTRODUCTION

The nonpharmacological management for treatment of hypertension (HTN) provides an excellent opportunity to the physician to coax his patients toward an ideal lifestyle which would have far reaching effects on his fitness, morbidity and mortality. These very simple guidelines have a positive effect on HTN but also on diabetes, coronary artery disease (CAD) and stroke. The ancillary benefits may be reduction in osteoarthritis, depression, Alzheimer's and even some type of cancers. It is interesting to note that each tenet of lifestyle change would work as much as a pharma drug of course without the side effects. The interventions are weight loss, exercise, low salt diet, tobacco cessation and stress reduction. This kind of lifestyle training will decrease the number of patients needing medicine, decrease the number of medication, and also decrease the incidence of end-organ damage. A successful nonpharmacological program would require just some time and commitment from the physician and patient (Box 1).

Box 1: Benefits of nonpharmacological treatment of hypertension.

- Reduces blood pressure in patients with or without hypertension
- May reduce the need for drug treatment
- Complement the action of antihypertensive drugs
- Occasionally allow the antihypertensive drugs to be stopped
- Have multiple additional benefits on risk reduction for diabetes mellitus, coronary artery disease, strokes and possible some cancers
- The effectiveness of each intervention may be as much as a single hypertension drug combination produces even better results

---

THE LOGIC BEHIND NONPHARMACOLOGICAL TREATMENT

For any medical treatment to be effective and universally applicable it should have three basic qualities—simple, accessible and affordable.[1]

1. Simple, so that the physician and the patient alike do not fear in learning and practicing it
2. Accessible, so that it can be implemented across the geographical spectrum to benefit the maximum number of people
3. Affordable, to be acceptable across the social spectrum and the cost does not become a limiting factor in continuance.

No other intervention in medicine can fulfill these tenets more aptly than lifestyle modification as a nonpharmacological treatment of disease. The principles are very simple principles of daily living, universally accessible requiring just commitment, and free of cost. The cost-benefit analysis of such an intervention would of course make us wonder at the over dependence on medicines.

An important aspect of nonpharmacological treatment of HTN is that the benefits go much beyond control of BP4. This positive change in lifestyle this is expected to bring down the incidence of diabetes, heart disease, stroke and even some types of cancer. In addition the fitness achieved in the process of lifestyle change leads to better mental and physical adjustment with the surroundings. Diet, exercise and weight loss have been shown to bring down morbidity and mortality across all spectrums of age, sex and social strata.[2] Another important difference between the drug treatment and nonpharmacological management of HTN is that the latter strategy is totally devoid of side effects. Whatever effects it has on the brain and the body are positive. In contrast to the drug therapy, as the patient gets into the habit of lifestyle change, there is less chance of withdrawal. This is in stark contrast with the medical therapy, whereas the duration of therapy increases, the patient compliance becomes poor. Most patients with established HTN would however need a combination of pharma and nonpharma management.[3] Herein, the important role of lifestyle change would be that these changes would augment the action of drugs. The possible mechanism of the synergistic action is by increasing the vasoreactivity, decreasing the salt load and decreasing the central sympathetic outflow.

TECHNIQUES FOR NON-PHARMACOLOGICAL TREATMENT OF HYPERTENSION, AND THE STRATEGIES TO FOLLOW (FIG. 1)

Lifestyle plays an important role in treating your high blood pressure (BP). With a healthy lifestyle, you might avoid, delay or reduce the need for medication (Table 1).[4]

Maintain an Ideal Weight

Obesity is a major contributor to HTN. Too much weight can result in sleep apnea which leads to resistant BP and its complications.

TABLE 1: Principles of nonpharmacological and pharmacological treatment of hypertension.

	Nonpharmacological management	Pharmacological management
Principles	Simple—anybody can understand	Complicated—needs medical expertise
Accessibility	Universally available	Varies with usage and patent patterns
Affordability	Affordable	New molecules—steep prices
Side effects	No side effects	Side effects common cause of withdrawal
Compliance	Compliance increases with time	Compliance decreases with time
Ancillary benefits	Holistic—across all organ systems	Almost none

Weight loss is the most effective strategy for controlling BP. Every small amount of weight helps reduce your BP. Each kilogram (about 2.2 pounds) of weight loss reduces your BP by about 1 mm Hg. In subjects with sustained weight loss, there is a fall in plasma insulin, plasma renin, cardiac output and BP. Just a 2 kg weight loss can decrease BP 5/3 mm Hg with a 42% decline in the frequency of BP.[5]

An ideal waist–hip ratio is also important. For men 0.9 and for women 0.8 would be an ideal ratio.

An ideal weight for your age and height is a reflection of your health. Maintain a body mass index of 22–25 kg/m^2.

- Know your weight and calorie goals. 8,000 calories = 1 kg weight is the simple equation. Aim is to create a calorie deficit
- For weight loss, an electronic weighing scale is essential with daily weight monitoring
- Each food comes with a calorie tag—learn to tag your food. Know your calories— research some food charts. Be a smart shopper. Read food labels when you shop and stick to your healthy-eating plan when you are dining out, too.

Physical Activity and Fitness

Regular physical activity can lower your BP by about 5–8 mm Hg. Regular exercise not only prevents the onset of HTN but also helps to better control it after the onset. Exercise increases the shear street on the vascular endothelium, resulting in release of vasodilator nitric oxide (NO).[6] The effect is more pronounced in young and the postexercise fall in BP may be sustained for 22 hours. Exercise training leads to a reduction in plasma renin and noradrenaline by 20% and 29%, respectively. The net result may be a decrease in BP by 8/6 mm Hg.

Continuity and persistence in exercise is the cornerstone for fitness. Exercise should be at least 30 minutes on almost everyday of the week.

- Keep walking. Introduce small minutes of walking throughout your daily routine. Count your activity/steps. This can be with a pedometer or a phone app. About 10,000 steps/day is the minimum goal. Aerobic activity like jogging and swimming can be added
- Aim to decrease your sitting time to 10% of your work-time. By decreasing your sitting by 50% you can decrease 50% disease. A standing desk is a good solution for desk jobs
- Keep changing your exercises to surprise your body. Push in some yoga. Play a sport; it gives you good balance and overall toning
- Core exercises like planks are essential for sustained results. Add some body weight exercises. To preserve the muscle mass and increase your BMR, add some strength exercises like push-ups and weight training (Table 2).

Eat a Healthy Diet

The Dietary Approaches to Stop Hypertension (DASH) diet—diet that is rich in whole grains,

TABLE 2: Recommendations to reduce blood pressure and cardiovascular risk factors.

Salt intake	Restrict to <5–6 g/day
Alcohol intake	Limit to <20–30 g/day (men); <10–20 g/day (women)
DASH diet	Increased vegetable, fruit, nuts; low dairy intake
BMI goal	<25 kg/m^2
Weight goal	Waist:Hip <0.9 (men); <0.8 (women)
Exercise goal	>30 min/day 5–7 days/week (moderate/dynamic exercise)
Tobacco	Quit tobacco and smoking

(BMI: body mass index; DASH: Dietary Approaches to Stop Hypertension)

fruits, vegetables and low-fat dairy products. The DASH diet has a market natriuretic effect and may cause a sustained BP fall of 12/6 mm Hg in hypertensives.[7]

It is not easy to change your eating habits, but with these tips, you can adopt a healthy diet:

- A good diet is the cornerstone to physical fitness. You cannot out-exercise a bad diet
- Sugar is the new tobacco—not only as a source of disease but also as an addiction. It is an addiction because of dopamine release and responsible for fat deposition due to insulin release. A zero-sugar diet is a basic tenant for your fitness goals
- Decrease the use of gluten (wheat). We use wheat 3–4 times in a day (aata, maida, sooji, daliya, noodles, bread, etc.). Gluten in the wheat promotes hyperglycemia and deposition of fat in internal organs. Start using alternates like maize, millet, corn, chana, etc. You can add salads and buttermilk to decrease the wheat in diet
- Take good amount of protein. This will prevent loss of muscle mass as you loose weight. The good vegetarian sources of protein are sprouted grains, pulses or rajma, paneer, tofu, dry-fruits (almond or walnut) and peanuts. In nonvegetarian, fish and eggs are a better source
- A potassium-rich diet can lessen the effects of sodium on BP. Fruits and vegetables, rather than supplements.

Reduce Sodium in your Diet

- High BP can be reduced by 5–6 mm Hg by small reduction in the salt intake[8]
- The prescribed limit of sodium intake is 2,300 mg/day. An ideal intake of sodium would be less than 1,500 mg/day
- To decrease sodium in your diet, consider these tips:
  - Read food labels. Processed food will contain added sodium and sodium preservatives. Check the food labels for low salt options
  - Don't add salt. Replace salt with herbs or spices to add flavor
  - Ease into it. The taste of salt is a learned taste. You can cut back slowly to allow your palate to adjust.

Limit the Amount of Alcohol You Drink

Recommendation of alcohol has been controversial due to its claimed effects on lipid profile. The present American College of Cardiology (ACC) recommendation suggests that whatever positive effect that alcohol may have on lipids is offset by its negative effect on BP. Cutting down on alcohol intake can decrease the BP by 4–5 mm Hg.[9] The upper limit is one drink/day for females and 2 drinks/day for males. One drink equals 12 ounces of beer, five ounces of wine or 1.5 ounces of 80-proof liquor.

Drinking more than recommended amounts of alcohol can raise BP by several points. It can also blunt the action of medications. Alcohol intake is thus an important factor to look for in resistant HTN.

Quit Smoking

Nicotine use has an acute and chronic effect on blood pressure. Each cigarette would raise the BP for minutes to hours. On chronic use it would contribute to atherosclerosis leading not only to HTN but also CAD and stroke. Quitting nicotine is an essential part of any health program.

Stress Reduction

Acute and chronic stress contributes to high BP.

- Say no to your stress triggers and avoid them. It can be a person, a situation, a place
- Try to talk things out. Do not sleep over a problem or argument
- Take time out for sports, hobbies and things you enjoy. Practice deep breathing

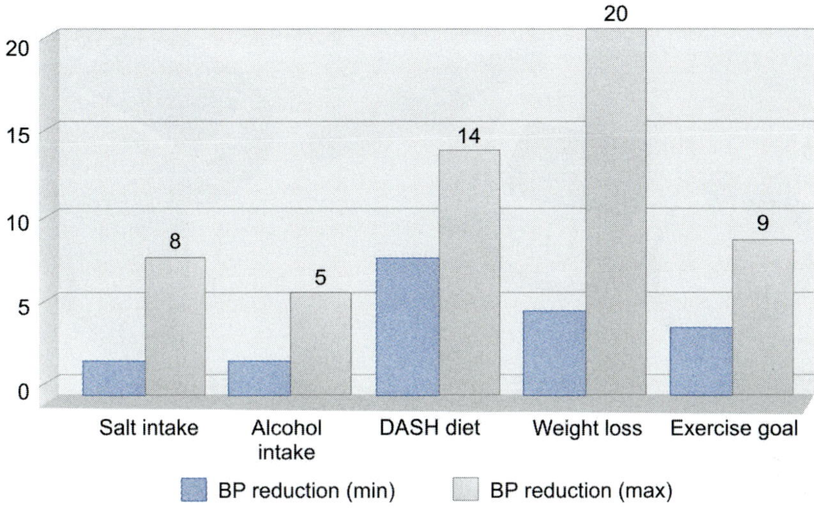

(BP: blood pressure; DASH: Dietary Approaches to Stop Hypertension)

Fig. 1: Effectiveness of nonpharmacological interventions on blood pressure.

- Practice gratitude. Expressing gratitude to others can help reduce your stress
- Change your expectations. Set your priorities and do not pursue things beyond your control
- Yoga, meditation and music decrease the sympathetic nervous activity and thus decrease the resting BP values.[4] The technique requires discipline and training for at least two 15-minutes sessions daily.

Home Blood Pressure Monitoring and Social Support

Home monitoring of BP helps to adhere to lifestyle and treatment plans and also rules out many cases of pseudohypertension. Family and support groups are important for diet plans, motivation and exercise adherence.

■ NONDRUG DEVICE INTERVENTIONS FOR HYPERTENSION

The RESPeRATE is a portable electronic device that promotes slow and deep breathing. RESPeRATE is approved by the Food and Drug Administration for reducing stress and lowering BP. It is available without a prescription. RESPeRATE paced breathing causes a decrease in systolic BP (SBP) 5–15 mm Hg.[10]

RESPeRATE uses chest sensors to measure your breathing, and then a computerized unit creates a melody for you to use to synchronize your breathing. The melody is supposed to help you slow your breathing with long exhalations.

The RESPeRATE is generally intended to be used at least 15 minutes a day, 3–4 days a week. Within a few weeks, the deep-breathing exercises can help lower both systolic and diastolic BP. You may need to keep doing the breathing exercises to maintain the BP lowering benefits (Fig. 2A).[11]

Zona Plus is a small computerized handheld device that is designed to help you lower your BP by guiding you through sets of handgrip exercises. This type of exercise (often called *isometric handgrip exercise)* has been found to be very effective at lowering BP.[12]

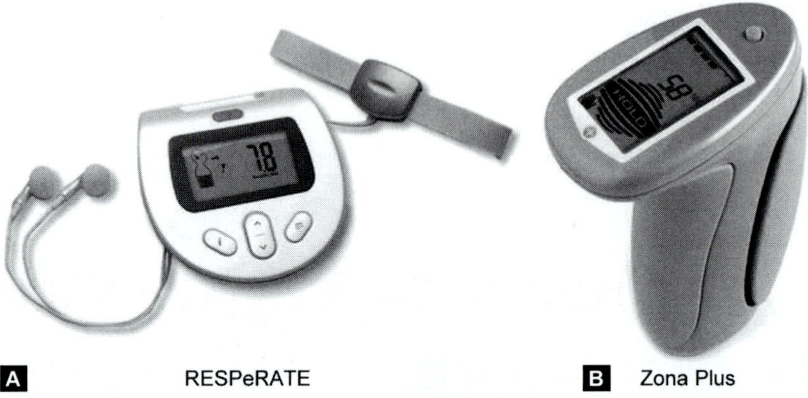

Figs. 2A and B: Devices to measure hypertension.

Studies show doing these exercises using the Zona Plus can reduce SBP by 6–8 mm Hg, and the makers of Zona Plus say that 9 out of 10 users have lower BP after 6–8 weeks using it. The device is to be used 12 minutes a day, 5 times a week.[13]

■ CONCLUSION

Nonpharmacological treatment of HTN is a strategy with positive ramifications on health which go beyond BP alone. These are simple and cost-effective strategies which each physician should try to install in his patient. This is important to bring down the socioeconomic burden of the disease. Nonpharmacological treatment may delay the use of drugs and have a synergistic effect when drug treatment is used for HTN.

"The greatest medicine of all is to teach people how not to need it."

■ REFERENCES

1. Achieving universal access to quality health services. [online] Available from: www.who.int/healthsystems/topics/health-law/chapter7.pdf [Last Accessed January, 2019].
2. van Dam RM, Li T, Spiegelman D, et al. Combined impact of lifestyle factors on mortality: prospective cohort study in US women. BMJ. 2008;337:a1440.
3. Whitworth JA. 2003 World Health Organization (WHO)/International Society of Hypertension (ISH) statement on management of hypertension. J Hypertens. 2003;21(11):1983-92.
4. Silverberg DS. Non-pharmacological treatment of hypertension. J Hypertens Suppl. 1990;8(4):S21-6.
5. Weinster RL, James LD, Darnell BE, et al. Obesity-related Hypertension: evaluation of separate effects of energy restriction and weight reduction on hemodynamic and neuroendocrine status. Am J Med. 1991;90(4):460-8.
6. Niebauer J, Cooke JP. Cardiovascular effects of exercise: role of endothelial shear stress.J Am Coll Cardiol. 1996;28(7):1652-60.
7. Appel LJ, Moore TJ, Obarzanek E, et al. A clinical trial of the effects of dietary patterns on blood pressure. DASH Collaborative Research Group. N Engl J Med. 1997;336(16):1117-24.
8. Moreira LB, Fuchs FD, Moraes RS, et al. Alcohol intake and blood pressure: the importance of time elapsed since the last drink. J Hypertens. 1998;16(2):175-80.
9. He FJ, Marciniak M, Visagie E, et al. Effect of modest salt reduction on blood pressure, urinary albumin, and pulse wave velocity in white, black, and Asian mild hypertensives. Hypertension. 2009;54(3):482-8.
10. Krum H, Schlaich M, Sobotka P, et al. Novel procedure- and device-based strategies in the management of systemic hypertension. Eur Heart J. 2011;32(5):537-44.
11. Mahtani KR, Nunan D, Heneghan CJ. Device-guided breathing exercises in the control of human blood pressure: systematic review and meta-analysis. J Hypertens. 2012;30(5):852-60.
12. Cruikshank J. Essential Hypertension. USA: People's Medical Publishing House; 2013. pp. 147-66.
13. Jackson EA. (2014). Assessing Alternative Approaches for Blood Pressure Control: A3BC Trial. NIH/NLM. USFDA Resources. University of Michigan. [online] Available from: https://clinicaltrials.gov/ct2/show/NCT02110381 [Last Accessed January, 2019].

Role of Yoga in Hypertension

SC Manchanda, Kushal Madan

INTRODUCTION

Hypertension is a major public health problem globally and is the single most important factor for high rate of cardiovascular mortality and morbidity.[1] In spite of several advances in the drug therapy, the prevention and management of hypertension has remained a major concern. The blood pressure is not properly controlled in majority of hypertensive patients especially in the developing countries.[2] Therefore, there is a need for an alternative simple cost-effective non-pharmacological technique. Yoga, an ancient Indian mind-body technique, may be such an alternative. Moreover, yoga may be especially useful to control stress which may be an important risk factor for development of hypertension. A recent review suggests that psychosocial stress and negative effective states are significant risk factors for hypertension.[3] Several psychosocial factors like job-related stress, job quality, job insecurity, wages, anger, depression, anxiety, aggression, personality, housing instability, social support and sleep quality have been shown to contribute to the development of hypertension. The exact mechanism of how stress causes hypertension is not clear but has been hypothesized that a complex inter-action of neurohormonal imbalance during stress may be a significant contributory factor (Flowchart 1).

WHAT IS YOGA?

Yoga is not a few postures (asanas) but a complete way of life. Yoga envisages health in totality on the principle of a healthy mind in a healthy body. There are several types of yoga but the commonly practiced is hatha yoga which includes stretching and physical postures (asanas), breathing exercises (pranayamas), and concentration techniques (meditation) designed to promote physical, mental, social and spiritual well being. Yoga also encourages a healthy lifestyle including healthy diet, and abstinence from tobacco and alcohol which are of proven benefit in management of hypertension.

PSYCHOPHYSIOLOGICAL RATIONALE FOR USE OF YOGA IN HYPERTENSION

Though the exact mechanisms underlying the apparent beneficial effects of yoga on hypertension are not well understood, mechanistic pathways are likely complex and interacting (Flowchart 2).[4] Yoga may impact hypertension

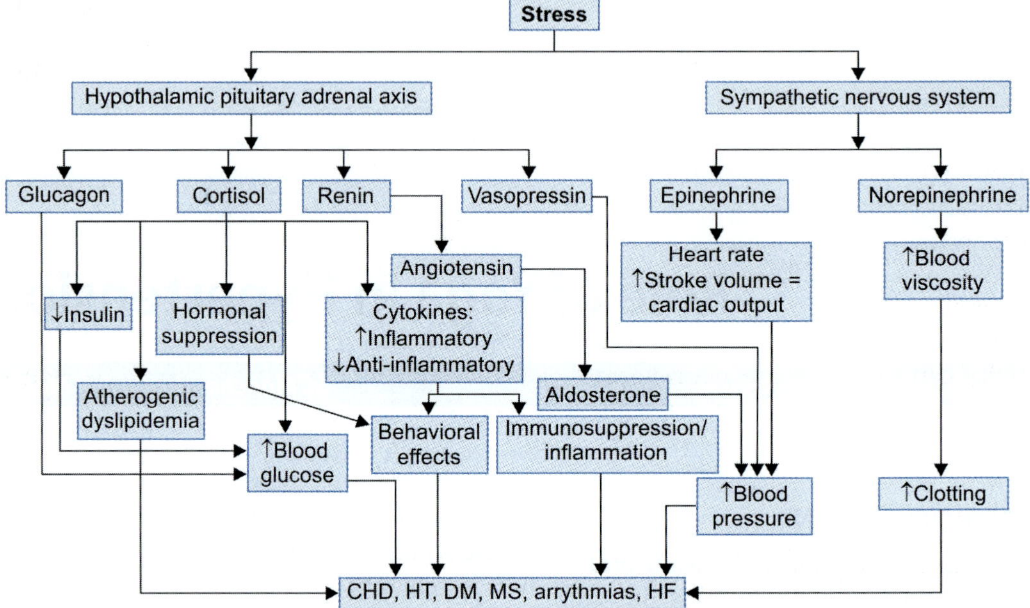

(CVD: cardiovascular disease; CHD: coronary heart disease; HT: hypertension; DM: diabetes mellitus; MS: metabolic syndrome; HF: heart failure).

Flowchart 1: Possible mechanisms of stress leading to cardiovascular disease.

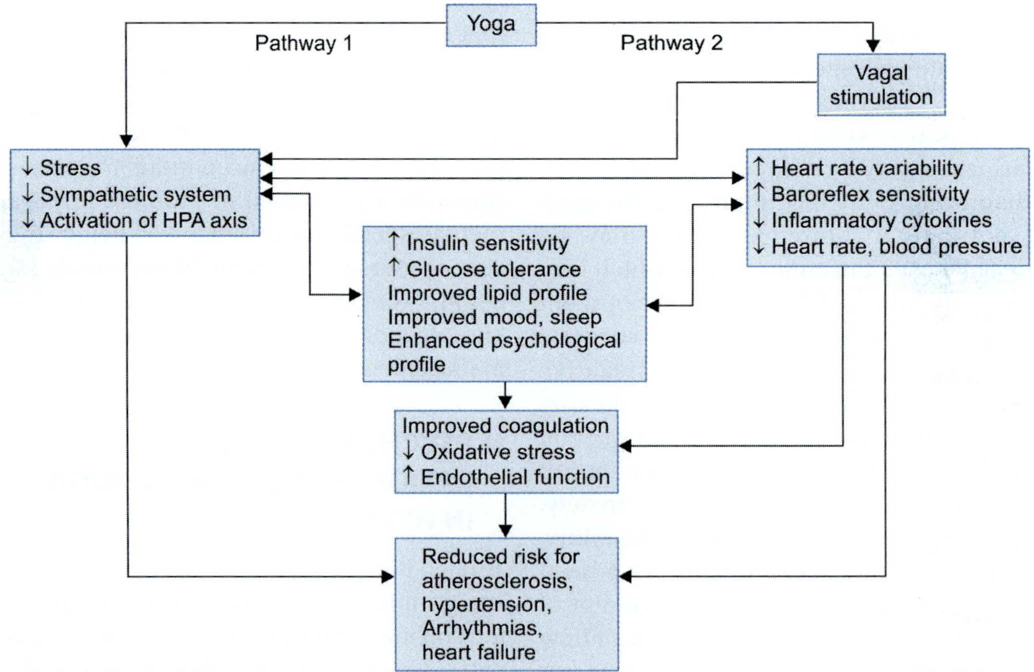

Flowchart 2: Psychophysiology of yoga in heart disease—possible mechanisms.

by lessening the negative impact of stress and improving several positive downstream effects on neuroendocrine status, metabolic and inflammatory responses. Yoga also has been shown to enhance well-being and reduce activation of hypothalamic pituitary adrenal axis and sympathovagal balance. Second mechanism may be that yoga practices shift the autonomic nervous system balance from sympathetic to parasympathetic possibly via vagal stimulation. Increased parasympathetic activity can also improve neurohormonal, hemodynamic, and inflammatory profiles like reduction in heart and respiratory rate, cortisol and catecholamine concentration, renin activity, skin conductance as well as increase in heart rate variability and improved baroreceptor activity.[5]

REVIEW OF PUBLISHED LITERATURE ON YOGA AND HYPERTENSION

Yoga has been shown to mitigate chronic fatigue, enhance endurance, improve organ and immune functions.[6] Yoga has also been demonstrated to be beneficial in several lifestyle-related chronic conditions like cardiovascular disease (CVD), diabetes, low back pain, asthma, depression, stress, anxiety, hypertension, etc. Large numbers of controlled, uncontrolled studies and meta-analysis regarding the role of yoga in hypertension have been reported and are reviewed in this article.

In 1969, Dateyet al. from India reported a significant reduction in blood pressure by Shavasana (a type of yogic activity for relaxation by autosuggestion).[7] Benson et al. from United States showed a significant decrease in systolic and diastolic blood pressure after practice of Transcendental Meditation (TM) 30 minutes twice a day.[8] However, these earlier studies were nonrandomized. Subsequently, several randomized controlled studies have been published (Table 1).[9-40] While majority have shown a modest but significant decrease in both systolic and diastolic blood pressure in patients with mild hypertension or prehypertension, a few have not reported any significant effect (Table 1). Some studies have employed ambulatory blood pressure and shown significant decreases in 24-hour mean

TABLE 1: Randomized control trials of yoga and hypertension.

Author and year	Number of subjects enrolled	Intervention	Duration	Results
Ponte et al. (2018)	42	Mindfulness meditation	20 weeks	Significant fall in ambulatory SBP and DBP
Thiyagarajan et al. (2015)	192	Yoga	12 weeks	Significant decrease in SBP, nonsignificant for DBP
Mashyal P et al. (2014)	32	Yoga and Laghu shankha prakshalana kriya	1 week	Reduction in BP, anxiety and fatigue. Increase in comfort and quality of sleep
Talbanos et al. (2014)	10	Integrative yoga program	3 months	Reduction in systolic and diastolic BP, anxiety and stress
Patil SG et al. (2014)	57	Yoga	3 months	Reduced BP and oxidative stress (malondialdehyde level) and increase in antioxidants (SOD, glutathione, vitamin C)

Continued

Continued

Author and year	Number of subjects enrolled	Intervention	Duration	Results
Hagins et al. (2014)	84	Yoga	–	Significant and modest reduction in 24 hours DBP and MBP as measured by ABPM
Blom et al. (2014)	101	MBSR	12 weeks	No effect on ambulatory BP
Wolff et al. (2013)	83	Yoga	12 weeks	Significant decrease in DBP with yoga at home
Pal et al. (2013)	258	Yoga	68 weeks	Significant decrease in SBP and DBP
Adhana et al. (2013)	30	Yogic breathing	3 months	Significant fall in SBP and DBP
Mizuno et al. (2013)	33	Yoga	–	Significant fall in SBP and DBP
Hughes et al. (2013)	56	MBSR	8 weeks	Significant fall in SBP and DBP
Dhameja et al. (2013)	60	Yoga	42 days	Significant fall in blood pressure and oxidative stress
Bhavanani et al. (2012)	29	Pranava pranayama	5 min	Significant fall in SBP and heart rate
Bhavanani et al. (2012)	22	Chandra nadi pranayama	5 min	Significant fall in SBP and heart rate
Chung et al. (2012)	129	Sahaja yoga	–	Significant fall in blood pressure and anxiety
Palta and Page et al. (2012)	20	MBSR	8 weeks	Significant fall in SBP and DBP
Agte et al. (2011)	52	Sudarshan kriya	2 months	Significant fall in DBP and oxidative stress and lipids
Subramanian et al. (2011)	94	Yoga + exercise +diet	8 weeks	Significant fall in blood pressure (with yoga, exercise and reduced salt intake)
Murthy et al. (2011)	104	Yoga + naturopathy	21 days	Significant fall in SBP, DBP, body weight and lipids
Cohen et al. (2011)	57	Iyengar Yoga	12 weeks	Significant fall in ambulatory SBP and DBP
Cade et al. (2010)	60 HIV infected	Yoga	20 weeks	Significant fall in SBP and DBP
Saptharishi et al. (2009)	113	Hatha Yoga	8 weeks	No significant decrease for systolic and diastolic blood pressure
Lee et al. (2009)	17	MBSR	8 weeks	Significant fall in SBP and DBP
Schneider et al. (2005)	98	Transcendental meditation	52 weeks	Significant fall in SBP and DBP
McCaffrey et al (2005)	53	Yoga	8 weeks	Significant decrease in SBP and DBP

Continued

Continued

Author and year	Number of subjects enrolled	Intervention	Duration	Results
Castillo-Richmond et al. (2000)	60	TM	12 weeks	Significant fall in SBP and DBP
Murugesan et al. (2000)	22	Yoga	11 weeks	Decrease of blood pressure equivalent to antihypertensive drug
Schneider et al. (1995)	74	TM	12 weeks	Decrease in SBP and DBP
Van Montfrans et al. (1990)	35	Relaxation	52 weeks	No change for SBP or DBP
Alexander et al. (1989)	31	TM	12 weeks	Decrease in SBP and DBP
Patel et al. (1975)	34	Yoga and biofeedback	52 weeks	Significant decrease in SBP and DBP

(BP: blood pressure; DBP: diastolic blood pressure; MDA: malondialdehyde; SBP: systolic blood pressure; SOD: superoxide dismutase)

arterial and diastolic pressure as compared to controls.[14] The effects are consistent with different types of yoga practices but the follow-up has been variable from few minutes to 68 weeks. Some randomized control trial have demonstrated that yoga is capable of producing long-term (52–68 weeks) beneficial effects in the treatment of hypertension.[17,33,40]

Meta-analysis and Systematic Reviews

As most of the studies regarding the efficacy of yoga in hypertension are small in number and have variable follow-up, a number of meta-analyses have been reported (Table 2).[41-48] One of the earlier meta-analysis which studied the effect of TM included nine randomized control trials and showed a modest but significant reduction in systolic blood pressure by 4.7 mm Hg and diastolic blood pressure by 3.2 mm Hg.[48] Okonta et al. (2012), in 10 randomized[47] and Hagins et al. in 17 studies[46] also observed a modest decrease, of systolic and diastolic blood pressure. Though different types of yogic practices showed a decrease but studies incorporating hatha yoga which included three basic components of yoga (asanas, pranayamas and meditation) showed a greater decrease in blood pressure. However, Wang et al. after analysis of six studies stated that there is no definite efficacy of yoga in hypertension because of low methodological quality.[45] Similarly, Tyagi[44] and Posadzki,[42] also reported that although majority of trials showed a decrease in blood pressure, a few did not show any effect. A recent systemic review and meta-analysis of blood pressure response to meditation and yoga in 13 randomized controlled studies showed that meditation and yoga appear to decrease both systolic and diastolic blood pressure.[41] Meditation appears to play a noticeable role in decreasing the blood pressure of subjects older than 60 years of age whereas yoga seems to contribute to the decrease of blood pressure in subjects less than 60 years of age.[41]

TABLE 2: Meta analysis and systemic review of yoga and hypertension.

Author and year	Type of study	Number of subjects enrolled	Intervention	Duration	Results
Park et al. (2017)	Review of 13 RCT	753	Meditation/yoga	8–12 weeks	Significant fall in SBP and DBP
Posadzki et al. (2014)	Review of 17 RCT		Yoga	Variable	11 RCT—reduction in SBP 8 RCT—reduction in DBP 5 RCT—no effect on SBP 8 RCT—no effect on DBP
Cramer et al. (2014)	Review and meta analysis of 7 RCT	452	Yoga	Variable	Low-quality evidence that yoga may be an adjunct in management of HTN
Tyagi et al. (2014)	Review of 39 cohort, 30 Non RCT, 48 RCT, 3 case report	6,693	Yoga	1 week–4 years	BP reduced in both normotensive and hypertensive subjects
Wang et al. (2013)	Review of 6 RCT	386	Yoga	Variable	Lower DBP and SBP
Hagins et al. (2013)	Review of 17 studies	–	Yoga	Variable	Significant fall in SBP and DBP
Okonta et al. (2012)	Review of 10 trials	–	Yoga	Variable	Significant fall in BP and glucose
Anderson et al. (2008)	Review of 9 RCT	–	TM	12–52 weeks	Significant fall in SBP and DBP

(SBP: systolic blood pressure; DBP: diastolic blood pressure; HTN: hypertension; RCT: randomized controlled trial; BP: blood pressure)

Thus, the majority of the randomized controlled studies demonstrate that yoga or meditation can reduce blood pressure significantly. Although the decrease in blood pressure in systolic and diastolic blood pressure is modest, this change may have a significant effect on reduction of strokes and coronary heart disease because it has been estimated that reducing systolic blood pressure by 3 mm Hg in general population has the potential to reduce stroke mortality by 8% and coronary heart disease by 5%.[49] Even the scientific committee of American Heart Association after reviewing the literature extensively concluded in 2013 that meditation decreased the blood pressure modestly.[50] They have suggested that it is reasonable for all individuals with blood pressure levels more than 120/80 mm Hg to consider meditation as an adjunct method to lower blood pressure when clinically appropriate (class IIb, LOE B). The safety and efficacy of yoga in managing hypertension has also been reported recently.[51] However, there are several limitations of the reported studies like small sample size, short follow-up and different methodologies of yoga. Hence, large multicenter well-controlled trials with uniform methodology and long follow-up are needed.

OTHER BENEFITS OF YOGA

Yoga has been shown to have several other benefits on risk factors which commonly accompany hypertension like diabetes mellitus, obesity, smoking, dyslipidemia, psychosocial stress, and inflammation.[52] A study has shown decrease of left ventricular hypertrophy by TM.[53] Few randomized studies have also shown a regression of early and advanced atherosclerosis.[54-56] In one secondary prevention study meditation has been shown to reduce risk for myocardial infarction, stroke, and mortality by 48%.[57] Arrhythmias and heart failure may also be improved with yoga meditation.[58,59]

CONCLUSION

Hypertension is a highly prevalent disorder and is a major risk factor for stroke, myocardial infarction and heart failure. In spite of phenomenal advances in the drug therapy, the control of hypertension is extremely low. Yoga, a simple, cost-effective, mind-body holistic technique, may be an alternative because yoga can improve the neurohumoral profile and relieves stress which may contribute to hypertension. Several randomized controlled trials demonstrate that yoga is a safe and effective technique in decreasing the blood pressure modestly in majority of subjects. In addition, yoga may reduce left ventricular hypertrophy and reduce risk factor for CVD. Hence, yoga, being a simple, cost-effective and safe technique, should be used either alone or as a complimentary technique in mildly elevated blood pressure or prehypertension. However, more large scale multicenter trials and larger number of patients utilizing the common protocol and long-term follow-up are needed.

REFERENCES

1. Lim SS, Vos T, Flaxman AD, et al. A comparative risk assessment of burden of disease and injury attributable to 67 risk factors and risk factor clusters in 21 regions, 1990-2010: a systematic analysis for the Global Burden of Disease Study 2010. Lancet. 2012;380(9859):2224-60.
2. Chow CK, Teo KK, Rangarajan S, et al. Prevalence, awareness, treatment, and control of hypertension in rural and urban communities in high-, middle-, and low-income countries. JAMA. 2013;310(9):959-68.
3. Cuffee Y, Ogedegbe C, Williams NJ, et al. Psychosocial risk factors for hypertension: an update of the literature. Curr Hypertens Rep. 2014;16(10):483.
4. Innes KE, Bourguignon C, Taylor AG. Risk indices associated with the insulin resistance syndrome, cardiovascular disease, and possible protection with yoga: a systematic review. J Am Board Fam Pract. 2005;18(6):491-519.
5. Selvamurthy W, Sridharan K, Ray US, et al. A new physiological approach to control essential hypertension. Indian J Physiol Pharmacol. 1998;42(2):205-13.
6. Raub JA. Psychophysiologic effects of Hatha Yoga on musculoskeletal and cardiopulmonary function: a literature review. J Altern Complement Med. 2002;8(6):797-812.
7. Datey KK, Deshmukh SN, Dalvi CP, et al. "Shavasan": A yogic exercise in the management of hypertension. Angiology. 1969 20(6):325-33.
8. Benson H, Rosner BA, Marzetta BR, et al. Decreased blood-pressure in pharmacologically treated hypertensive patients who regularly elicited the relaxation response. Lancet. 1974;1(7852):289-91.
9. Ponte Márquez PH, Feliu-Soler A, Solé-Villa MJ, et al. Benefits of mindfulness meditation in reducing blood pressure and stress in patients with arterial hypertension. J Hum Hypertens. 2018. [Epub ahead of print].
10. Thiyagarajan R, Pal P, Pal GK, et al. Additional benefit of yoga to standard lifestyle modification on blood pressure in prehypertensive subjects: a randomized controlled study. Hypertens Res. 2015;38(1):48-55.
11. Mashyal P, Bhargav H, Raghuram N. Safety and usefulness of Laghu shankha prakshalana in patients with essential hypertension: A self controlled clinical study. J Ayurveda Integr Med. 2014;5(4):227-35.
12. Tolbaños Roche L, Mas Hesse B. Application of an integrative yoga therapy program in cases of essential arterial hypertension in public healthcare. Complement Ther Clin Pract. 2014;20(4):285-90.
13. Patil SG, Dhanakshirur GB, Aithala MR, et al. Effect of yoga on oxidative stress in elderly with grade-I hypertension: a randomized controlled study. J Clin Diagn Res. 2014;8(7):BC04-7.
14. Hagins M, Rundle A, Consedine NS, et al. A randomized controlled trial comparing the effects of yoga with an active control on ambulatory blood pressure in individuals with prehypertension and stage 1 hypertension. J Clin Hypertens (Greenwich). 2014;16(1):54-62.
15. Blom K, Baker B, How M, et al. Hypertension analysis of stress reduction using mindfulness meditation and yoga:

results from the HARMONY randomized controlled trial. Am J Hypertens. 2014;27(1):122-9.

16. Wolff M, Sundquist K, Larsson Lönn S, et al. Impact of yoga on blood pressure and quality of life in patients with hypertension—a controlled trial in primary care, matched for systolic blood pressure. BMC Cardiovasc Disord. 2013;13:111.

17. Pal A, Srivastava N, Narain VS, et al. Effect of yogic intervention on the autonomic nervous system in the patients with coronary artery disease: a randomized controlled trial. East Mediterr Health J. 2013;19(5):452-8.

18. Adhana R, Gupta R, Dvivedii J, et al. The influence of the 2:1 yogic breathing technique on essential hypertension. Indian J Physiol Pharmacol. 2013;57(1):38-44.

19. Mizuno J, Monteiro HL. An assessment of a sequence of yoga exercises to patients with arterial hypertension. J Bodyw Mov Ther. 2013;17(1):35-41.

20. Hughes JW, Fresco DM, Myerscough R, et al. Randomized controlled trial of mindfulness-based stress reduction for prehypertension. Psychosom Med. 2013;75(8):721-8.

21. Dhameja K, Singh S, Mustafa MD, et al. Therapeutic effect of yoga in patients with hypertension with reference to GST gene polymorphism. J Altern Complement Med. 2013;19(3):243-9.

22. Bhavanani AB, Madanmohan, Sanjay Z, et al. Immediate cardiovascular effects of pranava pranayama in hypertensive patients. Indian J Physiol Pharmacol. 2012;56(3): 273-8.

23. Bhavanani AB, Madanmohan, Sanjay Z. Immediate effect of Chandra nadi pranayama (left unilateral forced nostril breathing) on cardiovascular parameters in hypertensive patients. Int J Yoga. 2012;5(2):108-11.

24. Chung SC, Brooks MM, Rai M, et al. Effect of Sahaja yoga meditation on quality of life, anxiety, and blood pressure control. J Altern Complement Med. 2012;18(6):589-96.

25. Palta P, Page G. Evaluation of a mindfulness-based intervention program to decrease blood pressure in low-income African-American older adults. J Urban Health. 2012;89:308-16.

26. Agte VV, Jahagirdar MU, Tarwadi KV. The effects of Sudarshan Kriya Yoga on some physiological and biochemical parameters in mild hypertensive patients. Indian J Physiol Pharmacol. 2011;55(2):183-7.

27. Subramanian H, Soudarssanane MB, Jayalakshmy R, et al. Non-pharmacological interventions in hypertension: A community-based cross-over randomized controlled trial. Indian J Community Med. 2011;36(3):191-6.

28. Murthy SN, Rao NS, Nandkumar B, et al. Role of naturopathy and yoga treatment in the management of hypertension. Complement Ther Clin Pract. 2011;17(1):9-12.

29. Cohen DL, Bloedon LT, Rothman RL, et al. Iyengar yoga versus enhanced usual care on blood pressure in patients with prehypertension to stage I hypertension: a randomized controlled trial. Evid Based Complement Alternat Med. 2011;2011:546428.

30. Cade WT, Reeds DN, Mondy KE, et al. Yoga lifestyle intervention reduces blood pressure in HIV-infected adults with cardiovascular disease risk factors. HIV Med. 2010;11(6):379-88.

31. Saptharishi L, Soudarssanane M, Thiruselvakumar D, et al. Community-based randomized controlled trial of non-pharmacological interventions in prevention and control of hypertension among young adults. Indian J Community Med. 2009;34(4):329-34.

32. Lee KA. Effects of Mindfulness Meditation on Blood Pressure, Stress and Well-being in the Hypertensive Middle Aged Women (MSc Thesis). Seoul, Republic of Korea: Duksung Womens' University; 2009.

33. Schneider RH, Alexander CN, Staggers F, et al. A randomized controlled trial of stress reduction in African Americans treated for hypertension for over one year. Am J Hypertens. 2005;18(1):88-98.

34. McCaffrey R, Ruknui P, Hatthakit U, et al. The effects of yoga on hypertensive persons in Thailand. Holist Nurs Pract. 2005;19(4):173-80.

35. Castillo-Richmond A, Schneider RH, Alexander CN, et al. Effects of stress reduction on carotid atherosclerosis in hypertensive African Americans. Stroke. 2000;31(3): 568-73.

36. Murugesan R, Govindarajulu N, Bera TK. Effect of selected yogic practices on the management of hypertension. Indian J Physiol Pharmacol. 2000;44(2):207-10.

37. Schneider RH, Staggers F, Alexander C, et al. A randomised controlled trial of stress reduction for hypertension in older African Americans. Hypertension. 1995;26(5):820-7.

38. Van Montfrans GA, Karemaker JM, Wieling W, et al. Relaxation therapy and continuous ambulatory blood pressure in mild hypertension: a controlled study. BMJ. 1990;300(6736):1368-72.

39. Alexander CN, Langer EJ, Newman RI, et al. Transcendental meditation, mindfulness, and longevity: An experimental study with the elderly. J Pers Soc Psychol. 1989;57(6): 950-64

40. Patel C. 12-month follow-up of yoga and bio-feedback in the management of hypertension. Lancet.1975;1(7898):62-4.

41. Park SH, Han KS. Blood pressure response to meditation and yoga: A systematic review and meta-analysis. J Altern Complement Med. 2017;23(9):685-95.

42. Posadzki P, Cramer H, Kuzdzal A, et al. Yoga for hypertension: a systematic review of randomized clinical trials. Complement Ther Med. 2014;22(3):511-22.

43. Cramer H, Haller H, Lauche R, et al. A systematic review and meta-analysis of yoga for hypertension. Am J Hypertens. 2014;27(9):1146-51.

44. Tyagi A, Cohen M. Yoga and hypertension: a systematic review. Altern Ther Health Med. 2014;20(2):32-59.

45. Wang J, Xiong X, Liu W. Yoga for essential hypertension: a systematic review. PLoS One. 2013;8(10):e76357.

46. Hagins M, States R, Selfe T, et al. Effectiveness of yoga for hypertension: systematic review and meta-analysis. Evid Based Complement Alternat Med. 2013;2013:649836.

47. Okonta NR. Does yoga therapy reduce blood pressure in patients with hypertension? an integrative review. Holist Nurs Pract. 2012;26(3):137-41.

48. Anderson JW, Liu C, Kryscio RJ. Blood pressure response to transcendental meditation: a meta-analysis. Am J Hypertens. 2008; 21(3):310-6.

49. Appel LJ. Lifestyle modification as a means to prevent and treat high blood pressure. J Am Soc Nephrol. 2003;14(7 Suppl 2):S99-102.

50. Brook RD, Appel LJ, Rubenfire M, et al. Beyond medications and diet: alternative approaches to lowering blood pressure: a scientific statement from the American Heart Association. Hypertension. 2013;61(6):1360-83.

51. Cramer H. The efficacy and safety of yoga in managing hypertension. Exp Clin Endocrinol Diabetes. 2016;124(2): 65-70.

52. Manchanda SC, Madan K. Yoga and meditation in cardio-vascular disease. Clin Res Cardiol. 2014;103(9):675-80.

53. Barnes VA, Kapuku GK, Treiber FA. Impact of transcendental meditation on left ventricular mass in African American adolescents. Evid Based Complement Alternat Med. 2012;2012:923153.

54. Manchanda SC, Mehrotra UC, Makhija A, et al. Reversal of early atherosclerosis in metabolic syndrome by yoga - a randomized controlled trial. J Yoga PhysTher. 2013;3: 132.

55. Ornish D, Brown SE, Scherwitz LW, et al. Can lifestyle changes reverse coronary heart disease? The Lifestyle Heart Trial. Lancet. 1990;336(8708):129-33.

56. Manchanda SC, Narang R, Reddy KS, et al. Retardation of coronary atherosclerosis with yoga lifestyle intervention. J Assoc Physicians India. 2000;48(7):687-94.

57. Schneider RH, Grim CE, Rainforth MV, et al. Stress reduction in the secondary prevention of cardiovascular disease: randomized, controlled trial of transcendental meditation and health education in Blacks. Circ Cardiovasc Qual Outcomes. 2012;5(6):750-8.

58. Lakkireddy D, Atkins D, Pillarisetti J, et al. Effect of yoga on arrhythmia burden, anxiety, depression, and quality of life in paroxysmal atrial fibrillation: the YOGA My Heart Study. J Am Coll Cardiol. 2013;61(11):1177-82.

59. Krishna BH, Pal P, Pal G, et al. A randomized controlled trial to study the effect of yoga therapy on cardiac function and N Terminal Pro BNP in heart failure. Integr Med Insights. 2014;9:1-6.

Diuretics and Hypertension

Anita Jaiswal Ektate, Neeta Rajram Narang, Virendra KR Chauhan

■ INTRODUCTION

As all monogenic forms of hypertension have sodium retention as one of the main mechanisms for the increase in blood pressure, increasing urinary sodium excretion is a logical and fundamental part of treatment of hypertension.[1] Consistent with this understanding, thiazide diuretics are listed in hypertension guidelines as one of the three equally weighted first-line antihypertensive options alongside CCB and blockers of the renin–angiotensin system (RAS). Diuretics have been used as antihypertensives since 1960 till date. Paradigms have shifted in antihypertension management, diuretics from being 3rd line to becoming one of the 1st line drugs in hypertension. Randomized controlled trials and meta-analyses have demonstrated that when compared with placebo or no treatment, blood pressure lowering by these antihypertensive drug classes is also accompanied by significant reductions of stroke and major cardiovascular events.[2] In spite of proven benefits, diuretics have not been used as first line drugs by clinicians due to fear of side effects mainly dyselectrolytemia.

■ DEFINITION

Drugs which increase urine formation by increasing urine volume (diuresis) or by increasing excretion of Sodium and water (natriuresis).

Mechanism

- *Extrarenal:*
  - ○ Increasing cardiac output: Digoxin and dopamine in congestive heart failure (CHF)
  - ○ Inhibiting antidiuretic hormone (ADH): H_2O, alcohol.
- *Renal:*
  - ○ Most diuretics inhibit Na^+ and H_2O reabsorption.

■ CLASSIFICATION

- *Based on the intensity of the diuretic effect*: Highly, moderately and weakly effective diuretics
- *Based on effect on K^+ excretion:* K^+ (and H^+)-losing and K^+ (and H^+)-sparing diuretics
- Based on the site and mechanism of diuretic action (Table 1 and Fig. 1).

High efficacy (up to 25% NaCl excretion):
- *Loop diuretics:*

TABLE 1: Diuretics mechanism, uses and side effects

Diuretic	Examples	Mechanism of Action	Uses	Side Effects

Loop diuretics	• Furosemide
	• Torsemide
	• Bumetanide
	• Ethacrynic acid
		• Acts on thick ascending part of loop of Henle
		• Inhibit Na^+-K^+-$2Cl^-$ cotransport and reabsorption
		• Increase NaCl excretion (up to 25% high efficacy)
		• Na^+ exchanges with K^+ in the DT → K^+ loss
		• Effective in very low GFR of <30 mL/min
			Edema: Cardiac (CHF), hepatic (cirrhotic ascites) and renal (nephrotic syndrome)
			• Acute pulmonary edema
			• Cerebral edema (mannitol preferred)
			• Acute hypercalcemia
			• Acute renal failure
			• Forced diuresis in drug poisoning (barbiturate)
			Hypertension (thiazides preferred):
			• Hyperkalemia mild
			• Along with massive blood transfusion
			• Anion overdose (Iodide, bromide and fluoride)
				Hypokalemia
				• *Clinical Features:*
				  ○ May Increase digoxin toxicity, arrhythmia,
				  ○ Muscle weakness, fatigue and cramps
				• *To prevent hypokalemia:*
				  ○ Use low dose
				    – KCl supplement (oral solution or IV infusion) or
				    – Combine with K sparing diuretic
				• *Advice:*
				  ○ *More intake of K containing food:* Coconut water and fruit juice.
				  ○ Hypochloremic alkalosis
				  ○ Dehydration
				  ○ Hyponatremia
				  ○ *Ototoxicity:* More likely with IV use, in RF, other ototoxic drugs

Continued

Continued

Diuretic	Examples	Mechanism of Action	Uses	Side Effects
Thiazide diuretics	• Chlorothiazide • Hydrochlorothiazide • Metolazone • Indapamide	*Acts on early part of distal tubules*: • Inhibit Na^+-Cl^- symporter and reabsorption • Increase NaCl excretion (5–10% medium efficacy) • Na exchanges with K^+ in the DT → K^+ loss → Hypokalemia • Not effective in very low GFR of <30 mL/min, may reduce GFR further	• Hypertension (hydrochlorothiazide, Indapamide) • *Edema*: cardiac, hepatic and renal • Less efficacious than loop diuretic • Useful for maintenance therapy • Hypercalciuria and renal Ca stones • Diabetes Insipidus (DI) (Nephrogenic responds better) • Metolazone useful even when GFR is as low as 15 mL/min	• Hypokalemia • May precipitate renal failure • Hyperuricemia • Hyperglycemia • Hyperlipidemia • Hypomagnesemia

Osmotic	Mannitol	Not mediated by any receptors or target site:
		• Expands ECF volume—increase RBF and GFR
		• Osmotic gradient in the tubular lumen—prevent reabsorption of mainly H_2O → dilute urine diuresis
		• Prevent Na^+ reabsorption—up to 20% NaCl excretion (acute effect)
		• May inhibit transport process in ascending loop of Henle
		• Classified as weak diuretic in some textbooks
		• Never used for chronic edema or as a natriuretic
			• *ARF*: Treatment and prevention
			  ○ To maintain GFR during major surgeries, trauma cases, severe jaundice, hemolytic reactions, etc.
			• *Cerebral edema*:
			  ○ To lower intracranial tension before brain surgery
			  ○ To lower intraocular tension-
			  ○ Acute glaucoma
			  ○ Before intraocular surgeries
			  ○ Forced diuresis in drug poisoning (FAD in barbiturate poisoning)
			  ○ To counteract low plasma osmolality after dialysis
				• Acute Intravascular volume expansion
				• Before diuresis starts, it exerts osmotic effect in the blood
				• Contraindicated in pulmonary edema, cardiac edema (CHF) and intracranial hemorrhage, and established renal failure
				• Thrombophlebitis
				• Headache (due to hyponatremia)
				• Nausea
				• If overdose → dehydration → hypernatremia.

Continued

Continued

Diuretic	Examples	Mechanism of Action	Uses	Side Effects

Potassium sparing diuretics	• Spironolactone
	• Amiloride
	• Triamterene
		Acts on cortical segment of distal tubules:
		• Competitive antagonist of aldosterone
		• Inhibit AIP → inhibit Na^+ reabsorption
		• Causes K' retention (K^+-sparing effect) → Hyperkalemia
		• Mild saluretic (natriuresis) 3% of NaCl
		• Never used alone as diuretic
		• Useful when combined with thiazide or furosemide
		• AIP—Aldosterone induced proteins
			• Edema more useful in cirrhotic and nephrotic syndrome—breaks resistance to thiazide or frusemide in refractory edema
			• To counteract K^+ loss due to thiazides, frusemide
			• *Hypertension*: combined with thiazide
			• Eplerenone is a new drug approved for HTN, No gynecomastia
			• CHF: as an adjunctive therapy it retards disease progression and reduces mortality RALES (Randomized Aldosterone Evaluation Study)
			• Primary hyperaldosteronism (Conn's syndrome)
				• Hyperkalemia
				  ○ Risk in CRF patients
				  ○ Patients taking ACE inhibitor (Enalapril) or ATRA (Losartan)
				  ○ potassium chloride KCl supplement
				• Related to steroid structure
				  ○ Gynecomastia,
				  ○ Impotence in males
				  ○ Hirsutism,
				  ○ Menstrual irregularities in females
				• *Miscellaneous*: Drowsiness, abdominal upset
				• Drug Interaction
				  ○ May increase digoxin levels in CHF
				  ○ NSAIDs (aspirin) decreases its effect

(ACE: angiotensin-converting enzyme; ATRA: angiotensin receptor antagonist; ARF: acute renal failure; CHF: congestive heart failure; ECF: extracellular fluid; FAD: forced alkaline diuresis; GFR: glomerular filtration rate; IV: intravenous; NSAIDs: nonsteroidal anti-inflammatory drug; RBF: renal blood flow)

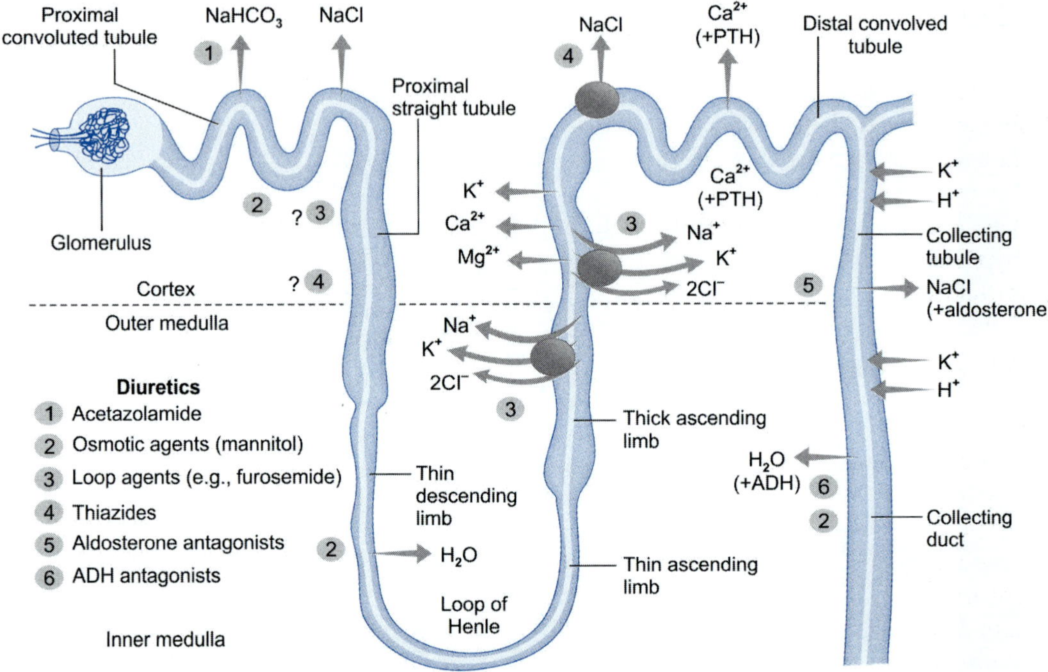

(ADH: antidiuretic hormone; PTH: parathyroid hormone)

Fig. 1: Tubule transport systems and site of action of diuretics.

- o Furosemide, torsemide and bumetanide (SO_2NH_2 group)
- o Ethacrynic acid.
- *Organic mercurials*: Mersalyl (now obsolete).

Medium efficacy (5–10% NaCl excretion):
- *Thiazides:* Hydrochlorothiazide, chlorothiazide, benzthiazide, hydroflumethiazide, clopamide and polythiazide
- *Thiazide like:* Chlorthalidone, metolazone, xipamide and indapamide.

Weak efficacy:
- *Carbonic anhydrase inhibitors (5% NaCl excretion):*
- Acetazolamide, methazolamide and dichlorphenamide
- *Potassium sparing diuretics (3% NaCl excretion):*
  - o Aldosterone antagonists spironolactone and eplerenone
  - o Directly acting: Amiloride and triamterene.

- *Osmotic diuretics (up to 20% NaCl excretion):*
  - o Mannitol, glycerol and isosorbide.

■ THE JNC 8 GUIDELINES

For Choice of Antihypertensives

- *Nonblack persons:*
  - o Angiotensin-converting enzyme (ACE) inhibitors
  - o Angiotensin receptor blocker (ARB)
  - o Calcium channel blocker (CCB)
  - o Thiazide-type diuretic.
- *Black persons (including those with diabetes):*
  - o Calcium channel blocker
  - o Thiazide-type diuretic.
- *Chronic kidney disease (regardless of race or diabetes status):*
  - o Angiotensin-converting enzyme inhibitor or ARB as initial or add-on antihypertensive therapy.

FOCUS ON HYPERTENSION

Thiazide and thiazide like diuretics have been preferred over other diuretics.

Difference of thiazide from loop diuretic:

- Longer duration of action
- Low ceiling diuretic
- Less effective in renal dysfunction and hypercalcemia.

Chlorthalidone is better than hydrochlorothiazide:

- More consistent reduction in cardiovascular events (Trials – HDFP, MRFIT, SHEP, ALLHAT)
- More reduction in left ventricular hypertrophy (Trials – MRFIT).

Low dose versus high dose:

- Low dose thiazides preferred as similar result in reduction of blood pressure and lesser risk of metabolic complications especially in elderly (Trials – SHEP, STOP-2, MRC, TOMHS).

SPECIAL CONSIDERATIONS

Diabetes Mellitus

In hypertensive patients with diabetes mellitus along with kidney disease, RAS inhibitors are the first-line treatment (Table 2). However, these patients are prone to fluid retention and are at significant risk of heart failure or renal impairment.[3] They are also likely to benefit from diuresis, despite the potential effect of some diuretics on metabolic parameters. This dichotomy is reflected in guidelines—ADA guidelines and Hypertension Canada guidelines support equally the prescription of diuretics and RAS inhibitors, but give preference to RAS inhibitors in presence of proteinuria or microalbuminuria. The most recent ESC/ESH guidelines have addressed this issue by recommending the initiation of treatment with a combination of a RAS inhibitor and a diuretic (or a CCB).[4]

Evidence that supports equal weight being given to treatment with diuretics and ACE inhibitors can be found in the Natrilix sustained release versus Enalapril Study in hypertensive type 2 diabetic patients with Microalbuminuria trial [(NESTOR); N = 565) of hypertensive patients with type 2 diabetes mellitus (T2DM).[5] In this study, Indapamide was more effective in patients with a marked fluid and sodium retention. Effects on microalbuminuria (urinary albumin: creatinine ratio) were equivalent, and

TABLE 2: Treatment (first line) as per different JNC protocol.

	Year	Initial antihypertensive
JNC 1	1977	Thiazide
JNC 2	1980	Diuretic
JNC 3	1984	Thiazide or β-blocker
JNC 4	1988	Diuretic or β-blocker or CCB or ACE inhibitor
JNC 5	1993	Diuretic or β-blocker
JNC 6	1997	Diuretic or β-blocker
JNC 7	2003	Thiazide for most without compel indication; compel indication use thiazide, ACE inhibitor, ARB, β-blocker or CCB
JNC 8	12/13	ACE inhibitor or ARB, CCB or diuretic; If CKD, then irrespective of diabetes or race status -ACE inhibitor or ARB preferred

(ACE: angiotensin-converting enzyme; ARB: angiotensin receptor blocker; CCB: calcium channel blocker; CKD: chronic kidney disease; DM: diabetes mellitus; JNC: Joint National Committee)

TABLE 3: Effect of blood pressure by chlorthalidone, hydrochlorothiazide and indapamide.

	Hydrochlorthiazide	Chlorthalidone	Indapamide
Half life	6–15 h	40–60 h	14–24 h
Duration of action	16–24 h	48–72 h	>24 h
Equipotency of office SBP	25 mg	12.5 mg	1.5 mg
Dose effect for office SBP	Yes	Mixed data	No

therefore, challenged the perception that RAS inhibitors should be the preferred treatment in the presence of microalbuminuria. However, a higher rate of hypokalemia (10.2 vs. 1.0%, respectively) was noted with indapamide than with enalapril.

Elderly

Two major trials support the preferred use of chlorthalidone and indapamide in the elderly due to reduced risk of stroke, cardiovascular events and heart failure (SHEP and ALLHA trials).

History of Stroke

ACE Inhibitors/ARB inhibitors are preferred. if among thiazide or thiazide like then indapamide has risk reduction benefits.

Salt-sensitive and Low-renin hypertension

Lastly, though not addressed in most guidelines, patients with salt-sensitive hypertension and/or low-renin hypertension have characteristics that lend themselves well to treatment with a diuretic. In most cases, low levels of renin are an indication that the RAS is suppressed because of volume overload and sodium retention. In such patients, as well as in salt-sensitive patients, treatment with diuretics, which reduce volume and increase sodium excretion, would be expected to be efficacious, whereas treatment with RAS inhibitors would be expected to suppress the RAS further. In fact, in the few clinical trials that

have looked at patients with low-plasma renin activity and/or salt sensitivity, effective blood pressure lowering strategies include HCTZ, chlorthalidone, indapamide, or spironolactone (Table 3).[6]

As salt-sensitive hypertension is especially common in black patients, older adults, and in patients with more severe blood pressure or with comorbidities, such as metabolic syndrome, diabetes mellitus, or chronic kidney disease and as low-renin hypertension is particularly common in African, Americans, the elderly, and patients with resistant hypertension, it is not surprising that diuretics have been shown to be particularly effective in these patient populations.

Indapamide or Chlorthalidone

In the Latin American Society of Hypertension guidelines, indapamide is preferred in patients with a history of stroke or transient ischemic attack; whereas in the most recent ACC/AHA hypertension recommendations, chlorthalidone is listed as the optimal choice.[7]

These recommendations are based on meta-analyses that highlight potential differences between chlorthalidone and indapamide. Both treatments had significant effects on stroke and on the composite endpoint (stroke and coronary heart disease). Similar results were obtained by the United Kingdom National Clinical Guideline meta-analysis for stroke (significant vs. placebo for both treatments) and all-cause mortality (only significant vs. placebo for indapamide).[8]

Coronary heart disease, however, was significantly reduced with indapamide, but not chlorthalidone.

LACUNES TO THINK OVER

- Hypokalemia may cause muscular spasms and then due to these spasms, patient may have symptoms and then due to symptoms and anxiety then patient may have increased hypertension
- Hyponatremia may cause disorientation and hence this by itself may cause missing of doses and increase in hypertension. Hence, the patient has to be monitored for this adverse effect
- Hyperuricemia (due to thiazides) may cause joint pain and due to these increased symptoms stress increases and hypertension increases.

CONCLUSION

Indapamide and Chlorthalidone are preferred over Hydrochlorothiazides. However, a comparative trial between Indapamide and Chlorthalidone is needed for superiority. Low dose diuretics should be considered especially in elderly patients to avoid metabolic complications. Spironolactone is most effective drug as add on drug for resistant hypertension.

REFERENCES

1. Padmanabhan S, Caulfield M, Dominiczak AF. Genetic and molecular aspects of hypertension. Circ Res 2015; 116:937–59.
2. Thomopoulos C, Parati G, Zanchetti A. Effects of blood pressure lowering on outcome incidence in hypertension. 1. Overview, meta-analyses, and meta-regression analyses of randomized trials. J Hypertens 2014; 32:2285–95.
3. Bahtiyar G, Gutterman D, Lebovitz H. Heart failure: a major cardiovascular complication of diabetes mellitus. Curr Diab Rep 2016;16:116
4. Williams B, Mancia G, Spiering W, Agabiti Rosei E, Azizi M, Burnier M, et al. 2018 ESC/ESH Guidelines for the management of arterial hypertension: the Task Force for the management of arterial hypertension of the European Society of Cardiology and the European Society of Hypertension: The Task Force for the management of arterial hypertension of the European Society of Cardiology and the European Society of Hypertension. J Hypertens 2018; 36:1953–2041.
5. Marre M, Puig JG, Kokot F, Fernandez M, Jermendy G, Opie L, et al. Equivalence of indapamide SR and enalapril on microalbuminuria reduction in hypertensive patients with type 2 diabetes: the NESTOR Study. J Hypertens 2004; 22:1613–22.
6. Kobalava ZD, Kotovskaya YV, Kravtsova OA. Plasma renin activity and potential of indapamide retard to improve control of hypertension. Kardiologiia 2015;55:21–6
7. Whelton PK, Carey RM, Aronow WS, Casey DE Jr, Collins KJ, Dennison Himmelfarb C, et al. 2017 ACC/AHA/AAPA/ABC/ACPM/AGS/APhA/ASH/ASPC/NMA/PCNA Guideline for the prevention, detection, evaluation, and management of high blood pressure in adults: a report of the American College of Cardiology/American Heart Association Task Force on Clinical Practice Guidelines. Hypertension 2018; 71:1269–1324
8. E. National Clinical Guideline Centre. Hypertension. The clinical management of primary hypertension in adults (NICE clinical guideline 127). London, United Kingdom. 2011.

Beta-blockers in Hypertension

Chandrasekhar Valupadas

INTRODUCTION

Hypertension is the most important and leading global risk factor for different chronic noncommunicable disease burden. In India, the prevalence of hypertension is more than one-fourth (29.8%) of the population with a little difference between urban (33%) and rural (25%) areas. Among them, only 38% (urban) and 25% (rural) are being treated where as only one-tenth and one-fifth hypertensive population have their blood pressure (BP) under control, respectively.[1]

Recently two studies in India, i.e. *Fourth National Family Health Survey* (n = 799,228) and *Fourth District Level Household Survey* (n = 1.3 million) demonstrated the true prevalence of hypertension in the country and reported that its prevalence is higher in men than women. Social determinants such as human expansion, greater urbanization, and social development with faulty lifestyles are important factors for the development of hypertension. Hypertension led to 1.63 million deaths in India as compared to million deaths in 1990. The disease burden in the form of disability-adjusted life years (DALYs) attributable to hypertension has increased from 21 million in 1990 to 39 million in 2016.[2]

SYSTEMS RESPONSIBLE FOR HYPERTENSION

Systems responsible for hypertension include—(a) sympathetic nervous system activation; (b) renin–angiotensin-aldosterone system (RAAS); and (c) structural and functional integrity of vasculature and endothelium. Any pathophysiologic abnormalities of these systems results in development of hypertension.

Endothelial dysfunction has greatly contributed to the pathogenesis of hypertension and this concept had gained support in recent years. Nitric oxide (NO) is a potent vasodilator responsible for vasodilation. In healthy individuals, the cardiovascular system is continuously exposed to NO-dependent vasodilator tone, which is decrease in hypertensive persons leading to vasoconstriction, atherothrombosis, inflammation and remodeling of vasculature.

Drugs which improve endothelial function are angiotensin-converting enzyme (ACE) inhibitors, statins, calcium channel blockers (CCBs), thiazolidinediones, estrogen, L-arginine and antioxidants etc. Newer β-blockers such as nebivolol, are now discovered to join the list that improve endothelial function.

■ NATURAL HISTORY OF UNTREATED HYPERTENSION AND TREATMENT OPTIONS

Untreated hypertension is a self-accelerating condition leading to arteriolar hypertrophy, coronary heart disease, heart failure (HF) and cerebral stroke. To pervert the perpetuation of hypertension and prevent the associated morbidity and mortality, it is important to treat hypertension to the recommended targets. There are various effective antihypertensive drugs such as ACE inhibitors, angiotensin receptor blockers (ARBs), CCBs, β-adrenoceptor blockers, α-adrenoceptor blockers, diuretics and endothelin receptor antagonists etc. The ideal characteristics and effects of various antihypertensives drugs to chose the near- ideal class of drug for different indications shown in the Table 1.[4]

■ BETA-ADRENERGIC RECEPTORS AND BLOCKERS

Beta-adrenergic receptor is a site on a cell membrane which interacts with epinephrine or norepinephrine to control heart rate and contractility, vasodilation of blood vessels, and other physiological processes in the body (Fig. 1). There are three known types of β-receptors; beta-1 (β1), beta-2 (β2) and beta-3 (β3) which are distributed in different tissues with various functions (listed in Table 2).

Beta-adrenergic Receptor Blockers

Beta-blockers, also known as β-adrenergic receptor blocking agents, are a class of antihypertensive drugs (listed in Table 3), which inhibit sympathetic neurotransmitters norepinephrine and epinephrine from binding to β-receptors. They reduce heart rate and myocardial contraction resulting in decreased cardiac output and BP (Fig. 2). They also reduce renin secretion by antagonizing β-receptors in the juxtaglomerular apparatus in the kidney.[5]

Newer β-blockers which have an additional property of vasodilation were discovered which decrease BP by reducing systemic vascular resistance, while maintaining cardiac output. The benefits of peripheral vasodilation is decrease in afterload and preload, which in turn results in reduced central aortic pressure and possibly reverse the adverse arterial remodeling.

TABLE 1: Effects of antihypertensive drugs in hypertension.

Effect	Ideal drug	Traditional β-blocker	Vasodilating β-blocker	α1-blocker	ACE inhibitor/ARB	Dihydropyridine CCB	Thiazide diuretic
Mean arterial BP	↓	↓	↓	↓	↓	↓	↓
Total peripheral resistance	↓	↑	↓	↓	↓	↓	↓
Cardiac output	0	↓	0	0	0	0	0
Heart rate	0/↓	↓	0/↓	↑	0	↑	0
SNS activation	↓	↓	↓	↑	↓	↑	↑
RAAS	↓	↓	↓	0	↓	↑	↑
Lipid metabolism	0/+	–	0	0/+	0	0	–
Glucose metabolism	0/+	–	0	0	0/+	0	–

(ACE: angiotensin-converting enzyme; ARB: angiotensin receptor blocker; BP: blood pressure; CCB: calcium channel blocker; RAAS: renin–angiotensin-aldosterone system; SNS: sympathetic nervous system)

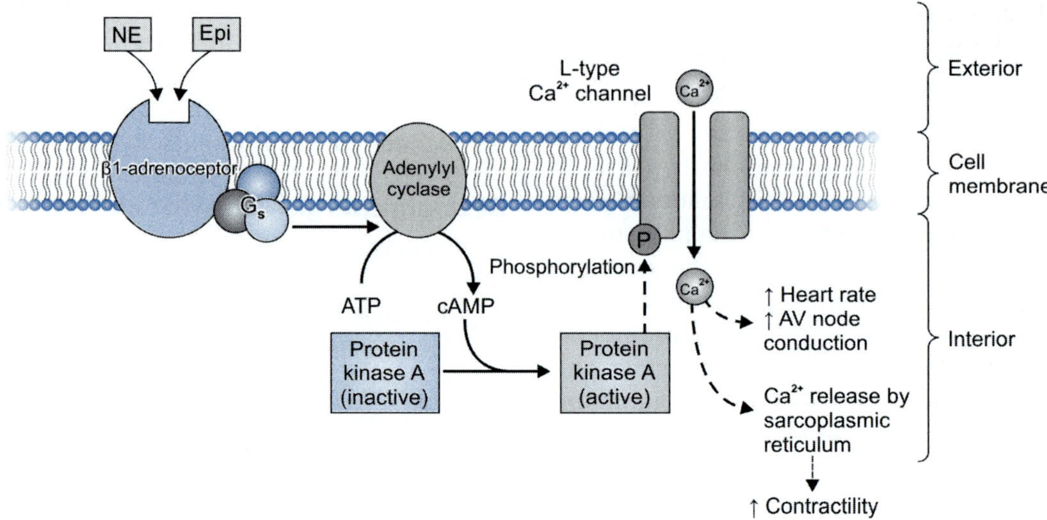

(AV: atrioventricular; ATP: adenosine triphosphate; cAMP: cyclic adenosine monophosphate)

Fig. 1: Mechanism of β1-adrenoceptor.

TABLE 2: Classification of β-adrenergic receptors.

Type	Tissue distribution	Functions
β1	Heart	Positively inotropic and chronotropic
	Kidney	Renin release
	Adipocytes	Lipolysis
β2	Lung and bronchial	Bronchodilation
	Vascular smooth muscle	Vasodilation
	Heart	Positively inotropic and chronotropic
	Uterus	Relaxation
	Bladder	Relaxation
	Eye	Increase aqueous hwmor formation
	Liver	Glycogenolysis
	Skeletal muscle	Glycogenolysis
	Sympathetic terminal	Norepinephrine release
β3	Adipocytes	Lipolysis
	Uterus	Relaxation
	Bladder	Relaxation
	Heart	Negatively inotropic

TABLE 3: Classification of β-adrenergic receptor blockers.

β-adrenergic receptor blockers	Examples
First generation (older, traditional, nonselective)	Propranolol, nadolol, timolol, penbutolol, sotalol, pindolol
Second generation (β1 selective)	Metoprolol, atenolol, acebutolol, bisoprolol, esmolol
Third generation (newer, with additional α blocking and/ or vasodilator property)	Labetalol, carvedilol, celiprolol, nebivolol, betaxolol

They also lack adverse effects on lipid and glucose metabolism and therefore they are more appropriate in the hypertension treatment in comparsion with older/ traditional β-blockers.

The pharmacokinetic and pharmacodynamic properties of various β-blockers are described in Table 4. Among different β-blockers, nebivolol has the highest β1 selectivity.[5]

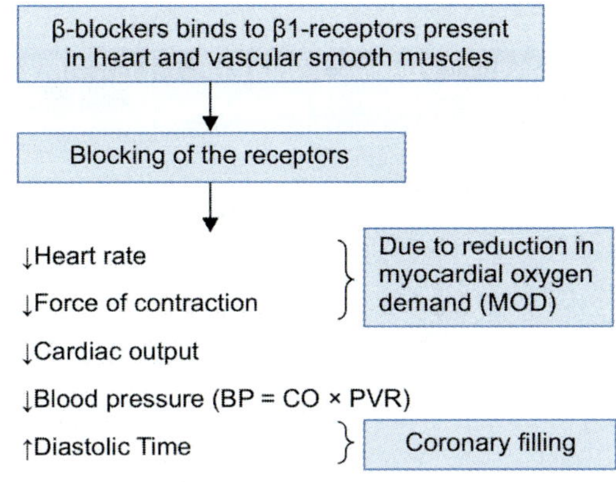

(BP: blood pressure; CO: cardiac output; PVR: peripheral vascular resistance)

Fig. 2: Mechanism of action of β-blockers in the heart.

The European Society of Hypertension (ESH)/European Society of Cardiology (ESC) 2013 guidelines[6] for the management of hypertension has classified in five major antihypertensive drug classes as an initial therapy in which β-blockers are one of them. The treatment of choice with β-blockers in various conditions of hypertension are listed in Table 5.

They do not differ for their overall ability in BP reduction but they do differ in their ability to protect against overall cardiovascular risk and events, such as stroke and myocardial infarction (MI). Hence, there could be compelling indication of β-blockers in co-morbid conditions with hypertension.

Contraindications of Beta-blockers

The β-blockers are contraindicated in:
- Bronchospastic disease
- Young patients due to documented impotence/loss of libido
- Diabetics because of impaired insulin sensitivity
- Obese and patients with impaired lipid profile, as it may worsen lipid profile and increase atherosclerotic effect
- Peripheral vascular disease

- Heart failure, as cardiac output is reduced and there is no improvement in left ventricular function
- Renal impairment, as it gets accumulated and dosage reduction is often necessary.

Side Effects of Beta-blockers

Nonselective β-blockers may give rise to adverse effects like asthma and intermittent claudication as a result of antagonism of β2-receptors. The β1-selective blockers are free of these adverse effects; however, at higher doses cardioselectivity will be lost. Patients who develop marked bradycardia and tiredness may tolerate drug with partial agonist activity, i.e. intrinsic sympathomimetic activity (ISA) such as pindolol.

Drug interactions of β-blockers are shown in Table 6.

Beta-blockers in Uncomplicated Hypertension

As per the Eighth Joint National Committee (JNC-8), β-blockers are no longer recommended as first-line therapy for uncomplicated hypertension. But they are still used in treating hypertension, especially in patients with coronary artery disease, arrhythmias and chronic HF. This is the greatest shift from first-line therapy in JNC-7 or earlier to fourth-line therapy in JNC-8, pending controversies and arguments for/and against β-blockers. Such controversies fit better for intra-class of β-blockers rather than entire class against other class of antihypertensives. Beta-blockers such as carvedilol and nebivolol found to be more beneficial for hypertension than the older β-blockers, but trial results with these newer agents are scanty.[7] However, in patients whose BP is not adequately controlled with a diuretic, ACE inhibitor/ARB and CCB, the addition of a β-blocker may improve BP control.

TABLE 4: Various properties of β-adrenoceptor blockers.

β-blockers	Dose (mg)	Lipo-philicity	Bioavailability (%)	First-pass metabolism	Plasma t½ (h)	Route of elimination	ISA	MSA
First generation								
Propranolol	40–480	High	3–40	Yes	3–5	Hepatic	No	Yes
Sotalol	160–480	No	90–100	No	6–12	Renal, hepatic	No	No
Timolol	10–40	Weak	50–75	Partial	4–5	Renal, hepatic	No	No
Pindolol	10–30	Weak	90	No	3–4	Renal, hepatic	Yes	No
Penbutolol	10–40	Yes	90	Yes	~5	Renal	Yes	No
Alprenolol	–	Moderate	–	Yes	2–3	–	Yes	No
Oxprenolol	80–160	Yes	20–70	Yes	1–2	Renal	Yes	No
Carteolol	–	No	–	Yes	7	–	Yes	No
Nadolol	40–80	No	30	No	14–24	Renal	No	No
Second generation								
Metoprolol	100–400	Yes	40–50	Yes	3–6	Hepatic	No	No
Atenolol	25–100	No	50–60	No	6–9	Renal	No	No
Acebutolol	400–1,200	No	40–60	Yes	3–4	Renal, hepatic	Yes	Yes
Bisoprolol	2.5–10	Weak	80	No	9–12	Renal, hepatic	No	No
Esmolol	*	No	–	No	<10 min	Renal	No	No
Betaxolol	10–40	Yes	89	Yes	14–22	–	No	No
Bevantolol	200–600	Moderate	–	–	–	–	No	–
Third generation								
Labetalol	300–600	Moderate	25	Yes	4–6	Hepatic	No	No
Carvedilol	3.125–25	Yes	25–30	Yes	7–10	Hepatic	No	Yes
Celiprolol	200–600	No	30–70	No	5	Renal	Yes	No
Nebivolol	5–40	High	12–96	Yes	10	Hepatic	No	No

*Useful in postoperative hypertension, 0.5–1 mg/kg loading dose over 1 minute followed by an infusion of 50 µg/kg/min (maximum 300 µg/kg/min).

(ISA: intrinsic sympathomimetic activity; MSA: membrane stabilizing activity)

Beta-blockers in Complicated Hypertension

- *Stroke*: Beta-blockers have only a modest effect on stroke, while other classes of antihypertensive drugs reduce mortality more than β-blockers.[8] For these reasons, other classes like diuretics, ACE inhibitors/ARBs, and CCBs are preferred as first-line therapy for hypertension as they are better tolerated than β-blockers

TABLE 5: Clinical conditions when β-blockers are indicated in hypertensive patient.

Conditions	Antihypertensive drugs
Previous stroke	Any BP-lowering agent
Previous MI	β-blockers, ACE inhibitors, ARBs
Angina pectoris	β-blockers, CCB
Heart failure	Diuretics, β-blockers, ACE inhibitors, ARBs, antialdosterone agents
Atrial fibrillation	β-blockers, nondihydropyridine CCB

(ACE: angiotensin-converting enzyme; CCB: calcium channel blockers; ARBs: angiotensin receptor blockers; BP: blood pressure; MI: myocardial infarction)

TABLE 6: Drug interactions with β-blockers.

Pharmacokinetic interactions	Pharmacodynamic interactions
• All salts, cholestyramine (decrease absorption) • Enzyme inducers (decrease plasma concentrations) • Cimetidine, hydralazine (increase bioavailability) • They impair clearance of lidocaine	• Digoxin • Calcium channel blocker (verapamil) • Calcium channel blocker (DHP) • NSAIDs • Adrenalin and other α-agonists

(DHP: dihydropyridine; NSAIDs: nonsteroidal anti-inflammatory drugs

- *Heart failure*: Beta-blockers have been shown to reduce mortality in patients with chronic HF. For stage B heart failure, β-blockers and ACE inhibitors should be used in all patients with a history of MI regardless of ejection fraction or presence of HF, this can also be recommended in patients without a history of MI, with a reduced EF, and no HF symptoms. For stage C heart failure, diuretics, salt restriction, ACE inhibitors and β-blockers like bisoprolol, carvedilol or metoprolol are also recommended. The combination of these β-blockers with ACE inhibitor/ARBs has been shown to reduce symptoms of HF, improve clinical status, and reduce the risk of death and hospitalization by 30–40%[9]

- *Angina pectoris*: The American College of Cardiology (ACC)/American Heart Association (AHA) 2007 guidelines on chronic stable angina recommend initiating and continuing β-blocker therapy indefinitely in all patients who have had MI, acute coronary syndrome, or left ventricular dysfunction, with or without HF symptoms, and/or ACE inhibitors with the addition of other drugs, as required, for BP control. The β1-selective agents without ISA are most frequently used and have less inhibition of the peripheral vasodilation and bronchodilation induced by the β2-receptors.[10] However, at higher doses, cardioselectivity may be lost. The β-blockers with ISA may not decrease heart rate and BP at rest, but reduces exercise heart rate and can be effective in few selective patients

- *Acute MI [unstable angina (UA)/non-ST elevated myocardial infarction (NSTEMI) and ST elevated myocardial infarction (STEMI)]*: Beta-blockers prevent recurrent ischemia, life-threatening ventricular arrhythmias, and improve survival in patients with prior MI. Unless contraindicated, the ACC/AHA 2014 guidelines for NSTEMI and 2013 guidelines for STEMI recommend indefinite β-blocker therapy (cardioselective β-blocker without ISA) in all patients with UA, NSTEMI and STEMI[11]

- *Cardiac arrhythmia*: Beta-blockers improve survival in patients who have had MI as they are able to reduce the incidence of sudden cardiac death. The ACC/AHA/ESC 2006 guidelines consider β-blockers to be safe and effective mainstay of antiarrhythmic drug therapy for the management of ventricular arrhythmias and prevention of sudden cardiac death[12]

- *Chronic kidney disease (CKD)*: Beta-blockers are recommended as second-line agents after RAAS blockers for controlling hypertension in patients with CKD and systolic HF. As compared to other antihypertensive agents, there are no demerits to use β-blockers for renal protection as vasodilatory β-blockers are renoprotective. In CKD, often three or more different antihypertensive drugs are required to control BP, which is crucial for the prevention of cardiovascular events. There is no evidence that β-blockers are inferior to diuretics or CCBs as second or third-line agents for renal protection and control of BP in patients with CKD[13]

- *Metabolic syndrome (diabetes and dyslipidemia)*: BP management in hypertensive patients with metabolic abnormalities is challenging, since many of the antihypertensive drugs adversely affect metabolism. The third-generation β-blockers, such as nebivolol, are effective in hypertension control and offer neutral or beneficial effects on metabolism, especially in obese and diabetic hypertensive patients.[14]

Clinical Trial Evidence and Current Research on Beta-blockers

Beta-blockers have substantial clinical trial evidence of benefit over placebo in hypertension, and are relatively inexpensive. Building on the availability of propranolol since 1976, more than a dozen additional β-blockers have been introduced for hypertension treatment.[15] This drug class effectively lowers BP and has been a recommended treatment option by the JNC in 2003.[16] Vasodilatory activity may be a key contributor to advantageous outcomes in hypertension.[17] In recent times, their role is becoming controversial especially after the

evidence from the Losartan Intervention For Endpoint Reduction (LIFE), Anglo-Scandinavian Cardiac Outcomes Trial (ASCOT), and Cochrane database review in 2004, which have been placed β-blockers to fourth line in the treatment of hypertension in UK, according to latest National Institute for Health and Clinical Excellence (NICE) guidelines. Concerns have also been raised by meta-analysis in which β-blockers were reported to have a suboptimal effect on reducing stroke risk and increasing the risk for new-onset diabetes are compared with other antihypertensive agents.[18] Also these reviews and meta-analysis were evaluated primarily for atenolol, a β-blocker without vasodilatory activity. However, β-blockers are a diverse group of drugs with different properties, and there is a need of more well-conducted clinical trials in this area.[8]

■ CONCLUSION

Beta-blockers probably make little or no difference in the reducing number of deaths among people on hypertension treatment; this effect appears to be similar to that of diuretics and ACE inhibitors/ARBs but not as good as CCBs. They reduce the incidence of strokes, an effect which is similar to that of diuretics but not as good as ACE inhibitors/ARBs and CCBs. They also make little or no difference to the number of heart attacks, which may not be different from that of diuretics, ACE inhibitors/ARBs, and CCBs. The evidence of β-blockers on effects like modest CVD reduction, little or no effects on mortality are inferior to other antihypertensive drugs generated from studies on one traditional β- blocker, atenolol and it is unjust to extrapolate data of one drug to its entire class. Among all β-blockers, vasodilatory β-blockers such as nebivolol are found to be more effective. Therefore, further research is needed to explore the differences between different subtypes of β-blockers.

■ REFERENCES

1. Anchala R, Kannuri NK, Pant H, et al. Hypertension in India: a systematic review and meta-analysis of prevalence, awareness, and control of hypertension. J Hypertens. 2014;32(6):1170-7.

2. Gupta R, Gaur K, Ram CV. Emerging trends in hypertension epidemiology in India. J Human Hypertens. 2018. [Epub ahead of print].

3. Oparil S, Zaman MA, Calhoun DA. Pathogenesis of hypertension. Ann Intern Med. 2003;139(9):761-76.

4. Ram CV. Beta-blockers in hypertension. Am J Cardiol. 2010;106(12):1819-25.

5. Gupta S, Wright HM. Nebivolol: a highly selective beta1-adrenergic receptor blocker that causes vasodilation by increasing nitric oxide. Cardiovasc Ther. 2008;26(3):189-202.

6. Mancia G, Fagard R, Narkiewicz K, et al. 2013 ESH/ESC Guidelines for the management of arterial hypertension: the Task Force for the management of arterial hypertension of the European Society of Hypertension (ESH) and of the European Society of Cardiology (ESC). J Hypertens. 2013;31(7):1281-357.

7. Guo G. Beta-blockers in uncomplicated hypertension: Is it time for retirement? October, 2015.

8. Wiysonge CS, Bradley HA, Volmink J, et al. Beta-blockers for hypertension. Cochrane Database Syst Rev. 2017;1:CD002003.

9. Yancy CW, Jessup M, Bozkurt B, et al. 2013 ACCF/AHA guideline for the management of heart failure: executive summary: a report of the American College of Cardiology Foundation/American Heart Association Task Force on practice guidelines. Circulation. 2013;128(16):1810-52.

10. Fihn SD, Blankenship JC, Alexander KP, et al. 2014 ACC/AHA/AATS/PCNA/SCAI/STS focused update of the guideline for the diagnosis and management of patients with stable ischemic heart disease: a report of the American College of Cardiology/American Heart Association Task Force on Practice Guidelines, and the American Association for Thoracic Surgery, Preventive Cardiovascular Nurses Association, Society for Cardiovascular Angiography and Interventions, and Society of Thoracic Surgeons. Circulation. 2014;130(19):1749-67.

11. Amsterdam EA, Wenger NK, Brindis RG, et al. 2014 AHA/ACC guideline for the management of patients with non-ST-elevation acute coronary syndromes: executive summary: a report of the American College of Cardiology/American Heart Association Task Force on Practice Guidelines. Circulation. 2014;130(25):2354-94.

12. Zipes DP, Camm AJ, Borggrefe M, et al. ACC/AHA/ESC 2006 Guidelines for Management of Patients with Ventricular Arrhythmias and the Prevention of Sudden Cardiac Death: a report of the American College of Cardiology/American Heart Association Task Force and the European Society of Cardiology Committee for Practice Guidelines (writing committee to develop Guidelines for Management of Patients with Ventricular Arrhythmias and the Prevention of Sudden Cardiac Death): developed in collaboration with the European Heart Rhythm Association and the Heart Rhythm Society. Circulation. 2006;114(10):e385-484.

13. Ritz E, Rump LC. Do β-blockers combined with RAS inhibitors make sense after all to protect against renal injury? Curr Hypertens Rep. 2007;9(5):409-14.

14. Marketou M, Gupta Y, Jain S, et al. Differential Metabolic Effects of Beta-Blockers: an Updated Systematic Review of Nebivolol. Curr Hypertens Rep. 2017;19(3):22.

15. Frishman WH. A historical perspective on the development of β-adrenergic blockers. J Clin Hypertens. 2007;9(4):19-27.

16. Chobanian AV, Bakris GL, Black HR, et al. Seventh report of the Joint National Committee on Prevention, Detection, Evaluation, and Treatment of High Blood Pressure. Hypertension. 2003;42(6):1206-52.

17. Beevers G, Lip GY, O'Brien E. ABC of hypertension: The pathophysiology of hypertension. BMJ. 2001;322(7291):912-6.

18. Bangalore S, Parkar S, Grossman E, et al. A meta-analysis of 94,492 patients with hypertension treated with beta blockers to determine the risk of new-onset diabetes mellitus. Am J Cardiol. 2007;100(8):1254-62.

Angiotensin-converting Enzyme Inhibitor in Hypertension

Bhivaji R Bansode

■ INTRODUCTION

Hypertension is silent killer, when symptomatic patients have always some complication. Timely intervention done in these patients can save the life of patient. Five classes of antihypertensive drugs and lifestyle modification are the sheath anchor in the management of hypertension. Five classes of drugs are:

1. Angiotensin-converting enzyme (ACE)/ angiotensin receptor blocker (ARB)
2. Calcium channel blocker
3. Diuretics
4. Beta-blockers
5. Vasodilator and renin inhibitors.

Among these drugs renin–angiotensin system (RAS) blockers are most useful antihypertensive drugs in patient with hypertension. The RAS participates in the pathophysiology of hypertension, congestive heart failure, myocardial infarction, and diabetic nephropathy. This realization has led to a thorough exploration of the RAS and the development of new approaches for inhibiting its actions. Here we discuss the physiology of the classical RAS and novel RAS components. We also discuss the basic pharmacology of important class of drugs that inhibit ACE, and their clinical utility.

■ HISTORY

Tiegerstedt and Bergman discovered in 1898 that a pressor substance was present in crude saline extracts of kidney; they called it renin. Goldblatt and his colleagues reported in 1934 that there was persistent hypertension in dogs due to constriction of the renal arteries. Braun-Menéndez and his colleagues in Argentina and Page and Helmer in the United States noted in 1940 that renin was an enzyme acting on a plasma protein substrate for catalyzing the development of the actual pressor material, a peptide called hypertensin by the former group and angiotonin by the latter group. Finally, angiotensin was the name given to pressor substance, and plasma substrate was named as angiotensinogen.

Decapeptide (Ang I) and an octapeptide (Ang II) are the two forms of angiotensin, which are formed by the proteolytic cleavage of Ang I by an enzyme called ACE; these two forms were identified in the mid-1950s. The more active form was the octapeptide. It was synthesized in 1957 by Schwyzer and Bumpus and then it was accessible for extensive research. It was reported in later research that the kidneys are a significant site of aldosterone action and that in humans angiotensin potently stimulates aldosterone production. In addition, with Na^+ depletion, there is increase in renin secretion. The RAS was therefore identified as a mechanism to stimulate synthesis and secretion of aldosterone and as a significant homeostatic mechanism for regulating blood pressure and composition of electrolytes.

Polypeptides, which either inhibited the Ang II formation or blocked Ang II receptors, were discovered in the early 1970s. These inhibitors demonstrated significant pathophysiological and physiological roles for the RAS and motivated the development of a new and broadly effective class of anti-hypertensive drugs, i.e. the orally active ACE inhibitors. Studies with the ACE inhibitors revealed RAS roles in pathophysiology of vascular disease, heart failure, hypertension, and renal failure.

CLASSICAL RENIN–ANGIOTENSIN SYSTEM

Through the actions of Ang II, the RAS participates in blood pressure regulation, aldosterone release, Na^+-reabsorption from renal tubules, electrolyte and fluid homeostasis, and cardiovascular remodeling. Ang II is derived from angiotensinogen in two proteolytic steps. First, the enzyme renin, released into the circulation from the juxtaglomerular (JG) cells in the kidneys, cleaves the decapeptide Ang I from the amino terminus of angiotensinogen (renin substrate). Then, an ACE, located on the endothelial cell lining of the vasculature, removes the carboxy-terminal dipeptide of Ang I to produce the octapeptide Ang II. Ang II acts by binding to two distinct heptaspanning G-protein-coupled receptors (GPCRs), AT1 and AT2.

New Paradigms in the Renin–Angiotensin System

The RAS has expanded from being solely an endocrine system to include a paracrine, autocrine or intracrine hormonal system with several new components and active pathways. The current understanding of the RAS involves local (tissue) RAS; alternative pathways for Ang II synthesis (ACE independent and renin independent); an ACE2/Ang (1–7)/Mas receptor axis that opposes the vasoconstrictor effects of ACE/Ang II/AT1 receptor axis; an Ang IV/AT4 receptor axis that is important in brain functions and cognition; multiple biologically active angiotensin peptides such Ang (1–9), Ang III, Ang (3–7), angiotensin A, and alamandine; multiple receptors for angiotensin (AT1, AT2, AT4; Mas; and MrgD); and the PRR.[1] Differential activation of these multiple arms of the RAS may underlie the pathophysiological outcome in cardiovascular and renal disease (Campbell, 2014; Santos, 2014).

Components of the Renin–Angiotensin System (Flowchart 1)

Renin

Renin is the major determinant of the rate of Ang II production; its secretion is regulated by several mechanisms. Renin is synthesized, stored, and secreted by exocytosis into the renal arterial circulation by the granular JG cells located in the walls of the afferent arterioles that enter the glomeruli. Renin is an aspartyl protease that cleaves the bond between residues 10 and 11 at the amino terminus of angiotensinogen to generate Ang I. The t1/2 of circulating renin is about 15 minutes.

Control of Renin Secretion

Renin is secreted by the granular cells within the JG apparatus and is regulated by the following pathways:
- The macula densa pathway
- The intrarenal baroreceptor pathway
- The β1 adrenergic receptor pathway.

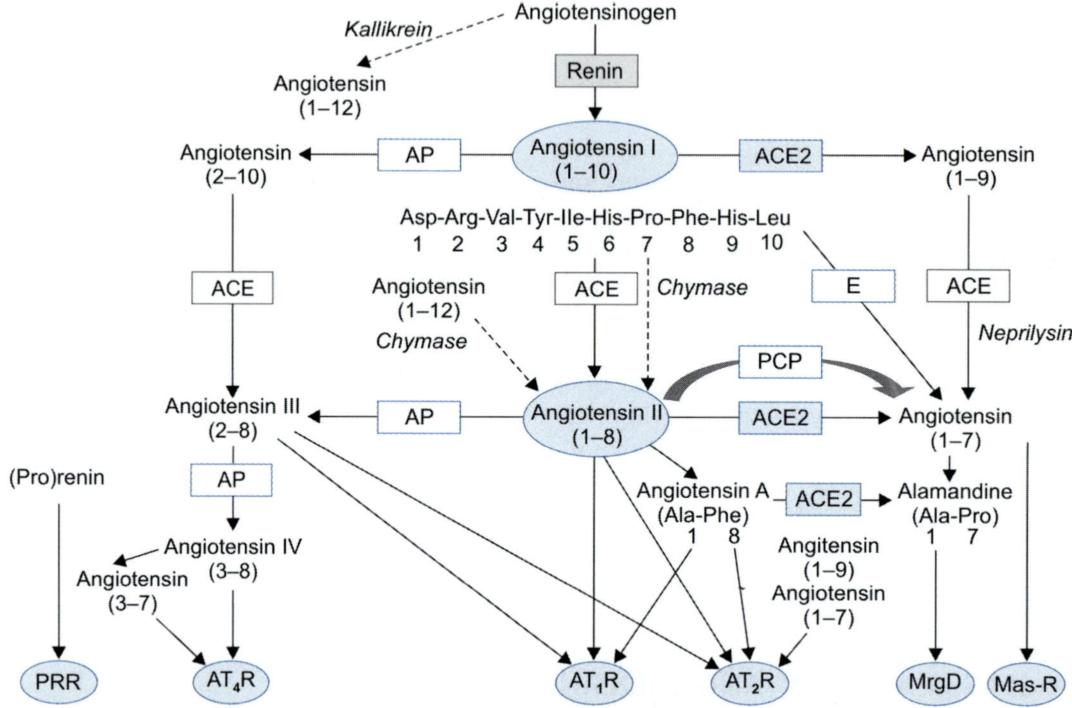

(ACE: angiotensin-converting enzyme; AP: aminopeptidase; E: endopeptidases; PCP: prolylcarboxypeptidase; RAS: drugs renin–angiotensin system)

Flowchart 1: Components of the RAS. The heavy arrows show the classical pathway, and the light arrows indicate alternative pathways. Receptors involved: AT1, AT2, AT4, Mas, MrgD and PRR.

Angiotensin II

Major physiological effects of Ang II have been shown in flowchart 2.

Angiotensin-converting enzyme 2 is not inhibited by the standard ACE inhibitors and has no effect on bradykinin. Reduced expression or deletion of ACE2 is associated with hypertension, defects in cardiac contractility, and elevated levels of Ang II (Flowchart 3). Inhibition of AT1 receptors by ARBs increases the expression of ACE2. Overexpression of the *ACE2* gene decreases blood pressure and prevents Ang II-induced cardiac hypertrophy in hypertensive rats. ACE2 is protective against diabetic nephropathy through the Ang (1–7)/Mas receptor pathway (Varagic et al., 2014). Ang (1–9), which is generated from Ang I by ACE2, may also have vasodilating and protective effects by activating AT2 receptors (Etelvino et al., 2014). In addition, ACE2 metabolizes Apelin peptides, serves as a receptor for the severe acute respiratory syndrome coronavirus, and has been reported to interact with and regulate amino acid transporters (Kuba et al., 2013).

◼ ANGIOTENSIN-CONVERTING ENZYME INHIBITORS

Pharmacological Effects

The ACE inhibitors inhibit the conversion of Ang I to Ang II. Inhibition of Ang II production lowers blood pressure and enhances natriuresis. ACE is an enzyme with many

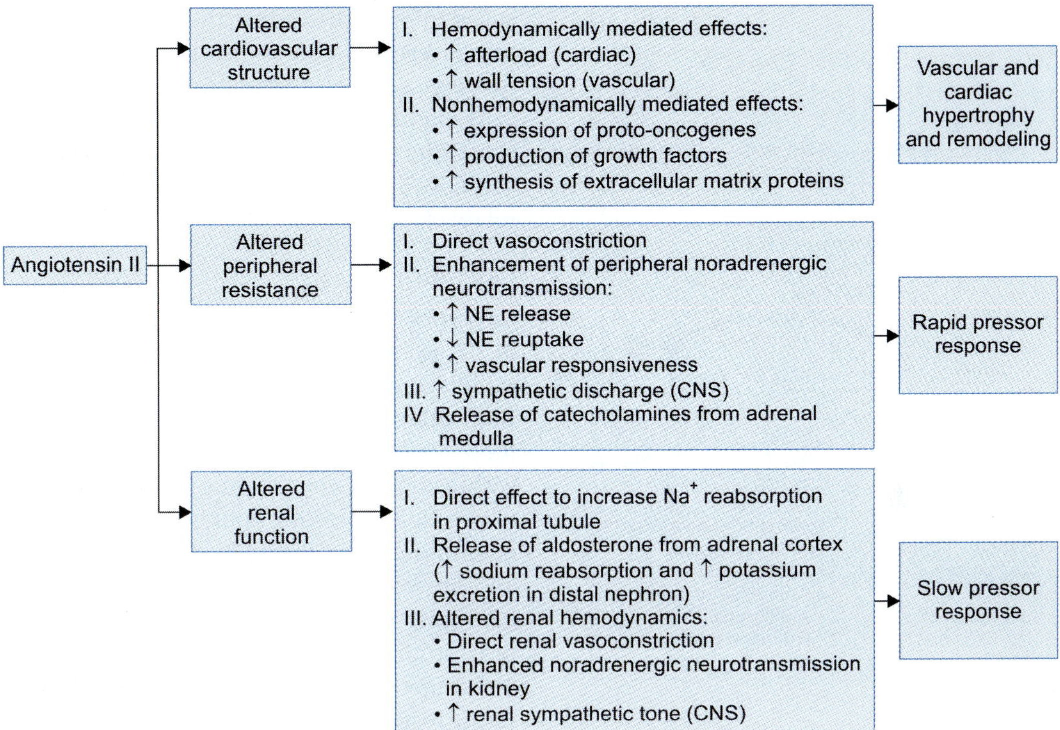

Flowchart 2: Physiological effects of Ang II.

substrates; thus, there are other consequences of its inhibition, including inhibition of the degradation of bradykinin, which has beneficial antihypertensive and protective effects.

The ACE inhibitors enhance the circulating levels of the natural stem cell regulator Ac-SDKP by 5-fold, which can also add to the cardioprotective effects of ACE inhibitors (Rhaleb et al., 2001). ACE inhibitors will enhance release of renin and rate of formation of Ang I by interfering with both the short-loop and the long-loop negative feedbacks on release of renin. Accumulating Ang I is directed down the alternative metabolic routes, which leads to enhanced vasodilator peptide production like Ang (1–9) and Ang (1–7).

Clinical Pharmacology

On the basis of the chemical structure, ACE inhibitors can be classified into three broad groups—(1) dicarboxyl-containing ACE inhibitors that are structurally related to enalapril (such as benazepril, lisinopril, moexipril, quinapril, ramipril, perindopril, and trandolapril); (2) the sulfhydryl-containing ACE inhibitors structurally related to captopril; and (3) the phosphorus-containing ACE inhibitors that are structurally related to fosinopril.[2]

All ACE inhibitors block the conversion of Ang I to Ang II and have similar therapeutic indications, adverse-effect profiles, and contraindications. Life-long treatment is generally required for hypertension, so in comparing the antihypertensive drugs, it is

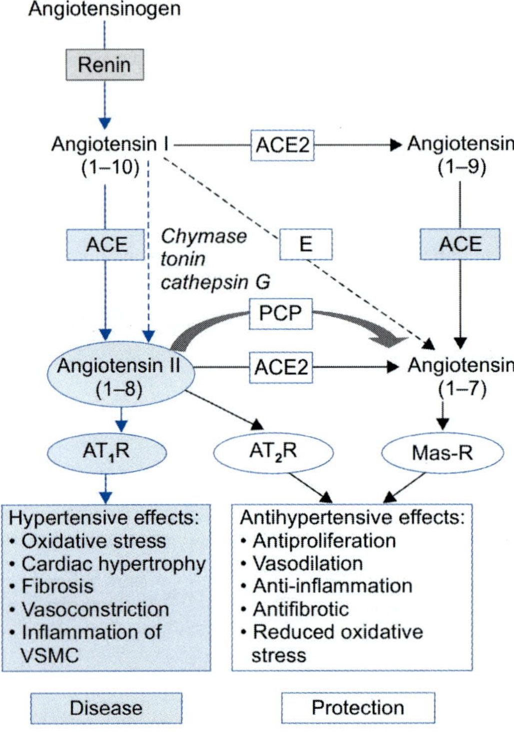

(ACE: angiotensin-converting enzyme; E: endopeptidase; PCP: prolylcarboxypeptidase; VSMC: vascular smooth muscle cells)

Flowchart 3: Schematic diagram of opposing arms in the RAS. Therapeutic interventions aim to inhibit the ACE/Angiotensin II/AT1 receptor axis (cyan) and enhance ACE2/Angiotensin (1–7)/Mas receptor axis (white).

important to consider the quality of life issues. Kidneys predominantly clear ACE inhibitors; trandolapril, fosinopril and quinapril, which show balanced elimination by the kidneys and liver, are the exceptions. Plasma clearance of most of the ACE inhibitors is substantially decreased by impaired renal function. In patients having renal impairment, dosage of these drugs should be decreased. Patients are rendered hyper-responsive to ACE inhibitor-induced hypotension by increase in plasma renin activity (PRA). In patients with elevated plasma levels of renin, such as in the patients with heart failure and during

salt depletion including the use of diuretic, initial doses of all the ACE inhibitors should be decreased. ACE inhibitors differ markedly in tissue distribution, and it is possible that this difference could be exploited to inhibit some local (tissue) RAS while leaving others relatively intact.

Captopril

Captopril is a potent ACE inhibitor with a Ki of 1.7 nM. Given orally, captopril is absorbed rapidly and has a bioavailability of about 75%. Bioavailability is reduced by 25–30% with food. Peak concentrations in plasma occur within an hour, and the drug is cleared rapidly, with a t1/2 of about 2 hours. Most of the drug is eliminated in urine, 40–50% as captopril and the rest as captopril disulfide dimers and captopril–cysteine disulfide. The oral dose of captopril ranges from 6.25 mg to 150 mg 2–3 times daily, with 6.25 mg thrice daily or 25 mg twice daily appropriate for the initiation of therapy for heart failure or hypertension, respectively.

Enalapril

Enalapril maleate is a prodrug that is hydrolyzed by esterases in the liver to produce enalaprilat, the active dicarboxylic acid. Enalaprilat is a potent inhibitor of ACE with a Ki of 0.2 nM. Enalapril is absorbed rapidly when given orally and has an oral bioavailability of about 60% (not reduced by food). Although peak concentrations of enalapril in plasma occur within an hour, enalaprilat concentrations peak only after 3–4 hours. Enalapril has a t1/2 of about 1.3 hour, but enalaprilat, because of tight binding to ACE, has a plasma t1/2 of about 11 hours. Elimination occurs through kidneys either as intact enalapril or enalaprilat. Daily oral dose of enalapril ranges from 2.5 mg to 40 mg daily. For initiating therapy, in case of heart failure 2.5 mg and for hypertension 5 mg daily is appropriate.

Enalaprilat

Enalaprilat is poorly absorbed orally, but in case if oral therapy is not appropriate, it is accessible for intravenous administration. The dosage is 0.625–1.25 mg given intravenously over 5 minutes for hypertensive patients. This dose can be repeated every 6 hours.

Lisinopril

Lisinopril is a lysine analog of enalaprilat. Lisinopril is itself active, unlike enalapril. In vitro, as compared to enalaprilat, lisinopril is a slightly more potent ACE inhibitor. Through oral administration, the absorption of lisinopril is slow, variable, and incomplete (approximately 30%); although absorption of lisinopril is not reduced by food. In plasma, peak concentrations are achieved in approximately 7 hours. It is excreted unchanged by the kidney with a plasma t1/2 of about 12 hours. Accumulation of lisinopril does not occur in tissues. Lisinopril oral dosage ranges from 5 mg to 40 mg daily (single or in divided dose); dose of 5 mg and 10 mg daily is appropriate for heart failure and hypertension therapy initiation, respectively. For patients with heart failure with hyponatremia or renal impairment, a daily dosage of 2.5 mg is recommended with close medical supervision.

Benazepril

Benazepril, which is a prodrug, is transformed into benazeprilat by the cleavage of the ester moiety by hepatic esterases. After oral administration, absorption of benazepril is rapid but incomplete (37%) as it reduced only slightly by food. Benazepril is almost entirely metabolized to the benazeprilat and to the glucuronide conjugates of benazeprilat and benazepril that are excreted into the bile and urine. In plasma, peak concentrations of benazepril are achieved in 0.5–1 hours and that of benazeprilat in 1–2 hours. The benazeprilat has an effective plasma half-life of 10–11 hours. Accumulation of benazeprilat does not occur in tissues except for the lungs. Benazepril's oral dosage is from 5 mg to 80 mg daily (in single or divided dose).

Fosinopril

Fosinopril is transformed into fosinoprilat by cleavage of the ester moiety by hepatic esterases. After oral administration, absorption of fosinopril is slow but incomplete (36%); rate is reduced by food, but extent remains unaffected. Fosinopril is mostly metabolized to the fosinoprilat (75%) and to glucuronide conjugate of fosinoprilat. In both, the urine and the bile, these are excreted. Peak plasma concentrations of fosinoprilat are achieved in approximately 3 hours. The effective plasma half-life of fosinoprilat is approximately 11.5 hours, which is a figure that is not significantly altered by impairment in renal function. Its oral dosage is from 10 mg to 80 mg daily (in single or divided dose). In the patients with Na^+ or water depletion or renal failure, initial dose is decreased to 5 mg daily.

Trandolapril

After oral administration, trandolapril is absorbed and produces the plasma levels of trandolapril (bioavailability 10%) and trandolaprilat (bioavailability 70%); its absorption is not reduced by food. As an ACE inhibitor, trandolaprilat is about eight times more potent as compared to trandolapril.

De-esterification products and glucuronides of trandolapril are recovered in feces (66%) and urine (33%, largely trandolaprilat). In plasma, peak concentrations of trandolaprilat are achieved in 4–10 hours.

Biphasic elimination kinetics are showed by trandolaprilat, with an initial half-life of approximately 10 hours (which is the significant component of elimination), which is followed by a longer half-life (that is due to slow dissociation of trandolaprilat from the tissue ACE). Both the renal insufficiency and the hepatic insufficiency decrease plasma clearance of the trandolaprilat. Oral dosage of trandolaprilat ranges from 1 mg to 8 mg daily (in single or divided dose). In patients taking diuretic or having renal impairment, the initial dose is 0.5 mg.

Quinapril

Quinapril, which is a prodrug, is transformed into quinaprilat by cleavage of the ester moiety. Oral absorption of quinapril is rapid; in 1 hour, peak concentrations are attained. The rate of oral absorption (60%) may be reduced by food—delayed peak; extent is not affected by food. Excretion of quinaprilat and the other minor metabolites of quinapril occur in urine (61%) as well as in feces (37%). In about 2 hours, peak concentrations of the quinaprilat in plasma are attained. In patients with diminished liver function, there is a reduction in conversion of quinapril to quinaprilat. The initial half-life of the quinaprilat is approximately 2 hours. Due to the high-affinity binding of the drug to tissue ACE, there can be a longer terminal t1/2 of approximately 25 hours. The quinapril's oral dosage ranges from 5 to 80 mg daily.

Ramipril

Orally administered ramipril is absorbed rapidly (peak concentrations in 1 hour; the rate but not extent of its oral absorption (50%–60%) is reduced by food. Ramipril is metabolized to ramiprilat by hepatic esterases and to inactive metabolites that are excreted predominantly by the kidneys. Peak concentrations of ramiprilat in plasma are achieved in about 3 hours. Ramiprilat displays triphasic elimination kinetics (t1/2 values: 2–4, 9–18, and more than 50 hours). This triphasic elimination is due to extensive distribution to all tissues (initial t1/2), clearance of free ramiprilat from plasma (intermediate t1/2), and dissociation of ramiprilat from tissue ACE (long terminal t1/2). The oral dosage of ramipril ranges from 1.25 mg to 20 mg daily (single or divided dose).

Moexipril

Antihypertensive activity of moexipril is because of its deesterified metabolite, i.e. moexiprilat. Absorption of moexipril occurs incompletely; the bioavailability of moexiprilat is approximately 13%. Food reduces bioavailability of moexiprilat. Peak concentration of moexiprilat in plasma is achieved in about 1.5 hours. The elimination half-life ranges from 2 hours to 12 hours. Recommended dosage range is from 7.5 mg to 30 mg daily (in single or divided doses). Among patients taking diuretics or having renal impairment, dosage range is halved.

Perindopril

Perindopril erbumine is a prodrug. Hepatic esterases transform 30–50% of the systemically available perindopril into perindoprilat. Food does not affect the oral bioavailability of perindopril (75%); however, food reduces bioavailability of perindoprilat by approximately 35%. Perindopril is metabolized to inactive metabolites and perindoprilat; these are excreted mainly by the kidneys. The time to peak plasma concentration of perindoprilat is 3–7 hours. Biphasic elimination kinetics is showed by perindoprilat, with half-life of approximately 3–10 hours (which is the significant component of elimination), and 30–120 hours (that is due to slow dissociation of perindoprilat from the tissue ACE). The recommended oral dosage range is 2–16 mg daily (in single or divided dose).

Therapeutic Uses of Angiotensin-converting Enzyme Inhibitors

The ACE inhibitors are used in the treatment of diabetic nephropathy, cardiovascular disease and heart failure.

Angiotensin-converting Enzyme Inhibitors in Hypertension

Angiotensin-converting enzyme inhibition reduces systemic vascular resistance and mean, diastolic, and systolic blood pressures in many hypertensive states except when primary aldosteronism causes high blood pressure. Prior to treatment, the initial change in blood pressure is positively correlated with Ang II plasma levels and PRA.[3] Some patients, however, may demonstrate a sizable decrease in blood pressure that is poorly correlated with pretreatment values of PRA. Enhanced tissue responsiveness to normal Ang II levels or increased local (tissue) production of Ang II may make some hypertensive patients sensitive to the ACE inhibitors despite normal PRA.

In hypertensive individuals treated with ACE inhibitors, the long-term fall in systemic blood pressure is noted that is accompanied by a leftward shift in the renal pressure–natriuresis curve and a decrease in total peripheral resistance (TPR) in which different vascular beds have variable involvement. The kidney is a notable exception. Since the renal vessels are extremely sensitive to Ang II's vasoconstrictor actions, ACE inhibitors enhance the flow of renal blood through efferent and afferent arterioles vasodilatation. Without an increase in glomerular filtration rate, increased renal blood flow occurs; therefore, the filtration fraction is decreased.

The ACE inhibitors lead to systemic arteriolar dilation and increase in the compliance of large arteries. This results in decrease of systolic pressure. There is generally little change in cardiac function in patients with uncomplicated hypertension, although the stroke volume and the cardiac output may rise slightly with sustained treatment. Cardiovascular reflexes and baroreceptor function are not compromised and there is little impairment in response to exercise and postural changes. Even if there is a significant reduction in blood pressure, heart rate and plasma catecholamine levels are usually only slightly increase, if at all. This may reflect a baroreceptor function alteration with enhanced arterial compliance and the loss of Ang II's normal tonic influence on the sympathetic nervous system.

The ACE inhibitors reduce but not seriously impair the secretion of aldosterone. Other steroidogenic stimuli such as adrenocorticotropic hormone and K^+ maintain the secretion of aldosterone at appropriate levels. These secretagogues' activity on the adrenal cortex's zone glomerulosa needs very small trophic or permissive amounts of Ang II that are always present because ACE inhibition is never complete. Excessive K^+ retention is found in patients with renal impairment, in those taking supplementary K^+, or in those taking other medications that decrease excretion of K^+.

In approximately 50% of patients with mild-to-moderate hypertension, the ACE inhibitors alone normalize blood pressure. The combination of an ACE inhibitor and a Ca^{2+} channel blocker, a $\beta 1$ adrenergic receptor blocker, or a diuretic will control 90% of patients with mild-to-moderate hypertension. Diuretics increase the antihypertensive response to ACE inhibitors by making the blood pressure of patients' renin dependent. For the management of hypertension, many ACE inhibitors are marketed in fixed-dose combinations along with a Ca^{2+} channel blocker or thiazide diuretic.

Use of Angiotensin-converting Enzyme Inhibitors in Left Ventricular Systolic Dysfunction

Unless contraindication is there, all patients with impaired left ventricular systolic function should be given ACE inhibitors regardless of whether or not they have symptoms of the overt heart failure. It is shown by many large clinical studies that ACE inhibition in patients with systolic dysfunction delays or prevents heart failure progression; reduces the incidence of myocardial infarction and sudden death; reduces hospitalization; and enhances quality of life. ACE inhibition generally decreases afterload and systolic wall stress and increases both cardiac index and cardiac output, as do indices of stroke volume and stroke work. Ang II reduces arterial compliance in systolic dysfunction, and this is reversed by inhibition of ACE. In general, the heart rate is decreased. Systemic blood pressure falls at the beginning, sometimes steeply, but tends to return to initial levels. There is a sharp fall in renovascular resistance and an increase in renal blood flow. Natriuresis results from enhanced renal hemodynamics, decreased stimulus to secretion of the aldosterone by Ang II, and decreased direct effects of the Ang II on kidney. There is a decrease in venous return to the right side of the heart due to contraction of excess volume of body fluids. There is a further reduction, which results from venodilation and increased capacity of the venous bed.

While Ang II possess little acute venoconstrictor activity, its long-term infusion helps to increase venous tone, perhaps through peripheral or central interactions with the sympathetic nervous system. In addition, the response to ACE inhibitors includes decreases in pulmonary capillary wedge pressure, pulmonary arterial pressure, and left atrial and ventricular filling volumes and pressures. Preload stress and diastolic wall stress are therefore reduced. Due to better hemodynamic performance, there is increased exercise tolerance and suppression of the sympathetic nervous system. Even when there is a reduction in systemic blood pressure, coronary and cerebral blood flows

are usually well maintained. ACE inhibitors decrease ventricular dilation in heart failure and tend to restore normal elliptical shape of the heart. ACE inhibitors can reverse ventricular remodeling through preload/afterload changes by prevention of growth effects of Ang II on the myocytes and by attenuation of cardiac fibrosis, which is induced by aldosterone and Ang II.

Use of Angiotensin-converting Enzyme Inhibitors in Acute Myocardial Infarction

In acute myocardial infarction, the useful effects of ACE inhibitors are especially large in case of diabetic and hypertensive patients. Unless there is a contraindication (such as severe hypotension or cardiogenic shock), use of ACE inhibitors should be initiated immediately during the acute phase of myocardial infarction.[4] It can be administered with aspirin, thrombolytics, and beta-adrenergic receptor antagonists (ACE Inhibitor Myocardial Infarction Collaborative Group, 1998). ACE inhibition should be continued for long term in high-risk patients (such as systolic ventricular dysfunction and large infarct).

Use of Angiotensin-converting Enzyme Inhibitors in Patients Who Are at High Risk of Cardiovascular Events

Treatment with ACE inhibitors greatly benefits patients at high risk of cardiovascular events (Heart Outcomes Prevention Study Investigators, 2000). ACE inhibition significantly reduces the rate of stroke, myocardial infarction, and death in patients with no ventricular dysfunction but with evidence of diabetes or vascular disease and one another risk factor for cardiovascular disease. ACE inhibition reduces cardiovascular disease death and myocardial infarction in patients with coronary artery disease but without heart failure (European Trial, 2003).

Use of Angiotensin-converting Enzyme Inhibitors in Diabetes Mellitus and Renal Failure

The leading cause of renal disease is diabetes mellitus. ACE inhibitors prevent or delay the progression of renal disease in patients with type 1 diabetes mellitus (TIDM) and diabetic nephropathy, enabling renoprotection as defined by changes in excretion of albumin. In T1DM, the renoprotective effects of ACE inhibitors are partly independent of reduction in blood pressure. Furthermore, ACE inhibitors may reduce the progression of retinopathy in T1DM and reduce the renal insufficiency progression in patients with a variety of nondiabetic nephropathies (Ruggenenti et al., 2010).

Several mechanisms are involved in ACE inhibitors' renal protective effects. Increased glomerular capillary pressure causes glomerular injury, and by reducing arterial blood pressure and dilating renal efferent arterioles, ACE inhibitors decrease this parameter. ACE inhibitors improve the filtering membrane's permeability selectivity, thereby decreasing the mesangium's exposure to proteinaceous factors that may stimulate the proliferation of mesangial cells and the production of matrix, which are the two processes that make a contribution to the expansion of the mesangium in case of diabetic nephropathy. As Ang II is a growth factor, decreases in Ang II's intrarenal levels may further leads to attenuation of mesangial cell growth and production of matrix. ACE inhibitors improve levels of Ang (1–7) by hindering its metabolism by ACE. Ang (1–7) binds to Mas receptors and has protective and antifibrotic effects (Santos, 2014). In the setting of diabetes, at the level of renal epithelial podocytes, activation of AT1 receptors leads to activation of protein kinase signaling cascades, cytoskeletal rearrangements, retraction of podocyte processes, and a reduction in proteins of the slit diaphragm, all resulting in increased permeability of the renal epithelium to proteins (proteinuria). ACE inhibitors reduce these effects of Ang II (Márquez et al., 2015).

Angiotensin-converting Enzyme Inhibitors in Scleroderma Renal Crisis

The use of ACE inhibitors considerably improves survival of patients with scleroderma renal crisis.

Adverse Effects of Angiotensin-converting Enzyme Inhibitors

In general, ACE inhibitors are well tolerated. The drugs do not change Ca^{2+} or uric acid plasma concentrations and may enhance insulin sensitivity and glucose tolerance in patients with insulin resistance and reduce lipoprotein(a) and cholesterol levels in proteinuric renal disease.

Hypotension

A steep drop in blood pressure in patients with high PRA may happen after the first dose of an ACE inhibitor. Patients with salt depletion, multiple antihypertensive drugs, or congestive heart failure should be treated with care.

Cough

Angiotensin-converting enzyme inhibitors induce a troublesome, dry cough that is mediated by accumulation of bradykinin, substance P or prostaglandins (PGs) in lungs, in 5–20% of the patients. Iron supplementation, thromboxane antagonism, and aspirin decrease cough induced by ACE inhibitors. Supplementation with thromboxane, aspirin and iron reduces cough caused by ACE inhibitors. Reducing the dose of ACE or switching to an ARB may be effective at times. The cough disappears after stopping ACE inhibitors, generally within 4 days.

Hyperkalemia

In patients with normal renal function, significant K^+ retention is rarely found. However, in patients with renal insufficiency or diabetes, or in patients taking K^+ supplements, K^+-sparing diuretics, beta-receptor blockers, or nonsteroidal anti-inflammatory drugs (NSAIDs), ACE inhibitors may cause hyperkalemia.

Acute Renal Failure

Angiotensin-converting enzyme inhibition can result in acute renal insufficiency in patients with bilateral renal artery stenosis; artery stenosis to a single remaining kidney; heart failure; or volume depletion due to diarrhea or diuretics.

Angioedema

In about 0.1–0.5% of the patients, rapid swelling is induced by ACE inhibitors in the nose, mouth, lips, tongue, throat, glottis or larynx. Disappearance of angioedema is noted within hours, after stopping the ACE inhibitors. In the meantime, the airway of the patient should be protected and epinephrine—an antihistamine—or a glucocorticoid should be administered, if necessary. As compared to Caucasians, there is a 4.5 times greater risk of ACE inhibitor-induced angioedema in African Americans. Although rarely, angioedema of the intestine (visceral angioedema), which is characterized by watery diarrhea, emesis and abdominal pain, also has been reported. Angioedema induced by ACE inhibitor is a class effect. No other drugs of the ACE inhibitor class should be prescribed for patients who develop this adverse event.

Fetopathic Potential

In pregnancy, it should be avoided. Fetal hypotension may cause the fetopathic effects.

Skin Rash

A maculopapular self-resolving rash (that can itch) can be caused by the ACE inhibitors; antihistamine may be required for the treatment.

Other Side Effects

Dysgeusia (a change in or loss of taste), glycosuria, neutropenia, hepatotoxicity and anemia are extremely rare but reversible side effects.

Drug Interactions

Bioavailability of the ACE inhibitors can be decreased by the antacids. Cough induced by ACE inhibitor can be worsen by Capsaicin. K^+ supplements and K^+-sparing diuretics may exacerbate hyperkalemia induced by the ACE inhibitors. NSAIDs (including aspirin) may decrease the antihypertensive response to the ACE inhibitors. Plasma levels of the digoxin and lithium and hypersensitivity reactions to the allopurinol can be increased by ACE inhibitors.

■ SUMMARY

Guidelines for using Angiotensin-Converting Enzyme Inhibitors

- ACE inhibitors should be taken 1 hour before meals on empty *stomach*. Follow the directions mentioned on the label on how often this medication should be taken. How long you need to take the medication, the number of doses you take each day, and the time allowed between doses will depend on the type of prescribed ACE inhibitor and your condition
- When taking ACE inhibitors, salt substitutes should not be used. These substitutes consist of potassium. Potassium is retained by ACE inhibitor medications in the body. One should learn how to

read food labels in order to select foods with low-potassium and low-sodium. A dietician can assist you in choosing the right food
- Over-the-counter NSAIDs such as *Aleve* and *Motrin* should be avoided. These drugs can lead the body to retain water and sodium and reduce an ACE inhibitor's effect. Before taking any anti-inflammatory drugs, consult with your doctor
- As recommended by your physician, your blood pressure and renal function should be regularly checked while taking this medicine
- Medication should never be stopped without consulting with doctor, even if a patient feels that it is not working. If you are taking ACE inhibitors for the heart failure, your symptoms of heart failure may not improve immediately. Long-term use of ACE inhibitors, however, helps in managing chronic heart failure and in decreasing the risk of worsening of your condition.

Can Angiotensin-converting Enzyme Inhibitors be Recommended in Pregnant Women?

Use of ACE inhibitors should be avoided during pregnancy, particularly during the 2nd and 3rd trimesters. During *pregnancy*, ACE inhibitors can reduce blood pressure and cause renal failure or elevated levels of potassium in the mother's blood. In the *newborn*, they can cause death or deformity.

Can Angiotensin-converting Enzyme Inhibitors be Recommended in Children?

Yes, ACE inhibitors can be prescribed to children. Children, however, are more sensitive to the effects of these drugs on the blood pressure. Therefore, they are having a high risk of severe side effects from this drug. Before providing this medication to children, parents should be encouraged to discuss with their pediatric cardiologist the potential benefits and risks.

■ REFERENCES

1. Larry JJ, Kasper D, Hauser S, et al. Principles of Internal Medicine, 19th edition. New York: McGraw Hill Medical education; 2015.
2. McInnes G. Therapeutics of Hypertension. New York: Elsevier; 2008.
3. Muruganathan A. Manual of Hypertension. New Delhi: Jaypee Brothers Medical Publishers (P) Ltd.; 2016.
4. Williams B. Drug treatment of hypertension. BMJ. 2003; 326(7380):61-2.

Angiotensin Receptor Blocker— Newer Insights

Nihar Mehta, Saurabh Dhariya

■ INTRODUCTION

In spite of the availability of numbers of drugs for hypertension, blood pressure (BP) still remains a poorly controlled parameter in most. There is always a search for potent and safer new antihypertensive drugs. Drugs that modulate the renin–angiotensin–aldosterone system (RAAS) are used because of their efficacy and excellent tolerability profile. Here we are elaborating about the role of angiotensin II receptor blockers in managing primarily hypertension and other uses.

Angiotensin-converting enzyme (ACE) inhibitors inhibit the conversion of angiotensin I (AT_1) to angiotensin II (AT_2) whereas angiotensin receptor blockers (ARBs) antagonize receptor binding of AT_2 to AT_1 receptors. Therefore, it is often assumed that the two drug classes have similar efficacy in cardiovascular disease prevention. There are several important differences between the two classes, which play a vital role in the fine-tuning of BP control. In the last few years, amongst the novel anti-hypertensive medications available, the one with the most promise is an ARB—Azilsartan.

■ MECHANISM OF ACTION

The most prominent actions of ARB are as follows:

- Generalized arterial vasodilatation
- Vasodilatation of efferent and afferent glomerular arterioles, particularly efferent arteriole, which leads to reduction in intraglomerular pressures and leads to decrease in glomerular filtration rate (GFR) and urine albumin excretion
- Inhibition of aldosterone secretion.

In addition to these effects ARBs reduce proteinuria by direct improvement in the permissive properties of the glomerulus, independent of changes in glomerular hemodynamics. ARBs have an antifibrotic action, which could contribute to the slowing of renal and cardiac disease progression. The fall in protein excretion induced by RAAS inhibitor may be associated with a reduction in serum lipid levels (Fig. 1).

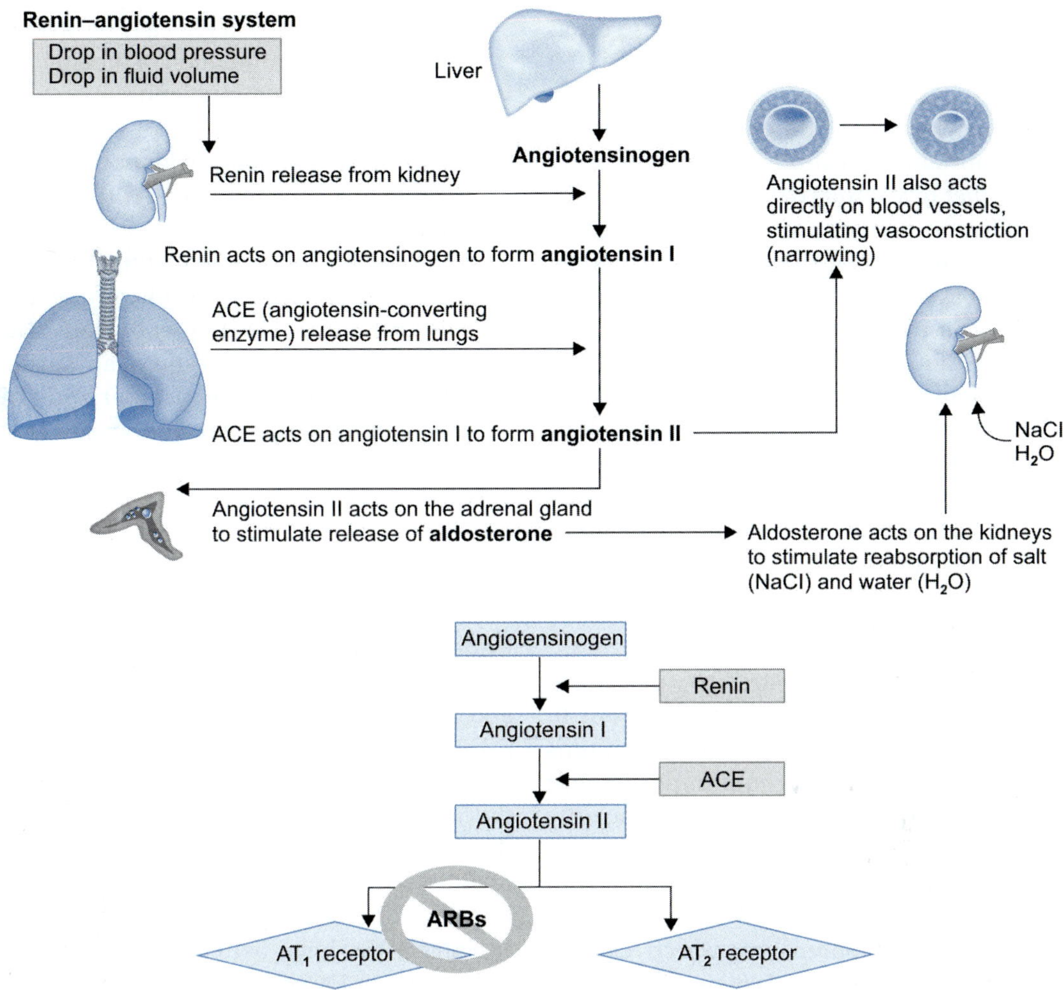

(ACE: angiotensin-converting enzyme)

Fig. 1: Angiotensin receptor blockers (ARBs) predominantly blocks angiotensin I (AT$_1$) receptors.

LIST OF ARBs WITH THEIR DOSING

Drug	Dose	Frequency/Day
Olmesartan	20–40 mg	1
Telmisartan	20–80 mg	1
Irbesartan	150–300 mg	1
Losartan	50–100 mg	1–2
Valsartan	80–320 mg	1
Candesartan	8–32 mg	1
Azilsartan	40–80 mg	1

USES OF ARBs

- *Hypertension*: ARBs have a pivotal role in controlling BP. They can be used as the first drug in treatment of naive patients; they can be used as monotherapy or combination therapy, and they have compelling indications in patients with associated comorbidities such as diabetes mellitus, chronic kidney disease, left ventricular dysfunction and postmyocardial infarction

- Left ventricular dysfunction—these drugs inhibit remodeling and preserve left ventricular function
- Postmyocardial infarction is one of the important indications for prevention of further myocardial damage
- It can be used as prevention or reduction of cardiovascular risk in high-risk patient such as diabetes mellitus with proteinuria
- *Other uses*:
  - Angiotensin receptor neprilysin inhibitor—sacubitril valsartan—for the management of heart failure with a reduced ejection fraction
  - Atrial fibrillation—telmisartan could have a role in prevention of atrial fibrillation.[1]

SIDE EFFECTS OF ARBs

- Hypotension appears to be more common with ARBs than ACE inhibitor. In ONTARGET trial, hypotensive symptoms severe enough to require permanent discontinuation occurred significantly more often with telmisartan. Weakness, dizziness and syncope result from excessive reduction in BP
- First-dose hypotension, which can be marked in hypovolemic patients with high baseline renin levels, can be minimized by not initiating therapy if the patient is volume depleted and by discontinuing prior diuretic therapy for 3–5 days
- A reduction in GFR, which is usually modest but may be severe can be seen in high risk patients who have bilateral renal arterial stenosis due to reduction in intraglomerular perfusion pressure
- Hyperkalemia seen usually in approximately 3.3%
- A dry, hacking cough has been described in 5–20% of patients treated with an ACE inhibitor, but it is very much less common in ARBs. Usually starts in 1–2 weeks of initiation of therapy. It typically resolves in 3–4 days of discontinuation of therapy
- Anemia due to erythropoietin suppression by ARBs
- *Angioedema*: Available evidence suggests the rate of angioedema with ARB therapy is low
- *Enteropathy with olmesartan*: In 2017, the United States Food and Drug Administration (FDA) reported that olmesartan could produce a "sprue-like enteropathy" characterized by severe chronic diarrhea and weight loss, occurring months to years after initiation of the drug.[2]

WHY AND HOW TO CHOOSE ARBs

Evidence exists for ACE inhibitor and ARBs in lowering BP, preventing cardiovascular events and preventing progression of nephropathy. Although there is no preference of ACE inhibitor over ARBs in BP reduction per say, the fact remains that ARBs are better tolerated than ACE inhibitor. The once-a-day dosing of ARBs also adds to the convenience and improves the adherence of patients. Some specific ARBs have beneficial effects such as losartan in lowering uric acid and candesartan in prevention of migraine. Therefore, ARBs are one of the most commonly used antihypertensive medications today (Table 1).

Amongst the various ARBs available, there are minor differences. A few studies have demonstrated that a greater percentage of patients treated with olmesartan achieved BP targets, compared to those who received initial doses of losartan, candesartan, valsartan and irbesartan, with a significant greater reduction of both clinical and ambulatory systolic and diastolic BP levels, after 1, 2, 4 and 8 weeks of therapy, both in naïve and previously treated patients and independent of the grade of hypertension.[3]

TABLE 1: Comparison between Angiotensin Converting Enzyme inhibitors and Angiotensin receptor blockers

Angiotensin-converting enzyme inhibitors	Angiotensin receptor blockers
Reduce the biosynthesis of angiotensin II (AT_2) produced by the action of ACE on angiotensin I (AT_1)	Reduce the activation of the AT_1 receptor more effectively than do ACE inhibitors
Do not inhibit the non-ACE angiotensin II generating pathways (escape pathway)	AT_1 inhibited irrespective of the biochemical pathway leading to the angiotensin II formation
ACE inhibitors increase the renin release. They are not associated with increased angiotensin II levels	ARBs also increase the renin release. Increased levels of angiotensin II are available to activate AT_2 receptors
• ACE inhibitors increase the levels of ACE substrates like bradykinin • Cough and angioedema are more common	• No effect on bradykinin metabolism • Cough and angioedema are less common

(ACE: angiotensin-converting enzyme)

■ AZILSARTAN

Azilsartan (EDARBI, Takeda) is an AT_2 receptor antagonist, approved by the FDA February 25, 2011 for the treatment of hypertension, alone, or in combination with other antihypertensive agents. Azilsartan is a selective AT_1 subtype AT_2 receptor antagonist. Effects mediated by the activation of AT_1 receptors include vasoconstriction, production and release of aldosterone, sodium reabsorption by the kidney, and activation of the sympathetic nervous system. The bioavailability of azilsartan is approximately 60% and is not affected by food. The time to peak plasma concentrations is within 1.5–3 hours after oral administration. Azilsartan is more than 99% protein bound and undergoes hepatic metabolism, primarily by CYP2C9. Renal clearance is approximately 2.3 mL/minute and the elimination half-life approximately 11 hours. Azilsartan of 80 mg is shown more effective control in BP as compared to 40 mg of olmesartan or 320 mg of valsartan in some trials.

■ RECENT TRIALS ABOUT ANGIOTENSIN RECEPTOR BLOCKER

- Two recent identically designed trials (one Italian and one European multinational) have compared the head-to-head efficacy and safety of the AT_2 receptor blocker olmesartan medoxomil and the angiotensin converting enzyme inhibitor ramipril, in elderly patients with essential hypertension. Olmesartan provides more effective BP control than ramipril in elderly hypertensive patients with and without metabolic syndrome[4]
- DETAIL study was done in subjects of diabetes exposed to telmisartan and enalapril. Systolic BP was reduced 6.9 mm Hg in the telmisartan group and 2.9 mm Hg in the enalapril group (95% CI, –8.5 to 0.5). Both groups experienced a decrease in GFR, but it was found that telmisartan was not inferior to enalapril in preventing the progression of renal disease[5]

- PRISMA Trial I, II is head-to-head comparison between ramipril and telmisartan. In this trial, dose of telmisartan and ramipril was 80 mg/day and 5–10 mg/day, respectively. This trial concluded that telmisartan is more effective than ramipril throughout the 24-hour period and during early morning[5]

- ONTARGET trial is a landmark trial, which confirms the role of telmisartan in reducing cardiac event rate in high-risk patients. Telmisartan was equivalent to ramipril for the primary outcome. Telmisartan shows lower possibility of bradykinin-mediated side effects than ramipril. Combination of these two drugs does not improve the outcome. Hence, to summarize, this trial RAAS blockade is necessary to reduce cardiac event and telmisartan is comparable to ramipril[6]

- PRoFESS (Prevention Regimen for Effectively Avoiding Second Strokes) is another randomized control trial that evaluated role of telmisartan in ischemia stroke. Therapy with telmisartan initiated soon after an ischemic stroke and continued for 2.5 years did not significantly lower the rate of recurrent stroke, major cardiovascular events, or diabetes[7]

- Transcend trial studied correlation between telmisartan and left ventricular mass. The researchers reported CV–related hospitalization in 30.3% of telmisartan participants and 33.0% of placebo participants [risk ratio (RR) = 0.92; 95% confidence interval (CI), 0.85–0.99]. Hypotensive symptoms occurred more often in participants in the telmisartan group (n = 29), compared with placebo (n = 16), though permanent discontinuation of the study medication occurred less often in the telmisartan group than in the placebo group (21.6% vs. 23.8%; p = 0.055). After 5 years of initiating telmisartan it reduces LVH in statistically significant number of patients and it reduces new onset LVH when compared with placebo[8]

- Latest review about choice of ARB in 2018 International Journal of Cardiology says "Olmesartan has a greater efficacy than irbesartan, valsartan, losartan and candesartan in reducing 24-hour ambulatory BP and diastolic BP after 8 weeks treatment". Similar results have been obtained in the BP CRUSH and the TRINITY [the TRIple therapy with olmesartan medoxomil, amlodipine, and hydrochlorothiazide (HCTZ) in hyperteNsIve patients studY] trials, which have demonstrated that both seated systolic and diastolic BP reductions were faster and greater with triple combination therapy of olmesartan, amlodipine and HCTZ, compared with those of dual combination therapies.[9]

■ CONCLUSION

Current evidence shows that ACE inhibitor and ARBs have similar efficacy in reducing BP. Fine-tuning our selection of ACE inhibitor and ARBs in more optimal treatment of hypertension could result in better control. ARBs are used as monotherapy or combination therapy in treatment of hypertension. They have a distinct advantage in hypertension associated with diabetes, chronic kidney disease, left ventricular dysfunction, or postmyocardial infarction. ARBs are well tolerated and the convenient once-a-day dosing of longer acting agents is a distinct advantage in terms of adherence and 24-hour BP control. Some evidence favors olmesartan amongst the ARBs. Azilsartan is a promising novel agent in our armamentarium to treat high BP.

■ REFERENCES

1. Pan G, Zhou X, Zhao J. Effect of telmisartan on atrial fibrillation recurrences in patients with hypertension: a systematic review and meta-analysis. Cardiovasc Ther. 2014;32(4):184-8.

2. Kalikar M, Nivangune KS, Dakhale GN, et al. Efficacy and tolerability of olmesartan, telmisartan, and losartan in patients of stage I hypertension: a randomized, open-label study. J Pharmacol Pharmacother. 2017;8(3):106-11.

3. Abraham HM, White CM, White WB. The comparative efficacy and safety of the angiotensin receptor blockers in the management of hypertension and other cardiovascular diseases Drug Saf. 2015;38(1):33-54.

4. Omboni S, Malacco E, Mallion JM, et al. Antihypertensive efficacy and safety of olmesartan medoxomil and ramipril in elderly mild to moderate essential hypertensive patients with or without metabolic syndrome: a pooled post hoc analysis of two comparative trials. Drugs Aging. 2012;29(12):981-92.

5. Akhrass PR, McFarlane SI. Telmisartan and cardioprotection. Vasc Health Risk Manag. 2011;7:673-83.

6. Fitchett D. Results of the ONTARGET and TRANSCEND studies: an update and discussion. Vasc Health Risk Manag. 2009;5(1):21-9.

7. Kikuchi K, Tancharoen S, Ito T, et al. Potential of the angiotensin receptor blockers (ARBs) telmisartan, irbesartan, and candesartan for inhibiting the HMGB1/RAGE axis in prevention and acute treatment of stroke. Int J Mol Sci. 2013;14(9):18899-924.

8. Yusuf S, Teo K, Anderson C, et al.; Telmisartan Randomised AssessmeNt Study in ACE iNtolerant subjects with cardiovascular Disease (TRANSCEND) Investigator. Effects of the angiotensin-receptor blocker telmisartan on cardiovascular events in high-risk patients intolerant to angiotensin-converting enzyme inhibitors: a randomised controlled trial. Lancet. 2008;372(9644):1174-83.

9. Oparil S, Williams D, Chrysant SG, et al. Comparative efficacy of olmesartan, losartan, valsartan, and irbesartan in the control of essential hypertension. J Clin Hypertens (Greenwich). 2001;3(5):283-91,318.

Alpha Blockers: Role in Hypertension

Dilip A Kirpalani

INTRODUCTION

Alpha-receptor antagonists are one of the class of antihypertensive medications used today. Albeit, they are not first-line agents in the treatment of essential hypertension, they are very useful as add-on drugs in difficult-to-treat hypertension.

There are two types of alpha-receptors, which exist on peripheral sympathetic nerve terminals—the alpha-1 receptors and alpha-2 receptors. The alpha-1 receptors are further divided into three homologous subtypes—(1) alpha-1A, (2) alpha-1B and (3) alpha-1D. The functions of the alpha-receptors are as follows:

- Vasoconstriction
- Smooth muscle contraction of the internal urethral sphincter
- Contraction of sphincters in the gastrointestinal (GI) tract
- Increased secretion from sweat and salivary glands
- Pupillary dilatation
- Relaxation of smooth muscles of the GI tract.

The alpha-2 receptors are subdivided into alpha-2A, alpha-2B and alpha-2C. The functions of Alpha-2 Receptors are the following:

- Inhibition of neurotransmitter release
- Decrease in central sympathetic outflow
- Increased platelet aggregation
- Decrease in insulin release.

CLASSIFICATION OF ALPHA-BLOCKERS

Alpha-receptor antagonist drugs are broadly subdivided into nonselective alpha-blockers and selective alpha-blockers. The selective alpha-blockers are further subdivided into alpha-1 blockers and alpha-2 blockers.

The alpha-1 selective blockers include prazosin, terazosin and doxazosin and these are the drugs, which are used for the management of chronic hypertension.

The alpha-2 receptor blockers will actually lead to an increase in blood pressure (BP). An example of this group of drugs is an old drug called yohimbine, which was used in the past for treatment of orthostatic hypotension.

The nonselective alpha-blockers are used only in the treatment of pheochromocytoma. These include phentolamine and phenoxybenzamine. These drugs are not used in the management of chronic hypertension as they can cause severe orthostatic hypotension and tachycardia as a result of their nonselectivity.

There is another group of drugs used in the management of chronic hypertension, which also works through alpha-receptors. These include the presynaptic alpha-2 receptor agonists, which cause antihypertensive effect by reducing central sympathetic outflow. Clonidine and moxonidine are two drugs, which belong to this group of antihypertensives.

Alpha-1 Receptor Antagonists in the Treatment of Hypertension

Alpha-blockers, which are used in the treatment of chronic hypertension, are the alpha-1 receptor antagonists and these drugs reduce BP by decreasing peripheral vascular resistance. These drugs act by blocking the alpha-1 receptors, which are present post-synaptically and they act mainly on the alpha-1B subtype of the alpha-1 receptor, which is present on vascular smooth muscle cell, thereby leading to a reduction in vasoconstriction.

The most commonly used alpha-blocker in the treatment of hypertension is prazosin. The dose of prazosin is 5–20 mg/day, which is usually given in two to three divided doses. This is a short-acting drug with a half-life of 3 hours and it has a 50% oral bioavailability. The advantage of this drug is that it causes little or no reflex tachycardia.

Doxazosin is another antihypertensive in this class, which is longer acting than prazosin. The dose of prazosin is 4–16 mg/day in one or two divided doses. The major problem with doxazosin is the "first-dose phenomenon", which means that there may be severe orthostatic hypotension after the first few doses but with time, this problem reduces.

Terazosin is the third drug in this group. Its dose is 5–20 mg/day in one or two divided doses. The advantage of terazosin is that it has a very high bioavailability when given orally and it is longer acting than prazosin with half-life of 9–12 hours.

BENEFITS OF ALPHA-1 RECEPTORS ANTAGONISTS IN HYPERTENSION

The TOMHS (Treatment of Mild Hypertension Study) and the GATES study showed that doxazosin is a very potent antihypertensive.[1,2]

In the ASOCIA study,[3] which involved over 3,500 patients, doxazosin achieved the target BP in 61% of patients at 16 weeks when it was used as an add-on therapy versus placebo. This study also showed that there was an average 19% fall in rate pressure product amongst the subjects after adding on doxazosin and an average 15% fall in pulse pressure amongst the subjects after adding on doxazosin, thereby showing that the alpha-blocker in adding to reducing BP was able to reduce myocardial oxygen demand.

There are various pleiotropic benefits of alpha-1 receptor antagonists as well. These are the following:

- Decrease in total cholesterol and decrease in low-density lipoprotein (LDL) cholesterol
- Improvement in insulin sensitivity
- Improvement in endothelial function
- Reduction in arterial stiffness.

Alpha-1 receptors antagonists are also the drugs of choice in elderly males with hypertension and benign prostatic hyperplasia because these drugs act on the smooth muscle in the prostate gland and on the smooth muscle in the urinary bladder neck, thereby leading to improvement in obstructive urinary symptoms.

In chronic kidney disease, alpha-1 receptors antagonists are excellent drugs as antihypertensives, particularly when two or more drugs are not bringing down the BP to target. This is because these drugs neither increase the serum potassium nor do they worsen glomerular filtration rate (GFR) and no major biochemical monitoring is required after initiation of alpha-blockers.[4]

Side Effects of Alpha-1 Receptors Antagonists

The alpha-blockers are known to cause postural hypotension. Hence, these drugs need to be used very cautiously in elderly people where there is already a high chance of getting postural hypotension. Whenever an alpha-blocker is initiated in an elderly person, it is a good idea to start with a very low dose and preferably at night-time with a very gradual up-titration of dose based on the BP response. In addition to this, the patient who is receiving the alpha-blocker should be instructed to get up very gradually from a recumbent position.

It is very important that the doctor checks both, the supine BP (or sitting BP) and standing BP in any patient who is receiving an alpha-1 receptor antagonist.

Miscellaneous Alpha-blockers

Carvedilol is a combined alpha and beta-blocker and it is a very good drug in the treatment of cardiac failure, although its antihypertensive potency is not very strong.

Labetalol is a combined alpha and beta-blocker, which is an excellent drug used for the treatment of hypertensive emergencies as it can be used parenterally as well. Labetalol is one of the safe antihypertensives for use in hypertension during pregnancy.

Alpha-2 Receptor Agonists

The presynaptic alpha-2 receptor agonists, namely, clonidine and moxonidine, act as antihypertensives by reducing central sympathetic outflow. Although they are not alpha-blockers, they have been briefly mentioned here, as they are excellent anti-hypertensives when used as add-on drugs in difficult-to-treat hypertension.[5]

Moxonidine has an additional agonistic action at the imidazoline-1 receptor in the rostral ventrolateral medulla and therefore causes lesser side effects such as sedation compared to clonidine.

■ CONCLUSION

Alpha-1 receptor antagonists are an excellent third-line or fourth-line agent for BP control in difficult-to-treat hypertension and resistant hypertension, particularly if hyperkalemia is an issue and aldosterone antagonist is contraindicated.

They have a great advantage in that they are both glucose neutral and lipid neutral and do not affect serum potassium or GFR. In addition, they have multiple pleiotropic benefits such as improvement in endothelial function and reduction in vascular stiffness.

The alpha-1 receptor antagonist could be a great add-on drug in a hypertensive who is already on the first-line agents such as calcium channel blocker, thiazide or thiazide-like diuretic and a renin–angiotensin–aldosterone system (RAAS) blocker and is yet not at target BP. These drugs have a good tolerability profile as well.

Hypertension guidelines across the world have not yet endorsed alpha-1 receptors antagonists in a major way. However, the need of the hour demands more drugs for the treatment of chronic hypertension and hence alpha-1 receptor antagonists must be included in hypertension guidelines, not necessarily as first or second-line agents but definitely as add-on agents in the treatment of chronic hypertension. In the treatment of elderly males with hypertension and benign prostatic hyperplasia, they should be used as first or second-line antihypertensive agents and it is important to watch out for postural hypotension in any patient who is receiving an alpha-1 receptor antagonist.

■ REFERENCES

1. The treatment of mild hypertension study. A randomized, placebo-controlled trial of a nutritional-hygienic regimen along with various drug monotherapies. The Treatment of Mild Hypertension Research Group. Arch Intern Med. 1991;151:1413-23.
2. Black HR, Keck M, Meredith P, et al. Controlled-release doxazosin as combination therapy in hypertension: The GATES study. J Clin Hypertens. 2006;8:159-66.
3. de Alvaro F, Hernández-Presa MA. Effect of doxazosin gastrointestinal therapeutic system on patients with uncontrolled hypertension: The ASOCIA Study. J Cardiovasc Pharmacol. 2006;47:271-6.
4. Kabra NK. Alpha Blockers and metabolic syndrome. J Assoc Physicians India. 2014;62:13-6.
5. Izzo Jr JL, Black HR, American Heart Association Council on High Blood Pressure Research. Hypertension Primer, 3rd edition. Philadelphia: Llppincott Williams & Wilkins; 2003. pp. 421-5.

Centrally Acting Antihypertensive Agents

Girish Mathur, Ashutosh Chaturvedi, Divyansh Mathur

■ INTRODUCTION

Hypertension is a leading public health concern in both economically developing and developed countries. It is an important modifiable risk factor for cardiovascular and cerebrovascular disease and death. Timely use of antihypertensive drugs reduces target organ damage and improves cardiovascular disease outcomes. There is a wide list of different classes of antihypertensive drugs, of which centrally acting blood pressure lowering drugs are considered to be an important group. Although still a complex and incompletely understood phenomenon, the central regulation of the sympathetic nervous system has a decisive role in the development and maintenance of high blood pressure in many patients of essential hypertension. Studies suggest that up to 30% of essential hypertension patients have a primary neurogenic cause leading to increased blood pressure.[1] As compared to the first generation of centrally acting antihypertensive drugs, the second generation agents like moxonidine and rilmenidine are considered superior owing to their selective binding at the vasomotor center and selective action at imidazoline-1 (I_1) receptors and thus finds an important place in treatment of hypertension.

■ CENTRAL REGULATION OF BLOOD PRESSURE

Activation of sympathetic nervous system plays an important role in the pathophysiology of development of essential hypertension.[2] The vasomotor center situated in the RVLM (rostral ventrolateral medulla) part of medulla along with hypothalamus, is a major determinant of sympathetic activation. Neurones which arise in the RVLM terminate in the sympathetic neurones of the intermediolateral column in the spinal cord and form the major excitatory pathway (Fig. 1).[3,4] Chronic and inappropriate stimulation of the sympathetic nervous system causes variety of pathophysiologic changes such as cardiac arrhythmias,[5] left ventricular hypertrophy,[6] impaired renal perfusion,[7] and atherosclerosis[8] leading to target organ dysfunction.

■ CENTRAL SYMPATHOLYTICS: MECHANISM OF ACTION

Centrally acting antihypertensive drugs cross blood–brain barrier and act by stimulating I_1 and/or central alpha-2-adrenoceptors in the RVLM and the nucleus of tractus solitarius (NTS). Various central sympatholytics are classified on the basis of action on these two

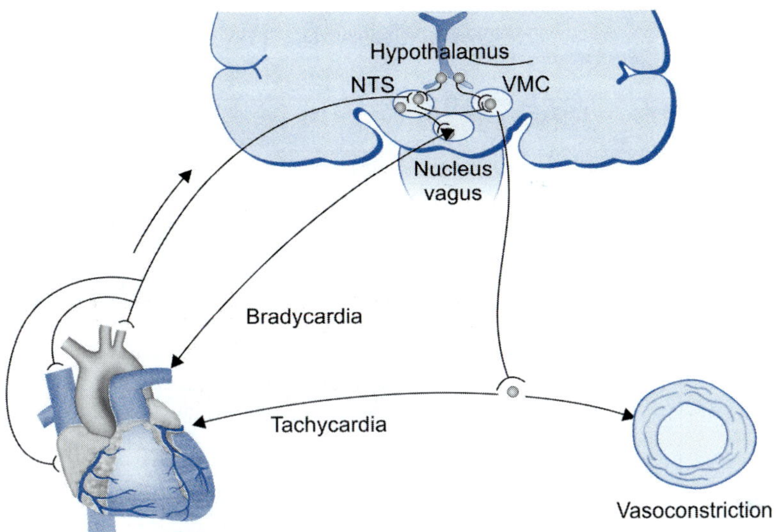

Fig. 1: Central regulation of blood pressure. The vasomotor center (VMC) in the rostral ventrolateral medulla (RVLM) controls the activity of the sympathetic neurones located in the intermediate lateral column of the spinal cord. Sympathetic neuronal impulses reaching the heart regulate myocardial contractility, heart rate and increase arteriolar tone.

TABLE 1: Centrally acting antihypertensive and their target central nervous system receptors.

Compound	Receptors
Methyldopa	α_2
Guanfacine	α_2
Guanabenz	α_2
Clonidine (mixed agonist)	$\alpha_2 + I_1$
Moxonidine	I_1
Rilmenidine	I_1

types of receptors (Table 1). The parent drug clonidine nonselectively stimulates both alpha-2 and I_1 receptors while methyldopa, guanfacine, and guanabenz stimulate alpha-2 receptors more than the I_1 receptors. The second generation agents like moxonidine and rilmenidine selectively stimulate I_1 receptors. The presence of alpha-2 receptors in the NTS, nucleus coeruleus and salivary glands along with RVLM results in side effects like dry mouth, sedation, and depression by ingestion of drugs acting through alpha-2 receptors. On the other hand, the I_1 receptors are almost exclusively present in the RVLM leading to much lesser central adverse effects by use of selective I_1 stimulator agents (Fig. 2).

The blood pressure lowering effect of centrally acting agents is based on decrease in noradrenaline levels and decreased peripheral resistance. The reduction in peripheral resistance is persistent with long-term treatment and also during exercise.[9] Reflex tachycardia does not develop in fact, heart rate may be somewhat reduced during the course of treatment. Cardiac output and renal blood flow remain unchanged with drugs in this class.[10] Centrally acting agents also decrease plasma renin activity[11] but tend to cause dose-dependent salt and fluid retention with long-term treatment which is reversible with diuretic therapy.

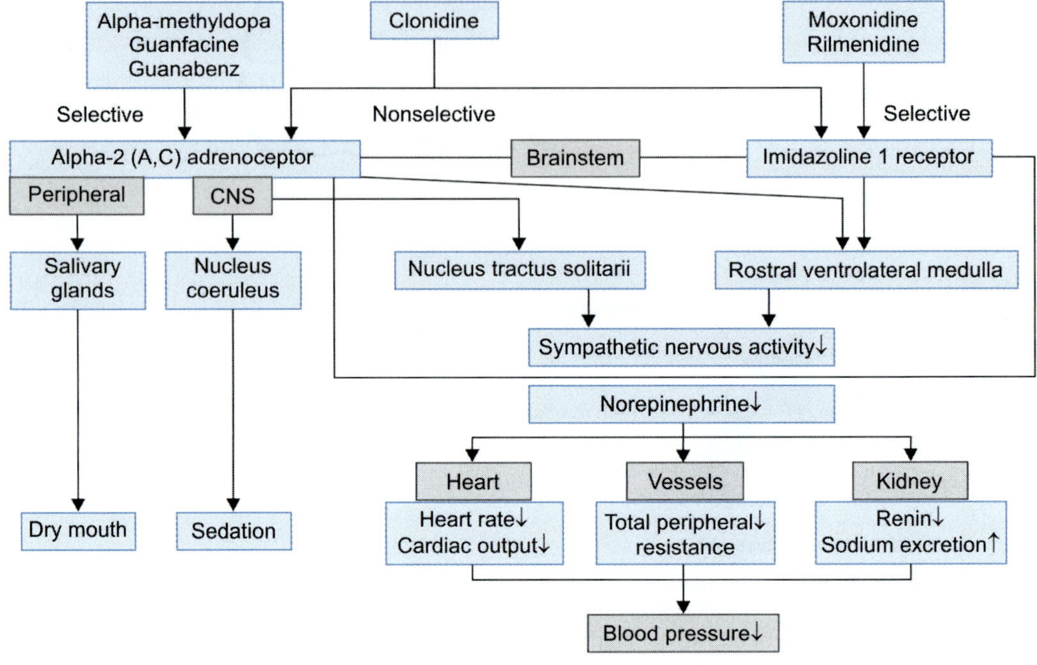

(CNS: central nervous system)

Fig. 2: Mechanism of action of different central sympatholytic agents.[12]

TABLE 2: Summary of pharmacokinetic properties of central sympatholytic drugs.

Drug	Half-life (hours)	Total dose range (mg/day)	Doses/day	Renal elimination (%)
Clonidine	6–16	0.2–1.2	2–3	40–60
Clonidine patch	14–26	0.1–0.6	Weekly	40–60
Methyldopa	1–2	250–2,000	2	70
Moxonidine	2–3	0.2–0.6	1–2	50–75
Rilmenidine	8.5	1–2	1	52–93
Guanabenz	6–14	8–32	2	<5
Guanfacine	10–30	1–3	1	50

The systemic half-life and onset of action varies among the different agents of this class which is attributable to differing receptor affinity and depository effects in deeper tissues. The newer agents, moxonidine, and rilmenidine encounter extensive renal clearance leading to requirement of dose adjustments in renal failure patients (Table 2).

■ CENTRAL SYMPATHOLYTICS: USES AND ADVERSE EFFECTS

Centrally acting agents are not recommended as a first-line therapy because of lesser effectiveness and inability to reduce mortality in clinical trials when used as monotherapy. They are mostly used as an adjunctive therapy along with other antihypertensive drugs particularly to check reflex sympathetic stimulation occurring with other drugs specially vasodilators. These are very useful for patients of labile hypertension with marked anxiety component. Clonidine, the parent drug of this class, has been shown to be an effective antihypertensive agent, especially in whites and older blacks.[13] Along with methyldopa, it is the only drug of this class having intravenous preparation available in few countries. It is also available as a transdermal delivery patch.[14]

Along with thiazide-type diuretics they are used for treating resistant hypertension and hypertension of pregnancy when beta-blockers are contraindicated. Centrally acting compounds are also safe to use in asthmatics and diabetics without hampering glycemic control.[15] In the perioperative period, clonidine is especially useful to control sympathetically driven hypertension along with benefits of analgesic-sparing and anesthetic effect also.

Currently, owing to their significant adverse effects like somnolence, dry mouth, and depression,[16,17] centrally acting agents are less frequently used nowadays. Other less common side effects include gastrointestinal symptoms, postural hypotension, weakness and fluid retention in body. Dry mouth of long standing duration may lead to increased risk of periodontal disease, dental caries, and oral candidiasis.[18] Simultaneous use of other sedative-hypnotic agents, antihistaminics, ethanol can exaggerate the sedative effect of central sympatholytics. Selective I_1 receptor agonists like moxonidine and rilmenidine are relatively better tolerated than other drugs.

■ CENTRALLY ACTING SYMPATHOLYTIC AGENTS

Clonidine

Clonidine is the most commonly used centrally acting sympatholytic drug. It has the fastest onset of action of 30–60 minutes and also the shortest duration of action most of the times which necessitates its frequent dosing.[19] The blood pressure reducing effect lasts for about 8–10 hours. Oral preparations are available in 0.1, 0.2, and 0.3-mg dosages and the recommended maximum dose is 2.4 mg/day. Oral clonidine is mainly used for resistant hypertension, hypertensive urgencies, post-menopausal syndrome, symptoms like hot flushes, and for sympathetically driven forms of hypertension along with restless leg syndrome.

Transdermal Clonidine Patch

It is available in 2.5, 5.0 and 7.5 mg dosages and is best absorbed by application over chest or upper arm.[20] It gives a constant clonidine delivery for about a week with peak effect being attained within 1–2 days. After removal of patch the effect lasts for 8–24 hours.[21] At comparable doses the clonidine patch relatively results in more fluid and salt retention than oral drug form.[14] Transdermal clonidine is particularly useful for labile hypertension requiring multiple and frequent drug administration, to control early morning blood pressure surges, and also in those patients who are unable to take oral drugs.

Blood Pressure Independent Uses of Clonidine

Clonidine has a variety of alternative uses apart from control of blood pressure. It can be used for opioid and alcohol withdrawal symptoms, migraine prophylaxis, post-traumatic stress disorder, and also in open angle glaucoma as a secondary treatment. It has also been found useful to treat diarrhea associated with short gut syndrome.[22] In perioperative period, it is used to improve anesthesia and analgesia and to manage postoperative sympathetic responses.[14]

Clonidine is also useful in cirrhosis patients with ascites to enhance dieresis and control sympathetic activity associated with heart failure.[23] In new onset atrial fibrillation it can also control the ventricular rate with a comparable efficacy to other commonly used antiarrhythmics. For the diagnosis of pheochromocytoma, 0.1 mg clonidine is given every hour for three doses and plasma norepinephrine levels are measured subsequently. If levels remain unchanged then diagnosis of pheochromocytoma is made while if levels decrease it suggests essential hypertension.[24]

Side Effects and Contraindications

Apart from dry mouth and sedation, headache, orthostatic hypotension, and impotence are potential adverse effects. Rebound hypertension is common with abrupt withdrawal of clonidine, more commonly if patient is also taking beta-blockers simultaneously. In this the blood pressure of patient commonly overshoots the pretreatment blood pressure.[25] This phenomenon is also called as discontinuation syndrome and should be managed by restarting clonidine. Rebound hypertension is less common with the transdermal form of clonidine. Transdermal patch can cause pruritus, erythema and pigmentation problems in 15–20% of patients. These skin reactions are believed to be due to active drug compound and not the patch specifically.[14] Clonidine overdose can cause paradoxical hypertension when central alpha-2 stimulation exceeds the peripheral alpha-2 stimulation.[26]

Well-known contraindications include sick-sinus syndrome and second degree and third degree atrioventricular block especially when used in chronic kidney disease patients.[27]

Methyldopa

Methyldopa was used very commonly up to late 1970s. It has a slow onset of action of 2–3 hours with half-life of about 12 hours. Orally it is available in 125, 250 and 500 mg dosages. The maximum dose is up to 3,000 mg. It is also available in intravenous form given at dose of 20–40 mg/kg/day in divided doses every 6 hourly.

Uses

Being nonteratogenic in nature, it is mainly used to treat hypertension of pregnancy as it does not hamper the maternal cardiac output and preserves the uterine and renal perfusion.[28] It can also be used in clonidine—intolerant patients[29] and in hypertensive emergencies.

Side Effects and Contraindications

Apart from class specific side effects methyldopa can cause autoimmune reactions, flu-like syndrome, Coombs-positive hemolytic anemia, lupus like disease, and occasionally drug-induced hepatitis.[30] All these side effects are mostly reversible with drug discontinuation.

The major contraindication is the presence of an active hepatic disease.

Guanfacine

The major advantage of guanfacine is its 24 hours duration of action allowing once daily dosing.[31] It is commonly prescribed in evening which controls the blood pressure during the early morning catecholamine surge and also plays out any potential sedating effect during sleep. Usual dose is 1 mg at bedtime with maximum dose limit of 3 mg.

Uses

It is mainly useful for patients who are clonidine intolerant.

Side Effects and Contraindications

It causes relatively lesser side effects than clonidine and withdrawal symptoms are also fewer. The risk of adverse effects increases with doses beyond 1 mg.

Guanabenz

Guanabenz has a longer duration of action and major advantage is less chances of fluid retention. Dose modification is also not required in renal failure patients.[32] Usual doses are 4 mg twice daily with maximum permissible dose of 64 mg per day. An additional advantage of this drug is that it reduces total cholesterol levels by 10–20% by inhibiting triglyceride and hepatic cholesterol production with stimulation of fatty acid oxidation.[33] The side effect profile is similar to the clonidine. Withdrawal syndrome, rebound hypertension, and hypersensitivity reactions can also occur. It is not safe to be used in pregnancy.

Moxonidine

The I_1 receptor agonist moxonidine is an effective drug to treat hypertension both as monotherapy and in combination therapy. Unlike clonidine it does not reduce the heart rate.[34] It has a plasma half-life of 2–3 hours only. It is available in 0.2 mg formulation and the maximum dose should not increase 0.6 mg per day with any single dose not exceeding 0.4 mg. Moxonidine is extensively cleared in kidneys, so its dose needs to be adjusted in renal failure as per glomerular filtration rate (GFR).[35] It should not be used in cases of severe renal failure with GFR below 30 mL/min.

Uses

It is mainly used as an add-on therapy to further lower blood pressure when combination therapy with other drugs is insufficient. Combining moxonidine with a beta-blocker increases the chances of rebound hypertension on withdrawing moxonidine. In addition to blood pressure reduction, moxonidine may also increase sodium excretion and improve glucose tolerance and insulin resistance.

Side Effects and Contraindications

Due to its selective action on I_1 receptors it is less likely to cause adverse effects like sedation and dry mouth than clonidine.

Headache, dizziness, nausea and tiredness are common side effects. It is contraindicated in bradycardia and bradyarrhythmias, heart failure, and severe renal impairment.

The MOXCON trial in heart failure patients was stopped prematurely due to increased number of deaths among moxonidine group than placebo group.[36]

Use in pregnancy is also discouraged as it passes into breast milk. Alcohol can potentiate the hypotensive effects of moxonidine.

Rilmenidine

It is an effective and well-tolerated drug to treat mild-to-moderate hypertension in monotherapy or when combined with other drugs.[37] Usual doses are 1–2 mg. Single tablet is recommended in morning and can be increased in evening also when target blood pressure is not achieved. It can be given safely to diabetics, elderly and also in renal failure without any dose adjustment. It does not affect heart rate because it increases the parasympathetic tone. Rilmenidine should never be stopped suddenly and should not be used in patients with severe depression. Concomitant use with monoamine oxidase inhibitors is discouraged.

Side effects are rare, not severe and also transient at usual doses. Common side effects are palpitations, insomnia, fatigue, dry mouth, cramps, skin rash, hot flushes and constipation.

MANAGEMENT OF ADVERSE EFFECTS OF CENTRALLY ACTING ANTIHYPERTENSIVES

The adverse effects related with central sympatholytics can be usually treated by withdrawal of the offending drug. To avoid and manage such side effects centrally acting agents should be given divided in such manner that total daily dose is achieved at lower but more frequent individual dosing. An alternative is to reduce the total daily dose of centrally acting agent and add drug from other drug classes available.

Sedating effects of these drugs can be managed with night-time dosing or with switching over to a less sedating drug while to deal with dry mouth occurring after taking these drugs, salivary substitutes can be added.

Clonidine intolerant patients may be switched over to transdermal patch form with which the adverse effects are less common.[14] Transdermal clonidine patch can cause skin reactions and contact dermatitis which are managed by using 0.5% topical hydrocortisone cream or an aerosolized spray of beclometasone which is more potent steroid. Also spray will allow the patch to adhere better than the hydrocortisone cream.[38]

CONCLUSION

Sympathetic nervous system plays an important role in pathogenesis of hypertension in a significant number of patients. Centrally acting sympatholytics continue to be an effective treatment option for hypertension in patients refractory or sensitive to the newer agents. Patients with resistant hypertension, diabetic, and/or renal failure patients respond well to these agents. Because of bothersome side effects their use has dramatically declined in last few years but still centrally acting agents, being very diverse in their actions, will remain as an important weapon in the armamentarium of clinicians to treat hypertension.

REFERENCES

1. Rahn KH, Barenbrock M, Hausberg M. The sympathetic nervous system in the pathogenesis of hypertension. J Hypertens Suppl. 1999;17(3):S11-4.
2. Kjeldsen SE, Schork NJ, Leren P, et al. Arterial plasma norepinephrine correlates to blood pressure in middle-aged men with sustained essential hypertension. Am Heart J. 1989;118(4):775-81.
3. Sun MK. Central neural organization and control of sympathetic nervous system in mammals. Prog Neurobiol. 1995;47(3):157-233.
4. Benedict CR. Centrally acting antihypertensive drugs: re-emergence of sympathetic inhibition in the treatment of hypertension. Curr Hypertens Rep. 1999;1(4):305-12.
5. Rosen MR, Danilo P Jr, Robinson RB, et al. Sympathetic neural and alpha-adrenergic modulation of arrhythmias. Ann N Y Acad Sci. 1988;533:200-209.
6. Long CS, Kariya K, Karns L, et al. Sympathetic activity: modulator of myocardial hypertrophy. J Cardiovasc Pharmacol. 1991;17(Suppl 2):S20-4.
7. DiBona GF: Sympathetic neural control of the kidney in hypertension. Hypertension.1992;9(Suppl 1):I28-35.
8. Kaplan JR, Pettersson K, Manuck SB, Olsson G. Role of sympathoadrenal medullary activation in the initiation and progression of atherosclerosis. Circulation. 1991;84(Suppl 6):VI23-32.
9. Dollery CT. Advantages and disadvantages of alpha 2-adrenoceptor agonists for systemic hypertension. Am J Cardiol.1988;61(7):1D-5D.
10. Goldberg M, Gehr M. Effects of alpha-2 agonists on renal function in hypertensive humans. J Cardiovasc Pharmacol.1985;7(Suppl 8):S34-7.
11. Mohammed S, Fasola AF, Privitera PJ, et al. Effect of methyldopa on plasma renin activity in man. Circ Res.1969;25(5):543-8.
12. Kazuomi K. Central sympathetic agents and direct vaso-dilators. In: Bakris GL, Sorrentino M (Eds). Hypertension: A Companion to Braunwald's Heart Disease, 3rd edition. Elsevier; 2018. pp. 254-60.
13. Materson BJ, Reda DJ, Cushman WC. Department of veterans affairs single-drug therapy of hypertension study. Revised figures and new data. Department of Veterans Affairs Cooperative Study Group on Antihypertensive Agents. Am J Hypertens.1995;8(2):189-92.
14. Sica DA, Grubbs R. Transdermal clonidine: therapeutic considerations. J Clin Hypertens (Greenwich). 2005;7(9): 558-62.

15. Foxworth JW, Reisz GR, Pyszczynski DR, et al. Oral clonidine in patients with asthma: no significant effect on airway reactivity. Eur J Clin Pharmacol. 1995;48(1):19-22.

16. van Zwieten PA, Thoolen MJ, Timmermans PB. The hypotensive activity and side effects of methyldopa, clonidine, and guanfacine. Hypertension.1984;6(5 Pt 2):II28-33.

17. Webster J, Koch HF. Aspects of tolerability of centrally acting antihypertensive drugs. J Cardiovasc Pharmacol. 1996;27(Suppl 3):S49-54.

18. Watson GE, Pearson SK, Bowen WH. The effect of chronic clonidine administration on salivary glands and caries in the rat. Caries Res. 2000;34(2):194-200.

19. Houston MC. Treatment of hypertensive emergencies and urgencies with oral clonidine loading and titration. A review. Arch Intern Med. 1986;146(3):586-9.

20. Hopkins K, Aarons L, Rowland M. Absorption of clonidine from a transdermal therapeutic system when applied to different body sites. In: Weber MA, Mathias CJ (Eds). Mild Hypertension: Current Controversies and Approaches. Darmstadt: Steinkopf Verlag; 1984. pp. 143-7.

21. MacGregor TR, Matzek KM, Keirns JJ, et al. Pharmacokinetics of transdermally delivered clonidine. Clin Pharmacol Ther. 1985;38(3):278-84.

22. Buchman AL, Fryer J, Wallin A, et al. Clonidine reduces diarrhea and sodium loss in patients with proximal jejunostomy: a controlled study. JPEN J Parenter Enteral Nutr. 2006;30(6):487-91.

23. Lenaerts A, Codden T, Meunier JC, et al. Effects of clonidine on diuretic response in ascitic patients with cirrhosis and activation of sympathetic nervous system. Hepatology. 2006;44(4):844-9.

24. Bravo EL, Tarazi RC, Fouad FM, et al. Clonidine-suppression test: a useful aid in the diagnosis of pheochromocytoma. N Engl J Med. 1981;305(11):623-6.

25. Hansson L, Hunyor SN, Julius S, et al. Blood pressure crisis following withdrawal of clonidine (Catapres, Catapresan), with special reference to arterial and urinary catecholamine levels, and suggestions for acute management. Am Heart J. 1973;85(5):605-10.

26. Domino LE, Domino SE, Stockstill MS. Relationship between plasma concentrations of clonidine and mean arterial pressure during an accidental clonidine overdose. Br J Clin Pharmacol.1986;291(1):71-4.

27. Byrd BF 3rd, Collins HW, Primm RK. Risk factors for severe bradycardia during oral clonidine therapy for hypertension. Arch Intern Med. 1988;148(3):729-33.

28. Khedun SM, Maharaj B, Moodley J. Effects of antihypertensive drugs on the unborn child: What is known, and how should this influence prescribing? Paediatr Drugs. 2000;2(6):419-36.

29. Chobanian AV, Bakris GL, Black HR, et al. Seventh report of the Joint National Committee on Prevention, Detection, Evaluation, and Treatment of High Blood Pressure. Hypertension. 2003;42(6):1206-52.

30. Carstairs KC, Breckenridge A, Dollery CT, et al. Incidence of a positive direct coombs test in patients on alpha-methyldopa. Lancet.1966;2(7455):133-5.

31. Oster JR, Epstein M. Use of centrally acting sympatholytic agents in the management of hypertension. Arch Intern Med. 1991;151(8):1638-44.

32. Meacham RH, Emmett M, Kyriakopoulos AA, et al. Disposition of 14C-guanabenz in patients with essential hypertension. Clin Pharmacol Ther. 1980;27(1):44-52.

33. Capuzzi DM, Cevallos WH. Inhibition of hepatic cholesterol and triglyceride synthesis by guanabenz acetate. J Cardiovasc Pharmacol. 1984;6(Suppl 5):S847-52.

34. Sica DA. Centrally acting antihypertensive agents: an update. J Clin Hypertens (Greenwich). 2007;9(5):399-405.

35. Kirch W, Hutt HJ, Plänitz V. The influence of renal function on clinical pharmacokinetics of moxonidine. Clin Pharmacokinet. 1988;15(4):245-53.

36. Cohn JN, Pfeffer MA, Rouleau J, et al. Adverse mortality effect of central sympathetic inhibition with sustained-release moxonidine in patients with heart failure (MOXCON). Eur J Heart Fail. 2003;5(5):659-67.

37. Reid JL. Rilmenidine: a clinical overview. Am J Hypertens. 2000;13 (6 Pt 2):106S-11S.

38. Ito MK, O'Connor DT. Skin pretreatment and the use of transdermal clonidine. Am J Med. 1991;91(1A):42S-9S.

Direct Vasodilators in Hypertension

Rajib Ratna Chaudhary

■ INTRODUCTION

Direct-acting vasodilators used as monotherapy in the management of hypertension were limited due to its side effects.[1] A better understanding of the pharmacological actions of the direct-acting vasodilators and the compensatory cardiovascular responses triggered by them has led to their use in combination with sympatholytics and diuretics, especially in resistant hypertension and hypertensive emergencies.[2] Few direct-acting vasodilators are used in clinical practice and they differ in their vasodilator potency. They have variable dilatory effects on the large arteries, smaller arteries, arterioles and capacitance vessels. We attempt to describe the clinically used direct-acting vasodilators in this review.

Hydralazine

Hydralazine has shown significantly decreased mortality when used as fixed dose combination with isosorbide dinitrate in cases of severe congestive heart failure. It is recommended in those hypertensives who cannot tolerate angiotensin-converting enzyme (ACE)-inhibitors.[3]

Hydralazine directly acts on arterioles with little effect on venous smooth muscle. The molecular mechanisms which is endothelium dependent and involve generation of nitric oxide (NO) and stimulation of cGMP, and a reduction in intracellular Ca^{2+} concentrations.[4] The sympathetic nervous system stimulation by hydralazine causes vasodilation, increased heart rate and contractility, increased plasma renin activity, and fluid retention. The blood pressure is lowered both in the supine and upright positions and due to dilatation of arterioles than veins so postural hypotension is not a problem.

Hydralazine is well absorbed orally. The bioavailability of the drugs is low (16% in fast acetylators and 35% in slow acetylators) due to acetylation of hydralazine in bowel and liver. The rate of acetylation is genetically determined. The acetylated compound is inactive so the dose necessary to produce a systemic effect is larger. The hydralazine pyruvic acid hydrazone is produced when hydralazine with circulating α-keto acids and this has a longer t½ than hydralazine. The bioavailability of hydralazine is determined by rate of acetylation.[5] The hypotensive effect of the drug reaches its peak within 30–120 minutes of oral intake. The effects of hydralazine can last as long as 12 hours although the plasma t½ is about 1 hour and there is no clear explanation for this.

Hydralazine is used in the treatment of hypertension not as a first-line drug due to side effect profile. The drug can be combined in low doses with diuretic and beta-blocker in the treatment of hypertension. Hydralazine used in elderly patients and in hypertensive with coronary artery disease may precipitate myocardial ischemia due to reflex tachycardia. The oral dosage of hydralazine is 25–100 mg twice daily. The maximum recommended dose of hydralazine is 200 mg/day.[6,7]

Adverse effects include headache, nausea, flushing, hypotension, palpitations, tachycardia and dizziness which is caused due to vasodilation. Angina pectoris and myocardial ischemia can occur by the baroreceptor reflex–induced stimulation of the sympathetic nervous system which increase O_2 demand. Parenteral administration of hydralazine is not advisable in elderly hypertensive patients with coronary artery disease. High-output congestive heart failure develops due to salt retention. Postural hypotension is not significant because of less action on veins, so venous return and cardiac output are not reduced. Drug-induced lupus syndrome is the most common due to immunological reactions. The side effects like serum sickness, hemolytic anemia, vasculitis, and rapidly progressive glomerulonephritis may occur after hydralazine therapy.

KATP Channel Openers: Minoxidil

Minoxidil was used as hypotensive agent in 1965. Minoxidil is a powerful vasodilator and its action resembles that of hydralazine, as direct arteriolar smooth muscle relaxant with little effect on veins. The peak concentrations of minoxidil in blood occur 1 hour after oral intake because formation of the active metabolite is delayed. The duration of action minoxidil is 24 hours, occasionally even longer with plasma t½ of 3–4 hours.

Sulfotransferase metabolized minoxidil into the active molecule, minoxidil NO sulfate which relaxes vascular smooth muscle by activating the ATP-modulated K^+ channel permitting K^+ efflux, and causes hyperpolarization and relaxation of smooth muscle.[8] The blood flow to skin, skeletal muscle, the gastrointestinal tract, and the heart is increased more than to the central nervous system. The disproportionate increase in blood flow to the heart may have a metabolic basis, in that administration of minoxidil is associated with a reflex increase in myocardial contractility and in cardiac output. [9]

Minoxidil can be used successfully in the treatment of severe hypertension that does not respond to other antihypertensive medications, especially in both adults and children patients with renal insufficiency.[10] Minoxidil should be used in combination with a diuretic to avoid fluid retention, with a sympatholytic drug to control reflex cardiovascular effects and a RAS inhibitor to prevent remodeling effects on the heart. Minoxidil is administered either once or twice a day, but some patients may require more frequent dosing for adequate control of blood pressure. The starting dose of minoxidil is as little as 1.25 mg daily which can be increased gradually to 40 mg in OD or BID daily doses.[11]

Adverse effects of minoxidil fall into three major categories—fluid and salt retention, cardiovascular effects, and hypertrichosis. Salt and water retention results from increased proximal renal tubular reabsorption, due to reduced renal perfusion pressure and to reflex stimulation of renal tubular α-adrenergic receptors. The cardiovascular effects are caused by baroreceptor-mediated activation of the sympathetic nervous system during minoxidil therapy and are similar to those seen with hydralazine; there is an increase in heart rate, myocardial contractility and myocardial O_2 consumption. Pericardial effusion is an uncommon but serious complication of minoxidil.

Mild and asymptomatic pericardial effusion is not an indication for discontinuing minoxidil. Effusions usually clear when the drug is discontinued but can recur if treatment with minoxidil is resumed. Flattened and inverted T waves are observed in the electrocardiogram following the initiation of minoxidil treatment.[12] Excess hair growth occurs in patients who receive minoxidil for a long duration due to K^+ channel activation and it occurs on the face, back, arms, and legs, and is particularly offensive to women. Other rare side effects of the drug are rashes, Stevens–Johnson syndrome, glucose intolerance, serosanguineous bullae, formation of antinuclear antibodies and thrombocytopenia.

Diazoxide

This K^+ channel opener dilator of arterioles was used in hypertensive emergencies for rapid reduction of BP in the past. It is rapidly administered by intravenous route in fractional doses (50–100 mg) repeated every 5–10 minutes, as needed. Slow intravenous injection or infusion is less effective because it binds tightly to plasma proteins before binding to vessel wall.

The duration of action is 6–24 hours because of tight binding to plasma and tissue proteins. It is employed in place of nitroprusside when regulated intravenous infusion or close monitoring is not possible. A side effect of diazoxide includes hypotension and has resulted in stroke and myocardial infarction. Diazoxide is used to treat hypoglycemia secondary to insulinoma.

Sodium Nitroprusside

Sodium nitroprusside has been known since 1850 and its hypotensive effect in humans was described in 1929. Nitroprusside is a nitrovasodilator that acts by releasing NO. NO activates the guanylyl cyclase–cyclic guanosine monophosphate–protein kinase G pathway, leading to vasodilation. The mechanism of release of NO from nitroprusside is not clear and likely that it involves both enzymatic and nonenzymatic pathways.[13,14]

Sodium nitroprusside is a nonselective vasodilator, and regional distribution of blood flow is little affected by the drug; so renal blood flow and glomerular filtration are maintained. Sodium nitroprusside usually causes only a modest increase in heart rate and an overall reduction in myocardial O_2 demand. Sodium nitroprusside is used in the management of hypertensive emergencies.

About 50 mg is added to a 500 mL bottle of saline/glucose solution, 0.02 mg/minute and titrated upward with the response—0.1–0.3 mg/minute if needed. Sodium nitroprusside decomposes at alkaline pH and on exposure to light—the infusion bottle should be covered with black paper. Nitroprusside is split to release cyanide. Cyanide is converted in liver to thiocyanate which is excreted slowly. The mean elimination t½ for thiocyanate is 3 days in patients with normal renal function and may be longer in patients with renal insufficiency. Excess thiocyanate may accumulate and produce toxicity if larger doses are infused for more than 1–2 days. Side effects are palpitation, nervousness, vomiting, perspiration, pain in abdomen, weakness, disorientation, lactic acidosis (caused by the released cyanide) and psychosis.

Fenoldopam

Fenoldopam is an agonist of dopamine D1 receptors causing dilation of peripheral arteries and natriuresis. The half-life of fenoldopam is 10 minutes. The dose of fenoldopam is (0.1 µg/kg/min) administered by continuous intravenous infusion, and the dose is then titrated upward every

15 or 20 minutes to a maximum dose of 1.6 µg/kg/minute or until the desired blood pressure is achieved. Side effects are reflex tachycardia, headache and flushing. Fenoldopam also increases intraocular pressure and should be avoided in patients with glaucoma.

■ CONCLUSION

The side effects of direct-acting vasodilators and advent of newer class of antihypertensives, limited its use as monotherapy in the management of hypertension. Pharmacological actions of the direct-acting vasodilators and the compensatory cardiovascular responses triggered by them has led to their use in combination with sympatholytics and diuretics, especially in resistant hypertension and hypertensive emergencies. In clinical practice few direct-acting vasodilators are used and they differ in their vasodilator potency and they have variable dilatory effects on the large arteries, smaller arteries, arterioles and capacitance vessels.

■ REFERENCES

1. New Drug Application (NDA): 008303. Company: NOVARTIS. (2017). Drug Name(s): Apresoline. FDA. Drugs@FDA: FDA Approved Drug Products. [online] Available from https://www.accessdata.fda.gov/scripts/cder/daf/index.cfm?event=overview.process&ApplNo=008303 [Last Accessed January 2019].
2. Perez MI, Musini VM. Pharmacological interventions for hypertensive emergencies. Cochrane Database Syst Rev. 2008;(1):CD003653.
3. Ferdinand KC, Elkayam U, Mancini D, et al. Use of isosorbide dinitrate and hydralazine in African-Americans with heart failure 9 years after the African-American Heart Failure Trial. Am J Cardiol. 2014;114(1):151-9.
4. Ellershaw DC, Gurney AM. Mechanisms of hydralazine induced vasodilation in rabbit aorta and pulmonary artery. Br J Pharmacol. 2001;134(3):621-31.
5. Shephard AM, McNay JL, Ludden TM, et al. Plasma concentration and acetylator phenotype determine response to oral hydrazine. Hypertension. 1981;3(5):580-5.
6. O'Malley K, Segal JL, Israili ZH, et al. Duration of hydralazine action in hypertension. Clin Pharmacol Ther. 1975;18(5 Pt 1):581-6.
7. Silas JH, Ramsay LE, Freestone S. Hydralazine once daily in hypertension. Br Med J (Clin Res Ed). 1982;284(6329):1602-4.
8. Leblanc N, Wilde DW, Keef KD, et al. Electrophysiological mechanisms of minoxidil sulfate-induced vasodilatation of rabbit portal vein. Clin Res. 1989;65(4):1102-11.
9. Ogilvie RI. Comparative effects of vasodilator drugs on flow distribution and venous return. Can J Physiol Pharmacol. 1985;63(11):1345-55.
10. Campese VM. Minoxidil: A review of its pharmacological properties and therapeutic use. Drugs. 1981;22(4):257-78.
11. Swales JD, Bing RF, Heagerty A, et al. Treatment of refractory hypertension. Lancet. 1982;1(8277):894-6.
12. Chi L, Uprichard AC, Lucchesi BR. Profibrillatory actions of pinacidil in a conscious canine model of sudden coronary death. J Cardiovasc Pharmacol. 1990;15(3):452-64.
13. Linder AE, McCluskey LP, Cole KR 3rd, et al. Dynamic association of nitric oxide downstream signalling molecules with endothelial caveolin-I in rat aorta. J Pharmacol Exp Ther. 2005;314(1):9-15.
14. Ramachandra R, Barrett CJ, Malpas SC. Nitric oxide and sympathetic nerve activity in the control of blood pressure. Clin Exp Pharmacol Physiol. 2005;32(5-6):440-6.

Combination Therapy in Hypertension

BA Muruganathan

▪ INTRODUCTION

Hypertension is considered as a chronic multifactorial disorder leading to patho-physiological changes in target organs over a period of time through diverse mechanisms. Recommended guidelines for blood pressure (BP) is less than 140/90 mm Hg in un-complicated conditions. Current evidence-based guidelines achieving the control of BP with single agent acting through one particular mechanism may not be possible. A meta-analysis of more than 40 studies has shown that combining two agents from any two classes of antihypertensive drugs increases the BP reduction much more than increasing the dose of one agent. Therapy with two drugs separately or with fixed combinations that include agents with complementary actions. Many combinations have been shown to improve cardiovascular outcome and include a diuretic with the renin–angiotensin–aldosterone system (RAAS) blocker. Choice of combination therapy depends upon the risk factors, presence of comorbidities like diabetes, renal dysfunction and the adverse effects and tailored according to individual patient.

▪ RATIONAL COMBINATION THERAPY FOR HYPERTENSION— FOUR WS

- When and where to use combination therapy?
- Why to use combination therapy?
- What and how to use (principles) combination therapy?

When to use Combination Therapy?

The combination therapy is recommended, when the BP is not under control and crucial with single drug. Reduction in systolic BP (SBP) by only 2 mm of Hg reduces the risk of cardiovascular events by 7–10%.

Current hypertension treatment guide-lines reflect the observation that most patients are not adequately controlled with a single agent and therefore combination treatment with antihypertensives from different classes is appropriate and recommended. If initial monotherapy fails to achieve the BP goal or when there are associated risk factors or target organ damage/complications or concomitant diseases/conditions for patients with stage 1 hypertension, combination therapy will be right choice.

Combination therapy is a first-line approach for patients with stage 2 hypertension and defined as SBP more than or equal to 160 mm Hg or diastolic BP (DBP) more than or equal to 100 mm Hg; it generally requires more aggressive treatment to achieve their BP goal and minimizes the long-term complications of hypertension.

Combination therapy may be considered as the initial therapy to treat BP that is more than 20/10 mm Hg over goal as it doubles the risk of stroke, ischemic heart disease and cardiovascular disease.

Why to use Combination Therapy?

Failure of Single-drug Regimen

Monotherapy is effective only in 25 % of the patients. Most drugs only reduce SBP 7–13 mm Hg and DBP 4–8 mm Hg. Single drug is not effective in controlling the BP because the high BP is due to multifactorial mechanism and the drug can also have counter regulatory mechanism. Simply up titrating the dose of treatment is unlikely to significantly improve response and can increase the side effects. Identifying best drug by substitution is time consuming.

Combination Therapy Advantages

Combination therapy covers more hypertension phenotypes and failure rate is less. In addition to achieving higher rates of BP control, initiating treatment with combination therapy rather than monotherapy may enable a patient to achieve their BP goal more quickly thereby reducing the long-term risk of hypertension-related complications. Reducing the time required to normalize BP may confer target organ protection since late or ineffective therapy cannot reverse progressive organ damage. Smaller dose of individual drugs minimize the side effects compared to single drug at full dose. Single pill and/or once daily administration would also greatly improve medication adherence and cost effectiveness (Flowcharts 1 and 2).

A recent survey has shown that patients receiving combination therapy have a lower drop-out rate than patients given any monotherapy. The tolerability profile of a drug, in some cases can be improved by addition of a second agent. The addition of an angiotensin-converting enzyme (ACE) inhibitor or angiotensin receptor blocker (ARB) to a diuretic, improve the tolerability of the diuretic by reducing the incidence and magnitude of hypokalemia.

Antihypertensive agents from different classes can have complementary effects may offset adverse reactions from each other such as a diuretic decreasing edema occurring secondary to treatment with a calcium channel blocker, adding an ACE inhibitor to a calcium channel blocker to reduce peripheral edema presumably through venodilation. Compelling indication(s) present that may benefit from different mechanisms of action of multiple antihypertensives.

Although the BP-reducing ability of antihypertensive drug classes and individual agents varies by only a few mm Hg, net effect more than sum of individual effect of two agents in combination varies considerably. Thus, combining an ACE inhibitor and a diuretic produces fully additive BP reduction, whereas the same ACE inhibitor added to an ARB results in additional BP reduction of only 2–3 mm Hg.

Wald et al. showed in a meta-analysis that BP reduction with drug combinations from two different classes is approximately five times greater than doubling the dose of one drug.

"Hypertensive patient's adequate BP control can be achieved by a combination therapy of at least two or more antihypertensive drugs from different classes" is the guidelines endorsed by the European Society of Hypertension/European Society

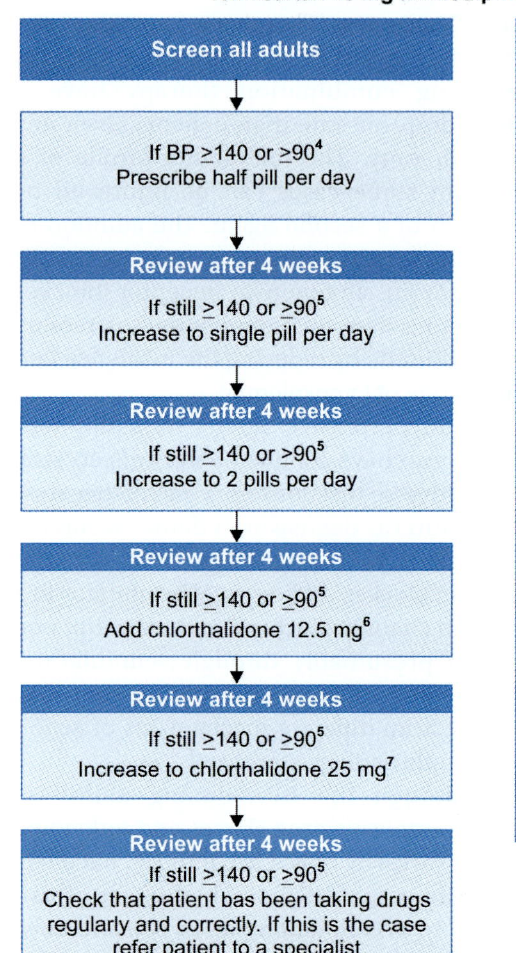

[1]Telmisartan 40 mg can be replaced with any once-daily angiotensin receptor blocker (ARB) (e.g., losartan 50 mg) or once daily angiotensin converting-enzyme inhibitor (ACE) (e.g. lisinopril 20 mg, ramipril 5 mg, perindopril 4 mg/L ACE inhibitor and ARB should not be given to women who are or who may become pregnant. Before initiating and several weeks after starting ACE inhibitors or ARBs check serum creatinine and potassium if possible.

[2]Amlodipine can be replaced with another once-daily dihydropyridine calcium channel blocker. Alternatively, amlodipine can be replaced with chlorthalidone 12.5 indapamide 1.25 mg. or indapamide SR 1.5 mg. If neither chlorthalidone nor indapamide is available, hydrochlorothiazide 25 mg can be used. If a diuretic is used instead of amlodipine, check serum potassium if possible and see 6 below.

[3]Medications can be used as individual agents, if single-pill combinations are not available.

[4]If BP <160 or <100, start same day and consider initiating entire tablet daily. If 140–159 or 90–99, check on a different day. and if still elevated, start.

[5]If systolic BP repeatedly <110. consider going to prior less intensive regimen.

[6]If a diuretic is used initially instead of amlodipine, then amlodipine or another once-daily dihydropyridine calcium channel blocker would be used at this step.

[7]Hypokalemia is more common using full-dose diuretic—consider regular lab monitoring. If a diuretic is used instead of amlodipine in the initial treatment, this consideration would apply in the protocol.

(BP: blood pressure)

Flowchart 1. Recommended single-pill combination hypertension treatment regimen.

of Cardiology (ESH/ESC) (Tables 1 and 2). The Joint National Committee 8 (JNC8) recommendation 9 advocates using two or more than two drugs to control hypertension, if required.

Evidence for Combination Therapy

Major drug combinations used in trials of antihypertensive treatment in a step-up approach or as a randomized combination (Table 3).

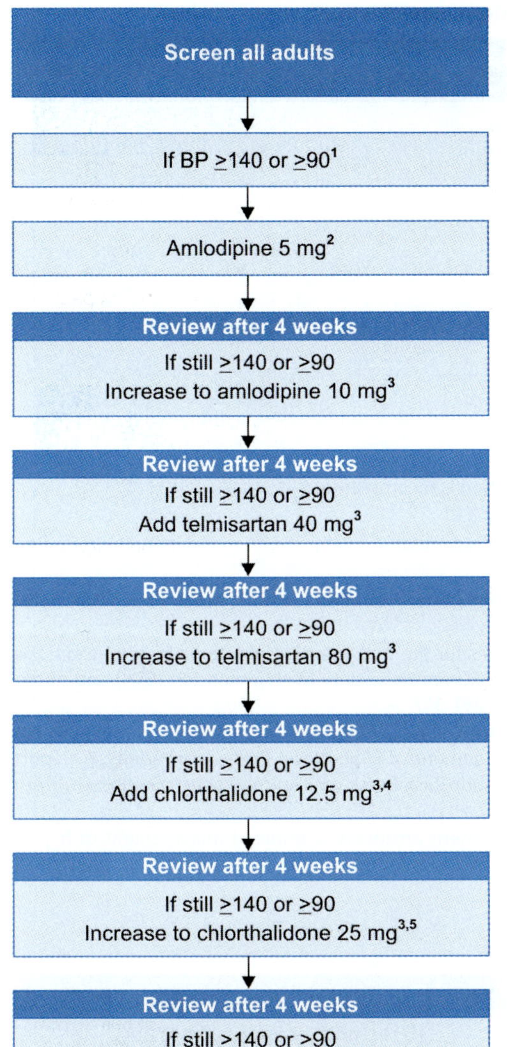

Provision for specific patients

- Manage diabetes as indicated by national protocol
- Aim for BP target of <130/80 for people with diabetes or otherwise at high risk
- Start statin and aspirin in people with prior heart attack or ischemic stroke
- Start beta-blocker in people with heart attack in past 3 years
- Consider statin in people at high risk

Lifestyle management advice for all patients

- Stop all tobacco use, avoid second-hand tobacco smoke
- Avoid unhealthy alcohol intake
- Increase physical activity to equivalent of brisk walk 150 min per week
- If overweight, lose weight
- Eat a heart-healthy diet:
  - Eat less than 1 teaspoon of salt per day
  - Eat ≥5 servings of vegetables/fruit per day
  - Use healthy oils
  - Eat nuts, legumes, whole grains and foods rich in potassium
  - Limit red meat to once or twice a week at most
  - Eat fish or other food rich in omega-3 fatty acids at least twice a week
  - Avoid added sugar

¹If <160/100, start same day and consider initiating 10 mg of amlodipine daily. If SBP 140–159 or DBP 90–99, check on a different day and if still elevated start.

²Smaller, fragile patients should be started on 2.5 mg per day. Alternatively, amlodipine can be replaced with a thiazide diuretic (e.g. chlorthalidone 12.5, indapamide 1.25 mg, or indapamide SR 1.5 mg; if neither chlorthalidone nor indapamide is available, hydrochlorothiazide 25 mg) or a once-daily angiotensin receptor blocker (ARB) (e.g. telmisartan 40 mg or losartan 50 mg) or once-daily angiotensin-converting enzyme (ACE) inhibitor inhibitor (e.g. lisinopril 20 mg, ramipril 5 mg. perindopril 4 mg). ACE inhibitor and ARB should not be given to women who are or who may become pregnant. Before initiating and several weeks after starting a thiazide diuretic, ACE inhibitor, or ARB, check serum creatinine and potassium if possible.

³If SBP repeatedly <100, consider going to prior, less intensive regimen.

⁴Indapamide can be used if chlorthalidone is not available (1.25 mg starting dose, 2.5 mg intensification; for indapamide SR 1.5 mg, do not increase dose at step 7). Hydrochlorothiazide can be used if neither of the other diuretic agents is available (25 mg starting dose, 50 mg intensification).

⁵Hypokalemia is more common using full dose diuretic—consider regular lab monitoring. If a diuretic is used instead of amlodipine in the initial treatment, this consideration would apply earlier in the protocol.

(DBP: diastolic blood pressure; SBP: systolic blood pressure)

Flowchart 2: Recommended single-agent hypertension treatment regimen.

TABLE 1: Guidelines of International Support for fixed-dose combination.

	China 2010	India 2013	Thailand 2015	ACC/AHA 2017	ESC/ESH 2013/2018	WHO HEARTS
Recommendations when to use single-pill combinations						
Substitute to separate pills for improving adherence	Yes	Yes	NR	Yes	Yes	NR
Recommendations when to use two BP-lowering drugs						
Uncontrolled on monotherapy	Yes	Yes	Yes	Yes	Yes	Yes
Initial treatment for selected patients e.g. >20/10 mm Hg from goal* and/or high CV risk	Yes	Yes	Yes	Yes	Yes	Yes

*Some referred to this as stage II HTN or marked BP elevation.

Note:
- For patients needing >1 BP-lowering drug, fixed-dose combination is recommended
- ACC/ AHA 2017 - [ARB or ACE inhibitor] [Thiazide/Thiazide like] [CCB]

(BP: blood pressure; CV: cardiovascular; HTN: hypertension; NR: not reported)

Source:
- Association of Physicians of India. Indian guidelines on hypertension (I.G.H)-III. 2013. J Assoc Physicians India. 2013;61:6-36
- Mancia G, Fagard R, Narkiewicz K, et al. 2013 ESH/ESC Guidelines for the management of arterial hypertension: the Task Force for the management of arterial hypertension of the European Society of Hypertension (ESH) and of the European Society of Cardiology (ESC). J Hypertension. 2013;31:1281-357
- Whelton PK, Carey RM, Aronow WS, et al. 2017 ACC/AHA/AAPA/ABC/ACPM/AGS/APhA/ASH/ASPC/NMA/PCNA Guideline for the Prevention, Detection, Evaluation, and Management of High Blood Pressure in Adults: A Report of the American College of Cardiology/American Heart Association Task Force on Clinical Practice Guidelines. J Am College Cardiol. 2017:24430
- Jaffe MG, Frieden TR, Campbell NRC, et al. Recommended treatment protocols to improve management of hypertension globally: A statement by Resolve to Save Lives and the World Hypertension League (WHL). J Clin Hypertens (Greenwich). 2018;20:829-36.

TABLE 2: Guidelines—focus on four combinations.

	Example combinations*	Dose option.s (mg)
ACE inhibitor and thiazide or thiazide-like diuretics	Lisinopril and hydrochlorothiazide	10 mg and 12.5 mg; 20 mg and 12.5 mg; 20 mg and 25 mg
ARB and CCB	Telmisartan and amlodipine	40 mg and 5 mg; 80 mg and 5 mg; 80 mg and 10 mg
ACE inhibitor and CCB	Lisinopril and amlodipine	10 mg and 5 mg; 20 mg and 5 mg; 20 mg and 10 mg
ARB and thiazide or thiazide-like diuretics	Telmisartan and hydrochlorothiazide	40 mg and 12.5 mg; 80 mg and 12.5 mg; 80 mg and 25 mg

*Indicative components—similar clinical performance cam be expected with other once-daily drugs from the same class to optimize choice.

(ACE: angiotensin-converting enzyme; ARB: angiotensin receptor blocker; CCB: calcium channel blocker)

Source:
- Kishore SP, Salam A, Rodger A, et al. Fixed-dose combinations for hypertension. Lancet. 2018;392:819-20.
- Salam A, Kanukula R, Esam H, et al. An application to include blood pressure lowering drug fixed dose combinations to the model essential medicines list for the treatment of essential hypertension in adults. [Accessed 2019 June 26]. Available at: https://www.who.int/selection_medicines/committees/expert/22/s12_FDC-antihypertensives.pdf

TABLE 3: Drug combinations used in trials of antihypertensive treatment.

Trial	Comparator	Type of patients	SBP difference (mm Hg)	Outcomes
ACE inhibitor and diuretic combination				
PROGRESS 296	Placebo	Previous stroke or TIA	−9	−28% strokes (p <0.001)
ADVANCE 276	Placebo	Diabetes	−5.6	−9% micro/macrovascular events (p = 0.04)
HYVET 287	Placebo	Hypertensives aged = 80 years	−15	−34% CV events (p <0.001)
CAPPP 455	BB + D	Hypertensives	+3	+5% CV events (p = NS)
Angiotensin receptor blocker and diuretic combination				
SCOPE 450	D + placebo	Hypertensives aged = 70 years	−3.2	−28% nonfatal strokes (p = 0.04)
LIFE 457	BB + D	Hypertensives with LVH	−1	−26% stroke (p <0.001)
Calcium antagonist and diuretic combination				
FEVER 269	D + placebo	Hypertensives	−4	−27% CV events (p <0.001)
ELSA 186	BB + D	Hypertensives	0	NS difference in CV events
CONVINCE 458	BB + D	Hypertensives with risk factors	0	NS difference in CV events
VALUE 456	ARB + D	High-risk hypertensives	−2.2	−3% CV events (p = NS)
ACE inhibitor and calcium antagonist combination				
Syst-Eur 451	Placebo	Elderly with ISH	−10	−31% CV events (p <0.001)
Syst-China 452	Placebo	Elderly with ISH	−9	−37% CV events (p <0.004)
NORDIL 461	BB + D	Hypertensives	+3	NS difference in CV events
INVEST 459	BB + D	Hypertensives with CHD	0	NS difference in CV events
ASCOT 423	BB + D	Hypertensives with risk factors	−3	−16% CV events (p <0.001)
ACCOMPLISH 414	ACE inhibitor + D	Hypertensives with risk factors	−1	−21% CV events (p <0.001)
BB and diuretic combination				
Coope and Warrender 453	Placebo	Elderly hypertensives	−18	−42% strokes (p <0.03)
SHEP 449	Placebo	Elderly with ISH	−13	−36% strokes (p <0.001)
STOP 454	Placebo	Elderly hypertensives	−23	−40% CV events (p = 0.003)
STOP 2 460	ACE inhibitor or CA	Hypertensives	0	NS difference in CV events
CAPPP 455	ACE inhibitor + D	Hypertensives	−3	−5% CV events (p = NS)

Continued

Continued

Trial	Comparator	Type of patients	SBP difference (mm Hg)	Outcomes
LIFE 457	ARB + D	Hypertensives with LVH	+1	+26% stroke (p <0.001)
ALLHAT 448	ACE inhibitor + BB	Hypertensives with risk factors	–2	NS difference in CV events
ALLHAT 448	CA + BB	Hypertensives with risk factors	–1	NS difference in CV events
CONVINCE 458	CA + D	Hypertensives with risk factors	0	NS difference in CV events
NORDIL 461	ACE inhibitor + CA	Hypertensives	–3	NS difference in CV events
INVEST 459	ACE inhibitor + CA	Hypertensives with CHD	0	NS difference in CV events
ASCOT 423	ACE inhibitor + CA	Hypertensives with risk factors	+3	+16% CV events (p <0.001)
Combination of two renin–angiotensin system (RAS) blockers/ACE inhibitor + ARB or RAS blocker + renin inhibitor				
ONTARGET	ACE inhibitor or ARB	High-risk patients	–3	More renal events
ALTITUDE 433	ACE inhibitor or ARB	High-risk diabetic patients	–1.3	More renal events

(ACE: angiotensin-converting enzyme; ARB: angiotensin receptor blocker; BB: beta-blocker; CA: calcium antagonist; CHD: coronary heart disease; CV: cardiovascular; D: diuretic; ISH: isolated systolic hypertension; LVH: left ventricular hypertrophy; NS: not significant; SBP: systolic blood pressure; TIA: transient ischemic attack)

How and What to be Used in Combination Therapy?

Combination therapy can either be fixed dose combinations or drugs added sequentially one after other. Combinations may be individualized according to the presence of comorbidities like diabetes mellitus (DM), chronic renal failure, heart failure (HF), thyroid disorders and for special population groups like elderly and pregnant females.

What is Required for Combination Therapy?

The primary hemodynamic parameters for BP regulation are intravascular volume, cardiac output and systemic vascular resistance (Flowchart 3). The RAAS and the sympathetic nervous system are the fine-tuners that continuously both regulate and calibrate these parameters.

Persistent hypertension can develop only in response to increase in cardiac output (CO) or a rise in peripheral vascular resistance.

■ PRINCIPLES OF COMBINATION

- Different mechanisms (cardiac output + peripheral resistance)
- Same mechanism, different pathway (cardiac output or peripheral resistance)
- Same mechanism, same pathway (cardiac output or peripheral resistance).

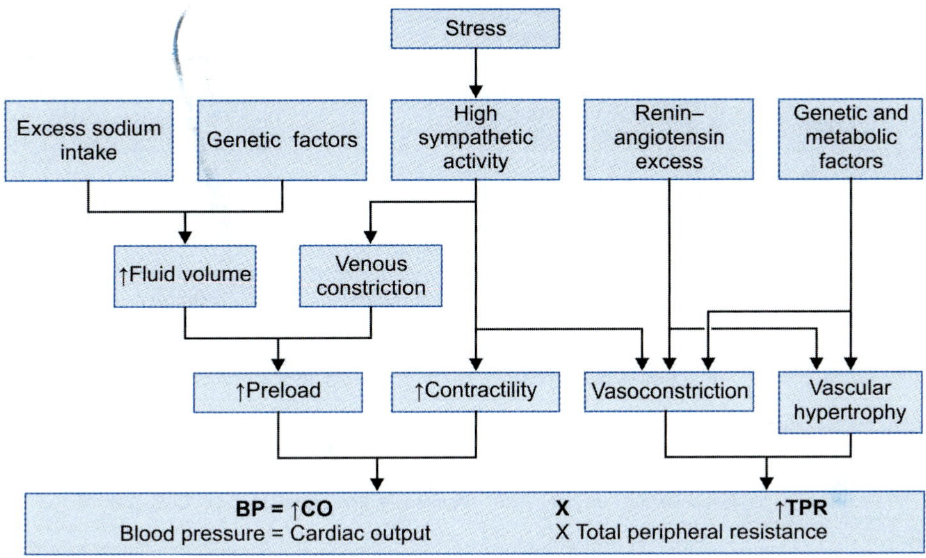

Flowchart 3: Interplay of various factors affecting cardiac output and peripheral resistance.

Different Mechanism

Beta-blockers	Ca blocker (DHP)
Decreased cardiac output	Decreased peripheral resistance

Preferred in:
- Coronary artery disease (CAD) and high BP
- Pregnancy and hypertension.

Not preferred in:
- Diabetic nephropathy
- Beta-blockers and nondihydropyridine (non-DHP) calcium channel blockers not to be combined.

Different Mechanism

Beta-blockers	Angiotensin inhibitor
Decreased cardiac output	Decreased peripheral resistance

Preferred in:
- CAD and postmyocardial infarction
- Left ventricular (LV) dysfunction, HF
- DM + CAD.

Not preferred in:
- To achieve targets
- Renal failure.

Not a good combination in pure hypertension.

Different Mechanism

Beta-blockers	Alpha-blockers
Decreased cardiac output	Decreased peripheral resistance

Preferred in:
- Accelerated high BP due to sympathetic over action
- CAD + benign prostatic hypertrophy
- Renal failure
- Renal + HF (carvedilol).

Not preferred in:
- Target organ protection.

Different Mechanism

Diuretic	Ca blocker (DHP)
Decreased cardiac output	Decreased Peripheral resistance

	Younger, <55 years			Older, >55 years	
Step 1	ARB/ACE inhibitor or newer **beta**-blockers			**CCB**	
Step 2	ARB/ACE inhibitor or newer beta-**blockers**			**CCB or diuretic**	
Step 3	ARB/ACE inhibitor or newer **beta**-blockers	+ CCB +	Diuretic		
Step 4	Add either alpha-blocker or spironolactone or other diuretic				

Note: Combination therapy involving B and D may induce more new onset diabetes compared with other combination therapies. Use β-blockers only in special situations. B = Newer β-blockers. Younger age: <55 years, Older: >55 years.

(ACE: angiotensin-converting enzyme; ARB: angiotensin II receptor blocker; CCB: calcium channel blocker).

Flowchart 4: Indian Guidelines for Hypertension III: Algorithm for recommended drug combination.

Preferred in:
- Isolated systolic hypertension in elderly
- Prevention of strokes.

Not preferred in:
- Target organ protection
- DM and nephropathy
- CAD.

Different Mechanism

Diuretic (K losing)	Angiotensin inhibitor
Decreased cardiac output	Decreased peripheral resistance

Preferred in:
- To achieve targets
- HF, LV dysfunction
- Diabetes.

Not preferred in:
- Elderly hypertension
- Severe renal failure.

Different Mechanism Summary

- β-blockers + Ca blockers
- β-blockers + ANG inhibitors
- β-blockers + α-blockers

- Diuretic + ANG inhibitors
- Diuretic + Ca blockers.

Same Mechanism, Different Pathways (Decreased Cardiac Output)

β-blockers	Diuretic
Decrease contractility	Decrease preload

Preferred in:
- Uncomplicated high BP without target organ disease.

Not preferred in:
- DM, metabolic syndrome and obese hypertensives.

Same Mechanism, Different Pathways (Decreased Peripheral Resistance)

Angiotensin I	Ca blockers
Vascular hypertrophy ↓	Vasoconstriction ↓

Preferred in:
- To achieve targets
- End organ protection

- DM, high BP + nephropathy
- CAD (non-DHP)
- Obese, metabolic syndrome
- Prevent future DM.

Not preferred in:

- Elderly hypertension.

Same Mechanism, Different Pathways (Decreased Peripheral Resistance)

Angiotensin inhibitor	Alpha-βlockers
Vascular hypertrophy ↓	Vasoconstriction ↓

Preferred in:

- For effective BP lowering
- Where angiotensin inhibitor and Ca blockers can't be combined
- With benign prostatic hypertrophy
- DM ± nephropathy.

Not preferred in:

- Elderly.

Same Mechanism, Different Pathways (Decreased Peripheral Resistance)

Ca blocker	Alpha-blockers
Decrease intracellular cardiac	Block alpha stimulation

Preferred in:

- Renal failure
- Benign prostate hypertrophy
- Bronchial asthma or peripheral vascular disease.

Not preferred in:

- Elderly
- CAD
- DM.

Same Mechanism, Different Pathways Summary

- β-blockers + diuretic (cardiac output)
- Ca blockers + ANG inhibitors (peripheral resistance)

- ANG inhibitors + α-blockers (peripheral resistance)
- Ca blockers + α-blockers (peripheral resistance).

Same Mechanism, Same Pathway

	Cardiac output
Diuretics	• Thiazide + loop diuretics • Thiazide + aldosterone inhibitors • Loop diuretics + aldosterone inhibitors
	Peripheral resistance
Ca blockers	DHP and non-DHP (CAD, bronchial asthma, arrhythmia, PVD)
Angiotensin I	ACE inhibitor and ARB, (nephropathy, chronic HF)

Other Combinations— Centrally-acting Drugs

Alpha methyldopa + hydralazine	Renal failure, pregnancy
Clonidine + diuretics	Severe hypertension and renal hypertension
Reserpine + diuretics	Still some patients are taking

Initial Combination Therapy Even in Stage I

CAD	β-blockers and ramipril
LV dysfunction	Specific β-blockers and ramipril
Heart failure	Specific β-blockers, ACE inhibitor and Aldo inhibitors
DM and CAD	Carvedilol and ramipril
Stroke (secondary prevention)	ACE inhibitor and indapamide
HF and RF (ACE inhibitor intolerance)	Hydralazine and nitrates

Combinations to be Avoided

β-blockers and diuretics	Diabetes
ACE inhibitor and ARB	Simple hypertension
β-blockers and clonidine	Bradycardia
β-blockers and non-DHP Ca Blockers	Bradycardia
β-blockers and ACE inhibitor or ARB	Simple hypertension
ACE inhibitor, ARB, and Aldo inhibitors	Hyperkalemia

Is single-pill combination (SPC) a better or free combination?

Single-pill (fixed-dose) combinations are often used to promote adherence by reducing pill burden and simplifying the treatment regimen. In a meta-analysis of nine studies comparing administration of SPCs or their separate components, the adherence rate was improved by 26% in patients receiving SPCs.

Single-pill combination formulations currently available, offers all the advantages- improved adherence, simplification of therapy, better efficacy and better tolerability, a wide range of dosages for the individual components offering good flexibility for dosage adjustment, and titration for optimal BP control. In addition, they are currently endorsed by international guidelines as the preferred strategy to combine BP-lowering drugs (Table 4).

■ COMBINATION OF TWO OR MORE DRUGS

If the target is not achieved by a two-drug combination at full doses, swapping to another two-drug combination can be considered or a third drug added. Preference should be given to the selection of an agent from a different class than the initial two drugs in the combination therapy. Addition of the third drug may be in the form of spironolactone (requires the assessment of renal functions and potassium), minoxidil, hydralazine, carvedilol and rest of the drugs depending on the specific conditions being treated. Centrally acting drugs should be the last option due to potential side effects.

To achieve BP targets up to 24–32% of patients will require three or more drugs as shown in clinical trials. This triple-drug combination the calcium channel blocker (CCB) amlodipine and the diuretic HCTZ combined with an ARB (valsartan and olmesartan) was shown to produce statistically greater BP reduction compared with any of their component two-drug combinations. Combinations of an ACE inhibitor or ARB,

TABLE 4: Comparison between different hypertension management strategies.

	Low-dose monotherapy	High-dose monotherapy	Free combination therapy	Single-pill combination therapy
Efficacy	–	+	++	++
Time to reach BP target	–	+	++	++
BP variability	–	–	+	+
Simplicity	+	+	–	+
Flexibility	+	+	+	+**
Compliance	+	+	–	+
Tolerability	+	–	+	++*

*Lower doses generally used in single-pill combinations.

**An increasing number of single-pill combinations are becoming available with a range of doses + = potential advantage.

(BP: blood pressure)

a CCB and a diuretic represent rational and effective treatment for a large percentage of patients. These are favored three-drug combinations in patients without conditions that mandate use of a drug from another class.

CONCLUSION

Combination therapy is indorsed by guidelines to treat hypertension and has become widely accepted by healthcare providers. The coherent use of drug combination is critical in achieving more rapid BP control and more effective organ protection. The choice of combination therapy is individualized depends upon the risk factors and presence of comorbidities. The physician should not have inertia of controlling BP and should have low threshold for combination therapy if BP is not controlled with single agent.

REFERENCES

1. Indian Guidelines on Hypertension (IGH) – III 2013.
2. ESH and ESC Guidelines 2013.
3. Salahuddin A, Mushtaq M, Materson BJ. Combination therapy for hypertension 2013: an update. J Am Soc Hypertens 2013;7(5):401-7.
4. Epstein BJ, Shah NK, Borja-Hart NL. Management of hypertension with fixed – dose triple combination treatments. Ther Adv Cardiovasc Dis. 2013;7(5):246-59.
5. Gradman AH. Strategies for combination therapy in hypertension. Curr Opin Nephrol Hypertens. 2012;21(5):486-91.
6. Hypertension published by the American Heart Association, 7272 Greenville Avenue, Dallas, TX 75231Hypertension Print ISSN: 0194-911X. Online ISSN: 1524-4563 Copyright © 2012 American Heart Association, Inc.
7. Recommended treatment protocols to improve management of hypertension globally: A statement by Resolve to Save Lives and the World Hypertension League (WHL) - Received: 11 March 2018 I Revised: 16 March 2018 I Accepted: 18 March 2018
8. Erdine S. Compliance with the treatment of hypertension: the potential of combination therapy. J Clin Hypertens (Greenwich). 2010;12(1):40-6.
9. Kalra S, Kalra B, Agrawal N. Combination therapy in hypertension: An update. Diabetol Metab Syndr. 2010; 2:44.
10. Wald DS, Law M, Morris JK, et al. Combination therapy versus monotherapy in reducing blood pressure: meta-analysis on 11,000 participants from 42 trials. Am J Med. 2009;122(3):290-300.
11. JENNIFER FRANK, MD, University of Wisconsin Department of Family Medicine, Appleton, Wisconsin. Managing hypertension using combination therapy. Am Fam Physician. 2008;77(9):1279-1286.
12. Ker J. Combination treatment for hypertension. SA Fam Pract. 2010;52(5):417-21
13. Rosenthal T, Gavras I. Fixed-drug combinations as first-line treatment for hypertension. Prog Cardiovasc Dis. 2006;48(6):416-25.

Interactions between Antihypertensive Drugs and Other Medications

Sekhar Chakraborty

■ INTRODUCTION

Hypertension remains a highly prevalent risk factor for cardiovascular disease, the worldwide prevalence of hypertension is increasing and blood pressure control in hypertensive population remains unacceptably poor. Approximately, 1 billion people are affected worldwide, which is a statistical figure of concern for any preventable and treatable disease. With the advent of different classes of antihypertensive pharmacotherapy, physicians have several therapeutic options including medications. To achieve the blood pressure (BP) targets, often combination therapy is being prescribed particularly in patients having high cardiovascular risk factors. Concomitant use of other medications to address other associated comorbidities like diabetes, dyslipidemia, obesity, renal disorder, stroke, chronic obstructive pulmonary disease (COPD), and cardiovascular diseases are also important, so far the antihypertensive drugs interactions are concerned. This chapter will venture to touch upon all these related issues.

Antihypertensive drug interactions can be viewed from different angles. Two major types of drugs interactions can be pointed out:

1. *According to the metabolism/action of the drug*:
   i. *Pharmacokinetic interaction*: By altering the absorption, distribution, or elimination of drugs, which ultimately affect the amount of drug at the site of action
   ii. *Pharmacodynamic interaction*: By altering the effect of any given amount of drug.
2. *According to the outcome of drug interaction*:
   i. Undesirable (hazardous)
   ii. Desirable (beneficial).

"Desirable" interactions are characterized by increased therapeutic benefits with minimal side effects.

"Undesirable" interactions are characterized by unacceptable side effects, which ultimately defeat the purpose of therapy.

■ STEPWISE APPROACH TO IDENTIFY DRUG INTERACTION

It is superfluous to mention that "recognition" remains the first step toward correction of any adverse interaction.

Recognition of Undesirable Interactions

- *First clue*: Loss of well-established blood pressure control or failure to achieve the blood pressure target
- Thorough review of all medications; be it self-prescribed or prescribed by any clinician, is required
- Acceleration of disease process or emergent of new illness in spite of getting optimal antihypertensive therapy.

Pharmacokinetic Interaction

- *Absorption*: Most of the antihypertensive drugs are taken orally. But it has been observed that presence of food or altered gut motility plays very limited role to affect the absorption of antihypertensive drugs. However, certain components of food, notably tyramine-rich cheeses can cause precipitous rise of blood pressure when taken along with monoamine oxidase (MAO) inhibitor
- *Distribution*: Distribution of anti-hypertensive drugs at the site of action has been well-studied by Mitchell et al. in 1970. The best possible example has been cited by demonstrating the interaction between tricyclic antidepressants (TCAs) and guanethidine, bethanidine or debrisoquine
- *Elimination*: Alteration of elimination process of antihypertensive drugs does not seem to be clinically relevant. However, a recent study has demonstrated that propranolol can reduce hepatic blood flow, thereby can reduce the clearance of some drugs, which are eliminated by liver, e.g. lignocaine.

Pharmacodynamic Interaction

Most of the drug interaction of antihyper-tensive is pharmacodynamics in nature.

- *Interaction of diuretics*: Diuretics remain one of the mainstay of treatment of hypertension since its inception in 1950s.

Its ability to control blood pressure or to restrict adverse effects may be enhanced by (desirable interaction):
  - Salt-restricted diet
  - Addition of potassium-sparing diuretics
  - Cautious use of cardiac glycosides
  - Concomitant diuretics therapy can enhance the efficacy and reduce side effects of sympathetic blockers.

It has been observed that excessive salt intake can nullify the effects of diuretics on blood pressure. As the salt restriction has got some efficacy that of diuretics, the concomi-tant use of salt restriction and diuretic therapy has shown additive effect on reduction of blood pressure. This consideration becomes more important when patients are getting sympathetic blockers simultaneously.

All adrenergic blockers cause sodium retention and these effects tend to raise blood pressure countering the antihypertensive action of these drugs and produce "pseudo-tolerance". The masked effect of adrenergic blockers can be revived by adding diuretics.

Generally, thiazides are diuretics of first choice when the estimated glomerular filtration rate (eGFR) is more than 30 mL/min/m^2. When the renal function deteriorates further, thiazides cannot work properly and loop diuretics are called upon. In extreme cases of fluid overloading, loop diuretics and metolazone (thiazide) are coprescribed to have the desirable effects but the possibility of inducing hypokalemia remains high.

A desirable intergroup pharmacodynamics interaction is exemplified by combination of a thiazide diuretic or loop with potassium-sparing diuretics to avoid hypokalemia. This combination therapy is useful in offsetting an adverse effect of thiazide and loop diuretics.

Simultaneous use of cardiac glycosides and diuretics can cause potentially fatal hypokalemia leading to cardiac arrhythmias. In this situation, potassium supplement is required. Clinician should be aware of potential hyperkalemia when potassium-retaining diuretics are used along with.

Thiazide diuretics can cause hyperglycemia, hyperuricemia and hypercalcemia. As the β-blocker can precipitate adult-onset diabetes and symptomatic gout, the combination of β-blockers and thiazide diuretics should not be preferred as initial therapy though diuretics remain the first choice as antihypertensive therapy.

- *Interaction with adrenergic-inhibiting drugs*: Adrenergic-inhibiting drugs can cause fluid retention by inhibiting sympathetic nervous system. Fluid retention tends to offset the antihypertensive efficacy of these drugs. Many such drugs also interfere with renal renin release. Combining diuretics with adrenergic-inhibiting drugs provide the following benefits:
  - Since all diuretics are potent stimulators of renin release, the combination of diuretic plus sympathetic-inhibiting drug frequently results in a plasma renin activity that is less than with the diuretic alone
  - Combining diuretics with antiadrenergic drugs can reduce fluid retention substantially.

  Sympathetic-inhibiting drugs than are most potent in preventing renin release:
  - β-blockers
  - Clonidine
  - Methyldopa
  - Reserpine
  - Guanethidine (it can increase plasma renin activity when it decreases arterial pressure. Similar property is also shown by bethanidine and debrisoquine).
- *Interaction with guanethidine and related drugs*: Guanethidine must be transported into adrenergic neurons to exert their

effect. The active transport mechanism that pumps adrenalin into sympathetic nerve ending is also used to transport guanidine compounds like guanethidine across the cell membrane. Guanethidine entering into the neuron depletes the storage of noradrenalin and paralyzes the neuron. In this way, it exerts its antihypertensive effect.

If this "noradrenalin pump" is inhibited, guanethidine cannot enter into the neurons and therefore cannot exert its antihypertensive property. As the TCAs are the potent inhibitors of this "noradrenalin pump", guanethidine has got an interaction with TCA. Chlorpromazine also inhibits this pump in the dose >150 mg/day but the degree inhibition is less profound compared to that of TCA.

Doxepin has less marked inhibition to this pump; therefore, it interacts with guanethidine only in significant high dose (e.g. 200 mg/day).

Phenothiazines, being fairly potent α-adrenergic blocking drugs, tend to reduce blood pressure and do not interact with guanethidine.

Pizotifen, used in migraine prophylaxis and mazindol, an anorexiant can interact with guanethidine by inhibiting noradrenalin pump mechanism.

Indirectly-acting sympathomimetic derivatives like amphetamine, ephedrine, pseudoephedrine, phenylpropanolamine, and phenylephrine compete with guanethidine for their uptake and storage. Simultaneous use of these drugs and guanethidine leads to therapeutic failure. These indirectly-acting sympathomimetics are commonly present in cold and cough formula, which is sold over-the-counter without prescription of doctors. Therefore, therapeutic failure of guanethidine-related drugs can happen when taken concurrently with cough formula.

- *Interaction with clonidine*: Clonidine can interact with TCA, e.g. desipramine but not with imipramine or amitriptyline.

Mechanism of this interaction is unknown but introduction of desipramine to a patient of hypertension controlled with clonidine shows rising of blood pressure within a week

- *Interaction with β-adrenergic blocking drugs*: Beta-adrenergic blocking drugs may be cardioselective or nonselective. In asthma and COPD, the amount of bronchodilators like salbutamol or terbutaline requirement is more when these patients receive nonselective β-blockers like propranolol. More cardioselective β-blockers like metoprolol, atenolol do not pose these problems.

Propranolol blunts the physiological response to hypoglycemia like palpitation, tachycardia, and tremors but sweating remains the same. Therefore, it develops "hypoglycemia unawareness".

Propranolol can intensify the hypoglycemic property of some oral hypoglycemic agents probably by inhibiting adrenergically-stimulated glycogenolysis.

Sometimes, propranolol can cause hypertension if circulating level of catecholamines is increased. It can be seen in drug-induced hypoglycemia, clonidine withdrawal, and in pheochromocytoma. It is due to α-adrenergic vasoconstriction unopposed by β-adrenergic vasodilatation.

- *Interaction with MAO inhibitor*: Ingestion of tyramine-rich food and beverages (cheese reaction) can cause precipitous rise of blood pressure when taken with MAO inhibitors due to liberation of large amount of catecholamines into circulation.

Similar mechanism can play when taken with cough formula containing ephedrine or pseudoephedrine. Frequent use of nasal decongestants can cause hypertension among young adults and children.

Monoamine oxidase inhibitors can interact with sulfonylureas or pethidine and can cause precipitous rise in blood pressure.

Levodopa also produces undesirable side effects causing hypertension with MAO inhibitors due to interference with the storage and release of dopamine and noradrenalin.

- *Interactions with vasodilators*: Direct-acting vasodilator, hydralazine, can cause tachycardia and palpitation due to increased sympathetic tone being augmented reflexly by direct vasodilation. The antihypertensive property of hydralazine is offset by this reflex sympathetic overactivity. When it is combined with propranolol, not only its sympathetic overactivity is decreased but also its antihypertensive property is enhanced.

Prazosin exerts its vasodilatory property by blocking postsynaptic α-adrenoceptors and its antihypertensive property is enhanced by β-blockers.[1]

Addition of diuretic to a vasodilator can often be a successful therapeutic option by reducing salt retention.

- *Multiple antihypertensive drugs combination*: Hypertensive patients often require more than one antihypertensive drug to control the blood pressure and to achieve the target. Multiple drug therapy may invite drug interaction between different groups of antihypertensive medications. The hexagonal structure depicted below represents different drug combinations (Fig. 1).[2-5] Any antihypertensive drug of one group may be combined with another agent except a few instances:[6-9]
    - Most important combination therapy, which has been discarded, is the combination between angiotensin-converting enzyme (ACE) inhibitors and angiotensin receptor blocker (ARB). After the publication of the Ongoing Telmisartan Alone and in Combination with Ramipril Global

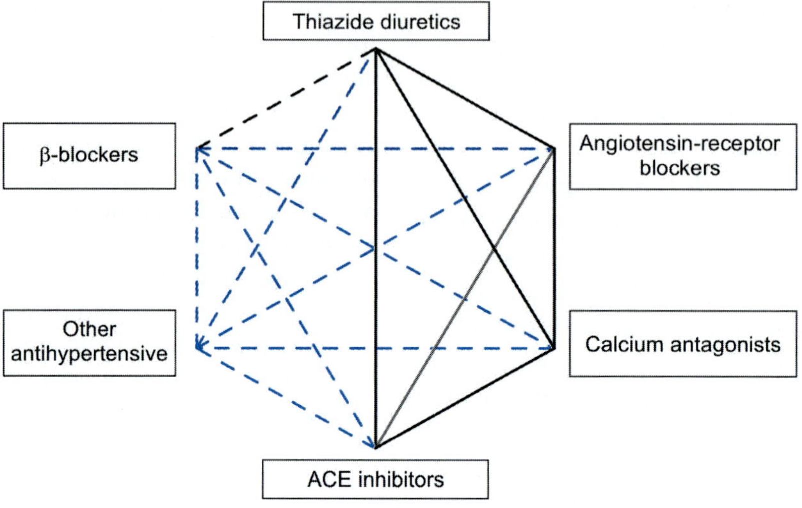

(ACE: angiotensin-converting enzyme)

Fig. 1: Current development of fixed-dose combinations.

Endpoint Trial (ONTARGET), it has been observed that this combination does not provide any extra benefit as synergistic or additive effect so far the optimum renin–angiotensin–aldosterone system (RAAS) blockade is concerned. Moreover, it may cause dangerous hyperkalemia and worsening of renal function in the background of acute renal failure

o Combination of β-blocker and nondihydropyridine calcium channel blockers should not be combined in the view of drug-induced bradycardia

o Alpha-blockers can cause postural hypotension, particularly in elderly. It should not be combined with others drugs, which can cause hypovolemia particularly diuretics

o Combination of ACE inhibitors or ARB can be combined with diuretics in a fashion that both acting together can prevent hypokalemia or hyperkalemia

o Combination of ACE inhibitors or ARB with calcium channel blockers (CCBs) may reduce pedal edema, which is a known side effect of CCB

o Loop diuretics should not be combined with aminoglycoside inhibitors or nonsteroidal anti-inflammatory drugs (NSAIDs) because it may cause worsening of renal function

o Loop diuretics or thiazide diuretics may potentiate the hypokalemia induced by long-acting corticosteroids.

■ CONCLUSION

Numerous permutations and combinations of different antihypertensive drugs and also other pharmacological agents are possible. Among them, some interactions are desirable, some are undesirable. Apart from the interactions mentioned above, other interactions are possible, which remains beyond the scope of this article. Rather than became enmeshed in a quagmire of infrequent and poorly understood interactions, an effort has been made to describe the best understood interactions only. My sincere intention remains to assist in the treatment of hypertensive diseases by the clinicians to reduce unwanted side effects as far as possible and to gain considerable benefits by using multiple drug regimens.

■ REFERENCES

1. Brogden RN, Heel RC, Speight TM, et al. Prazosin: a review of its pharmacological properties and therapeutic efficacy in hypertension. Drugs. 1977;14:163-97.
2. Dustan HP, Tarazi RC, Bravo EL. Dependence of arterial pressure on intravascular volume in treated hypertensive patients. N Engl J Med. 1972;286:861-6.
3. Koch-Weser J. Drug interactions in cardiovascular therapy. Am Heart J. 1975;90:93-116.
4. Morrelli HF. Drug interactions in hypertension: advantageous and adverse. Hospital Formulary. 1976;7:213-6.
5. Nies AS. Adverse reactions and interactions limiting the use of antihypertensive drugs. Am J Med. 1975;58:495-503.
6. Nies AS, Shand DG, Branch RA. Hemodynamic drug interactions. Cardiovasc Clin. 1974;6:43-53.
7. Pinder RM, Brogden RN, Speight TM, et al. Doxepin up-to-date: a review of its pharmacological properties and therapeutic efficacy with particular reference to depression. Drugs. 1977;13:161-218.
8. Simpson FO. Antihypertensive drug therapy. Drugs. 1973; 6:333-63.
9. Stafford JR, Fann WE. Drug interactions with guanidinium antihypertensives. Drugs. 1977;13:57-64.

Hypertensive Heart Disease

Pradip Sarkar, Soumitra Kumar

■ INTRODUCTION

High blood pressure (BP) is the most important risk factor for disabilities and death globally.[1] It increases varieties of cardiovascular diseases including stroke, heart failure (HF), coronary artery disease (CAD), peripheral vascular disease and cardiac arrhythmias including atrial fibrillation (AF). Essential hypertension accounts for the majority of adult individuals with hypertension which is almost 90% and remaining 10% accounts for secondary hypertension.

There is no universally accepted definition for "Hypertensive Heart Disease". The first classification, as proposed by the New York Heart Association (NYHA), equated hypertensive heart disease to HF in a patient with hypertension.[2] Later on, in most of the literatures the definition was limited to the presence of hypertensive left ventricular hypertrophy (LVH), diastolic dysfunction, or purely hemodynamic disturbances.[3] The Spanish Society of Cardiology proposed another definition and classification system for hypertensive heart disease, which included LV systolic dysfunction, myocardial ischemia and rhythm abnormalities in addition to LVH and diastolic dysfunction.[4]

Without sticking to any particular definition, in this chapter we will review the variable and complex set of effects of chronically elevated arterial blood pressure on heart itself.

■ EPIDEMIOLOGY

Adjusting for age and other HF risk factors, the hazard for developing HF in hypertensive patients was about 2-fold in men and 3-fold in women, in comparison to the normotensive subjects in the Framingham Heart Study. Considering LV mass as a continuous variable, there is a direct and progressive relationship between absolute amount of LV mass and cardiovascular risk.[5] As a discrete categorical variable, LVH increases the risk of HF, CAD, ventricular arrhythmia, sudden cardiac death (SCD) and stroke.[5,6]

■ PATHOPHYSIOLOGY

Prolonged and uncontrolled elevation of BP leads to a variety of pathophysiological changes in myocardium, coronary arteries and conducting tissues of the heart. These changes lead to the development of LVH, LV diastolic dysfunction, LV systolic dysfunction, CAD and various conduction abnormalities which ultimately manifest clinically as HF, angina, myocardial infarction (MI), arrhythmias—especially AF, and even SCD.

Left Ventricular Hypertrophy

Left ventricular hypertrophy in hypertensive patient is an adaptive response to chronic hemodynamic overload. Sustained high BP leads to an increase in wall stress which increases myocardial oxygen demand. In response to elevated wall stress there is also increase in LV wall thickness as well as overall LV mass, thereby resulting in reducing wall stress but development of concentric hypertrophy. On the other hand, increase in blood volume may lead to increase in chamber diameter causing eccentric hypertrophy. Development of LVH is affected by some other factors such as angiotensin II, norepinephrine, epinephrine and increased sympathetic drive. Hypertensive patients often concomitantly have other risk factors such as diabetes and obesity which are also risk factors for the development of LVH independent of high BP.[7]

Diastolic Dysfunction

Diastolic dysfunction is the main cause of symptomatic HF in hypertensive patients.[8] LVH causes persistently elevated LV end-diastolic pressure. This leads to elevated left atrial pressure and volume, which causes pulmonary venous congestion. This clinically manifests initially as exercise intolerance. Ischemia is also an important risk factor for the development of diastolic dysfunction. Hypertension itself accelerates atherosclerosis and endothelial dysfunction. Increase in LV mass without a proportional proliferation of capillaries in the myocardial vascular bed results in miss-match between coronary circulation and myocardial oxygen demand. In initial phase, the patients are asymptomatic during resting state, but a slight elevation in systemic vascular resistance occurs during exercise or slight change in circulating volume,

makes the stiff hypertrophied left ventricle incapable of handling the extra pressure/volume. This leads to progressive decline in LV function.

Systolic Dysfunction

As per the Framingham Heart Study report, severe systolic dysfunction occurs in about 3–6% of hypertensive individuals.[9] Hypertensive LV hypertrophy or remodeling is certainly followed by chamber dilation, if not treated appropriately. An eccentric pattern of hypertrophy is a strong risk factor for the development of LV systolic dysfunction. LV remodeling which is initially compensatory is followed by progressive worsening of cardiac function (Fig. 1).

Once the systolic dysfunction ensues, there is gradual decrease in systolic BP. The patients who were hypertensive to begin with, may become normotensive or even hypotensive, with the progression of LV systolic dysfunction. This phenomenon is known as "Decapitated Hypertension". Thus LV systolic dysfunction may be a powerful antihypertensive mechanism. These patients are difficult to manage, because they are intolerant to many HF medications such as angiotensin-converting enzyme (ACE) inhibitors, beta-blockers which reduce systolic BP further.

From clinical point of view, hypertensive heart disease is categorized in four ascending degrees, based on clinical and pathophysiologic impact of hypertension on heart (Fig. 2).[10]

- Degree I: Isolated LV diastolic dysfunction without LV hypertrophy
- Degree II: LV diastolic dysfunction with concentric LV hypertrophy
- Degree III: Clinical HF (dyspnea and pulmonary edema with preserved ejection fraction, HFpEF)
- Degree IV: Dilated cardiomyopathy with HF and reduced ejection fraction (HFrEF).

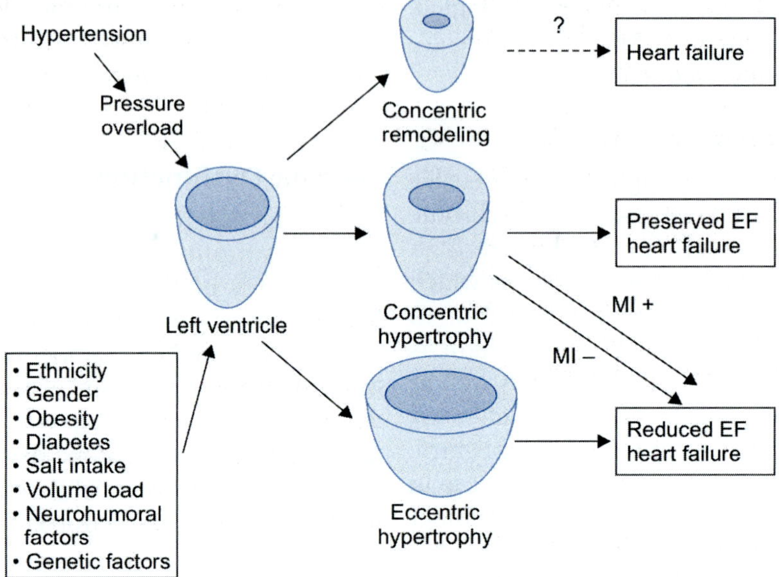

(EF: ejection fraction; MI: myocardial infarction)

Fig. 1: Pathways of left ventricular remodeling progression secondary to systemic hypertension.

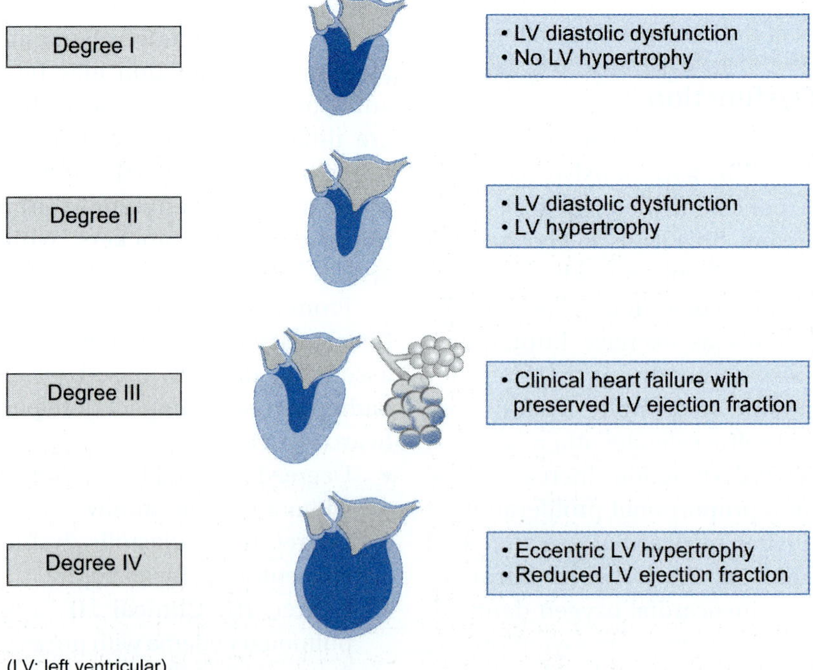

(LV: left ventricular)

Fig. 2: Stages of hypertensive heart disease.

This conventional concept of hypertensive remodeling was described by William Osler, almost 120 years ago.[11] He described that the hypertensive response, which were initially compensatory, were followed by progressive worsening of symptoms that was due to 'degeneration and weakening of the heart muscles'. Nowadays hypertensive heart disease is considered as a complex disease mediated not only by hemodynamic factors like LV pressure and volume overload, but also by interplay of several nonhemodynamic factors.[12] These include genetic and neurohormonal factors, ethnicity, gender, obesity and diabetes mellitus (Fig. 1).[12]

Several genes have been identified to influence the LV mass independent of BP.[13] Most of them involve renin–angiotensin–aldosterone system—*ACE* gene, X-linked angiotensin II type 2 receptor gene, angiotensinogen gene, aldosterone synthase gene. Other genes involve human type A natriuretic peptide receptor gene, gene involving Na^+-K^+ exchanger activity.

Increased fibrosis plays a central role in transition from LVH to HF. Oxidative stress which is a common feature of hypertension is likely to play some role in the process of promoting cardiomyocyte apoptosis and fibrosis. Another factor influencing this pathophysiological process is dysregulation of interaction between matrix metalloproteinases (MMPs) and their natural inhibitor—tissue inhibitors of matrix metalloproteinases (TIMPs). MMPs increase the degradation of extracellular matrix and fibrillar collagen. In the failing heart, they accelerate the degradation of normal type collagens which are replaced by poorly cross-linked collagens. This promotes LV dilation.

The prevalence of LV hypertrophy is higher in blacks than in whites. But whether it is independent of hypertension is uncertain as the prevalence of hypertension is also higher in blacks.

As compared with the nondiabetic subjects, diabetic patients exhibit higher LV wall thickness and mass even after adjusting BP and body mass index.[14] Hypertension and diabetes exert additive effect in LV mass.

Obesity is also an independent risk factor for LV hypertrophy.

Left Atrial Abnormalities

Increased LV stiffness secondary to chronic high BP leads to elevated LA pressure and over time, increased LA size and thickness. These structural changes predispose the patient to the development of AF. Thus, absence of atrial contribution to the LV filling, superimposed with diastolic dysfunction may precipitate overt HF.

Valvular Heart Disease

Hypertension is thought to accelerate the sclerosis of aortic valve. Aortic root dilation caused by chronic severe hypertension may cause aortic regurgitation.

Myocardial Ischemia

Hypertension is an established risk factor for CAD. Shear stress and endothelial dysfunction associated with hypertension impairs endothelial nitric oxide production which causes accelerated atherosclerosis.

Arrhythmia

Apart from AF as described earlier other arrhythmias observed in patient with hypertensive heart disease are ventricular premature beats and ventricular tachycardia.[15] Risk of SCD is also high.[16] Mechanisms implicated in the pathogenesis of ventricular arrhythmia in hypertensive heart disease are poor perfusion, inhomogeneity of myocardium, myocardial fibrosis, altered cellular structure, and metabolism and fluctuating afterload.

PROGNOSIS AND THERAPEUTIC APPROACHES

Mortality and morbidity are high among patients with hypertensive heart disease when compared with individual without it and it is dependent on the specific cardiac pathology.[17] Development of LVH is clearly associated with increased cardiovascular mortality, including SCD. Patients with diastolic dysfunction associated with hypertension even if it is asymptomatic are at increased risk of mortality and cardiovascular events. Mortality in patient with systolic dysfunction is also high.

Left ventricular mass regression is promoted by effective control of BP which has been shown to improve survival.[18] BP reduction with most classes of antihypertensive medications is associated with LV mass regression. However, pure vasodilators like hydralazine and minoxidil are exceptions. They reduce BP without promoting LV mass regression.[19] In addition to BP reduction, some other factors like inhibition of renin–angiotensin–aldosterone system may also contribute to LV mass regression. In a meta-analysis the overall reduction in LV mass index was shown to differ significantly, with different group of antihypertensive medications. After adjusting for decrease in BP and duration of treatment, LV mass decreased most with angiotensin receptor blockers (13%). This was followed by calcium channel blockers (11%), ACE inhibitors (10%), diuretics (8%) and beta-blockers (6%).[20]

Heart failure with diastolic dysfunction (HFpEF) and heart failure with systolic dysfunction (HFrEF) are treated as per standard therapeutic approach. In patients with AF anticoagulation should be considered.

FUTURE PERSPECTIVE

Cyclosporine, a pharmacological inhibitor of calcineurin, has been shown to block myocardial hypertrophy. As cyclosporine is less likely to be clinically useful in nontransplant patient, it is likely that new classes of calcineurin inhibitors will become available to modulate such responses like hypertrophy.[21]

Angiotensin 1 receptor blockade appears to improve the balance between MMPs and TIMPs. TIMPs may not be used clinically as they are very short acting, but synthetic inhibitors of MMPs are under development.[22]

A large-acid phosphoprotein adhesion molecule osteopontin promotes fibroblast growth and function. Future researches may lead to the development of therapies that directly target the osteopontin modulation.[23]

Agents that increase BNP level may promote LV mass regression. Neural endopeptidase is a natural deactivator of BNP. Omapatrilat is an inhibitor of neutral endopeptidase. It is shown to promote regression of LV mass and myocardial fibrosis in experimental animal.[24]

Gene therapy is also a potential therapeutic approach. Target genes are ACE, angiotensinogen gene, AT1 receptor antisense gene.[25]

Direct inhibition of TGF-β has been shown to improve diastolic dysfunction in pressure overload rat model with hypertension, by inhibiting myocardial fibrosis.[26]

REFERENCES

1. WHO. A Global Brief on Hypertension. Geneva: World Health Organization; 2013.
2. New York Heart Association, Criteria Committee, Ferrer MI. Nomenclature and Criteria for Diagnosis of Diseases of the Heart and Great Vessels/the Criteria Committee of the New York Heart Association, 8th edition. Boston: Little Brown; 1979. p. 12.
3. Mitchell JA, Ventura HO, Mehra MR. Early recognition and treatment of hypertensive heart disease. Curr Opin Cardiol. 2005;20(4):282-9.
4. Gonzalez-Maqueda I, Alegria-Ezquerra E, Gonzalez-Juanatey, et al. Hypertensive heart disease: a new clinical classification (VIA). Eur Soc Cardiol. 2009;7(20).

5. Levy D, Garrison RJ, Savage DD, et al. Prognostic implications of echocardiographically determined left ventricular mass in the Framingham Heart Study. N Engl J Med. 1990;322(22):1561-6.

6. Bikkina M, Larson MG, Levy D. Asymptomatic ventricular arrhythmias and mortality risk in subjects with left ventricular hypertrophy. J Am Coll Cardiol. 1993;22(4): 1111-6.

7. Devereux RB, Roman MJ. Left ventricular hypertrophy in hypertension: stimuli, patterns, and consequences. Hypertens Res. 1999;22(1):1-9.

8. Gandhi SK, Powers JC, Nomeir AM, et al. The pathogenesis of acute pulmonary edema associated with hypertension. N Engl J Med. 2001;344(1):17-22.

9. Devereux RB, Bella JN, Palmieri V, et al. Left ventricular systolic dysfunction in a biracial sample of hypertensive adults: The Hypertension Genetic Epidemiology Network (HyperGEN) Study. Hypertension. 2001;38(3):417-23.

10. Iriarte M, Murga N, Sagastagoitia D, et al. Classification of hypertensive cardiomyopathy. Eur Heart J. 1993;14(Suppl J):95-101.

11. Nadruz W. Myocardial remodeling in hypertension. J Hum Hypertens. 2015;29(1):1-6.

12. Osler W. The Principles and Practice of Medicine, 1st edition. Appleton: New York, London: D. Appleton & Company; 1892.

13. Deschepper CF, Boutin-Ganache I, Zahabi A, et al. In search of cardiovascular candidate genes: interactions between phenotypes and genotypes. Hypertension. 2002;39(2 Pt 2):332-6.

14. Murarka S, Movahed MR. Diabetic cardiomyopathy. J Card Fail. 2010;16(12):971-9.

15. Ghali JK, Kadakia S, Cooper RS, et al. Impact of left ventricular hypertrophy on ventricular arrhythmias in the absence of coronary artery disease. J Am Coll Cardiol. 1991;17(6):1277-82.

16. Jouven X, Desnos M, Guerot C, et al. Predicting sudden death in the population: the Paris Prospective Study I. Circulation. 1999;99(15):1978-83.

17. Kannel WB, Cobb J. Left ventricular hypertrophy and mortality—results from the Framingham Study. Cardiology. 1992;81(4-5):291-8.

18. Muiesan ML, Salvetti M, Rizzoni D, et al. Association of change in left ventricular mass with prognosis during long-term antihypertensive treatment. J Hypertens. 1995; 13(10):1091-5.

19. Sen S, Tarazi RC, Khairallah PA, et al. Cardiac hypertrophy in spontaneously hypertensive rats. Circ Res. 1974;35(5):775-81.

20. Klingbeil AU, Schneider M, Martus P, et al. A meta-analysis of the effects of treatment on left ventricular mass in essential hypertension. Am J Med. 2003;115(1):41-6.

21. Nagata K, Somura F, Obata K, et al. AT1 receptor blockade reduces cardiac calcineurin activity in hypertensive rats. Hypertension. 2002;40(2):168-74.

22. Li H, Simon H, Bocan TM, et al. MMP/TIMP expression in spontaneously hypertensive heart failure rats: the effect of ACE- and MMP-inhibition. Cardiovasc Res. 2000;46(2):298-306.

23. Matsui Y, Jia N, Okamoto H, et al. Role of osteopontin in cardiac fibrosis and remodeling in angiotensin II-induced cardiac hypertrophy. Hypertension. 2004;43(6):1195-201.

24. Maki T, Nasa Y, Tanonaka K, et al. Direct inhibition of neutral endopeptidase in vasopeptidase inhibitor-mediated amelioration of cardiac remodeling in rats with chronic heart failure. Mol Cell Biochem. 2003;254(1-2):265-73.

25. Glueck SB, Dzau VJ. Physiological genomics: implications in hypertension research. Hypertension. 2002;39(2 Pt 2): 310-5.

26. Kuwahara F, Kai H, Tokuda K, et al. Hypertensive myocardial fibrosis and diastolic dysfunction: another model of inflammation? Hypertension. 2004;43(4):739-45.

Hypertension and Diabetes: Treatment Aspects

Siddharth N Shah

INTRODUCTION

In India, diabetes and hypertension are the growing health problems. As we all know hypertension is a major risk factor for cardiovascular (CV), cerebrovascular and renal disease. Moreover, when hypertension occurs in diabetes, it accelerates the progression of both microvascular and macrovascular complications. Mortality also gets increased by more than 7-fold. This deadly duo is a well-known risk factor for cardiovascular disease (CVD). Atherosclerotic cardiovascular disease (ASCVD) is the costliest complication, which accounts for rapidly increase in the prevalence in developed as well as in developing countries and have emerged as the leading cause of premature mortality.[1]

INCIDENCE OF DIABETES AND HYPERTENSION[2]

Hypertension is twice as prevalent in diabetics as in non-diabetic individuals. In patients with type 1 diabetes mellitus (T1DM), hypertension develops at the onset of diabetic nephropathy while in type 2 diabetes mellitus (T2DM), >50% patients are hypertensive at the time of diagnosis.

The estimated number of people with hypertension is increasing worldwide and is expected to increase from 972 million in 2000 to 1.56 billion by 2025. In diabetes, estimated number of people worldwide is expected to increase from 382 million in 2012 to 592 billion in 2030. Forty-eight percent of the anticipated absolute global increase of 186 million people with diabetes is projected to occur in India and China alone.

EVIDENCE

Studies related to diabetes and hypertension worldwide:[2]

- In the UKPDS study, each 10 mm Hg decrease in mean systolic blood pressure (BP) was associated with relative risk reduction of 12% for any complication of diabetes, 15% for deaths related to diabetes, 11% for myocardial infarction and 13% for microvascular complications. The study also shows improved insulin resistance with metformin and decreased macrovascular events
- The HOT (Hypertension Optimal Treatment study) showed that diabetics with high BP, will need 2–3 drugs to control their BP

- The Systolic Hypertension in the Elderly Program (SHEP) and other studies like Hypertension Detection and Follow-up Program (HDFP), Systolic Hypertension in Europe (Syst-Eur), Normotensive Appropriate Blood Pressure Control in Diabetes (ABCD) and Heart Outcomes Prevention Evaluation (HOPE) provide firm evidence that even small BP reductions translate to significant decrease in both micro and macrovascular complications in persons with type 2 diabetes (T2D)
- The ADVANCE (Action in Diabetes and Vascular Disease; Preterax and Diamicron MR Controlled Evaluation) study showed that intensive control of BP resulted in reduction in composite micro and macrovascular complications by 9%, coronary events by 14% and renal events by 21%
- The Advance Collaborative Group study demonstrating the benefit of an Angiotensin-Converting Enzyme (ACE) inhibitor and indapamide in a fixed combination, strongly suggesting that the BP goal (<130/80 mm Hg) was beneficial
- The ACCORD (Action to Control Cardiovascular Risk in Diabetes) trial was unable to find a significant reduction in incidence of major CV events in patients with diabetes whose SBP was lowered to an average of 119 mm Hg compared with patients whose SBP remained at an average of 133 mm Hg
- The ONTARGET (Telmisartan, Ramipril, or Both in Patients at High Risk for Vascular Events) study compared between telmisartan and ramipril in patients with diabetes and vascular events
- The Anglo-Scandinavian Cardiac Outcomes Trial (ASCOT), the largest study of hypertension conducted in Europe. In a population of hypertensive adults at moderate risk of developing CVD, a regimen starting with amlodipine and adding perindopril as required reduced the risk of strokes by about 25%, coronary events and procedures by 15%, CV deaths by 25% and new cases of diabetes by 30% compared with standard treatment of atenolol plus a diuretic
- Thus, from various trials we interpret that there is an improved CV outcome and reduced progression of microvascular complications such as nephropathy and retinopathy by tight control of BP in diabetic patients.

◼ DIABETIC NEPHROPATHY AND HYPERTENSION[2]

- In type 1 diabetes (T1D), hypertension begins with the onset of nephropathy (microalbuminuria stage). A history of hypertension in the parents and increased erythrocyte sodium-lithium counter transport and DD Iso form of the *ACE* gene, which is linked to increased ACE generation are markers of genetic susceptibility to hypertension and nephropathy
- In T2D, about 50% already have obesity and age-related essential hypertension. Hypertension is present in more than 90% of diabetics with impaired renal function. Increased systolic BP is a significant risk factor for microalbuminuria and rapid progression of nephropathy
- Overall diabetic kidney disease is a potent risk factor for macrovascular disease, namely atherosclerosis, myocardial infarction, heart failure and cerebrovascular events.

■ STRATEGY FOR MANAGEMENT OF HYPERTENSIVE DIABETIC PATIENTS[2]

- Proper blood sugar control
- Achieve target level of BP control for diabetic patients
- Early detection of both diabetes and hypertension complications, manage them to delay their progression and improve patient's quality of life.

Non-drug Therapy

The multifactorial approach, based on the following non pharmaco-therapeutic interventions are:

Nutrition

Blood pressure of diabetic patients more sensitive to salt intake and this sodium sensitivity is found even in absence of nephropathy. A decreased salt intake is important for diabetic patients with hypertension.

Reducing Salt (Sodium) Intake

Aim for less than 3–5 grams per day. However, the daily average salt consumption in Indian scenario is 8–9 grams per day.

Ways to Reduce Sodium Intake

- Food items without added salt
- Unsalted nuts, seeds, beans
- Avoid adding salt and canned vegetables to homemade dishes
- Unsalted and sodium free, fat-free broths and soups
- Use fresh poultry, lean meat and fish
- Rinse canned foods to reduce sodium
- Low sodium, low fat cheeses
- Add spices and herbs to enhance taste
- Add fresh lemon juice instead of salt to fresh vegetable salad.

Benefits of Moderate Sodium Reduction

The benefits of moderate sodium reduction in diet are summarized in box 1.

Medical Nutrition Therapy in diabetics[3]

Medical nutrition therapy (MNT) is individualized in diabetic patients with two basic dimensions such as dietary quality and energy restriction. Trials showed that Mediterranean

---

Box 1: Benefits of sodium reduction in diet.

- Improvement in large artery compliance (Gates et al., 2004)
- Enhancement of efficacy of antihypertensive drugs (Slagman et al., 2011; Aziza et al., 2013
- Reduction of diuretic-induced potassium loss (Ram et al., 1981)
- Regression of left ventricular hypertrophy (Rodriguez et al., 2011)
- Reduction in proteinuria (Agarwal, 2012)
- Reduction in urine calcium excretion (Carbone et al., 2003)
- Decrease in osteoporosis (Martini et al., 2000)
- Decreased prevalence of stomach cancer (Fock et al., 2008)
- Decreased prevalence of stroke (Joossens and Kesteloot, 2008)
- Decreased prevalence of cataract (Cumming et al., 2000)
- Protection against onset of hypertension (Whelton PK, 2014)

Know What to Eat

- Dietary Approaches to Stop Hypertension (DASH) diet is an eating plan, rich in fruits, vegetables, whole grains, fish, poultry, nuts, legumes and low-fat dairy. These foods are high in key nutrients such as potassium, magnesium, calcium, fibre and protein. The DASH diet can lower BP because it has less salt and sugar.
- 4–5 servings of fruits and vegetables/6–8 servings of whole grain / saturated fat 6% of total calories/total cholesterol of <150 mg/day

eating pattern reported modest weight loss and improved glycemic control. The other diet pattern such as low-carbohydrate, low-glycemic index and high-protein diets and the DASH diet all improve glycemic control, but the effect of the Mediterranean eating pattern appears to be the greatest.

Weight Reduction[2]

The prevention and correction of overweight / obesity (BMI >25) is a prudent way of reducing the risk of hypertension, diabetes and indirectly reducing coronary artery disease; it goes with dietary changes. Loss of weight by 1 kg decreases BP by approximately 1 mm Hg.

Exercise Promotion

Physical activity

F Frequency - at least Five days per week

I Intensity   - Moderate

T Time   - 30–45 minutes

T Type   - Cardiorespiratory Activity

            - Walking, jogging

            - Cycling (including stationary)

            - Non-competitive swimming

            - Yoga, Tai chi

Exercise should be prescribed as an adjunctive to pharmacological therapy

Behavioral Changes

Reduction of stress, cessation of smoking, moderation of alcohol drinking, modification of personal life-style, yoga and transcendental meditation could be beneficial.

Diabetes Self-Management Education and Support[3]

"The First Duty of the Physician is to Educate the Masses not to Take Medicine"
-Sir William Osler

The function of Diabetes Self-Management Education and Support (DSMES) is to establish and implement the principles of diabetic care. This program is a cost-effective intervention in the healthcare systems which involves face-to-face contact in a group or individual sessions with trained educators. It should occur at the time of diagnosis, annually and when there is a rise in complications. The role is to promote medication adherence, healthy eating and physical activity and increase self-efficacy. Thereby, DSMES significantly improves clinical and psychological outcomes, improves glycemic control, reduces hospital admissions, improves patient knowledge and reduces the risk of all-cause mortality. It is recommended that all people with T2D should be offered access to ongoing DSMES programs.

■ SELF-CARE[2]

Blood Pressure Monitoring

In order to overcome the limitations of the office blood pressure (OBP) measurement, two methods are widely used in clinical practice:
1. Home blood pressure monitoring (HBPM)
2. 24 hours ambulatory blood pressure monitoring (ABPM).

The patient is taught about self-care, i.e. HBPM and keep a log-book of his BP readings. 24 hours ABP monitoring is a precise method to quantify BP levels and to diagnose hypertension and also it is used as a marker of CV morbidity and mortality.

Glucose Monitoring

Self-monitoring of blood glucose (SMBG) is becoming an important component in improving glycemic control in diabetes. It helps in adjustment of a treatment regimen in response to blood glucose level and provide information on glucose excursions and hypoglycemia related to drugs, insulin and lifestyle changes like dietary intake and exercise.

Role of ABPM in Diabetic Patients[4,5]

- ABPM is advisable in all diabetic patients with high-normal BP
- Diabetic patients are more likely to have
  - White-coat hypertension
  - Masked hypertension
  - Non-dipping
  - Reverse dipping
  - Morning BP surge
- High prevalence of masked hypertension in diabetic patients is associated with higher risk of brain and kidney damage and possible cardiac damage, which further increase CV complications
- White-coat hypertension in diabetic patients appears to be associated with a lower risk than sustained hypertension
- Non-dipping and reverse dipping may reflect autonomic dysfunction and it might be used as a clinical marker of diabetic autonomic neuropathy
- ABPM provides information on heart rate at the time of BP measurements all over the 24 hours, and a rough estimate of heart rate variability. The reduced heart rate variability is the index of diabetic neuropathy
- ABPM also provides information on pulse pressure (difference between systolic and diastolic BP), when increased is considered as a surrogate marker of stiffening of arterial walls.

Target BP in DM[2,6]

- On the basis the Eighth Joint National Committee on Prevention, Detection, Evaluation and Treatment of High Blood Pressure (JNC 8), the American Diabetes Association (ADA) and American Association of Clinical Endocrinologists (AACE) have recommended that BP should be measured at every routine visit. In all diabetic population it is mandatory to measure the BP in supine, sitting and standing positions to exclude the possibility of autonomic neuropathy
- Most patients with diabetes and hypertension should be treated with a BP goal of less than 130/80 mm Hg
- In patients with high risk of CVD BP should be less than 130/80 mm Hg
- The aim is to maintain low BP which the patient can tolerate without postural hypotension and without compromise on critical vascular beds as well as quality of life.

Ideal Antihypertensive Drug in DM[2]

- Must decrease BP to ≤130/80 mm Hg
- Must reduce the renin-angiotensin-aldosterone system (RAAS) activity, improve endothelial dysfunction
- Must prevent, improve or arrest proteinuria
- Must prevent and protect from coronary artery disease (CAD), chronic kidney disease (CKD), congestive heart failure (CHF)
- Must be favorable on glycemic control
- Must improve the dyslipidemia—not worsen it
- Must not worsen peripheral arterial disease
- Must not cause impotence
- Must not decrease eGFR and increase serum creatinine
- Must not increase uric acid, serum potassium
- Can be easily combined with other drugs

- An ideal agent should not increase insulin resistance
- Well tolerated, cost effective.

Effects of Antihypertensives on Diabetes[2,6]

There are three class of RAS modulating agents are available: Angiotensin converting enzyme (ACE) inhibitors, Angiotensin receptor blockers (ARBs) and Renin inhibitors. ACEIs and ARBs are suitable first line antihypertensive in diabetics. It has renal protective effect in incipient nephropathy, reduce insulin resistance and may improve glycemia in diabetes and patients with the metabolic syndrome.

Why ACEI is preferred in DM?

Improves insulin sensitivity

- Reverse vascular and ventricular remodeling
- Reverse left ventricular hypertrophy (LVH)
- Cardioprotection
- Renal protection
- Favorable glucose lipid metabolism.

The ACE inhibitors in the **HOPE trial** and ARBs in the **ONTARGET trial** have emphasized the importance of RAAS blockade to reduce the risk of microvascular and macrovascular complications in diabetes. Therefore, ACE inhibitors in T1D are recommended as the first line drug therapy while ARBs may be used in patients who have T2D or who are intolerant to ACE inhibitors.

Calcium channel blockers have been shown to be useful as monotherapy and in combination with ACEI in the **ASCOT trial**. The combination of amlodipine and perindopril was associated with significantly less incidence of new onset diabetes as compared to the combination of β-blocker and diuretic.

Thiazide diuretics and β-blockers have metabolic side-effects such as increasing insulin resistance or direct diabetogenesis, which make them less appropriate as first line agents. Beta-blockers also potentially mask hypoglycemic symptoms.[7] But cardio-selective β-blockers like long acting metoprolol, nebivolol and carvedilol can be used in hypertensive-diabetic population with evidence of coronary artery disease and congestive cardiac failure.

Antidiabetic Drugs[2]

- The antidiabetic agents like metformin and thiazolidinediones reduce insulin resistance
- The sodium-glucose cotransporter-2 (SGLT2) inhibitors cause osmotic diuresis leading to BP reduction and reduced the rate of CV events
- The glucagon-like peptide-1(GLP-1) receptor agonists and dipeptidyl peptidase-4 (DPP-4) inhibitors have been demonstrated to exert their effects directly through the activation of their receptors on the cardiac and vascular tissues or centrally positioned receptors to reduce the BP
- Insulin causes salt and water retention, increases body weight and it causes growth of tissues as an anabolic hormone.

■ CONCLUSION

Diabetes mellitus and hypertension are comorbid illnesses, in both developing and developed countries. The presence of one increases the risk of having the other and increase the risk of ASCVD events. So, every diabetes patient need measuring of BP in every visit. Hypertensive patients need to be screened for diabetes and dyslipidemia regularly. HBPM could be an ideal way in monitoring BP in hypertensive patients in general and diabetic patients in particular to ensure that the patient does not progress to develop CV and renal complications.

■ REFERENCES

1. Reddy KS, Yusuf S. Emerging epidemic of cardiovascular disease in developing countries. Circulation. 1998;97(6): 596-601.
2. Muruganathan A., M.D Diabetes and hypertension-Common soil hypothesis, Cardio-diabetes update 2017.
3. Davies MJ, D'Alessio DA, Fradkin J, et al. Management of hyperglycaemia in type 2 diabetes, 2018. A consensus report by the American Diabetes Association (ADA) and the European Association for the Study of Diabetes (EASD). Diabetologia. 2018;61(12):2461-98.
4. Grossman E. Ambulatory blood pressure monitoring in the diagnosis and management of hypertension. Diabetes care. 2013;36(Suppl 2):S307-11.
5. Leitão CB, Canani LH, Silveiro SP, et al. Ambulatory blood pressure monitoring and type 2 diabetes mellitus. Arquivos brasileiros de cardiologia. 2007;89(5):347-54.
6. American Diabetes Association Standards of Medical Care in Diabetes-2018.
7. Shah SN. Indian Guidelines on Hypertension -III 2013. Supplement to JAPI. 2013;(2):28-9.

Brain and Hypertension

Harish Jayakumar, Bhanu Kesavamurthy, Avathvadi Venkatesan Srinivasan, Sujatha Sudarsan

■ INTRODUCTION

Hypertension is the most prevalent cardio-vascular risk factor associated with increased incidence of stroke and neurological diseases. Systolic blood pressure (SBP) increases steadily throughout adulthood, whereas diastolic blood pressure (DBP) peaks at about 60 years of age in men and 70 years in women and falls gradually thereafter. As age advances, the SBP tends to increase more than the DBP. The systolic and DBP are higher in men than in women belonging to young and middle-aged group. The increase in blood pressure (BP) is steeper in women 0.6–1.2 mm Hg/year during adulthood compared to 0.4–0.8 mm Hg/year in men belonging to age of 30 years to the middle of the 70–79 years age group.[1] After the age of 70, BP of women is equal to or higher than that of men. Elevated BP is the strongest modifiable risk factor for stroke, both ischemic and hemorrhagic.

■ COMORBIDITIES ASSOCIATED WITH BRAIN DAMAGE IN HYPERTENSION

- *Dyslipidemia*: Lipoprotein elevation has a deleterious effect on brain homeostasis in patients with hypertension

- *Salt intake, alcohol, smoking*: Increased salt intake was associated with greater risk of stroke and cardiovascular disease. Slight intake of alcohol may reduce the risk of stroke by 30%, but excess intake significantly increases the risk of stroke. In hypertensive smokers, a dose response relationship is observed. A reformed smoker has the same risk as a nonsmoker[2]
- *Other comorbidities*: Diabetes, chronic kidney disease, coronary artery disease, obstructive sleep apnea—all these comorbidities either worsen or are worsened by persistent hypertension, thereby increasing the risk of brain damage.

■ PATHOPHYSIOLOGY OF BRAIN DAMAGE IN HYPERTENSION

Small Vessel Disease

Brain damage due to persistent hypertension can be explained based on microvascular and macrovascular remodeling. In patients with primary hypertension, the resistance arteries show a greater media thickness, elevated media to lumen ratio, without significant changes in total amount of wall tissue (eutrophic remodeling). Whereas in secondary hypertension and severe primary hypertension, there is hypertrophic remodeling along with hyperplasia and vascular smooth muscle hypertrophy.

Cerebral autoregulation is a physiological phenomenon which couples cerebral metabolic demand with cerebral perfusion. Although metabolic mechanisms seem to predominate in cerebral autoregulation, vessel myogenic responses have a major role. Chronic hypertension alters cerebral autoregulation and is associated with changes in cerebral microvascular structure. Eutrophic remodeling is observed in cerebral small arteries with increased media to lumen ratio along with capillary rarefaction. High central pulsatility which reflects high BP has been demonstrated in small vessels in the brain. Walls of the cerebral small vessels get exposed to such high pressure fluctuations as in other systemic large vessels thereby increasing the cerebral pulse pressure. This transmission of high pressure to small vessels results in hyaline degeneration known as Fischer's lipohyalinosis and fibrinoid necrosis. This also underlies the pathology of cognitive impairment.

Large Vessel Disease

Large artery stiffening has been attributed to cause cerebral lacunar infarcts and large white matter hyperintensities. Large artery remodeling is characterized by increased intima-media thickness (IMT) (about 15% to 40%), lumen enlargement in proximal elastic arteries, and no change in lumen diameter of distal muscular arteries.[3] This is due to compensation by the arterial walls to normalize circumferential wall stress due to high BP.

Middle cerebral artery (MCA) pulsatility has been found to be the strongest physiological correlate of leukoaraiosis, independent of age. This supports the notion that large artery stiffening results in increased

arterial pulsatility with direct transmission to small vessels and thereby resulting in leukoaraiosis.

PULSE WAVE ENCEPHALOPATHY

Bateman et al. described a possible mechanism of brain damage several years back. Increased pressure pulsatility possibly causes an excessive turnover of cerebrovascular fluid thereby resulting in structural and functional changes in cerebral circulation. This torrential circulation is directly transmitted to small vessels thereby damaging the ependymal lining and ependymal damage resulting in white matter hyperintensities.

ISCHEMIC AND HEMORRHAGIC STROKE

Ischemic strokes due to hypertension are related to both small vessel disease as well as atherosclerosis. Atherosclerosis is focal at places where arteries bend and branch. Normally, in a laminar flow, the total fluid energy is in the form of pressure energy. But when the vessel wall is disturbed this pressure energy gets converted to kinetic energy and plaques tend to develop in areas of shear stress. Lacunar infarctions are limited to small infarctions due to occlusion of arterioles and their small branches. Lacunar strokes and hypertensive hemorrhage occurs most commonly in basal ganglia, thalamus, internal capsule, cerebellum and brainstem.

Hypertensive hemorrhage can be divided into two major subtypes—hemorrhagic infarct and parenchymal hematoma. Hypertensive hemorrhage is defined as heterogeneous hyperintensity surrounded by a zone of infarction. It is subdivided into two types: Type 1—scattered petechiae around an infarcted zone; and Type 2—condensed petechiae around an infarcted zone. Parenchymal hematoma is also subdivided into two types: Type 1—homogenous hyperdensity hematoma of size less than 30% of the infarct area with mild mass effect; and Type 2—hematoma of size more than 30% of the ischemic zone with a significant mass effect.

POSTERIOR REVERSIBLE ENCEPHALOPATHY SYNDROME AND HYPERTENSIVE ENCEPHALOPATHY

Cerebral blood flow is autoregulated by dilatation during low blood flow and constriction during high blood flow. Autoregulation is broken down when the mean arterial BP is 150–160 mm Hg. Rapidly developing high BP breaks down the blood brain barrier (BBB) allowing interstitial extravasation of plasma and macromolecules. It has been suggested that posterior brain is particularly susceptible to hyperperfusion and BBB breakdown due to possible little sympathetic innervation in the posterior fossa.[4] Endothelial dysfunction due to systemic inflammatory state has also been considered as an alternate pathophysiological mechanism.

COGNITION

Persistent hypertension influences cognitive decline through a variety of mechanisms including eutrophic remodeling causing adaptive vascular changes. There is dysregulation of cerebral autoregulation, increased predisposition of atheroma formation, reduction in blood supply and decline in perfusion. This hypoperfusion causes discreet and subtle areas of cerebral infarction and diffuse ischemic changes in the deeper regions of the brain and periventricular regions. This underlies the mechanism of vascular dementia. Several of these mechanisms also overlap with the development of Alzheimer's dementia. The most common cognitive domain to be affected was observed to be executive domain.[5]

ECLAMPSIA

Pre-eclampsia is a multifactorial multisystem disorder characterized by symptom onset at >20 weeks' gestational age with 24-hour proteinuria ≥30 mg/day or, new onset hypertension with a SBP >140 mm Hg or DBP ≥90 mm Hg and disappearance of all these abnormalities before the end of the 6th week postpartum. Eclampsia is when pre-eclampsia is associated with seizures. Theoretical mechanisms include impaired nitric oxide synthase activity, exaggerated immune responses, prostaglandin imbalances, angiogenic imbalances, immune maladaptation and genetic factors.[6]

MANAGEMENT OF HYPERTENSION IN BRAIN DISEASES

Acute Ischemic Stroke

Elevated BP is a common finding in the acute phase of ischemic stroke and is associated with poor clinical outcomes. In the first 24 hours, up to 70–80% of ischemic strokes have supine BP >140/90 mm Hg and up to 15% have SBP >184 mm Hg.[7] BP changes in the peri-stroke phase with abnormal nocturnal BP have been identified in >75% of patients after the event[8] and peaks and troughs of consistently elevated BP have been observed prior to the event. Ten days after stroke, spontaneous reduction of SBP (20 mm Hg) and DBP (10 mm Hg) have been observed. The status of the blood vessels is one of the critical determinants of BP evolution which is particularly influenced by the autonomic regulation by the left ventromedial prefrontal cortex (VMPFC)—parasympathetic and the right VMPFC—sympathetic.[9]

Persistently elevated BP in the acute stage leads to further worsening and evolving brain swelling which may cause further worsening of the ischemic core and hemorrhagic transformation. Antihypertensive treatment should be administered with great caution to avoid hypotension, as the potentially salvageable area—the penumbra requires adequate blood supply to restore function after thrombolytic therapy. Only a gradual and a moderate BP decrease of <20% within 24 hours should be targeted. Rapid and large reduction of BP in early acute stage is associated with poor outcomes. A target of SBP between 140 and 159 mm Hg and DBP between 90 and 99 mm Hg is associated with very good long-term functional recovery. In a Cochrane review[10] and recent randomized control trials (RCT) Rapid Intervention with Glyceryl trinitrate in Hypertensive stroke Trial (RIGHT)[11] and Efficacy of Nitric Oxide in Stroke (ENOS)[12], administration of antihypertensive therapy within 4–6 hours of onset of symptoms is associated with excellent functional outcomes.

Recommendations from Safe Implementation of Thrombolysis in Stroke-Monitoring Study (SITS-MOST)[13] on management of BP in acute ischemic stroke:

- In patients excluded from thrombolytic therapy:
  - SBP <220 mm Hg and DBP <120 mm Hg: Do not treat unless accompanied with aortic dissection, acute myocardial infarction, pulmonary edema and acute renal failure
  - SBP >220 mm Hg and/or DBP >121–140 mm Hg: Treat until reaching SBP 220 and DBP 120 (should not exceed 20% of initial BP) with
    - IV labetalol 10–20 mg over 1–2 minutes, may be repeated once every 10 minutes, maximum of 300 mg
      - Continuous infusion of IV nicardipine 5 mg/h, dose may be increased every 5–15 minutes by 0.25 mg/h (maximum dose 15 mg/h) until target.

  - DBP >140 mm Hg
    - Continuous infusion of IV sodium nitroprusside 0.5 µg/kg/min or
    - Nitroglycerin 5 mg IV followed by 1–4 mg/hour infusion.
- In patients treated with thrombolytic therapy:
  - Before the administration of recombinant tissue plasminogen activator (rTPA) if BP >185 mm Hg:
    - IV labetalol 10–20 mg over 1–2 minutes, may be repeated once every 10 minutes, maximum of 300 mg
    - Continuous infusion of IV nicardipine 5 mg/h, dose may be increased every 5–15 minutes by 0.25 mg/h (maximum dose 15 mg/h) until target.

  After rTPA, monitor BP every 15 minutes for the first 2 hours, then every 30 minutes for the following 8 hours, and then every 1 hour in the following 16 hours.

  - If SBP >185 mm Hg and/or DBP >110 mm Hg (one of the following):
    - IV labetalol 10–20 mg over 1–2 minutes, may be repeated once every 10 minutes, maximum of 300 mg or continuous IV infusion 2–8 mg/min.
  - If SBP >230 mm Hg and/or DBP >121–140 mm Hg (one of the following):
    - IV labetalol 10–20 mg over 1–2 minutes, may be repeated once every 10 minutes , maximum of 300 mg or continuous IV infusion 2–8 mg/min
    - Continuous infusion of IV nicardipine 5 mg/h, dose may be increased every 5–15 minutes by 0.25 mg/h (maximum dose 15 mg/h) until target.
  - If above therapy is unsuccessful and/or DBP >140 mm Hg—IV continuous infusion of IV sodium nitroprusside 0.5 µg/kg/min to titrate according to BP.

Acute Hemorrhagic Stroke

Acute elevation of BP in the first 24 hours, known as the acute hypertensive response, occurs in 90% of the intracerebral hemorrhage (ICH) cases. Pre-existing hypertension with SBP ≥140 mm Hg or ≥160 mm Hg is found in 73% and 60% ICH cases, respectively. High BP in the acute phase is associated with hematoma expansion, mortality, and severe morbidity and is a risk factor and a marker for intracerebral bleeding and subsequent intracranial hypertension.

For patients with SBP between 150 and 220 mgHg and with no contraindication for BP lowering, American Society of Hypertension (ASA) and European Stroke Organisation (ESO) have recommended reduction to SBP <140 mm Hg. For ICH patients with SBP >220 mm Hg, more aggressive BP reduction is imperative.

Drugs effective in reduction of BP in ICH:

- *Labetalol*: 5–20 mg IV bolus every 15 minutes, up to 2 mg/h infusion
- *Nicardipine*: 5–15 mg/h infusion
- *Nitroglycerin*: 5–100 mg/min IV infusion
- *Esmolol*: 500 µg/kg IV bolus or 25–300 µg/kg/min IV infusion
- *Urapidil*: 12.5–25mg IV bolus or 5–40 mg/h infusion
- *Enalaprilat*: 1.25–5 mg every 6 hours IV Push
- *Hydralazine*: 10–20 mg IV bolus
- *Nipride*: 0.1–10 µg/kg/min IV infusion.

Posterior Reversible Encephalopathy Syndrome

Until recently, posterior reversible encephalopathy syndrome (PRES) was considered to produce bilateral and symmetric posterior parietal and occipital edema. Recently, four radiological patterns of PRES have been described.[14]

1. Holohemispheric watershed pattern
2. Superior frontal sulcus pattern
3. Dominant parietal-occipital pattern
4. Partial expression of three primary patterns.

Management includes ruling out other causes, management of hypertension, seizures and removal of offending factor.

Initial aim is to reduce BP to about 100–105 mm Hg which should be achieved within 2–6 hours (not exceeding 25% from the initial BP). More aggressive lowering will lead to ischemic events.

Imaging features that are associated with poor prognosis and irreversibility includes:

- Low apparent diffusion coefficient values in the lesions
- Evidence of hemorrhage
- Brainstem involvement.

Drugs commonly used are labetalol and nicardipine.

- *Nicardipine:* Initial 5 mg/h infusion can increase by 2.5 mg/h every 5–15 minutes
- *Labetalol:* Initial 10–20 mg IV over 2 minutes, may be repeated once every 10 minutes, maximum of 300 mg
- *Hydralazine:* 1.7–3.5 mg/kg divided in 4–6 doses
- *Nitroglycerin:* Initial 5 µg/min, can increase by 5 µg/min every 3–5 minutes. If no desired response is achieved at 20 µg/min, increments of 10 µg/min can be tried
- *Enalaprilat:* 1.25 mg IV Push Q6th hourly, not more than 48 hours
- *Fenoldopam:* Initial 0.01–1.6 µg/kg/min IV, increase or reduce by 0.05–0.1 µg/kg/min not more frequently than 15 minutes.

Management of seizures in PRES includes use of benzodiazepines, phenobarbital, fosphenytoin, midazolam, propofol and thiopental. Other management includes withdrawal of immunosuppressive or chemotherapy agent, correction of hypomagnesemia, general measures such as airway management and ventilator support, dialysis if needed.

Eclampsia

Key principles include prevention of maternal hypoxia, treatment of hypertension, prevention of recurrent seizure and evaluation for prompt delivery. Antihypertensive therapy is initiated when DBP >105–110 mm Hg or SBP ≥160 mm Hg. Acute therapy includes labetalol or hydralazine as first-line agents. Recently Cochrane review has suggested oral nifedipine as an acceptable alternative to parenteral labetalol or hydralazine. Target BP should be 130–150 mm Hg SBP and 80–100 mm Hg DBP, and no more than 25% should be achieved within 2 hours. Magnesium sulfate given for treatment of seizures has very little effect on BP.

Cognition

Three large scale RCTs have assessed the potential role of antihypertensive therapy in the prevention of cognitive impairment. The Systolic Hypertension in the Elderly Program (SHEP) study had found that thiazide diuretics reduce the risk of stroke, but not of cognitive decline.[15] In the Systolic Hypertension in Europe (Syst-Eur) trial,[16] it was found that isolated systolic hypertension when treated with nitrendipine, enalapril and hydrochlorothiazide reduced dementia risk by 50% in 2 years. A pooled analysis of different trials showed significant association of antihypertensive treatment with reduction in the risk of dementia.[17] Though evidence from several studies show benefit, some studies have shown the opposite in elderly patients. This subject thus remains to be unexplored and the optimal BP and choice of drugs remains to be validated.

■ CONCLUSION

Hypertension has a significant role in altering brain homeostasis through different mechanisms. Understanding of the various pathophysiology behind the development and progression of brain disease in hypertension highlights the importance of controlling BP. It is essential for practicing physicians to understand the implications of uncontrolled hypertension and how it can affect the morbidity and mortality of patients with brain disease.

■ REFERENCES

1. Lawes CM, Vander Hoorn S, Law MR, et al. Blood pressure and the global burden of disease 2000. Part 1: estimates of blood pressure levels. J Hypertens. 2006;24(3):413-22.
2. Wannamethee SG, Shaper AG, Whincup PH, et al. Smoking cessation and the risk of stroke in middle-aged men. JAMA. 1995;274(2):155-60.
3. Laurent S, Boutouyrie P. The structural factor of hypertension: large and small artery alterations. Circ Res. 2015;116(6):1007-21.
4. Fugate JE, Rabinstein AA. Posterior reversible encephalopathy syndrome: Clinical and radiological manifestations, pathophysiology, and outstanding questions. Lancet Neurol. 2015;14(9):914-25.
5. Scuteri A, Nilsson PM, Tzourio C, et al. Microvascular brain damage with aging and hypertension: pathophysiological consideration and clinical implications. J Hypertens. 2011;29(8):1469-77.
6. Uzan J, Carbonnel M, Piconne O, et al. Pre-eclampsia: pathophysiology, diagnosis, and management. Vasc Health Risk Manag. 2011;7:467-74.
7. Qureshi AI. Acute hypertensive response in patients with stroke pathophysiology and management. Circulation. 2008;118(2):176-87.
8. Tomii Y, Toyoda K, Suzuki R, et al. Effects of 24-hour blood pressure and heart rate recorded with ambulatory blood pressure monitoring on recovery from acute ischemic stroke. Stroke. 2011;42(12):3511-7.
9. Hilz MJ, Devinsky O, Szczepanska H, et al. Right ventromedial prefrontal lesions result in paradoxical cardiovascular activation with emotional stimuli. Brain. 2006;129 (Pt 12):3343-55.
10. Bath P, Krishnan K. Interventions for deliberately altering blood pressure in acute stroke. Cochrane Database Syst Rev. 2014;(10):CD00003.
11. Ankolekar S, Fuller M, Cross I, et al. Feasibility of an ambulance-based stroke trial, and safety of glyceryl trinitrate in ultra-acute stroke: the rapid intervention with glyceryl trinitrate in Hypertensive Stroke Trial (RIGHT, ISRCTN66434824). Stroke. 2013;44(11):3120-8.
12. Woodhouse L, Scutt P, Krishnan K, et al. Effect of hyperacute administration (within 6 hours) of transdermal glyceryl trinitrate, a nitric oxide donor, on outcome after

stroke: subgroup analysis of the Efficacy of Nitric Oxide in Stroke (ENOS) Trial. Stroke. 2015;46:3194-201.

13. Wahlgren N, Ahmed N, Dávalos A, et al. Thrombolysis with alteplase for acute ischaemic stroke in the Safe Implementation of Thrombolysis in Stroke-Monitoring Study (SITSMOST): an observational study. Lancet. 2007;369(9558):275-82.

14. Bartynski WS, Boardman JF. Distinct imaging patterns and lesion distribution in posterior reversible encephalopathy syndrome. AJNR Am J Neuroradiol. 2007;28:1320-7.

15. SHEP Cooperative Research Group. Prevention of stroke by antihypertensive drug treatment in older persons with isolated systolic hypertension: final results of the Systolic Hypertension in the Elderly Program (SHEP). JAMA. 1991; 265(24):3255-64.

16. Staessen JA, Fagard R, Thijs L, et al. Randomised double-blind comparison of placebo and active treatment for older patients with isolated systolic hypertension. The Systolic Hypertension in Europe (Syst-Eur) Trial Investigators. Lancet. 1997;350(9080):757-64.

17 Staessen JA, Richart T, Birkenhäger WH. Less atherosclerosis and lower blood pressure for a meaningful life perspective with more brain. Hypertension. 2007;49(3):389-400.

Pediatric and Adolescent Hypertension

V Padma

■ INTRODUCTION

In children and adolescents, high blood pressure (HBP) is an entity that was rarely found previously. Nowadays, it has become a serious challenge because of increase in the risk of end-organ damage, which comprises of ventricular hypertrophy, coronary artery calcifications, and increase in carotid intima-media thickness.[1,2] HBP present in childhood is an unprecedented predictor of the adult hypertension.[3,4] It is therefore vital to identify high blood pressure (BP) early in childhood, for preventing accelerated vascular aging and subsequent cardiovascular-related diseases.

Efforts were made to align the classification system of pediatric and adolescent hypertension with the Seventh Report of the Joint National Committee on Prevention, Detection, Evaluation and Treatment of High Blood Pressure (JNC-7). This was achieved through the "Fourth Report on the Diagnosis, Evaluation, and Treatment of High Blood Pressure in Children and Adolescents" (Fourth Report) published in 2004.[5] Though many countries and organizations are following their own childhood BP reference values, such as Canada's 2016 guidelines[6] and the European 2016 guidelines,[7] Fourth Report[5] has been used across many countries globally, including the United States and China.

Stage I hypertension can be diagnosed when BP of a child is more than the 95th percentile but less than or equal to the 99th percentile plus 5 mm Hg of the BP of healthy child of the same age. If the BP is between 90th and 95th percentile, it can be in category of prehypertension. If a discrepancy with respect to classification is caused by systolic and diastolic pressures, then by using the higher value the condition of the child should be categorized (Table 1).

■ PATHOPHYSIOLOGY

Blood pressure depends on the balance between cardiac output and vascular resistance. A rise in either or both of these variables in absence of compensatory reduction in the other causes increased BP. The following factors affect the BP in any individual.

Factors affecting cardiac output:[9]

- Baroreceptors
- Extracellular volume
- Effective circulating volume—atrial natriuretic hormones, mineralocorticoids and angiotensin
- Sympathetic nervous syndrome.

Factors that affect vascular resistance include the following:[9]

TABLE 1: Ninety-fifth blood pressure percentiles for 50th and 75th height percentiles in children and adolescents.[8]

Age, year	95th BP percentile for girls, mm Hg		95th BP percentile for boys, mm Hg	
	50th height percentile	75th height percentile	50th height percentile	75th height percentile
1	104/58	105/59	103/56	104/58
6	111/74	113/74	114/74	115/75
12	123/80	124/81	123/81	125/82
17	129/84	130/85	136/87	138/87

- Pressors—angiotensin II, calcium (intracellular), catecholamines, sympathetic nervous system and vasopressin
- Depressors—atrial natriuretic hormones, endothelial relaxing factors, kinins, prostaglandin E2, and prostaglandin I2
- Changes in electrolyte homeostasis, particularly changes in sodium, calcium, and potassium concentrations, affect some of these factors.

A defect in any of the various mechanisms of sodium homeostasis could result in sodium and thereby water retention, ultimately resulting in hypertension.

A rise in intracellular calcium concentration, results in increased vascular contractility, release of renin, synthesis of epinephrine and sympathetic nervous system activity causing increased BP.

In an obese child, hyperinsulinemia may cause rise in BP due to sodium reabsorption and increased sympathetic tone.

■ ETIOLOGY

Hypertension can either be primary (or essential) or secondary. In general, the younger the child and the higher the BP, the greater the chances that hypertension is secondary to one of the identifiable causes (Table 2). A secondary cause of hypertension most likely would be found before puberty whereas after puberty, hypertension is likely to be primary (or essential).

■ EPIDEMIOLOGY

The prevalence of systemic hypertension in children is increasing in developed countries, in view of the growing population of children with obesity.[11] However, the true incidence of hypertension in the pediatric population is not known, due to somewhat arbitrary definition of hypertension and in part to incomplete BP screening during routine pediatric clinical visits. It was found on survey that only two-thirds of routine pediatric visits had BP measurements and in 20% of overweight or obese children, there was no BP screening during their regular visits.[12] Also, in 75% cases of hypertension and 90% cases of prehypertension, it was found that further investigations were not carried out.[13]

Recent evidence shows that the roots of adult hypertension lie in childhood, and that childhood BP predicts BP in the adult.[14,15] Because of differences in genetic and environmental factors, incidences vary from country to country and even from region to region in the same country.

■ PROGNOSIS

Obese children have approximately a 3-fold higher risk for hypertension than nonobese children.[16] HBP is a precursor of complications like heart attacks and stroke. About 41% of children with HBP have left ventricular hypertrophy (LVH).[17] Increase in abdominal girth correlates to elevated BP.[18]

TABLE 2: Common causes of hypertension by age.[10,11]

Infants	Children		Adolescents
	1–6 years	7–12 years	
• Thrombosis of renal artery or vein • Congenital renal anomalies • Coarctation of aorta • Bronchopulmonary dysplasia	• Renal artery stenosis • Renal parenchymal disease • Wilms tumor • Neuroblastoma • Coarctation of aorta	• Renal parenchymal disease • Renovascular abnormalities • Endocrine causes • Essential hypertension	• Essential hypertension • Renal parenchymal disease • Endocrine causes

■ HISTORY

Clues about the cause of hypertension are provided by well-taken history, which helps in selection of specific investigations. There are no specific presenting symptoms and signs in case of neonates. Unless the hypertension is severe, the presenting symptoms and signs are absent in most of the older children.

Relevant information comprises of bronchopulmonary dysplasia; history of umbilical artery catheterization; prematurity; failure to thrive; family history of heritable diseases (such as hypertension, neurofibromatosis); history of head or abdominal trauma; episodes of pyelonephritis (which is perhaps suggested by unexplained fevers) that may lead to renal scarring; medications (e.g. steroids, pressor substances, cold remedies, tricyclic antidepressants, and medications for attention deficit hyperactivity disorder); sleep history, particularly snoring history; history of diet, comprising licorice, caffeine, and salt consumption; and habits (e.g. drinking alcohol, smoking and ingesting illicit substances).

In neonates, the signs and symptoms that indicate the possibility of hypertension comprise irritability or lethargy, congestive heart failure, seizure and respiratory distress.

In older children, the signs and symptoms indicating the possibility of hypertension consist of all of the above, and the following blurred vision, fatigue, epistaxis, headache and bell palsy.

■ EXAMINATION

Measurement and Recording of Blood Pressure

In every child more than 3 years of age, it is important to measure BP every year by auscultatory method. In children in whom auscultatory BP measurement is difficult to do, then oscillometric and doppler techniques can be used. Measurements that are obtained by oscillometry that is more than 90th percentile should be repeated with auscultation. For obtaining proper information about BP, measurements should be repeated over time.

For the accuracy of measurement of the BP, size of the cuff should be proper. At least 40% of the arm circumference of the patient—at a point midway between the olecranon process and the acromion process—should be covered by the width of the rubber bladder inside the cloth cover. About 80–100% of the arm's circumference should be covered by the length of the bladder in the cuff.

The child should be in relaxed and comfortable position, preferably sitting. Back should be supported and feet on the floor. Examination of infants and young children should be done in supine position. Inflation of cuff should be done at a pressure of about 20 mm Hg more than that at which radial pulse disappears. It should then be deflated at a rate of 2–3 mm Hg/second. Table 1 explains the interpretation of BP values.

Stage I HBP patients should be seen again within 1–2 weeks. If the patients of stage II hypertension are symptomatic, they should be re-evaluated within 1 week or sooner. For diagnosing the so called white-coat hypertension, ambulatory monitoring of BP is generally desirable.

Identification of Signs of Secondary Hypertension

One should identify the signs of secondary hypertension on physical examination. For the assessment of potential causes of the hypertension, following should be assessed:

- Thyromegaly may lead to an evaluation for hyperthyroidism
- Growth retardation may indicate chronic renal failure
- Tachycardia may lead to the diagnosis of hyperthyroidism, pheochromocytoma, and neuroblastoma
- Difference of BP between the upper extremities and the lower extremities points to coarctation of the thoracic aorta
- Café au lait spots may indicate neurofibromatosis
- Epigastric or abdominal bruit may indicate renal artery stenosis or coarctation of the abdominal aorta
- Body mass index may lead to the diagnosis of metabolic syndrome
- Acanthosis nigricans may suggest metabolic syndrome
- An abdominal mass may suggest polycystic kidney disease and Wilms tumor
- Virilization or ambiguity may lead to an evaluation for adrenal hyperplasia
- von Hippel-Lindau syndrome, Stigmata of Bardet-Biedl, Williams syndrome, or Turner syndrome.

Laboratory Studies

In the case of patients of hypertension, one should start from simple tests to complex noninvasive tests and then finally invasive tests should be performed.

- The complete blood cell count may lead to the diagnosis of anemia because of chronic renal disease
- Increase in serum creatinine concentration suggests renal disease
- Hypokalemia may lead to the diagnosis of hyperaldosteronism
- High plasma renin activity is diagnostic of renal vascular hypertension, including the coarctation of the aorta. Low plasma renin activity suggests Liddle syndrome, glucocorticoid-remediable aldosteronism, or apparent mineralocorticoid excess
- High values of plasma aldosterone concentration indicate hyperaldosteronism
- High catecholamines concentration (e.g. norepinephrine, epinephrine, or dopamine) may lead to the diagnosis of neuroblastoma or pheochromocytoma
- A positive result for protein or blood, on urine dipstick testing, may be indicative of renal disease
- For the evaluation of patient of chronic pyelonephritis, urine cultures should be used
- High excretion of catecholamines and catecholamine metabolites in urine (metanephrine) suggest neuroblastoma or pheochromocytoma
- Levels of urine sodium indicate intake of dietary sodium. It can be used as a marker to follow a patient after dietary modifications are attempted
- For evaluating metabolic syndrome in obese children, oral glucose-tolerance tests and fasting lipid panels are done.

Echocardiography and Ultrasonography

Chronic hypertension leads to LVH. Chronicity of the hypertension is confirmed by the findings of LVH on echocardiography. Evaluation of left ventricular function should also be done.

For the assessment of suspected aortic coarctation, echocardiography is necessary. It is necessary to examine the aortic arch and its branches in precise anatomical detail.[19]

Abdominal Ultrasonography

Renal scarring indicates that there is excessive release of renin. It can reveal structural anomalies or tumors of renal vasculature or kidneys. Renal masses may suggest a Wilms tumor and extrarenal masses may indicate neuroblastoma. Asymmetry in renal size is indicative of renal artery stenosis or dysplasia.

Other Investigations

- Renal angiography
- Twenty-four hour ambulatory BP monitoring
- Doppler studies.

■ TREATMENT CONSIDERATIONS

For the treatment of hypertension, the cause should be recognized and corrected to the extent possible. In a symptomatic infant, remediable causes of hypertension such as coarctation of the aorta should be identified. Therapeutic modalities are reserved for those children who have irremediable causes of essential hypertension or hypertension.[20]

Nonpharmacological Therapy

Nonpharmacological treatment may be sufficient in children with mild or moderate hypertension to reduce BP within normal limits. This strategy prevents the need for drugs that could have adverse effects and involve a degree of hard-to-achieve compliance in children.

In all the overweight children with hypertension, weight reduction should be a goal regardless of the etiology. There is a close correlation between hypertension and obesity, especially in adolescents.[16]

Unless there is a contraindication, isotonic and aerobic exercises show a direct beneficial effect on BP.

Potassium supplementation in adults can decrease BP and in hitherto unknown ways reduce ventricular hypertrophy.

Low diet limited in fat and salt is also noted to be useful.

Pharmacological Therapy

Indications for pharmacologic treatment are secondary hypertension, symptomatic hypertension, diabetes, hypertensive target organ damage, and hypertension, which persist even after taking nonpharmacologic measures.[21]

American Academy of Pediatrics (AAP) guidelines (2017) for treatment of pediatric and adolescent hypertension recommend the following:

First-line agents may comprise:

- Thiazide diuretic
- Long-acting calcium channel blocker
- Angiotensin receptor blocker (ARB) or angiotensin-converting enzyme (ACE) inhibitor.

In chronic kidney disease (CKD) or diabetes—ACE inhibitor or ARB are recommended.

In the case of hypertensive children and adolescents who could not get treated by lifestyle changes, especially those who have symptomatic hypertension, Stage II hypertension without a clearly modifiable factor, or LVH on echocardiography, pharmacologic treatment should be started by clinicians.[22] Pharmacologic treatment in such

TABLE 3: Drugs with their indications and contraindications.

Drug class	Indications	Contraindications
Angiotensin-converting enzyme inhibitors/angiotensin II receptor blockers	• Chronic kidney disease • Diabetes mellitus • Congestive heart failure	• Bilateral renal artery stenosis • Renal artery stenosis in solitary kidney • Hyperkalemia • Pregnancy
Calcium channel blockers	Post-transplantation	Congestive heart failure
Beta-blockers	Coarctation of the aorta	Asthma
Potassium-sparing diuretics	• Hyperaldosteronism • Chronic renal failure	Chronic renal failure
Loop diuretics	Congestive heart failure	
Vasodilators	Life-threatening conditions	

cases includes an ARB, ACE inhibitor, thiazide diuretic, or long-acting calcium channel blocker (Table 3).

■ MANAGEMENT OF HYPERTENSIVE CRISIS

Hypertensive crisis occurs due to an acute illness (such as acute renal failure or postinfectious glomerulonephritis), exacerbated moderate hypertension, or excessive ingestion of psychogenic substances or drugs.

The clinical manifestations may be those of seizures, cerebral edema, pulmonary edema, renal failure, or heart failure. It is important to accurately assess BP in every patient who presents with seizure, especially when there is no seizure disorder in that patient.

Anticonvulsant medications are generally ineffective in treating a seizure occurring as a result of hypertensive crisis. A fast-acting antihypertensive drug must be used to treat seizures due to severe hypertension.

Following are the drugs that are presently used for the treatment of hypertensive emergencies.

- *Nicardipine*: 1–3 µg/kg/minute intravenous (IV) infusion
- *Sodium nitroprusside*: 0.53–10 µg/kg/minute IV infusion to start
- Labetalol, 0.2–1 mg/kg/dose up to 40 mg/dose as an IV bolus or 0.25–3 mg/kg/hour IV infusion.

The aim of the therapy is to lower BP to the normal limits. Clinicians should know about the adverse effects and therapeutic effects of these drugs. In order to prevent an excessively rapid reduction in BP that can lead to the underperfusion of vital organs, patients must be carefully monitored.

■ CONSULTATIONS

In case pheochromocytoma is suspected, a pediatric endocrinologist should be consulted. Surgical removal of the tumor is indicated, in case of confirmation of diagnosis. If metabolic syndrome is diagnosed, a pediatric endocrinologist should also be consulted.

For the management of aortic coarctation, a pediatric and/or an interventional pediatric cardiologist should be consulted.

The DASH (Dietary Approaches to Stop Hypertension) eating plan should be reviewed with the patient's family by the nutritionist who can give more suggestions for sodium reduction and weight loss.

■ REFERENCES

1. Daniels SR, Pratt CA, Hayman LL. Reduction of risk for cardiovascular disease in children and adolescents. Circulation. 2011;124:1673-86.

2. Ingelfinger JR. The child or adolescent with elevated blood pressure. N Engl J Med. 2014;370:2316-25.

3. Chen X, Wang Y. Tracking of blood pressure from childhood to adulthood: a systematic review and meta-regression analysis. Circulation. 2008;117:3171-80.

4. Tirosh A, Afek A, Rudich A, et al. Progression of normotensive adolescents to hypertensive adults: a study of 26,980 teenagers. Hypertension. 2010;56:203-9.

5. National High Blood Pressure Education Program Working Group on High Blood Pressure in Children Adolescents. The fourth report on the diagnosis, evaluation, and treatment of high blood pressure in children and adolescents. Pediatrics. 2004;114:555-76.

6. Dionne JM, Harris KC, Benoit G, et al. Hypertension Canada's 2017 guidelines for the diagnosis, assessment, prevention, and treatment of pediatric hypertension. Can J Cardiol. 2017;33:577-85.

7. Lurbe E, Agabiti-Rosei E, Cruickshank JK, et al. 2016 European Society of Hypertension guidelines for the management of high blood pressure in children and adolescents. J Hypertens. 2016;34:1887-920.

8. National High Blood Pressure Education Program Working Group on High Blood Pressure in Children and Adolescents. The fourth report on the diagnosis, evaluation, and treatment of high blood pressure in children and adolescents. Pediatrics. 2004;114(2 Suppl 4th Report):555-76.

9. Gruskin AB. Factors affecting blood pressure. In: Drukker A, Gruskin AB (Eds). Pediatric Nephrology: Pediatric and Adolescent Medicine. 3rd edition. Basel, Switzerland: Karger; 1995. p. 1097.

10. Kapur G, Ahmed M, Pan C, et al. Secondary hypertension in overweight and stage 1 hypertensive children: a Midwest Pediatric Nephrology Consortium report. J Clin Hypertens (Greenwich). 2010;12(1):34-9.

11. Roulet C, Bovet P, Brauchli T, et al. Secular trends in blood pressure in children: A systematic review. J Clin Hypertens (Greenwich). 2017;19(5):488-97.

12. Shapiro DJ, Hersh AL, Cabana MD, et al. Hypertension screening during ambulatory pediatric visits in the United States, 2000-2009. Pediatrics. 2012;130(4):604-10.

13. Hansen ML, Gunn PW, Kaelber DC. Underdiagnosis of hypertension in children and adolescents. JAMA. 2007;298(8):874-9.

14. Sun SS, Grave GD, Siervogel RM, et al. Systolic blood pressure in childhood predicts hypertension and metabolic syndrome later in life. Pediatrics. 2007;119(2):237-46.

15. Banker A, Gupta-Malhotra M, Rao PS. Childhood hypertension: a review. J Hypertens. 2013;2(4):128.

16. Dhuper S, Buddhe S, Patel S. Managing cardiovascular risk in overweight children and adolescents. Paediatr Drugs. 2013;15(3):181-90.

17. Hanevold C, Waller J, Daniels S, et al. The effects of obesity, gender, and ethnic group on left ventricular hypertrophy and geometry in hypertensive children: a collaborative study of the International Pediatric Hypertension Association. Pediatrics. 2004;113(2):328-33.

18. Leung LC, Sung RY, So HK, et al. Prevalence and risk factors for hypertension in Hong Kong Chinese adolescents: waist circumference predicts hypertension, exercise decreases risk. Arch Dis Child. 2011;96(9):804-9.

19. Rao PS, Carey P. Doppler ultrasound in the prediction of pressure gradients across aortic coarctation. Am Heart J. 1989;118(2):299-307.

20. [Guideline] University of Michigan Health System. Essential hypertension. Ann Arbor (MI): University of Michigan Health System; 2009 Feb.

21. Meyers RS, Siu A. Pharmacotherapy review of chronic pediatric hypertension. Clin Ther. 2011;33(10):1331-56.

22. Schaefer F, Litwin M, Zachwieja J, et al. Efficacy and safety of valsartan compared to enalapril in hypertensive children: a 12-week, randomized, double-blind, parallel-group study. J Hypertens. 2011;29(12):2484-90.

Emerging Antihypertensive Drugs

Santanu Guha, Sidhartha Mani

Arterial hypertension is a complex process. A new study asserts that in 2010 hypertension was the leading risk factor for global disease burden.[1] Various effective treatments are available for hypertension. However, even with considerable improvements in diagnostic modalities and therapeutic interventions, recent observational studies have revealed persistently low rates of blood pressure control among hypertensive population.[2] Novel therapies to treat resistant hypertension, and reduce the associated cardiovascular risk factors are thus still required.

The armamentarium of antihypertensive treatment comprises calcium-channel blockers, β-blockers, diuretics and inhibitors of the renin–angiotensin-aldosterone system (RAAS).

In such a scenario where new drugs were necessary to control resistant cases, RAAS pathway was being progressively recognized as an useful target. In 2007, the first drug Aliskiren of a new drug class, direct renin inhibitor was approved. This drug 150–300 mg causes an upstream RAAS blockade by blocking the catalytic site of renin. Aliskiren decreases plasma renin activity in contrast to other renin–angiotensin-aldosterone related drugs. Clinical data suggests that aliskiren has similar antihypertensive efficacy to that of the other major antihypertensive drugs and also a similar safety profile to placebo. Aliskiren in combination with other molecules again showed significant blood pressure and proteinuria reductions. Compared to hydrochlorothiazide, ramipril, valsartan, amlodipine, irbesartan or losartan monotherapies (Gradman et al. 2005; Oparil et al. 2007; Schmieder et al. 2009; Uresin et al. 2007; Andersen et al. 2008; Solomon et al. 2009; Brown et al. 2011; Duprez et al. 2008), aliskiren monotherapy has shown similar or slightly higher antihypertensive efficacy.[3-10] In a pooled analysis of three trials, overall systolic blood pressure was lower with aliskiren than with ramipril.[11] How aliskiren fares in treating major cardiovascular events and preventing end-organ damage are being investigated in the "ASPIRE HIGHER" program. In the "ASPIRE HIGHER" program initial studies like Aliskiren Observation of Heart Failure Treatment (ALOFT), Aliskiren in the Evaluation of Proteinuria in Diabetes (AVOID), Aliskiren for GEriatric LowEring of SyStolic hypertension (AGELESS) showed favorable results, Aliskiren Study in Post-MI Patients to Reduce Remodeling (ASPIRE) and Aliskiren and Valsartan Versus Placebo in

Lowering NT-proBNP in Patients Stabilized Following an Acute Coronary Syndrome (AVANT-GARDE) studies showed contrasting results. Subsequently, the Aliskiren Trial in Type 2 Diabetes Using Cardiorenal Endpoints (ALTITUDE) study among diabetic patients with proteinuria and being treated with angiotensin converting enzyme (ACE) inhibitors/angiotensin-receptor blockers (ARBs) had to be terminated early because of safety concerns and lack of beneficial effects. More recent trials like Aliskiren Trial on Acute Heart Failure Outcomes (ASTRONAUT) showed that, addition of aliskiren to standard therapy in patients hospitalized for heart failure with reduced ejection fraction (HFrEF), did not reduce cardiovascular death or heart failure rehospitalization. The results of ongoing studies, e.g. Aliskiren Trial to Minimize OutcomeS in Patients with HEart failuRE (ATMOSPHERE) trial are awaited. Aliskiren, however, has a favorable tolerability profile in the hypertensive population, including the elderly.

Calcium antagonists are now widely used for the treatment of various types of hypertension. Cilnidipine (FRC-8653) is a newly synthesized third generation dihydropyridine type of organic calcium channel blocker that has been developed as a slow-onset and long-lasting antihypertensive drug in Japan, and have a potent inhibitory action on the peripheral neuronal N-type calcium channel in addition to L-type calcium channels. Thus, in addition to its vasodilatory action, cilnidipine suppresses cardiac sympathetic overactivity and is renoprotective. In clinical studies, cilnidipine has demonstrated its antihypertensive effects particularly in patients with severe hypertension or with complications such as diabetes, chronic kidney disease (CKD) and cerebrovascular disease. Cilnidipine has shown to improve some hypertensive conditions closely associated with sympathetic activation such as nocturnal hypertension, morning hypertension Ambulatory Blood Pressure Control and Home Blood Pressure (Morning and Evening) Lowering by N-Channel Blocker Cilnidipine (ACHIEVE-ONE) trial, white-coat hypertension, mental and cold stress.[12] Benidipine hydrochloride (benidipine, CAS 91599-74-5) is known to inhibit the T-type as well as L- and N-type calcium channels. Benidipine has a sustained antihypertensive effect, independent of its blood concentration since it binds to dihydropyridine receptors via a "membrane approach." Benidipine dilates glomerular afferent and efferent arterioles equally through inhibition of T-type Ca channels. Thus, it may cause a decrease of intraglomerular pressure as well as suppression of proteinuria. The inhibitory effect of benidipine on T-type calcium channels also results in aldosterone suppression in the adrenal glands and reducing oxidative stress caused by aldosterone. Thus, the aldosterone-inhibitory and antioxidant activities of benidipine would result in renoprotection and suppression of CKD progression. Certain trials demonstrate that benidipine has a more potent antihypertensive effect than cilnidipine and also a renoprotective effect, indicating the high usefulness of benidipine in hypertensive patients with diabetes. Benidipine also improves arterial compliance gradually and safely without any adverse effect.

Another latest antihypertensive molecule approved in 2010–2011 by FDA was the angiotensin II type 1 receptor (AT1R) blocker azilsartan. The approval of azilsartan medoxomil in 2011 increased the number of currently available agents in this class to eight. Azilsartan medoxomil is an AT1R blocker with peroxisome proliferator-activated receptor γ activity. Azilsartan was approved based on randomized trials involving almost 6,000 patients with mild-to-severe hypertension,[13,14] where it was found that an 80 mg dose of azilsartan was more effective than placebo or other active comparator molecules (valsartan 320 mg or olmesartan medoxomil 40 mg) in lowering 24 h mean blood pressure. The antihypertensive effect persisted even after 26 weeks of administration. However, there is insufficient long-term morbidity and mortality data. Fimasartan is the most recent, angiotensin II receptor antagonist approved for treatment of hypertension. Fimasartan, is a pyrimidin-4(3H)-one derivative of losartan with its imidazole ring been replaced, thus enabling higher potency and longer duration than losartan. Predominant elimination pathways of fimasartan include fecal elimination and biliary excretion with less than 3% urinary excretion in 24 h. Fimasartan is primarily catabolized by cytochrome P450 isoform 3A pathway and there is no significant drug interaction. Fimasartan, at a dosage range of 60–120 mg once daily, showed 24 h antihypertensive effect duration. Fimasartan showed an excellent safety profile in large scale, population-based observational study with additional anti-inflammatory and organ-protecting effects been shown in various preclinical studies.

With such a modest advancement in therapeutic options, some novel molecules or new formulations are currently in clinical studies.[15]

These are the following drugs:
- LCI699, an aldosterone synthase inhibitor
- LCZ696, an dual AT1R blocker and neutral endopeptidase inhibitor
- Daglutril, dual endothelin-converting enzyme and neutral endopeptidase inhibitor
- PS-433540, a dual AT1R and endothelin A receptor blocker
- PL-3994, a natriuretic peptide receptor agonist
- AR9281, a soluble epoxide hydrolase inhibitor
- Lercanidipine, a modified release calcium-channel antagonist
- Clonidine, controlled release centrally acting α2-adrenergic agonist
- Longer-acting phosphodiesterase type 5 (PDE5) inhibitors.

Aldosterone acts as a downstream effector of some deleterious angiotensin II effects, and plays important role in resistant hypertension,[16] have promoted the use of aldosterone antagonists in patients with hypertension. Spironolactone and eplerenone, both act on the mineralocorticoid receptor with comparable blood-pressure-lowering effects. Spironolactone is associated with an increased rate of progesterone-dependent and testosterone-dependent adverse effects. Aldosterone antagonists can lead to reactive increase in aldosterone levels, triggering the undesired mineralocorticoid receptor dependent effects (such as sodium/hydrogen exchanger or sodium/potassium exchanger activation) and mineralocorticoid receptor-independent effects (such as JNK kinase and phospholipase C activation) causing inflammation hypertrophy, and fibrosis. LCI699 could represent a first-in-class aldosterone synthase inhibitor which can prevent these effects. Initial results in 14 patients with primary aldosteronism showed that twice-daily administration of 0.5 mg or 1.0 mg of LCI699 for 4 weeks lowered 24 h ambulatory systolic blood pressure and supine plasma aldosterone concentrations.[17] A dose of 1 mg once daily, or 0.5 mg twice daily of LCI699 reduced ambulatory systolic and diastolic blood pressure as well as mean sitting systolic blood pressure.[18] This daily 1 mg dose achieved a similar blood-pressure reduction to that of 50 mg eplerenone twice daily (the highest approved dose). The frequency of hyperkalemia was low and similar to other treatment groups.[18] Further studies are needed to demonstrate whether aldosterone synthase inhibitors can deliver organ-protective effects like mineralocorticoid receptor antagonists apart from blood pressure control.

The PL-3994 [natriuretic peptide receptor A agonists (NPRA)] is presently in the clinical phase of investigation in patients with heart failure and hypertension. PL-3994, dose-dependently increased cyclic GMP levels, reduced blood pressure, and induced natriuresis on the day following treatment in healthy volunteers in the phase I trials.[19] Similar results were shown in a phase IIa study in patients with adequately controlled essential hypertension.[20] In this study, patients treated with ACE inhibitors experienced the largest blood-pressure-reducing effect, which suggested synergism between NPRA agonism and ACE blockade.[20]

Soluble epoxide hydrolase was identified as a novel therapeutic target for blood pressure control because its inhibition had a blood pressure-lowering effect in spontaneously hypertensive rats.[21] Inhibition of this enzyme also had antiproliferative effects.[22] In patients with hypertension and diabetes mellitus, higher levels of soluble epoxide hydrolase activity were observed.[23] AR9281 is the first soluble epoxide hydrolase inhibitor that is being tried under clinical trials. This agent, being lipophilic, can be administered per oral.

Stimulation of AT2R opposes many aspects of AT1R stimulation by mediating vasodilatory, antiproliferative, and anti-inflammatory effects.[24] The nonpeptide AT2R agonist compound 2,146 has been used to investigate the direct effects of pharmacological AT2R stimulation. This compound improved myocardial function independently of blood pressure,[25] and suppressed inflammation and NF-κB activity.[26]

Neutral endopeptidase, a metallo-peptidase, takes part in metabolism of various vasodilatory and vasoconstrictive substances, most important being natriuretic peptides leading to various effects on blood pressure.[27] However, if this enzyme is inhibited along with concomitant vasoconstrictor blockade, reduced degradation of vasodilatory substrates might lead to a net vasodilatory effect. The dual ACE-neutral endopeptidase inhibitor *omapatrilat* showed encouraging results in terms of efficacy in hypertension and heart failure in Omapatrilat Cardiovascular Treatment Assessment Versus Enalapril (OCTAVE) and Omapatrilat Versus Enalapril Randomized Trial of Utility in Reducing Events (OVERTURE) trials. However, they showed an increased incidence of angioedema compared to ACE inhibitor enalapril alone.[28,29] Consequently, attention was shifted to dual AT1R and neutral endopeptidase antagonism. The first-in-class, LCZ696 achieved a blood pressure reduction comparable to an AT1R blocker (valsartan) in a phase II, placebo-controlled, and active treatment-controlled clinical trial in patients with mild-to-moderate grade of essential hypertension.[30] The two highest doses of LCZ696 (200 mg and 400 mg) achieved a larger reduction in sitting systolic and diastolic blood pressures than comparable doses of valsartan (160 mg and 320 mg) in 8 weeks of treatment. The 400 mg dose of LCZ696 also resulted in superior pulse-pressure reduction compared with valsartan. No angioedema was reported in this study.[30]

AT1R and endothelin A receptor blockade is another tested modality. Endothelin, one of the most potent vasoconstrictors, has prominent roles in inflammation, oxidative stress, atherosclerosis, fibrogenesis, salt and water homeostasis, and pulmonary hypertension.[31-33] Thus, several endothelin receptor antagonists have been tried in the treatment of hypertension. In the DAR-311 (DORADO) trial, a selective endothelin A antagonist darusentan achieved encouraging blood pressure reductions in patients with resistant hypertension,[34] and a greater reduction in mean 24 h blood pressure (both systolic and diastolic) compared to placebo or the sympatholytic antihypertensive agent guanfacine in the DAR-312 (DORADO-AC) trial.[35] However, adverse effects like peripheral edema due to salt and water retention was a limitation of endothelin A receptor blockers.[34-37] However, these findings raise the question of whether dual-specificity AT1R and endothelin A receptor antagonists (such as PS433540, currently under clinical investigation) could prove more effective and better tolerated than specific endothelin A receptor antagonists. PS433540 (at doses of 200 mg, 400 mg and 800 mg) reduced systolic and diastolic blood pressures more effectively in a phase IIb, randomized, double-blind, placebo-controlled trial, with the highest dose achieving better blood pressure reduction than the AT1R blocker irbesartan. In addition, compared with irbesartan, triple drug combination lowered blood pressure by 40/25 mm Hg, which was significantly greater than that achieved by treatment with two drug combinations of valsartan and hydrochlorothiazide, valsartan and amlodipine, or amlodipine and hydrochlorothiazide.[38]

Dual endothelin-converting enzyme (ECE) and neutral endopeptidase inhibitors, such as SLV 338, are in preclinical trials. SLV 338 treatment was well tolerated in stroke prone, spontaneously hypertensive rats, and was associated with improved survival and lowered stroke incidence. However, the treatment did not show significant effects on blood pressure.[39]

Currently, a single pharmacologic agent is sufficient to achieve target blood pressure control in approximately one-third of patients with hypertension; another one-third requiring two drugs, while the rest needs at least three agents.[40]

Combination therapy is more useful because one agent typically blocks the counter-regulatory system activity triggered by the other[41] and might sometimes attenuate its adverse effects.

A triple combination of olmesartan (40 mg), amlodipine (10 mg) and hydrochlorothiazide (25 mg) was approved in 2010 on the basis of the Triple Therapy with Olmesartan Medoxomil, Amlodipine, and Hydrochlorothiazide in Hypertensive Patients (TRINITY) results in patients with hypertension.[42] The triple combination treatment was more effective than the double drug arms, e.g. olmesartan- hydrochlorothiazide, amlodipine-hydrochlorothiazide and olmesartan-amlodipine.[42]

Few combination therapies involving aliskiren include aliskiren *plus* hydrochlorothiazide (approved in 2008), aliskiren *plus* amlodipine, and aliskiren *plus* amlodipine *plus* hydrochlorothiazide (both approved in 2010). The aliskiren *plus* amlodipine combination achieved greater blood pressure reduction than either component alone in patients with mild-to-severe hypertension after 8 weeks of treatment.[43] The approval of aliskiren (300 mg) in a fixed-dose triple drug combination therapy with amlodipine (10 mg) and hydrochlorothiazide (25 mg) was on the basis of the results of a double-blind, active-treatment-controlled trial in patients with moderate-to-severe hypertension showing a greater mean blood-pressure reduction than the two-drug combinations.[42] In the ALTITUDE trial, which was designed to determine effects of adding aliskiren (300 mg once daily) to conventional treatment (including AT1R antagonist or an ACE inhibitor) in patients with type 2 diabetes mellitus, to reduce cardiovascular and renal morbidity and mortality.[44] However, this trial was halted prematurely because of no apparent benefits and an increase in adverse events.[45] These data suggest that the combination of aliskiren with an AT1R antagonist or an ACE inhibitor should not be used.

We can thus remain optimistic regarding approval of newer antihypertensive drugs in recent future. Further research in search of novel drugs and treatment modalities in this field should however continue with new momentum.

■ REFERENCES

1. Kotseva K, Wood D, De Backer G, et al. Cardiovascular prevention guidelines in daily practice: a comparison of EUROASPIRE I, II, and III surveys in eight European countries. Lancet. 2009;373(9667):929-40.

2. Lim SS, Vos T, Flaxman AD, et al. A comparative risk assessment of burden of disease and injury attributable to 67 risk factors and risk factor clusters in 21 regions, 1990–2010: a systematic analysis for the Global Burden of Disease Study 2010. Lancet. 2012;380(9859):2224-60.

3. Gradman AH, Schmieder RE, Lins RL, et al. Aliskiren, a novel orally effective renin inhibitor, provides dose-dependent antihypertensive efficacy and placebo-like tolerability in hypertensive patients. Circulation. 2005;111(8):1012-8.

4. Uresin Y, Taylor AA, Kilo C, et al. Efficacy and safety of the direct renin inhibitor aliskiren and ramipril alone or in combination in patients with diabetes and hypertension. J Renin Angiotensin Aldosterone Syst. 2007;8(4):190-8.

5. Oparil S, Yarows SA, Patel S, et al. Efficacy and safety of combined use of aliskiren and valsartan in patients with hypertension: a randomised, double-blind trial. Lancet. 2007;370(9583):221-9.

6. Schmieder RE, Philipp T, Guerediaga J, et al. Long-term antihypertensive efficacy and safety of the oral direct renin inhibitor aliskiren: a 12-month randomized, double-blind comparator trial with hydrochlorothiazide. Circulation. 2009;119(3):417-25.

7. Andersen K, Weinberger MH, Egan B, et al. Comparative efficacy and safety of aliskiren, an oral direct renin inhibitor, and ramipril in hypertension: a 6-month, randomized, double-blind trial. J Hypertens. 2008;26(3):589-99.

8. Solomon SD, Appelbaum E, Manning WJ, et al. Effect of the direct Renin inhibitor aliskiren, the Angiotensin receptor blocker losartan, or both on left ventricular mass in patients with hypertension and left ventricular hypertrophy. Circulation. 2009;119(4):530-7.

9. Brown MJ, McInnes GT, Papst CC, et al. Aliskiren and the calcium channel blocker amlodipine combination as an initial treatment strategy for hypertension control (ACCELERATE): a randomised, parallel-group trial. Lancet. 2011;377(9762):312-20.

10. Duprez D, Davis P, Botha J. The AGELESS study: the effect of aliskiren versus ramipril alone or in combination with hydrochlorothiazide and amlodipine in patients 65 years of age with systolic hypertension. Circulation. 2008;118:886-7.

11. Verdecchia P, Angeli F, Mazzotta G, et al. Aliskiren versus ramipril in hypertension. Ther Adv Cardiovasc Dis. 2010;4(3):193-200.

12. Yamagishi T. Beneficial effect of cilnidipine on morning hypertension and white-coat effect in patients with essential hypertension. Hypertens Res.. 2006;29(5):339-44.

13. White WB, Weber MA, Sica D, et al. Effects of the angiotensin receptor blocker azilsartan medoxomil versus olmesartan and valsartan on ambulatory and clinic blood pressure in patients with stages 1 and 2 hypertension. Hypertension. 2011;57(3):413-20.

14. Bakris GL, Sica D, Weber M, et al. The comparative effects of azilsartan medoxomil and olmesartan on ambulatory and clinic blood pressure. J Clin Hypertens (Greenwich). 2011;13(2):81–8.

15. New Medicines Database. PhRMA [online] Available from http://www.phrma.org/newmeds/results.php?skin=phrma&drug=&indication=38&company= &status= (2011). [Last accessed August, 2019].

16. Lane DA, Shah S, Beevers DG. Low-dose spironolactone in the management of resistant hypertension: a surveillance study. J Hypertens. 2007;25(4):891-4.

17. Amar L, Azizi M, Menard J, et al. Aldosterone synthase inhibition with LCI699: a proof-of-concept study in patients with primary aldosteronism. Hypertension. 2010;56(5):831-8.

18. Calhoun DA, White WB, Krum H, et al. Effects of a novel aldosterone synthase inhibitor for treatment of primary hypertension: results of a randomized, double-blind, placebo- and active-controlled phase 2 trial. Circulation. 2011;124(18):1945-55.

19. Jordan R, Stark J, Huskey S, et al. Phase 1 study of the novel A-type natriuretic receptor agonist, PL-3994, in healthy volunteers. Presented at the 12th scientific meeting of the Heart Failure Society of America. [online] Available from http://www.palatin.com/pdfs/HFSA%20Poster11-17%20Handout.pdf. [Last accessed August, 2019].

20. Sica D, Jordan R, Fischkoff SA. (2009) Phase IIa study of the NPR-agonist, PL-3994, in healthy adult volunteers with controlled hypertension. Presented at the 13th scientific meeting of the Heart Failure Society of America. [online] Available from http://www.palatin.com/pdfs/Palatin%20HSFA%2709_PO%28220%29%20HR.pdf. [Last accessed August, 2019.

21. Imig JD, Zhao X, Capdevila JH, et al. Soluble epoxide hydrolase inhibition lowers arterial blood pressure in angiotensin II hypertension. Hypertension. 2007;39(2 Pt 2):690-4.

22. Davis BB, Thompson DA, Howard LL, et al. Inhibitors of soluble epoxide hydrolase attenuate vascular smooth muscle cell proliferation. Proc Natl Acad. Sci USA. 2002;99(4):2222-7.

23. Chen D, Whitcomb R, MacIntyre E, et al. Pharmacokinetics and pharmacodynamics of AR9281, an inhibitor of soluble epoxide hydrolase, in single- and multiple-dose

studies in healthy human subjects. J. Clin. Pharmacol. 2012;52(3):319-28

24. Steckelings UM, Kaschina E, Unger T. The AT2 receptor—a matter of love and hate. Peptides. 2005;26(8):1401-9.

25. Kaschina E, Grzesiak A, Li J, et al. Angiotensin II type 2 receptor stimulation: a novel option of therapeutic interference with the renin–angiotensin system in myocardial infarction? Circulation. 2008;118(24):2523-32.

26. Rompe F, Artuc M, Hallberg A, et al. Direct angiotensin II type 2 receptor stimulation acts anti-inflammatory through epoxyeicosatrienoic acid and inhibition of nuclear factor κB. Hypertension. 2010;55(4):924-31.

27. Campbell DJ. Vasopeptidase inhibition: a double-edged sword? Hypertension. 2003;41(3):383-9.

28. Tabrizchi R. Omapatrilat. Bristol-Myers Squibb. Curr Opin Investig Drugs. 2001;2(10):1414-22.

29. Packer M, Califf RM, Konstam MA, et al. Comparison of omapatrilat and enalapril in patients with chronic heart failure: the Omapatrilat Versus Enalapril Randomized Trial of Utility in Reducing Events (OVERTURE). Circulation. 2002;106(8):920-6.

30. Ruilope LM, Dukat A, Böhm M, et al. Blood-pressure reduction with LCZ696, a novel dual-acting inhibitor of the angiotensin II receptor and neprilysin: a randomised, doubleblind, placebo-controlled, active comparator study. Lancet. 2010;375(9722):1255-66.

31. Kirkby NS, Hadoke PWF, Bagnall AJ, et al. The endothelin system as a therapeutic target in cardiovascular disease: great expectations or bleak house? Br J Pharmacol. 2008;153(6):1105-19.

32. Dhaun N, Pollock DM, Goddard J, et al. Selective and mixed endothelin receptor antagonism in cardiovascular disease. Trends Pharmacol. Sci. 2007;28(11):573-9.

33. Feldstein C, Romero C. Role of endothelins in hypertension. Am J Therapeutics. 2007;14(2):147-53.

34. Weber MA, Black H, Bakris G, et al. A selective endothelin receptor antagonist to reduce blood pressure in patients with treatment-resistant hypertension: a randomised, double blind, placebo-controlled trial. Lancet. 2009;374(9699):1423-31.

35. Bakris GL, et al. Divergent results using clinic and ambulatory blood pressures: report of a darusentan-resistant hypertension trial. Hypertension. 2010;56(5):824-30.

36. Sica DA. Endothelin receptor antagonism: what does the future hold? Hypertension. 2008;52(3):460-1.

37. Webb DJ. DORADO: Opportunity postponed: lessons from studies of endothelin receptor antagonists in treatment-resistant hypertension. Hypertension. 2010;56(5):806-7.

38. Calhoun DA, Lacourcière Y, Chiang YT, et al. Triple antihypertensive therapy with amlodipine, valsartan, and hydrochlorothiazide: a randomized clinical trial. Hypertension. 2009;54(1):32-9.

39. Wengenmayer C, Krikov M, Mueller S, et al. Novel therapy approach in primary stroke prevention: simultaneous inhibition of endothelin converting enzyme and neutral endopeptidase in spontaneously hypertensive, stroke-prone rats improves survival. Neurol Res. 2011;33(2): 201-7.

40. Düsing R. Optimizing blood pressure control through the use of fixed combinations. Vasc Health Risk Manag. 2010;6:321-5.

41. Sica DA. Rationale for fixed-dose combinations in the treatment of hypertension: the cycle repeats. Drugs. 2002;62(3):443-62.

42. Chrysant SG. Single-pill triple-combination therapy: an alternative to multiple-drug treatment of hypertension. Postgrad Med. 2011;123(6):21-31.

43. Littlejohn TW 3rd, Trenkwalder P, Hollanders, et al. Long-term safety, tolerability and efficacy of combination therapy with aliskiren and amlodipine in patients with hypertension. Curr Med Res Opin. 2009;25(4):951-9.

44. Parving HH, Brenner BM, McMurray JJ, et al. Aliskiren trial in type 2 diabetes using cardio-renal endpoints (ALTITUDE): rationale and study design. Nephrol Dial Transplant. 2009;24(5):1663-71.

45. Novartis. Novartis announces termination of ALTITUDE study with Rasilez®/Tekturna® in high-risk patients with diabetes and renal impairment. Novartis Global [online], http:// www.novartis.com/newsroom/media-releases/en/2011/1572562.shtml (2011).

Concordance and the Treatment of Hypertension

Michaela M Watts, Fraz A Mir

■ INTRODUCTION

Case History

A 48-year-old woman with apparently resistant hypertension was prescribed multiple antihypertensive agents. These comprised ramipril 10 mg od, bisoprolol 10 mg od, amlodipine 10 mg od, spironolactone 25 mg od, indapamide 2.5 mg od, doxazosin XL 4 mg od and methyldopa 250 mg tds.

She attended the hypertension clinic in the morning and underwent "directly-observed therapy", i.e. nurse-led administration of her prescribed medication and measurement of her blood pressure response. Her baseline average seated blood pressure was 168/102 mm Hg, with a heart rate of 96 bpm.

The HPLC-MS/MS[1] (high-performance liquid chromatography-tandem mass spectrometry) of a urine sample taken immediately prior to her directly-observed therapy revealed that none of the prescribed drugs was detectable.

Her 24-hour ambulatory blood pressure monitoring (ABPM) following step-wise administration of ramipril 10 mg, amlodipine 10 mg and indapamide 2.5 mg revealed a daytime average of 134/78 mm Hg (night-time average 115/69 mm Hg).

Adherence encompasses numerous health-related behaviors that extend beyond simply taking prescribed drugs. Defining adherence as to the extent to which the patient follows medical instructions is a helpful starting point.[2] However, the term "medical" may be insufficient in describing the range of interventions used to treat chronic diseases such as hypertension. In addition, the term "instructions" implies that the patient is passive, an acquiescent recipient of expert advice rather than an active collaborator in treatment. Adherence to any regimen reflects behavior of one type or another. Seeking medical attention, filling prescriptions, taking medications as prescribed, attending follow-up appointments, and modifying lifestyle choices that address self-management of diabetes, cessation of smoking, unhealthy diet, and insufficient levels of physical activity are all examples of therapeutic behaviors.

Therefore, the definition of adherence (to long-term therapy) as the extent to which a person's behavior—taking medication, following a diet and/or executing lifestyle changes—corresponds with agreed recommendations from a healthcare provider seems appropriate.

In 2003, the World Health Organization (WHO) emphasized that there is a need to differentiate adherence from compliance.[3] The main difference is that adherence requires the patient's agreement to the recommendations. The WHO said that patients should be active partners with health professionals in their own care and that good communication between patient and clinician is mandatory for effective clinical practice. Indeed, this shared decision making process via which patients and clinicians make treatment decisions together is known as "concordance".

▪ FIVE INTERACTING DIMENSIONS AFFECTING CONCORDANCE (TABLE 1)

The common belief that patients are solely responsible for "adhering" to their therapy is misleading and most often reflects a misunderstanding of how other factors affect people's behavior and capacity to adhere to their treatment. Concordance is a multidimensional phenomenon determined by the interplay of five sets of factors, of which patient-related factors are just one determinant.

TABLE 1: Concordance and treating hypertension.

Factors	Factors affecting adherence	Interventions to improve adherence
Socioeconomic-related factors	(–) Poor socioeconomic status, illiteracy, unemployment, limited drug supply and high cost of medication	Family preparedness, patient health insurance, uninterrupted supply of medicines, sustainable financing, affordable prices and reliable supply systems
Healthcare team/health system-related factors	(–) Lack of knowledge and training for healthcare providers on managing chronic diseases, inadequate relationship between healthcare provider and patient, lack of knowledge and inadequate time for consultations, and lack of incentives and feedback on performance (+) Good relationship between patient and physician	Training in education of patients on use of medicines; good patient-physician relationship; continuous monitoring and reassessment of treatment; monitoring adherence; nonjudgmental attitude and assistance; uninterrupted ready availability of information; rational selection of medications; training in communication skills; delivery, financing, and proper management of medicines; and pharmaceuticals: developing drugs with better safety profile, participation in patient education programs and developing instruments to measure adherence for patients
Condition-related factors	(+) Understanding and perceptions about hypertension	Education on use of medicines
Therapy-related factors	(–) Complex treatment regimens; duration of treatment; and low drug tolerability, adverse effects of treatment (+) Monotherapy with simple dosing schedules; less frequent dose; fewer changes in antihypertensive medications; and newer classes of drugs with less side effects: angiotensin II antagonists and calcium channel blockers	Simplification of regimens

Continued

Continued

Factors	Factors affecting adherence	Interventions to improve adherence
Patient-related factors	(–) Inadequate knowledge and skill in managing the disease symptoms and treatment, no awareness of the costs and benefits of treatment, nonacceptance of monitoring (+) Perception of the health risk related to the disease, active participation in monitoring and participation in management of disease	Behavioral and motivational intervention, good patient-physician relationship, self-management of disease and treatment, self-management of side effects, memory aids and reminders

Key: (+), factors having a positive effect on adherence; (–), factors having a negative effect on adherence.

Source: WHO. (2003). Adherence to long-term therapies: Evidence for action. [online] Available from: http://www.who.int/chp/knowledge/publications/adherence_full_report.pdf [Last Accessed March, 2019].

Socioeconomic-related Factors

Socioeconomic status has not consistently been found to be an independent predictor of adherence; however, in developing countries, low socioeconomic status may put patients in the position of having to choose between competing priorities. Such priorities for patients include demands to direct their limited available resources to meet and care for the needs of other family members.

Other factors reported to have a significant effect on concordance are—illiteracy, low level of education, unemployment, lack of effective social support networks, unstable living conditions, long distance from treatment center, expense of transport, costly medication, changing environmental situations, culture and lay beliefs about illness and treatment and family dysfunction.

Healthcare Team and System-related Factors

A good patient-provider relationship may improve concordance. However, there are many factors that have a negative effect. These include poorly developed health services, poor medication distribution systems, lack of knowledge and training for healthcare providers on managing chronic diseases such as hypertension, overworked healthcare providers, short consultations, poor capacity of the system to educate patients about their condition and provide them with timely follow-up, and lack of knowledge on adherence and of effective intervention for improving it.

Condition-related Factors

Condition-related factors represent particular illness-related demands faced by the patient. Some strong determinants of adherence are those directly related to the severity of symptoms. In general, hypertensive patients have little or no symptoms, which increase the difficulty in convincing the patient that they need life-long treatment. This is particularly the case when medications used to treat hypertension cause side effects. The severity of disease and the availability of effective treatments are also factors. Their impact depends on how they influence patients' risk perception, the importance of following treatment, and the priority placed on adherence. Unless patients understand the risks they face from nonadherence, they are unlikely to engage in a successful process of concordance.

Therapy-related Factors

There are many therapy-related factors that can affect adherence. Most notable are those related to the complexity of the medical regimen, previous treatment failures and/or side effects (discussed above), frequent changes in treatment, and the immediacy of beneficial effects.

Vrijens, et al. 2008,[4] explored once a day antihypertensive medication taking in 5,000 patients (Fig. 1). The above graph demonstrates the time course of various dosing parameters. By around 6 months, only about two-thirds of patients were still taking their medication; even less were taking it as prescribed originally. The resulting shortfalls in drug exposure could be a common cause of low rates of blood pressure control and high variability seen in response to prescribed drugs.

Randomized trials have shown that a polypill combining a statin with antihypertensive drugs and aspirin improves adherence rates and reduces cardiovascular risk.[5] However, in contrast to conditions such as HIV, and asthma where combination therapies have widespread approval, the idea of a polypill for cardiovascular disease prevention, while seemingly popular among patients, has proved to be less so among specialist physicians. Explanations include negative perceptions about the lack of flexibility in dosing and also concern about the loss of autonomy in clinical decision making. Until recently, there has been little enthusiasm from pharmaceutical companies to develop polypills because of perceived low financial margins, despite there being a huge target population. The tide seems to be turning, however, with the recent approval of a polypill, which contains aspirin, ramipril and atorvastatin in more than 30 countries across both Latin America and Europe. The availability and use of an affordable polypill would be universally welcome to help achieve the WHO target of reducing the number of deaths from noncommunicable diseases by 25% by 2025.

Patient-related Factors

Patient-related factors represent the resources, knowledge, attitudes, beliefs, perceptions and expectations of the patient. Patients' knowledge and beliefs about their

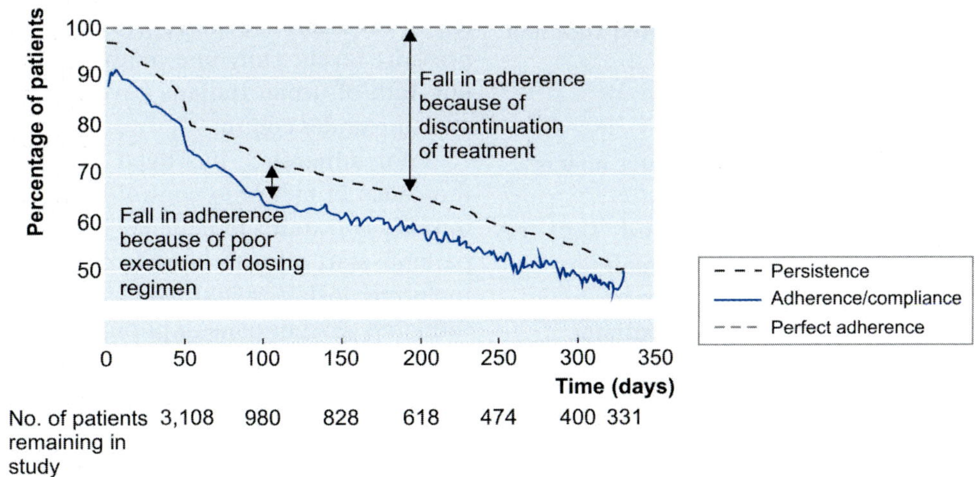

Fig. 1: Time course of adherence/compliance parameters (execution/persistence).

hypertension, motivation to manage it, confidence in their ability to engage in illness-management behaviors including lifestyle choices, and expectations regarding the outcome of treatment and the consequences of poor adherence, and interact to influence adherence behavior.

In 2005, a study reviewed the qualitative research on drug taking in a wide range of medical conditions and found that patients often actively decided not to take drugs (intentional nonadherence) rather than unintentionally omitting them.[6] In a systematic review of qualitative research looking at people's perspectives on hypertension and drug taking, many participants perceived stress to be the primary cause of their hypertension and associated symptoms. Participants intentionally adjusted their drug dose, took drugs sporadically and stopped altogether, often without seeking medical advice beforehand. Reasons given for reducing their treatments included a perception that their blood pressure had improved because of a reduction in symptoms, and that they felt the drugs were unnecessary when they were under less stress, they had a dislike of taking drugs, worried about risks of addiction or tolerance and also side effects.

Patient-related factors reported to affect adherence are:

- Forgetfulness
- Psychosocial stress
- Anxieties about possible adverse effects
- Low motivation
- Inadequate knowledge and skill in managing their disease and treatment
- Lack of self-perceived need for treatment
- Lack of perceived effect of treatment
- Negative beliefs regarding the efficacy of the treatment
- Lack of perception of the health risk related to their hypertension
- Misunderstanding of medication instructions

- Lack of engagement in monitoring of their blood pressure
- Low treatment expectations
- Low attendance at follow-up appointments
- Anxiety over the complexity of the drug regimen
- Feeling stigmatized by the disease.

■ CONCORDANCE AND HYPERTENSION

We live in a rapidly changing environment. Throughout the world, health is being forged by the same powerful forces—an aging worldwide population, rapid urbanization and global increase in unhealthy lifestyles. Increasingly, we are seeing that both wealthy and resource-poor countries are facing the same challenges. One of the most striking examples of this significant shift is the fact that noncommunicable diseases have overtaken infections as the world's leading cause of death. Indeed, the biggest modifiable risk factor and threat to human life globally is now thought to be hypertension.

Despite the wide availability of effective treatments and therapeutic interventions, studies have shown that in many countries less than a quarter of patients who are treated for hypertension achieve optimum blood pressure levels. Only one-tenth of rural and one-fifth of urban Indians have their blood pressure under control.[7]

Poor adherence has been identified as the cause of failure to control hypertension in up to two-thirds of patients. Usually, most patients start off with lifestyle modifications including losing weight, smoking cessation, reducing alcohol consumption, eating fresh fruits and vegetables high in potassium, regular exercising, etc. Taken together, these interventions can reduce blood pressure significantly. The challenge, however, is to maintain such a healthy lifestyle long-term; lifestyle modifications should be reiterated regularly, regardless of whether or not the patient is on antihypertensive medications.

In addition to prevention of death, stroke, and myocardial infarction, other costly consequences of untreated hypertension can also be prevented or minimized by effective treatment.[8,9] Examples include reduction in risk of cardiac failure, incidence of dementia, preservation of renal function and prevention of blindness in diabetic patients. It is apparent that in many countries, poorly controlled blood pressure represents not only a significant health burden but consequently, an important economic liability.[10,11] It is clear, therefore, that improving concordance could represent both an important potential source of health and economic advancement.

■ ASSESSING AND TACKLING CONCORDANCE: THE CAMBRIDGE PERSPECTIVE

Patients do not always take their medicines exactly as prescribed and healthcare professionals seldom inquire about drug adherence, thereby missing opportunities to provide vital information and support. Historically, "tagging" medicines with measurable drugs (e.g. barbiturates) was acceptable ethically. Nowadays, antihypertensive drugs can be detected in blood and urine samples (see above case). However, the use of such techniques can risk undermining the clinician-patient relationship and it is important that the clinician informs the patient prior to the sample collection. In order to make it easier for the patient to report nonadherence, asking the question in a way that does not apportion blame and explains the rationale behind, it is crucial. It is useful to ask about a specific time period such as "in the past week" and about their medicine-taking behaviors (e.g. reducing the prescribed dose, stopping and starting medicines, or taking "medicine holidays"). Also, the physician may use records of prescription reordering, pharmacy records, and return of any unused medicines to identify potential nonadherence.

Helpful interventions include suggesting that patients keep a "diary", encouraging patients to monitor their blood pressure at home and simplifying the dosing regimen. For the elderly or those less physically able, the use of liquid preparations, alternative packaging, or using a multicompartment medicines system should be considered.

As above, while hypertensive patients largely have no symptoms, side effects from antihypertensive drugs are not uncommon. This in turn leads to less adherence.[12] Of all modern antihypertensive agents, angiotensin receptor blockers have the most favorable side effect profile and are most likely to be tolerated. If nonadherence persists, it should be discussed how the patient would like to address it with an informed discussion of the benefits, disadvantages and long-term effects—do they really understand and appreciate the concept and level of risk to their health because of nonadherence? The clinician should consider adjusting the dosage of the medication—often patients can tolerate smaller doses of multiple agents rather than high doses of one or two; consideration for switching to another medicine with a different range of side effects can also be effective. Contemplate what other strategies might be used (e.g., timing of medicines). Often clinicians underestimate the significant cost burden of patients paying for their prescriptions.

■ DIRECTLY OBSERVED THERAPY

Suboptimal adherence with antihypertensive medication is an underestimated contributing factor in apparent treatment-resistant hypertension. Resistant hypertension supposedly has a prevalence of approximately 10%.[13] Such patients have a higher cardiovascular risk and poorer prognosis. In the experience of the authors, once secondary causes have been excluded, truly resistant hypertension is much rarer and constitutes a minority of patients. One strategy being increasingly employed to assess concordance in the field of hypertension, and thereby exclude resistant hypertension, is directly observed therapy (DOT). This is adapted from the approach applied so successfully in the treatment for tuberculosis. Patients are observed taking their antihypertensive medications under direct supervision at a "DOT" clinic. Patients attend early in the morning un-medicated. They are fitted with a 24-hour ABPM for ease of repeated measurement and each of their antihypertensive drugs is administered by a healthcare professional using a step-wise algorithm.

Typically, the "ACD" rule of the British Hypertension Society/National Institute of Clinical Excellence (NICE) is followed (Flowchart 1).[14] This is derived, in part, from research conducted in Cambridge. The patient remains in clinic under observation for 4–6 hours. ABPM recordings continue for the next 24 hours. Comparisons are then made between pre-and post-DOT clinic readings. Research suggests that up to 50% of patients undergoing DOT with apparently treatment-resistant hypertension are shown to be nonadherent to treatment.[15] Hence, the DOT clinic can be a highly effective method of

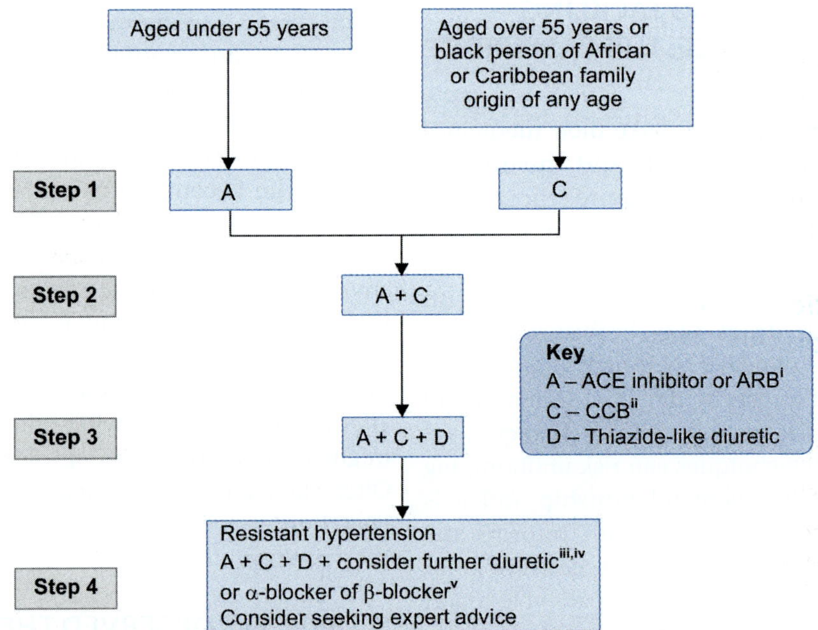

Key: (i) Choose a low-cost ARB. (ii) A CCB is preferred but consider a thiazide-like diuretic if a CCB is not tolerated or the person has edema, evidence of heart failure or is at high risk of heart failure. (iii) Consider a low dose of spironolactone or higher doses of a thiazide-like diuretic. (iv) At time of publication (August 2011), spironolactone did not have a United Kingdom market authorization for this indication. Informed consent should be obtained and documented. (v) Consider an alpha-blocker or beta-blocker, if further diuretic therapy is not tolerated, or is contraindicated or ineffective.

(ACE: angiotensin converting enzyme; ARB: angiotensin receptor blockers; CCB: calcium channel blockers)

Flowchart 1: Treatment algorithm for hypertension.

Source: National Clinical Guideline Centre. Hypertension: the clinical management of primary hypertension in adults. Clinical Guideline 127. Methods, evidence and recommendations. August 2011.

identifying and engaging with truly resistant hypertensive patients.

■ CONCLUSION

Concordance with therapeutics is one of medicine's most demanding challenges. It requires time, patience, excellent communication and a functional relationship between clinician and patient. A variety of methods can be employed to both assess and tackle patient adherence to therapy and thereby identify truly "resistant hypertensives". Nonadherence to therapy is an important cause of suboptimal blood pressure control but few practical tools exist to detect it. The use of a simple urine-based assay to evaluate the prevalence of nonadherence to antihypertensive treatment could be employed to guide further investigations and interventions. The Leicester group in 2014 found that out of a cohort of 208 hypertensive patients referred with inadequate blood pressure control at least 25% were found to be totally, or partially, nonadherent to their prescribed antihypertensive treatment.

Implications for Clinicians and Education about Hypertension

Some of the evidence discussed in this chapter adds gravity to the criticism of educational interventions that assume poor adherence to treatment is due to patients' deficiencies or failings, either in their knowledge or actually remembering to take drugs. The participants in some of the qualitative studies did not simply have a knowledge deficit but believed in alternative explanations for their hypertension and actively omitted to take their medication.

This may explain in part why educational interventions, which simply aim to inform patients about the "current" or "conventional" medical view, have proved to be ineffective.

Clinicians and any educational interventions must recognize and integrate patients' concerns and viewpoints. Patients should be given an honest and accurate depiction of the likely benefits and adverse effects with their prescribed treatments. Safety of long-term use of drugs should be emphasized; including that treatment is not thought to accumulate or "build up" in the body or cause a physical dependence or addiction. This is different to existing educational interventions, which seek to only highlight the importance of continuous uninterrupted tablet taking.

The possibility of symptoms and negative experiences should be acknowledged. Hypertensive patients will often report symptoms but they have not been found to be a reliable indicator of variations in blood pressure levels. Patients should be informed that their risk of cardiovascular disease is increased regardless of whether they have symptoms and that treatment is effective. "Stress" should be placed in the context of other modifiable risk factors for hypertension; however, it should be noted that relieving stress alone is unlikely to normalize blood pressure and that antihypertensive treatment is recommended at times of both "high" and "low" stress.

Nonintentional factors, for example "forgetting" and "being busy" were cited by many patients as reasons for nonadherence. However, there is some evidence from trials that reminder interventions may be beneficial. Indeed, a number of trials exploring the impact of mobile phone apps, self-administration techniques as well as nurse involvement are ongoing. The corollary seems to be that the greater the number and intensity of interventions, the better the adherence to treatment. Finally, in the recent literature there was an absence of robust evidence that educational interventions for hypertension need to be tailored to a particular cultural or ethnic group; it is more important to take account of common understandings and experiences across the world.[16]

■ REFERENCES

1. Tomaszewski M, White C, Patel P, et al. High rates of non-adherence to antihypertensive treatment revealed by high-performance liquid chromatography-tandem

2. Glynn L, Fahey T. Cardiovascular medication: improving adherence. Clin Evid (Online) 2011;2011:0220.

3. WHO. (2003) Adherence to long-term therapies: Evidence for action. [online] Available from: http://who.int/chp/knowledge/publications/adherence_full_report.pdf [Last Accessed March, 2019]

4. Vrijens B, Vincze G, Kristanto P, et al. Adherence to prescribed antihypertensive drug treatments: longitudinal study of electronically compiled dosing histories. BMJ. 2008;336(7653):1114-7.

5. Polypills: an essential medicine for cardiovascular disease. Lancet. 2017;389(10073):983-1074.

6. Pound P, Britten N, Morgan M, et al. Resisting medicines: a synthesis of qualitative studies of medicine taking. Soc Sci Med. 2005;61:133-55.

7. Anchala R, Kannuri NK, Pant H, et al. Hypertension in India: a systematic review and meta-analysis of prevalence, awareness, and control of hypertension. J Hypertens. 2014;32(6):1170-7.

8. Singer RB. Stroke in the elderly treated for systolic hypertension. J Insur Med. 1992;24:28-31.

9. Thompson DW, Furlan AJ. Clinical epidemiology of stroke. Neurol Clin. 1996;14:309-5.

10. Forette F, Seux ML, Staessen JA, et al.; Systolic Hypertension in Europe Investigators. The prevention of dementia with antihypertensive treatment: new evidence from the Systolic Hypertension in Europe (Syst-Eur) study. Arch Intern Med. 2002;162:2046-52.

11. Bergström J, Alvestrand A, Bucht H, et al. Progression of renal failure in man is retarded with more frequent clinical follow-ups and better blood-pressure control. Clin Nephrol. 1986;25:1-6.

12. Andrade JP, Vilas-Boas F, Chagas H, et al. Epidemiological aspects of adherence to treatment of hypertension. Arq Bras Cardiol. 2002;79:375-84.

13. Judd E, Calhoun DA. Apparent and true resistant hypertension: definition, prevalence and outcomes. J Hum Hypertens. 2014;28(8):463-8.

14. National Clinical Guideline centre. Hypertension: the clinical management primary hypertension in adults. Clinical Guideline 127. Methods, evidence and recommendations. August 2011.

15. Hameed MA, Tebbit L, Jacques N et al. Non-adherence to antihypertensive medication is very common among resistant hypertensives: results of a directly observed therapy clinic. Journal of Human Hypertension volume 30, pages 83–89 (2016)

16. Marshall IJ, Wolfe CD, McKevitt C. Lay perspectives on hypertension and drug adherence: systematic review of qualitative research. BMJ. 2012;345:e3953.

■ SUGESTED READINGS

1. Al-Roomi KA, Heller RF, Wlodarczyk J. Hypertension control and the risk of myocardial infarction and stroke: a population-based study. Med J Aust. 1990;153:595-9.

2. Berenson GS, Srinivasan SR, Bao W, et al. Association between multiple cardiovascular risk factors and atherosclerosis in children and young adults. The Bogalusa Heart Study. New Engl J Med. 1998;338:1650-6.

3. Borghi C, Bacchelli S, Esposti DD, et al. Effects of the administration of an angiotensin- converting enzyme inhibitor during the acute phase of myocardial infarction in patients with arterial hypertension. SMILE Study Investigators. Survival of Myocardial Infarction Long- term Evaluation. Am J Hypertens. 1999;12:665-72.

4. Burt VL, Whelton P, Roccella EJ, et al. Prevalence of hypertension in the US adult population. Results from the Third National Health and Nutrition Examination Survey, 1988-1991. Hypertension. 1995;25:305-13.

5. Collins R, MacMahon S. Blood pressure, antihypertensive drug treatment and the risks of stroke and coronary heart disease. Brit Med Bull. 1994;50:272-98.

6. Collins R, Peto R, MacMahon S, et al. Blood pressure, stroke, and coronary heart disease. Part 2, Short-term reductions in blood pressure: overview of randomised drug trials in their epidemiological context. Lancet. 1990;335:827-38.

7. Efficacy of atenolol and captopril in reducing the risk of macrovascular and microvascular complications in type 2 diabetes: UKPDS 39. UK Prospective Diabetes Study Group. BMJ. 1998;317:713-20.

8. Haynes RB. Determinants of compliance: the disease and the mechanics of treatment. Baltimore, MD: Johns Hopkins University Press; 1979.

9. Hennekens CH, Braunwald E. Clinical trials in cardio-vascular disease: a companion to Braunwald's heart disease. Philadelphia: WB Saunders; 1999.

10. Hershey JC, Morton BG, Davis JB, et al. Patient compliance with antihypertensive medication. Am J Public Health. 1980;70:1081-9.

11. Horne R. Patients' beliefs about treatment: the hidden determinant of treatment outcome? J Psychosom Res. 1999;47:491-5.

12. Luscher TF, Vetter H, Siegenthaler W, et al. Compliance in hypertension: facts and concepts. J Hypertens. 1985;3: S3-9.

13. Marmot MG, Poulter NR. Primary prevention of stroke. Lancet. 1992;339:344-47.

14. Medical Research Council Working Party. Medical Research Council Trial of treatment of hypertension in older adults. Principal results. BMJ. 1992;304:405-12.

15. Morisky DE, Levine DM, Green LW, et al. Five-year blood pressure control and mortality following health education for hypertensive patients. Am J Public Health. 1983;73:153-62.

16. National High Blood Pressure Education Program, National Heart, Lung, and Blood Institute. The Sixth Report of the Joint National Committee on Prevention, Detection, Evaluation and Treatment of High Blood Pressure. Bethesda, MD. National Institutes of Health. 1997.

17. Peterson JC, Adler S, Burkart JM, et al. Blood pressure control, proteinuria, and the progression of renal diseases. The Modification of Diet in Renal Disease Study Group. Ann Intern Med. 1995;123:754-62.

18. Rand CS. Measuring adherence with therapy for chronic diseases: implications for the treatment of heterozygous familial hypercholesterolemia. Am J Cardiol. 1993;72:68D-74D.

19. Rose LE, Kim MT, Dennison CR, et al. The contexts of adherence for African Americans with high blood pressure. J Adv Nurs. 2000;32:587-94.

Genetics and Hypertension

Genetic Approaches to Hypertension: Relevance to Human Hypertension

Barjinderjit K Dhillon, Chirag Uppal, Ramanpreet Kaur, Renu Moti Pandita, Navjot Bajwa, Gurpreet S Wander

■ INTRODUCTION

Blood pressure (BP) is the pressure of circulating blood on the walls of blood vessels and calculated by cardiac output and total resistance. It is expressed in terms of the systolic pressure over diastolic pressure. The condition when diastolic BP (DBP) is more than or equal to 140 mm Hg and systolic BP (SBP) is more than or equal to 90 mm Hg is referred as a hypertension and it is a bigger health issue associated with global mortality and morbidity among individuals of all age groups. The prevalence of hypertension was found to be 26% in year 2005 and it has been expected to reach 60% by the year 2025. According to data of World Health Organization (WHO), around 40% of patients above the age of 25 were suffering from hypertension in year 2008. The world health statistics 2012 revealed that 48% of worldwide deaths are due to cardiovascular disease among this, hypertension was the leading cause of death. It has been reported to be involved in the pathogenesis of various other diseases like kidney failure, heart attack, stroke, atherosclerosis and many more. Worldwide, it is the leading cause of disease stress.[1]

It is well established that hypertension is caused by both genetic and environmental factors and their complex interactions. It is caused by numerous modifiable and nonmodifiable factors. The modifiable factors that are associated with hypertension include excessive salt intake, obesity, low potassium and folic acid intake, excess alcohol, sedentary lifestyle, dyslipidemia, obstructive sleep apnea, increased triglycerides, hyperuricemia, increased atrial stiffness, systemic proinflammatory state, under nutrition in childhood, smoking, vitamin D deficiency, nonsteroidal inflammatory drugs and long-term exposure to noise, and psychological stress. The nonmodifiable factors include genetic predisposition, family history, ethnic origin, and low birth weight.[2]

■ GENETIC FACTORS AND HYPERTENSION

The term "complex trait" refers to any phenotype that does not exhibit classic Mendelian inheritance but results from the interactions between multiple genes and environmental factors. BP was inherited as a "graded character", and it is a complex non-Mendelian trait. Thus, it is a multifactorial disorder and among these factors, genetic factors have been reported to play a critical role in disease advancement. An individual with one or both hypertensive parents is at an increased risk of disease developing throughout his/her age. Numerous epidemiological studies have reported that around 30% of variations in BP among different ethnic groups are attributable to genetic abnormalities.[3] Recent advances in molecular genetics have enabled us to link the genetic polymorphism with essential hypertension (EH). Interaction between several environmental and genetic factors elicits the hypertensive responses.[1] Studies on human twins, families, and animal models suggested that 30–60% of the BP variation is controlled by the genes.

Recently numerous bioinformatics tools and advanced genetic technology including single nucleotide polymorphism (SNP), exome sequencing, non-RNA arrays, and genome wide association studies have identified numerous loci that are involved in the pathogenesis of hypertension.

Common genetic variants found during human genome project and HapMap have been highlighted by genome-wide association studies (GWAS). Around 280 genetic variants have been associated with risk of high BP, as well as other traits such as coronary artery disease, for which hypertension may be on the causal pathway.[4-7] Although the contribution of each SNP to SBP and DBP values is typically very small, when combined together their cumulative impact is more revealing.

ECE1 gene is a candidate gene on chromosome 1 that has been reported to play role in BP regulation. A study on patients of European ancestry has identified five gene polymorphisms associated with hypertension.[8] In addition, another study presented an evidence of genetic linkage between angiotensin gene and hypertension after identifying significant difference in plasma angiotensin levels among different subjects with different angiotensinogen (AGT) genotypes.[9]

Numerous genes like *HYT3, AGTR1A, ADD1, HYT6, CYP3A5, HYT4, GNB3, HYT2, NOS2A, MEX3C, HYT5* and *PTGIS* have been reported to be associated with disease development. Overlapping signals between BP and other cardiovascular risk factor by GWAS includes B-Cell *CLL*/lymphoma 2 *(BCL2)*, carbamoyl-phosphate synthetase 1 *(CPS1)* and melatonin receptor 1B *(MTNR1B)*, *rs79598313/KDF1* (keratinocyte differentiation factor 1) and *APOE* (apolipoprotein E) locus which often coexist. Whereas GWAS for BP and coronary artery disease includes *APOE*, endothelin receptor type A *(EDNRA)* and SWAP switching B-Cell complex subunit 70 *(SWAP70)*. Locus for vascular endothelial growth factor A *(VEGFA)* and *CPS1* were observed in GWAS overlap signals for BP and renal function association. According to the various studies, polymorphism in these genes either increases the risk of an individual to disease development or these alterations might result in increasing drug resistance.[10,11]

In recent years, there has been an increased interest in epigenome-wide association studies (EWAS). Similarly to GWAS, it is utilizing SNPs, quantifiable epigenetic markers, DNA methylation to identify loci, which can differentiate between cases and controls.[10] Recently, *NPR3, SLC4A7*, and genes have explored and it has been found that the BP-raising allele at the *NPR3* (natriuretic peptide receptor C) locus was correlated with chromatin change, increased *NPR3* expression, increased vascular smooth muscle cell proliferation, angiotensin II-induced calcium flux, and cell contraction .

Monogenic Forms of Hypertension

A monogenic hypertension syndrome is controlled by single genes and thus it follows the Mendelian law of inheritance. All the monogenic form of hypertension is caused by the abnormalities in genes regulating the salt and water reabsorption.[8] Familial hyperaldosteronism (FH) type 1 was the first identified monogenic hypertension syndrome. Now a number of monogenic forms are present like Liddle syndrome, Gordon's syndrome and apparent mineralocorticoid excess (AME), etc. (Flowchart 1).[2]

- *Liddle's syndrome:* It is autosomal dominant syndrome that causes excessive reabsorption of sodium and water in the renal collecting tubules. This disturbance in sodium and water levels causes hypertension. Polymorphism in the genes encoding β and Υ subunits of epithelial sodium channel (ENaC) was reported to be associated with this syndrome. *Nedd4-2* decreases the expression of ENaC by targeting the channel for degradation but these alterations disrupt the interaction between these two and cause increased surface expression of ENaC that leads to increased renal absorption of water and sodium (Flowchart 1)
- *Mineralocorticoid receptor (MR) activating mutation:* A heterozygous gain of function mutation, *S810L* has been in reported in the *MR* gene. The alterations have been reported to be associated with early onset of severe hypertension, i.e. before an age of 20 years. Increased renal salt reabsorption, increased BP, and suppression of aldosterone secretion have been observed in these patients
- *Apparent mineralocorticoid excess syndrome:* It is an autosomal recessive disorder that has been found to be associated with early onset of moderate or severe hypertension. Among hypersensitive patients, insufficient levels of 11β-hydroxysteroid dehydrogenase enzyme (deactivates cortisol) were detected due to alterations in the gene that encodes the enzyme.

Polygenic (Essential) Form of Hypertension

These forms of hypertension are controlled by the combination of several genes. Renin–angiotensin–aldosterone system (RAAS) is the most studied polygenic form of hypertension. RAAS system is prominently controlled by *AGT* gene. Several inhibitors of renin–angiotensin system are widely used for the treatment of hypertension.[2] The number of candidate genes has been presented and out of them AGT is undeniably the most potent gene controlling the disease. By definition, polygenic hypertension has no traceable cause. Most likely, it is familial or is an outcome of interaction between genetic

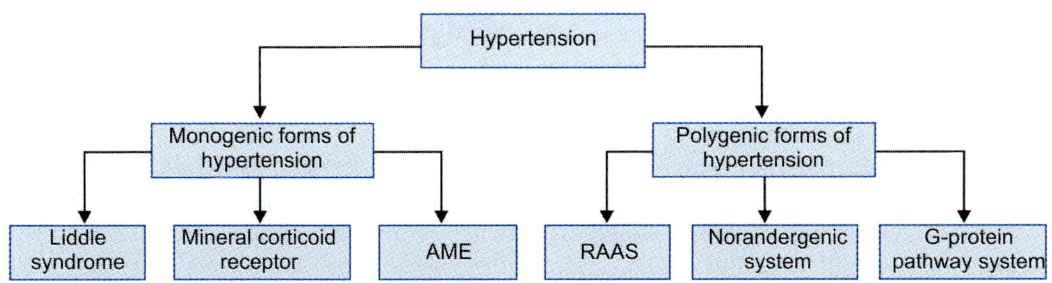

(AME: apparent mineralocorticoid excess; RAAS: renin–angiotensin–aldosterone system)

Flowchart 1: Subtypes of hypertension.

and environmental factors (Flowchart 1). Biological systems that have been reported to be associated with polygenic form of hypertension are as follows:

- *Renin–angiotensin–aldosterone system:* One of the most commonly studied system in hypertensive patients is RAAS. AGT gene has been reported to be frequently altered in RAAS system. In a meta-analysis, it has been found the *M235T* polymorphism in AGT gene is most commonly involved in the pathogenesis of hypertension. Genetic alterations in RAAS including angiotensin (*AG7*), angiotensin-converting enzyme (ACE), angiotensin II receptor type 1 (*AT1R*), and aldosterone synthase (*CYP11B2*) genes have been found to be associated with hypertension. Two variants, i.e. *T344C* and *A6547G* in *CYP11B2* have been reported to be associated with hypertension among women. These genes alter the RAAS system; affecting BP and salt-water homeostasis[7]
- *G-proteins or signal transduction pathway system:* G-proteins translate the signals from cell surface to the cell to initiate the intracellular effect of hormones and peptides. These pathways are influenced by hormones and neurotransmitters and act to control the BP. *C825T* alteration in β3 subunit of G protein has been linked with increased risk of cardiovascular diseases, including obesity, diabetes, hypertension and dyslipidemia
- *Norandergenic system:* The system affects the BP by cardiac output and peripheral resistance regulation. *ADRBI*, β1 adrenergic receptor polymorphism has been found to be involved in the disease development. *S49G* and *R389G* are associated with BP. In addition, β2 receptor gene polymorphism, i.e. *R16G, Q27G*, and *T164I* were significantly associated with hypertension.

ASSOCIATION OF EPIGENETIC FACTORS WITH HYPERTENSION

The epigenetics modifications such as DNA methylation, histone proteins modifications, and noncoding RNAs (miRNAs) play critical role in controlling the physiological processes.[12] Thus, abnormalities in epigenetics can elicit development of hypertension. According to the study by *Smolarek et al. (2010)*, higher stages of hypertension results from the lower levels of DNA methylation. Moreover, the smokers with hypertension are known to have low levels of DNA methylation giving the best example of gene-environment interaction. Similarly, LPS induced-histone modifications have been reported to increase the expression of genes like *ACE1* leading to hypertension. This epigenetic phenomenon can be identified as potential targets for the development of novel antihypersensitive therapies.[13]

PHARMACOGENOMIC OF HYPERTENSION

Genetics plays important role in determining the individual response to antihypersensitive treatment. Pharmacokinetic and pharmacogenetic studies have enabled, identification of specific targets for antihypertensive medications such as *SLC12A2* (loop diuretics), *CACNA1C* and *CACNB4* (calcium channel blockers), within the pathway itself such as *NOS3* (nitric oxide donors), targets under investigation *EDN1* (endothelin 1), *NPR1* and *NPR3* (natriuretic peptide analogs), and *ENPEP* (aminopeptidase A inhibitors) by in silico anaylsis (e.g. SIFT and Polyphen). In other words, genetic associations for genes that are the targets of current antihypertensive drugs, provide a hope that other newly discovered genes for BP may also have the potential to discover new drugs for treatment of hypertension in the future. Hence, the knowledge of pharmacogenomics will help with the designing of personalized medication regimes.[14]

■ FUTURE PERSPECTIVES AND TRANSLATION OF GENETIC FINDINGS

The heritability of hypertension is highly appreciated and thus prompts us to understand both the monogenic and polygenic forms of genetic factors, which will help in developing the novel approaches in terms of diagnostics, risk assessment of the end points such as stroke and cardiovascular diseases and reducing healthcare costs. As large clusters of genes and their gene–gene interaction control the etiology of hypertension, thus annotating the single gene or genetic factor is still challenging.[15]

Deciphering the genes controlling hypertension has enabled us to apply the biotechnological tools for the management of hypertension. Gene therapy is one of the most powerful tool that has been discovered to compensate the hypoactivity or hyperactivity of a defective gene.[16] Technically, gene therapy involves the construction of a target gene in vitro and then introducing that gene in living system (cells or lab rats) to increase or decrease the expression of abnormal gene. For example, intravenous application of endothelial nitric oxide gene (eNOS) in the 7-week-old spontaneously hypertensive rat (SHR) attenuated the SBP rises between 2 and 12 weeks after injection along with high cyclic guanosine monophosphate (cGMP) levels.[3]

The translation of genetic findings from GWAS into the clinical practice remains restricted. However, the case for statins in the treatment of high low-density lipoprotein (LDL)-cholesterol provides anticipation for the probable use of GWAS-identified BP genes as pharmaceutical targets for antihypertensive drug development. Although statins were developed in the last century, a recent GWAS identified that the gene (*HMGCR*) encoding the statins' target protein, 3-hydroxy-3-methylglutaryl coenzyme A reductase, was associated with plasma LDL-cholesterol levels. Although, the development of novel drugs based on GWAS findings will take some time. Data from the National Human Genome Research Institute's repository of GWAS and Informa Healthcare's Pharmaprojects of drug development has been analyzed by Sanseau and collaborators (2012), they have found that 92 genes were associated with drugs that had indications for diseases that differed from their mapped GWAS traits.[17] A region on chromosome 12 that was associated with DBP response to hydrochlorothiazide has been identified and validated by GWAS of antihypertensive pharmacogenomics. This region includes *LYZ*, *YEATS*, and *FRS2* genes that had not been previously involved in hypertension or response to diuretics.[18] For example, genetic variants of several genes from the RAAS (*ACE, AGT, AGTR1, AGTR2,* and *REN*) have been widely investigated for their associations with BP response to ACE inhibitors and angiotensin II receptor blockers). Variants of β1-adrenergic receptor (*ADRB1*) from the sympathetic nervous system and its associated regulatory protein (*GRK4*) have shown significant interaction effects with β-blocker on BP lowering.[19] All these studies provide light on the potential power of the GWAS approach in antihypertensive pharmacogenomics.

This not only supports the role of genetic factors in determining individual's response to antihypertensive medications, but it also highlights the necessity and importance of utilizing multiple ethnicities to identify genetic variants responsible for varied BP response to treatment. These findings suggest that GWAS data may help us identify novel uses for existing drugs, response to antihypertensive medications and individual genetic risk score (GRS). Besides, each BP-associated variant only has a small effect individually, a GRS can recognize the larger combined effects of all variants.

CONCLUSION

To sum up, there is no doubt that within the next few years we will have new approaches that are being sought to help explain the specific gene variants that contribute to hypertension. A broad investigation of the genome and environmental exposure, research of gene-gene interactions is necessary to provide more effective risk quantification and to identify the pathophysiological factors contributing to BP regulation. In addition, the future for BP genomics research is promising with the formation of global GWAS meta-analysis consortia, the evolution of epigenetics, and the onset of next-generation sequencing technology. Advances in gene therapy like CRISPR-Cas system, using effective vector delivery system would have a bright option to correct the target genes. Moreover, advances in pharmacogenomics of antihypertensive drugs may be used to develop novel personalized treatments for hypertension. The global health impact of hypertension is substantial and decoding the genes controlling hypertension will enable us to apply the biotechnological tools for the management of hypertension. All advancements in the genomic architecture of hypertension will help to check the increasing load of cardiovascular disease at global levels.

REFERENCES

1. Murray CJ, Lopez AD. Evidence-based health policy—lessons from the Global Burden of Disease Study. Science. 1996.;274(5288):740-3.
2. Sarkar T, Singh NP. Epidemiology and genetics of hypertension. J Assoc Physicians India. 2015;63(9):61-98.
3. Butler MG. Genetics of hypertension. Current status. J Med Liban. 2010;58(3):175-8.
4. Wellcome Trust Case Control Consortium. Genome-wide association study of 14,000 cases of seven common diseases and 3,000 shared controls. Nature. 2007;447: 661-78.
5. Ehret GB, Ferreira T, Chasman DI, et al. The genetics of blood pressure regulation and its target organs from association studies in 342,415 individuals. Nat Genet. 2016;48(10):1171-84.
6. Warren HR, Evangelou E, Cabrera CP, et al. Genome-wide association analysis identifies novel blood pressure loci and offers biological insights into cardiovascular risk. Nat Genet. 2017;49:403-15.
7. Padmanabhan S, Delles C, Dominiczak AF. Genetic factors in hypertension. Arch Med Sci. 2009;5(2A):S212-9.
8. Funke-Kaiser H, Reichenberger F, Köpke K, et al. Differential binding of transcription factor E2F-2 to the endothelin-converting enzyme-1b promoter affects blood pressure regulation. Hum Mol Genet. 2003;12(4):423-33.
9. Caulfield M, Lavender P, Farrall M, et al. Linkage of the angiotensinogen gene to essential hypertension. N Eng J Med. 1994;330(23):1629-33.
10. Patel RS, Masi S, Taddei S. Understanding the role of genetics in hypertension. Eur Heart J. 2017;38(29):2309-12.
11. Ng FL, Warren HR, Caulfield MJ. Hypertension genomics and cardiovascular prevention. Ann of Translational Medicine. 2018;6(15):291.
12. Kato N, Loh M, Takeuchi F, et al. Trans-ancestry genome-wide association study identifies 12 genetic loci influencing blood pressure and implicates a role for DNA methylation. Nat Genet. 2015;47(11):1282-93.
13. Smolarek I, Wyszko E, Barciszewska AM, et al. Global DNA methylation changes in blood of patients with essential hypertension. Med Sci Monit. 2010;16(3):CR149-55.
14. Zhao Q, Kelly TN, Li C, et al. Progress and future aspects in genetics of human hypertension. Curr Hypertens Rep. 2013;15(6):676-86.
15. Ahn SY, Gupta C. Genetic Programming of Hypertension. Front Pediatr. 2018;5:285.
16. Paulis L, Franke H, Simko F. Gene therapy for hypertension. Expert opinion on biological therapy. 2017;17(11):1345-61.
17. Sanseau P, Agarwal P, Barnes MR, et al. Use of genome-wide association studies for drug repositioning. Nat Biotechnol. 2012;30:317-20.
18. Turner ST, Bailey KR, Fridley BL, et al. Genomic association analysis suggests chromosome 12 locus influencing antihypertensive response to thiazide diuretic. Hypertension. 2008;52:359-65.
19. Vandell AG, Lobmeyer MT, Gawronski BE, et al. G protein receptor kinase 4 polymorphisms: beta-blocker pharmacogenetics and treatment-related outcomes in hypertension. Hypertension. 2012;60:957-64.

Interventional Interventions in Hypertension

Renal Denervation and Hypertension

VT Shah

■ INTRODUCTION

Systemic hypertension is a common chronic disease with major burden to healthcare system and individuals worldwide. Major cardiac and cerebral adverse events including stroke and myocardial infarction and its association with uncontrolled hypertension are well recognized. Even with use of multidrug therapy, blood pressure (BP) control is often not achieved. Moreover, adverse effects of antihypertensive drugs interfere patients' daily life and ultimately results in noncompliance to treatment which is being recognized as one of the leading contributor to insufficient BP control. Hence, alternative treatment modalities have been probed and analyzed. In recent years, renal sympathetic nervous system (SNS) and its involvement in the pathogenesis of systemic hypertension have been refocused. Catheter based radiofrequency denervation of the renal SNS has emerged as potential treatment for resistant hypertension in humans with favorable results. This chapter includes overview of anatomy and physiology of the renal SNS, review of early clinical trials, consequences and effects of renal sympathetic denervation (RDN).

■ ANATOMY AND PHYSIOLOGY OF RENAL SYMPATHETIC NERVOUS SYSTEM

The kidneys are heavily innervated with renal efferent and afferent nerves to receive and send signals to the central nervous system. Neuronal system of kidney has impact on BP by both efferent and afferent sympathetic fibers. Efferent sympathetic fibers found in the adventitia of the renal arteries invade all peripheral segments of the renal cortex and communicates signals to the central nervous system via afferent sympathetic fibers (Fig. 1).

Afferent signals from kidney and baroreceptors as well as from the hypothalamus, cortex and limbic system go to autonomic centers in the medulla oblongata and mid brain. Postintegration of these signals, autonomic centers transmit efferent signals to sympathetic preganglionic neurons in the intermediolateral column (T10 to T12, L1 to L2) which extend via splanchnic nerves to postganglionic neurons situated in prevertebral ganglia. Postganglionic neurons come in proximity to kidney via adventitia of the renal arteries. As the nerves traverse deeper into the kidney, they begin to divide further which form a network of fibers which

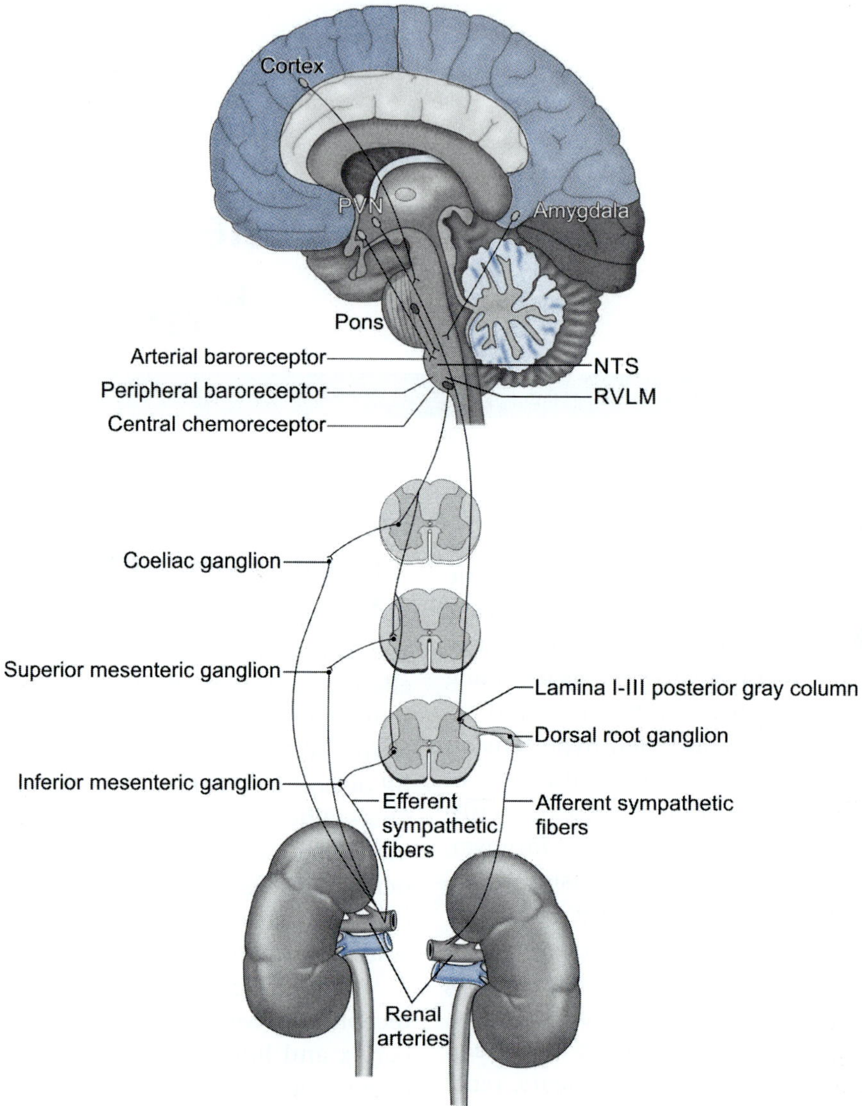

Fig. 1: Renal sympathetic nervous system.

supply all parts of the kidney, including the renal tubular cells, juxtaglomerular apparatus and vasculature.[1]

Stimulation of the renal sympathetic nerves (efferent fibers) causes norepinephrine release which leads to activation of the adluminal basolateral Na^+/K^+ adenosine triphosphatases (ATPase), which results in sodium and water reabsorption by the renal tubular epithelial cells, renin release by the granular cells of the juxtaglomerular apparatus and vasoconstriction of renal arterioles by contraction of smooth muscle cells (Fig. 2). Intensity of the sympathetic signal is also important in regard to its response, such that low frequency stimulates renin secretion, while sodium reabsorption and renal vascular tone get stimulated with higher frequencies

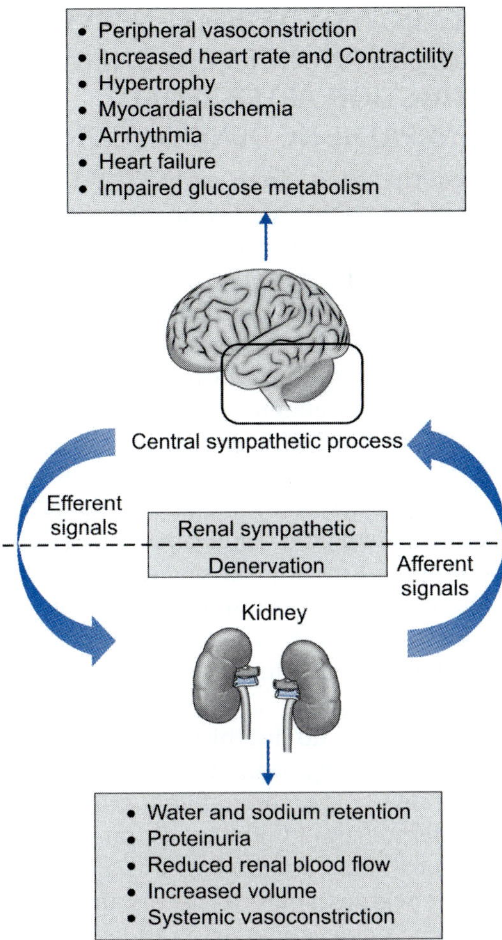

Fig. 2: Effect of sympathetic hyperactivity.

respectively.[2] In conclusion, efferent renal sympathetic activation raises BP directly by salt and water retention in kidney, while indirectly by renin release which stimulates the production of angiotensin II. SNS has remarkable effect on goal BP regulation by kidney, in the same way kidney has influence on overall sympathetic tone.

Afferent fibers are less abundant compared to efferent and they have an inhibitory effect on both ipsilateral and contralateral efferent renal sympathetic nerve activity. Unilateral disturbances of salt and water excretion are maintained by contralateral kidney, via communications of afferent fibers.

EARLY TRIALS IN HUMANS— SURGICAL SYMPATHECTOMY

Before modern pharmacotherapy, interventions for malignant hypertension were limited. In the early 1940s, radical sympathectomy was trailed in which both the splanchnic nerve and thoracic dorsal sympathetic chain were sectioned resulting in interruption of sympathetic outflow, decreased peripheral resistance and lowering in BP.[3] Reduction in BP was also observed without compromising renal function in long-term follow-up studies of sympathectomy. However, side effects including postural hypotension, sensory and sexual dysfunction and depression were associated with this highly invasive procedure.[3] With high operative mortality and significant side effects, sympathectomy was abandoned as effective antihypertensive drugs emerged. However, early clinical studies of sympathectomy provided proof-of-concept evidence that renal denervation may be an effective strategy for the treatment of hypertension by specifically interrupting renal sympathetic.

CATHETER-BASED RENAL SYMPATHETIC DENERVATION— EARLY CLINICAL TRIALS

Invention of use of catheter-based technology using radiofrequency energy to selectively resect renal nerves resumed interest in further research on RDN for the treatment of hypertension. Several clinical trials were conducted to explore radiofrequency RDN in humans in last decade. SYMPLICITY HTN-1 study which used catheter radiofrequency RDN, demonstrated significant reduction in office systolic blood pressure (SBP) at 1 month ($\approx$14 mm Hg) and 12 months ($\approx$27 mm Hg), which was also maintained at 36 months.[4] While, SYMPLICITY HTN-2 study demonstrated reduction in office BP (-32/-12 mm Hg) with RDN in randomized control design.[5] Overall, both SYMPLICITY HTN-1 and HTN-2 studies concluded that radiofrequency catheter RDN was relatively safe and effective for reducing BP and its maintenance, however lack of placebo control group and significant concerns about treatment compliance were limitations of both studies.

SYMPLICITY HTN-3 was a prospective, single-blind, randomized, sham-controlled trial which enrolled 535 patients at total 88 sites. This study failed to show a significant reduction of SBP in patients with resistant hypertension 6 months after renal-artery denervation as compared with a sham-control.[6] However, significant procedural issues were identified in this study, which resulted in inadequate denervation. Moreover, majority of untrained operators and lack of tests to assess degree of denervation influenced study outcomes. With realization that multiple sites were required for adequate and effective RDN, development of multiple electrode instruments with competence of creating multiple ablations simultaneously were achieved.

Other similar clinical trials have also demonstrated conflicting results of radio-frequency catheter-based RDN, which are mentioned in Table 1.[7] Even though majority of these studies propose that RDN is efficacious in BP reduction, design and execution of these studies were challenged and thus effectiveness of catheter based RDN remains to be confirmed.

RADIANCE-HTN SOLO a multicenter, randomized, double-blind, sham-controlled, 2-cohort study was conducted using endo-vascular ultrasound energy by Paradise system (Recor medical, USA) or a sham procedure, reported promising results as shown in Table 1.[7]

CRYO-RDN first-in-man study was presented at recently held EURO-PCR (May-2019) meeting using a novel cryoablation catheter which showed promising results, while randomized controlled trials are ongoing.

■ REGROWTH OF RENAL NERVES AND RETURN OF RENAL NERVE FUNCTION AFTER RENAL SYMPATHETIC DENERVATION

Long-term results from early SYMPLICITY trials indicated that both sympathetic efferent and sensory afferent renal nerves regrow after RDN. Preclinical trials of RDN in normotensive Sprague Dawley rats demonstrated complete restoration of nerve growth at 12-week and suggested communication of denervated kidney to contralateral kidney, which may explain lack of efficacy in hypertensive models with unilateral or partial RDN.[8] Moreover, rat studies suggested enhanced nerve regrowth after denervation via freezing as compared to surgical section indicating method of denervation may affect nerve regrowth. Regrowth of renal nerves has also been demonstrated in pig and sheep models with radiofrequency catheter-based RDN.[9] In humans, there is no clear histological evidence of renal nerve regrowth after catheter based RDN, however anatomic nerve growth has been demonstrated post renal transplant.[10] Preclinical and certain clinical trials clearly indicate regrowth of renal nerves after RDN, however complete reservation and functional restoration in hypertension is ambiguous.

■ OTHER EFFECTS OF DENERVATION THERAPY

Heart Rate Reduction

Clinical trial of 136 patients with renal denervation demonstrated heart rate reduction of 2.6 ± 0.8 bpm and 2.1 ± 1.1 bpm at 3 months and 6 months, respectively with more than 90% response rate for heart rate or BP reduction.[11] High resting heart rate is a risk factor for cardiovascular diseases including arterial hypertension, coronary artery disease and heart failure. Considering heart rate as an important marker for cardiovascular risk, it may be used as an outcome to RDN.

TABLE 1: Change in BP in response to RDN in major clinical trials.

Human trials	Experimental design	Catheter type, ablations per renal artery	BP primary end point, duration	Change in office SBP/DBP
SYMPLICITY HTN-1 2009	Open-labeled	Symplicity flex	Office BP	RDN (n = 88) −32/−14 mm Hg*
	No control	4 ablations (max 6)	36 months	
SYMPLICITY HTN-2 2010	RCT	Symplicity flex	Office BP	RDN (n = 49) −32/−12 mm Hg*†
	Control-drug alone	4 ablations (max 6)	6 months	Drug alone (n = 51) +1/0 mm Hg
	No change in medication			
SYMPLICITY HTN-3 2014	RCT	Symplicity flex	Office BP	RDN (n = 353) −14/−7 mm Hg*
	Single-blind, sham-control	2 ablations (max 6)	6 months	Sham (n = 171) −12/−5 mm Hg*
	No change in medication			
Oslo RDN 2014	RCT	Symplicity flex	Office systolic BP	RDN (n = 10) −8/−2 mm Hg
	Double-blind, sham-control	8 ablations (range 6–11)	6 months	Control (n = 10) −28/−11 mm Hg*
	Control-SSHAT			
DENERHTN 2015	RCT	Symplicity flex	Day-time SBP	RDN (n = 53) −15/−9 mm Hg*†
	Single-blind, sham-control	5.5 ablations (max 6)	6 months	Control (n = 53) −9/ 6 mm Hg*
	Control-SSHAT			
PRAGUE-15 2015	RCT	Symplicity flex	Office SBP	RDN (n = 54) −12/−7 mm Hg*
	Single-blind, sham-control	5 ablations (max 6)	6 months	Sham (n = 52) −14/−7 mm Hg*
	No change in medication			
RESET 2016	RCT	Symplicity flex	24-h systolic AMBP	RDN (n = 33) −4/−2 mm Hg
	Open-label, sham-control	5.5 ablations (max 6)	6 months	Sham (n = 36) −2/3 mm Hg
	Intensified drug treatment			

Continued

Continued

Human trials	Experimental design	Catheter type, ablations per renal artery	BP primary end point, duration	Change in office SBP/DBP
INSPIRED	RCT	EnligHTN; multi-electrode	Systolic AMBP	RDN (n = 9) −22/−13 mm Hg*†
2017	Control-drug alone	11 ablations	6 months	Drug alone (n = 6) +1/0 mm Hg
	No change in medication			
SPYRAL HTN OFF-MED	RCT	Spyral; multi-electrode	AMBP	RDN (n = 37) −10/−5 mm Hg*†
2018	Single-blind, sham-control	20 ablations including proximal branches	3 months	Sham (n = 41) −2/0 mm Hg
	Off medication			
SPYRAL HTN-ON-MED	RCT	Spyral; multi-electrode	AMBP	RDN (n = 40) −10/−5 mm Hg*†
2018	Single-blind, sham-control	20 ablations including proximal branches	6 months	Sham (n = 42) −3/−2 mm Hg
	On medication			
Radiance-HTN SOLO	RCT	Paradise; multi-electrode	Day-time AMBP	RDN (n = 74) −11/−6 mm Hg*†
2018	Single-blind, sham-control	5.4 emissions	2 months	Sham (n = 72) −4/−1 mm Hg
	On medication			

*Significantly different to baseline.

†Significantly different to control.

(AMBP: 24-hr ambulatory BP monitoring; CKD: chronic kidney disease; RCT: randomized controlled trial; SSHAT: standardized stepped-care antihypertensive treatment; BP: Blood pressure; RDN: renal sympathetic denervation; SBP: Systolic blood pressure; DBP: disystolic blood pressure)

Improved Exercise Tolerance

Cardiovascular risk and mortality are associated with extreme rise in BP and heart rate during exercise. Moreover, slow rate of reduction in SBP post exercise is also associated with adverse cardiovascular outcomes. RDN significantly reduces exercise induced rise in BP by 21 mm Hg at peak work rate and by 31 mm Hg at rest in resistant hypertension patients which ultimately improve exercise tolerance.[12]

Improved Peripheral Circulation

Rise in pulse wave reflection and amplified pulse wave velocity are signals of adverse cardiovascular outcomes. Increased pressure on the heart, brain and kidney (central BP) is better predictor of cardiovascular risk as compared to peripheral BP. Antihypertensive drugs have different effects on central and peripheral BP. Renal denervation reduces central pulse pressure as well as peripheral pulse pressure along with reduction in pulse wave velocity. The level of improvement in vascular stiffness after RDN is associated with the degree of stiffness at baseline.[13]

Attenuation of Heart Failure

Excessive stimulation of the SNS is one of the aggravating factors for heart failure. Moreover, renin-angiotensin-aldosterone system stimulation and activation of α-adrenergic receptor in the proximal tubules during heart failure results in water and salt retention, which may lead to cardiorenal syndrome.[14] Hypertensive heart diseases are also associated with cardiac myocyte hypertrophy and interstitial fibrosis which may hamper left ventricular filling.

Clinical trials have demonstrated reduction in left ventricular mass index and improvement in left ventricular filling pressure with renal denervation therapy for resistant hypertension.[15] Reduction in myocardial hypertrophy suggests role of renal denervation in reversing the heart failure with conserved ejection fraction that occurs due to hypertrophy.[16]

Improved Sleep Apnea and Arrhythmias

Uncontrolled hypertension is associated with sleep apnea and both are predictors for development of treatment resistant atrial fibrillation. Renal denervation reduces hypoxia and sleep apnea and improves the efficacy of pulmonary vein isolation.[17] Reduction in number of sleep apnea episodes achieved by renal denervation reduces atrial fibrillation and potential associated cardiovascular risk. Moreover, direct attenuation of sympathetic outflow during sleep apnea could prevent the arrhythmias and other adverse cardiovascular outcomes observed in such patients.

Renal Effects

Chronic kidney disease can be either reason or complication of hypertension and can result in resistance to antihypertensive treatments. Trials of renal denervation have demonstrated reduction in severity of microalbuminuria and macroalbuminuria in resistant hypertension patients which highlight renoprotective effects and potential cardiovascular risk reduction.[18] Small trials of chronic kidney disease have exhibited beneficial role renal denervation, however large prospective trails are required to confirm that RDN can decrease BP and improve cardiovascular outcomes in similar conditions.

Metabolic Disease

Sympathetic activation is associated with increased insulin state which predicts development of type-2 diabetes mellitus. Moreover, significant correlation has been identified between sympathetic activation and obesity, metabolic syndrome and resistant hypertension. In a subgroup of metabolic syndrome patients, improvement in fasting glucose, fasting insulin and fasting C-peptide levels have been observed after RDN.[19] However, data on potential use of RDN therapy for the treatment of metabolic syndrome in normotensive patients is lacking and needs further investigation.

CONCLUSION

Renal sympathetic denervation has been studied since decades, however with invention of radiofrequency catheter-based RDN, controlled denervation is possible with minimal surgical adverse effects. Effectiveness of RDN in severe resistant hypertension patients have been exhibited, however in patients with mild-to-moderate hypertension it is unknown. Moreover, renal denervation has potential as treatment modalities for other sympathetic tone associated cardiovascular, renal or metabolic conditions. Preclinical and clinical trials have identified potential benefits and associated challenges; however large scale prospective clinical trials are suggested to confirm the same. Future techniques and instrumental advances may explore further suitability of this procedure and identify the way forward of treatment in different clinical conditions in large population.

REFERENCES

1. Bertog SC, Sobotka PA, Sievert H. Renal denervation for hypertension. JACC Cardiovasc Intervent. 2012;5(3):249-58.
2. Koepke JP, DiBona GF. Functions of the renal nerves. Physiologist. 1985;28(1):47-52.
3. Smithwick RH. Surgical treatment of hypertension. Am J Med. 1948;4(5):744-59.
4. Krum H, Schlaich MP, Sobotka PA, et al. Percutaneous renal denervation in patients with treatment-resistant hypertension: final 3-year report of the Symplicity HTN-1 study. Lancet. 2014;383(9917):622-9.
5. Esler MD, Krum H, Obotka PA, et al. Renal sympathetic denervation in patients with treatment-resistant hypertension (The Symplicity HTN-2 Trial): a randomised controlled trial. Lancet. 2010;376:1903-9.
6. Bhatt DL, Kandzari DE, O'Neill WW, et al. A controlled trial of renal denervation for resistant hypertension. N Engl J Med. 2014;370:1393-401.
7. Singh RR, Denton KM. Renal denervation: a treatment for hypertension and chronic kidney disease. Hypertension. 2018;72(3):528-36.
8. Rodionova K, Fiedler C, Guenther F, et al. Complex reinnervation pattern after unilateral renal denervation in rats. Am J Physiol-Regulat Integrat Comparat Physiol. 2016;310(9):R806-18.
9. Cohen-Mazor M, Mathur P, Stanley JR, et al. Evaluation of renal nerve morphological changes and norepinephrine levels following treatment with novel bipolar radiofrequency delivery systems in a porcine model. J Hypertens. 2014;32(8):1678.
10. Gazdar AF, Dammin GJ. Neural degeneration and regeneration in human renal transplants. N Engl J Med. 1970;283(5):222-4.
11. Ukena C, Mahfoud F, Spies A, et al. Effects of renal sympathetic denervation on heart rate and atrioventricular conduction in patients with resistant hypertension. Int J Cardiol. 2013;167(6):2846-51.
12. Ukena C, Mahfoud F, Kindermann I, et al. Cardiorespiratory response to exercise after renal sympathetic denervation in patients with resistant hypertension. J Am Coll Cardiol. 2011;58(11):1176-82.
13. Brandt MC, Reda S, Mahfoud F, et al. Effects of renal sympathetic denervation on arterial stiffness and central hemodynamics in patients with resistant hypertension. J Am Coll Cardiol. 2012;60(19):1956-65.
14. DiBona GF. Physiology in perspective: The Wisdom of the Body. Neural control of the kidney. Am J Physiol-Regulat Integrat Comparat Physiol. 2005 ;289(3):R633-41.
15. Brandt MC, Mahfoud F, Reda S, et al. Renal sympathetic denervation reduces left ventricular hypertrophy and improves cardiac function in patients with resistant hypertension. J Am Coll Cardiol. 2012;59(10):901-9.
16. Zile MR, Little WC. Effects of autonomic modulation: more than just blood pressure. J Am Coll Cardiol. 2012;59:910-2.
17. Pokushalov E, Romanov A, Corbucci G, et al. A randomized comparison of pulmonary vein isolation with versus without concomitant renal artery denervation in patients with refractory symptomatic atrial fibrillation and resistant hypertension. J Am Coll Cardiol. 2012;60(13):1163-70.
18. Schmieder RE, Schrader J, Zidek W, et al. Low-grade albuminuria and cardiovascular risk. Clin Res Cardiol. 2007;96(5):247-57.
19. Mahfoud F, Schlaich M, Kindermann I, et al. Effect of renal sympathetic denervation on glucose metabolism in patients with resistant hypertension: a pilot study. Circulation. 2011;123(18):1940-6.

Baroreceptor Stimulation and Hypertension

Anjan Lal Dutta, Soumik Chaudhuri

■ INTRODUCTION

Hypertension is one of the major cardio-vascular risk factors in the world and is the leading preventable cause of death.[1] It is a significant public health problem and as per recent estimates, there are currently more than 207 million people in India living with hypertension,[2] with the number exceeding more than one billion people worldwide, and is estimated to be reached 1.5 billion by 2025.[3] The development of the myriad groups of antihypertensive drug therapy has contributed significantly in the rate of reduction of cardiovascular events.[4] Although, the general awareness and implementation of hypertensive control has steadily risen over the last couple of decades, they still remain away from perfect,[5] focusing on the need to identify more novel and effective approaches.

Antihypertensive drugs belong to a number of different classifications and bring to bear their effects through mechanisms that may be unique or even synergistic at times. However, despite the optimal usage of single or multiple antihypertensive agents, there remains a small group of hypertensive patients (5–15%), in whom the blood pressure (BP) remains uncontrolled.[6] This is the set that is commonly referred to as resistant hypertension. As a percentage, 5–15% may not seem like a very large subgroup. But when one factors in the high prevalence of hypertension in the population, the absolute number of resistant hypertensives assumes a much more significant proportion. Thus, the pressing need for alternative approaches to hypertension control has gained traction over the last several years. Interventional management of hypertension initially gained ground in the mid-20th century but then was slowly abandoned as the initial euphoria did not materialize into tangible results in the field. However, scientific interest has slowly returned over the past decade and the two most durable candidates seem to be carotid baroreceptor stimulation and renal sympathetic denervation, with promising preliminary results in the treatment of resistant hypertension. However, the latter is in thick controversy regarding its efficacy. More improvisation in the future may change the scenario.

The carotid baroreflex is an integral part of BP homeostasis. Carotid baroreceptors can perceive the intra-arterial BP and adjust the sympathetic tone in an opposite direction. High BP will lead to baroreceptor activation which will then result in a markedly attenuated sympathetic tone, whereas an augmented sympathetic tone compensates for a decrease in BP. For a long period of time, the carotid baroreflex was considered to be a "short-term buffer" viz. it helped in regulating any precipitous and transient fluctuations of BP around a "set-point", and its role in the long-term management of BP had not been adequately expounded.[7] However, recent data disputes this perennial belief, and strongly alludes to the potential capability of the carotid baroreflex system to exert prolonged and sustainable effects on BP, thus reviving interventional activation of the carotid baroreflex as a means for long-term management of resistant hypertension.

■ ANATOMY OF THE BAROREFLEX ARC

The carotid baroreflex circuit is the most significant part of the arterial baroreflex system. Despite the presence of baro-receptors in the peripheral circulation (heart, pulmonary vasculature and the aortic arch), there is an overwhelming level of evidence that has confirmed the crucial role played by the carotid baroreceptors on buffering of BP.

Carotid baroreceptors are stretch-sensitive mechanosensors, located at the right and left carotid sinus. Information from the carotid baroreceptors travel via afferent fibers in the carotid sinus nerve (a branch of cranial nerve IX; glossopharyngeal) and the associated sensory cell bodies exist in the petrosal ganglia. The aortic arch baroreceptors transmit their afferent sensations through the aortic depressor nerve (a branch of cranial nerve X; vagus) with sensory cell bodies that are located in the nodose ganglia. These afferent signals then reach the nucleus tractus solitarii (NTS) that is situated in the

dorsal medulla and is a "reception center" of impulses from arterial baroreceptors. These signals are then transmitted to the caudal ventrolateral medulla (CVLM), which acts as the "conversion center", since it processes and converts the excitatory signals originating from peripheral baroreceptors to efferent inhibitory signals that travel to the rostral ventrolateral medulla (RVLM). The RVLM is the "coordinating center" since the sympathetic outflow from here traverses to the intermediolateral cell columns in the spinal cord and furthermore onto effector organs (blood vessels and heart), regulating the sympathetic tone in the vasculature.[8] An overview of the integrated baroreceptor system is shown in Figure 1.

■ BAROREFLEX SENSITIVITY: WHAT AND WHY?

Baroreflex sensitivity (BRS) is a surrogate marker of the cardiovascular system and is the response of the autonomic effector system to a given change in arterial pressure. BRS may be assessed by a number of different ways, both noninvasive (computer-assisted spectral imaging and oscilloscopy, valsalva maneuver, and lower body negative pressure chamber techniques) and invasive ones [muscle sympathetic nerve activity (MSNA)].[9] Changes in BP set off counter-regulatory changes in heart rate, mediated through the baroreflex. The heart rate in response to a spectrum of pressures changes may be plotted as in Figure 2. There is a sigmoidal relationship and the linear portion of the curve is analyzed by regression to determine slope and BRS. A high BRS signifies there is a larger fall in heart rate, in response to a given pressure elevation. The BRS is low when the slope is flat, i.e. heart rate response to a change in MAP is minimal.

Reduced BRS (i.e. a flatter slope) can be seen in a number of conditions, viz., obesity,

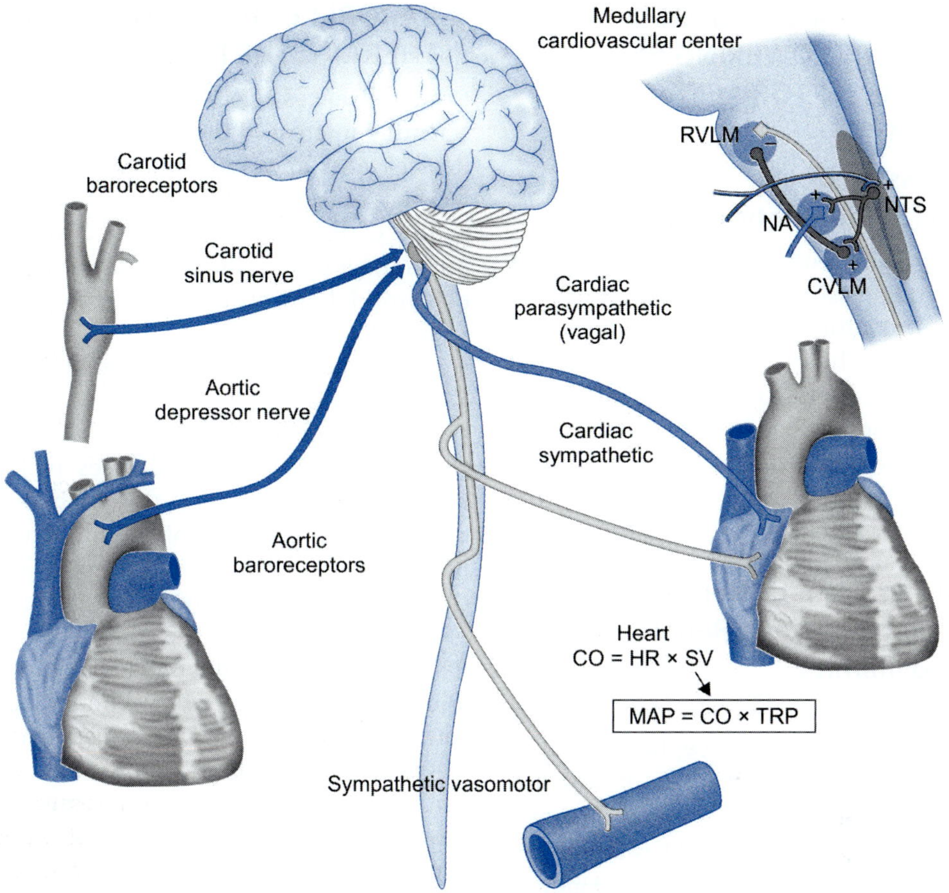

(CO: cardiac output; CVLM: caudal ventrolateral medulla; HR: heart rate; MAP: mean arterial pressure; NA: nucleus ambiguous; NTS: nucleus tractus solitaris; RVLM: rostral ventrolateral medulla; SV: stroke volume; TRP: total peripheral resistance)

Fig. 1: Outline of the central integration of arterial baroreceptor input.

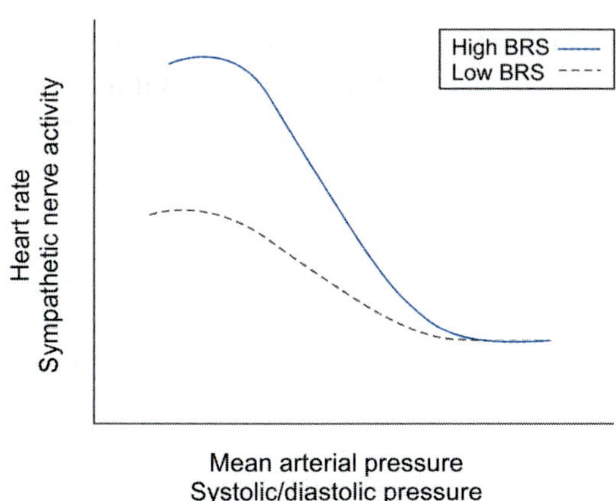

Fig. 2: Baroreflex sensitivity (BRS).

aging, hypertension, diabetes and coronary artery disease, which are carrying a much poorer prognosis.[10] In postmyocardial infarction, reduced BRS may predict the likelihood of fatal arrhythmias and cardiac mortality.[11] Similarly, in congestive heart failure, a reduced BRS predicts high risk of sudden cardiac death.[11] Significantly, regular exercise can improve BRS and is thus protective against age-related decline in baroreflex function. This improvement is "dose-dependent", clearly underlining the benefit of regular exercise.

MECHANISMS OF BLOOD PRESSURE LOWERING BY BARORECEPTOR ACTIVATION THERAPY

Suppression of Central Sympathetic Outflow

Physiological baroreceptor activation by rise in arterial pressure leads to suppression of central sympathetic outflow and consequent reduction in heart rate and BP. Chronic baroreceptor activation has a consistent and sustained effect in inhibiting central sympathetic outflow, thus lowering BP. This effect is beyond pharmacological adrenergic mechanisms alone.[12]

Renal Sympathetic Nerve Activity, Renin Secretion and Renal Hemodynamics

An important factor in the chronic hypotensive effects of baroreceptor activation therapy (BAT) is the inhibition of pressure-dependent renin release. A small decrease in GFR that occurs during BAT is dependent upon inhibition of both the direct and indirect (angiotensin-mediated) effects of the renal nerves on reabsorption of sodium. Thus, BAT provides the most significant clinical benefit in hypertensive patients with sympathetic activation and a renin–angiotensin–aldosterone system that is amenable to neural modulation.[13]

Effect on Cardiac Autonomic Activity

Baroreceptor activation therapy restores cardiac BRS and improves heart rate variability. Reduced parasympathetic activity plays a crucial role in the impairment of cardiac BRS and heart rate variability and this is optimized by baroreceptor activation devices.[14]

BARORECEPTOR ACTIVATION THERAPY: THE DEVICE

Recent advances in technology have rekindled scientific interest in baroreceptor activation devices and may hold an alluring key in resistant hypertension. A US-based company called *CVRx* was the first to develop an implantable device (Rheos) for the stimulation of carotid baroreceptors. Its components included:

- An implantable pulse generator (IPG)
- Bilateral carotid sinus leads
- Programmer system.

The next generation devices included the Barostim Neo and the Mobius HD devices. The typical implantation site of a Rheos device is shown in Figure 3. During the procedure, the optimal placement of the electrodes on the carotid sinus is dependent upon reductions in heart rate and arterial pressure while stimulating the carotid baroreceptor.[15] Once confirmed, the electrodes are sutured around the carotid sinuses. The pulse generator is externally programmable using radiofrequency control, allowing for modulations in current delivery, both intermittent and continuous. The second-generation Barostim neo employs a miniaturized electrode and is less invasive. Furthermore, it is implanted only on one side.

THE EVIDENCE FOR BARORECEPTOR ACTIVATION THERAPY

Rheos Trials

- The Device-Based Therapy in Hypertension Trial (DEBuT-HT) was a non-randomized trial, held in multiple centers, that assessed the safety of BAT.[16,17] Forty five patients were recruited for this trial and the primary inclusion criteria included resistant hypertension; some of

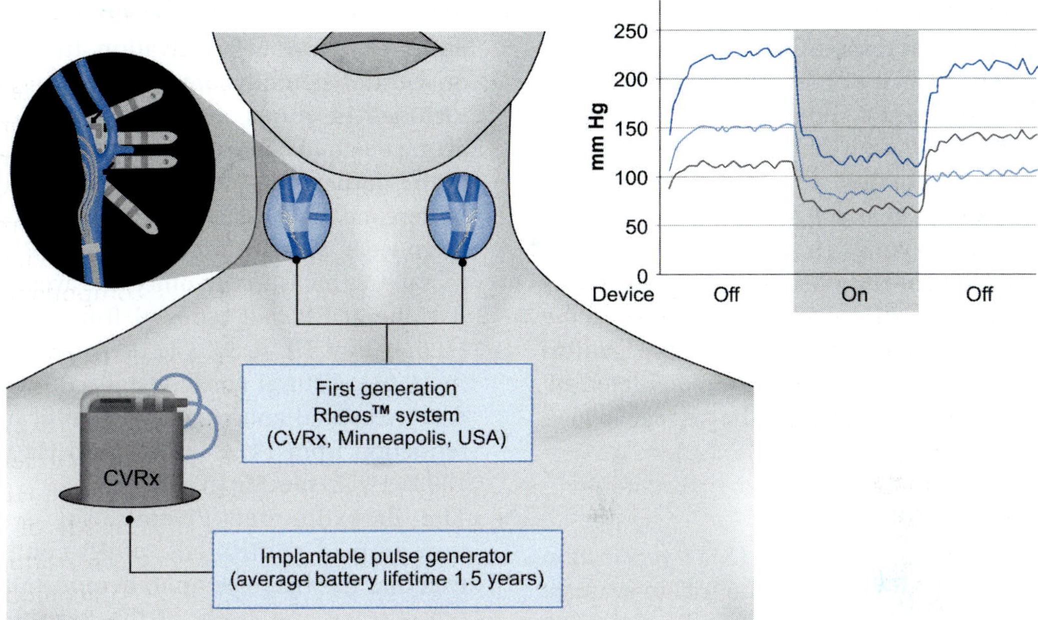

Fig. 3: Typical implantation of a Rheos device.

TABLE 1: Office-based blood pressure response in the DEBuT-HT trial.

No. of patients	Time	Systolic reduction of BP	Diastolic reduction of BP	p-value
37	3 months	21 ± 4 mm Hg	12 ± 2 mm Hg	<0.001
26	1 year	30 ± 6 mm Hg	20 ± 4 mm Hg	<0.001
17	2 years	33 ± 8 mm Hg	22 ± 6 mm Hg	<0.002

these patients were then monitored and followedup, till 2 years. The mean office-based BP was reduced at all follow-up points, as compared to baseline values. This is summarized in Table 1.

These reductions were, however, much more modest in the ambulatory BP measurement groups and significant at only 1-year and 2-year follow-ups.[17]

- The Rheos Pivotal Trial was a randomized controlled, double-blind trial that included 265 patients with resistant hypertension, randomized in a 2:1 ratio. Group A (n = 181) received immediate activation (1 month after implant) while the activation of the device was delayed in the second group (B) (n = 84) till 7 months postimplant. At 6 months, 42% of patients in group A had a systolic BP less than 140 mm Hg (office-based BP measurement) as compared to 24% in group B. At 1 year, when both groups had now been on activated BAT for either 12 or 6 months, more than 80% of patients had a decrease in systolic BP of at least 10 mm Hg and approximately half of the study size had systolic BP at or below 140 mm Hg. A significant proportion of the participants ($\approx$ 75%) had however received unilateral, rather than bilateral, carotid stimulation.[18]

- After completion of the Rheos Pivotal Trial, 276 of the total 322 patients were monitored in a long-term, follow-up. A clinically significant response to BAT treatment was defined as sustained systolic BP less than or equal to 140 mm Hg (below 130 mm Hg in patients with diabetes or renal disease), or a reduction of 20 mm Hg or more following at least 6 months of BAT. Almost 88% of patients (n = 244) had a clinically significant response. BP was determined by office-based BP measurements. In the patients who showed an initial clinical response, more than 55% maintained BP reductions throughout the average follow-up of 28 months.[18]

Barostim neo Trial

- The Barostim neo trial (XR-1 verification study) was a single-group trial to evaluate the efficacy and safety of the Barostim neo device[19] (formerly known as the XR-1). The trial included a total of 30 patients and was conducted at seven centers, the majority being in Europe (6 centers). Resistant hypertension was defined as systolic BP (resting) over 140 mm Hg despite taking at least three antihypertensive drugs, which must include one diuretic. There were 14 male patients and 16 female patients, most of whom were obese and middle-aged (≈57 years) and were taking an average of six medications for hypertension. The mean baseline BP was 171.7 (±20.2) mm Hg systolic/99.5 (±13.9) mm Hg diastolic. The Barostim neo device was then activated 2 weeks after implantation and BP was measured using an office-based device. The average reduction in BP readings was 26.0 (±4.4) mm Hg systolic and 12.4 (±2.5) mm Hg diastolic (p <0.001) at a follow-up point of 6 months and 43% of patients maintained a systolic BP less than or equal to 140 mm Hg
- A small observational study in Germany, published in 2015, followed up 25 of the original 30 patients who received

the Barostim neo, and examined the effect of baroreflex activation therapy on central hemodynamics.[20] The study included 14 women and 11 men, with an average age of 61 years. About one-third of the participants (9/25) had previously undergone renal denervation and most of them were obese. After 6 months of BAT therapy, as measured in office, the average peripheral BP had reduced from 109.9 (±20.4) mm Hg to 97.3 (±18.5) mm Hg (p <0.01). Central aortic systolic BP was also measured and showed a significant reduction from 147.2 (±27.8) mm Hg to 130.2 (±25.2) mm Hg (p <0.01)

- The Barostim neo Pivotal trial is a randomized-controlled, multi-center trial that has been set up to demonstrate the efficacy and safety of the Barostim neo system in management of resistant hypertension. It aims to include more than 300 patients in the United States. The primary efficacy endpoint is a systolic BP reduction of 12.5 mm Hg, with a superiority margin of, at least, 5 mm Hg for the Barostim neo treatment group (BAT plus optimal medical management) as compared to patients in the control group (optimal medical management only).[19] Whether the Barostim neo treatment will reduce morbidity or mortality has not yet been demonstrated conclusively.

Mobius HD devices

- The CALM-FIM EUR study was a prospective, open-label study done at six European centers. The inclusion criteria included patients with resistant hypertension (the systolic BP cut-off here was ≥160 mm Hg, despite being on at least three antihypertensive agents, one of which had to be a diuretic). The Mobius HD devices were implanted unilaterally in the internal carotid artery. It is to note that the primary endpoint in this study, at 6 months, was safety, i.e. incidence of serious adverse events. Efficacy, i.e. changes in office and 24-hour ambulatory BP, was a secondary endpoint.[21] Thirty patients were successfully implanted the device between December, 2013 and February, 2016. Mean age was 52 years, there was an equal sex distribution and average antihypertensive use was 4 drugs. There were five serious adverse events (in four patients) at 6 months—hypotension, wound infection, worsening hypertension and intermittent claudication. The efficacy endpoints are summarized in Table 2.

Thus, it was concluded that in patients with resistant hypertension, baroreceptor amplification through IPG or endovascular methods (viz. Mobius HD device) could significantly lower BP levels with an acceptable safety profile. However, randomized and double-blinded studies would have to be performed before any definitive guidelines may be issued.

ADVERSE EFFECTS OF BARO-RECEPTOR ACTIVATION THERAPY

Procedural adverse effects include wound site infection and complications, hypoglossal

TABLE 2: Efficacy of the CALM-FIM EUR study.

	Office blood pressure	Ambulatory blood pressure
Mean systolic BP	184 mm Hg	166 mm Hg
Reduction in systolic BP at 6 months	24 mm Hg (13–34)	21 mm Hg (14–29)
p-value	0.0003	<0.0001
Mean diastolic BP	109 mm Hg	100 mm Hg
Reduction in diastolic BP at 6 months	12 mm Hg (6–18)	12 mm Hg (7–16)
p-value	0.0001	<0.0001

nerve damage (temporary and permanent), surgical complications, and chronic pain in the glossopharyngeal nerve region. Some patients complain of a sensation of tingling in the neck, which decreases over time. A few patients may experience BAT-related hypertensive crises and even strokes.[22]

Assessment of renal function, post 1-year of BAT, shows a mild increase in serum creatinine and an insignificant reduction in estimated glomerular filtration rate (e-GFR), implying that it does not appear to affect kidney function significantly.[23]

CONCLUSION

Baroreceptor activation therapy has shown encouraging initial results, achieving and maintaining a consistent, sustained and safe reduction in BP levels of patients with resistant hypertension. The initial doubts regarding safety (from the first-generation Rheos devices) have been addressed by the more compact and advanced Barostim neo device. The individual tailoring of therapy, which is adjustable and fully reversible, makes it an attractive therapeutic approach and for obvious reasons the patient is fully compliant with therapy, unlike drug regimens. Management of resistant hypertension has always been a challenge and these patients were at high risk for consequences of unchecked arterial hypertension. A combination of traditional drug therapies, lifestyle modifications, and newer interventions like Baroreceptor Activation, hold the key. Randomized controlled trials are currently ongoing and their outcomes will surely shape the role of BAT in the future.

REFERENCES

1. Mills KT, Bundy JD, Kelly TN, et al. Global disparities of hypertension prevalence and control: a systematic analysis of population-based studies from 90 countries. Circulation. 2016;134:441-50.

2. Gupta R, Xavier D. Hypertension: the most important non-communicable disease risk factor in India. Indian Heart J. 2018;10:565-72.

3. Kearney PM, Whelton M, Reynolds K, et al. "Global burden of hypertension: analysis of worldwide data". Lancet. 2005;365(9455):217-23.

4. Pierdomenico SD, Lapenna D, Bucci A, et al. Cardiovascular outcome in treated hypertensive patients with responder, masked, false resistant, and true resistant hypertension. Am J Hypertens. 2005;18:1422-8.

5. Egan BM, Zhao Y, Axon RN. "US trends in prevalence, awareness, treatment, and control of hypertension, 1988–2008," JAMA. 2010;303(20):2043-50.

6. Papadopoulos DP, Papademetriou V. Resistant Hypertension: Diagnosis and Management. J Cardiovasc Pharmacol Ther. 2006;11(2):113-8.

7. Cowley AW Jr, Liard JF, Guyton AC. Role of baroreceptor reflex in daily control of arterial blood pressure and other variables in dogs. Circ Res. 1973;32: 564-76.

8. Thrasher TN. Unloading arterial baroreceptors causes neurogenic hypertension. Am J Physiol Regul Integr Comp Physiol. 2002;282;4:R1044-53.

9. Benarroch EE. The arterial baroreflex: functional organization and involvement in neurologic disease. Neurology. 2008;71:1733-8.

10. Lanfranchi PA, Somers VK. Arterial baroreflex function and cardiovascular variability: interactions and implications. Am J Physiol Regul Integr Comp Physiol. 2002;283:R815-26.

11. La Rovere MT, Pinna GD, Raczak G. Baroreflex sensitivity: measurement and clinical implications. Ann Noninvasive Electrocardiol. 2008;13:191-207.

12. Lohmeier TE, Hildebrandt DA, Dwyer TM, et al. Prolonged activation of the baroreflex decreases arterial pressure even during chronic adrenergic blockade. Hypertension. 2009;53:833-8.

13. DiBona GF, Kopp UC. Neural control of renal function. Physiol Rev. 1997;77:75-197.

14. Reed MJ, Robertson CE, Addison PS. Heart rate variability measurements and the prediction of ventricular arrhythmias. Quart J Med. 2005;98:87-95.

15. Tordoir JHM, Scheffers I, Schmidli J, et al. An implantable carotid sinus baroreflex activating system: surgical technique and short-term outcome from a multi-center feasibility trial for treatment of resistant hypertension. Eur J Vasc Endovasc Surg. 2007;33:414-21.

16. Alnima T, Scheffers I, De Leeuw PW, et al. Sustained acute voltage-dependent blood pressure decrease with prolonged carotid baroreflex activation in therapy-resistant hypertension. J Hypertens. 2012;30(8):1665-70.

17. Scheffers IJ, Kroon AA, Schmidli J, et al. Novel baroreflex activation therapy in resistant hypertension: results of a European multi-center feasibility study. J Am Coll Cardiol. 2010;56(15):1254-8.

18. Bakris GL, Nadim MK, Haller H, et al. Baroreflex activation therapy provides durable benefit in patients with resistant hypertension: results of long-term follow-up in the Rheos Pivotal Trial. J Am Soc Hypertens. 2012;6(2):152-8.

19. Hoppe UC, Brandt MC, Wachter R, et al. Minimally invasive system for baroreflex activation therapy chronically lowers blood pressure with pacemaker-like safety profile: results from the Barostim neo trial. J Am Soc Hypertens. 2012;6(4):270-6.

20. Wallbach M, Lehnig LY, Schroer C, et al. Effects of baroreflex activation therapy on arterial stiffness and central hemodynamics in patients with resistant hypertension. J Hypertens. 2015;33(1):181-6.

21. Spiering W, Williams B, Van der Heyden J, et al. Endovascular baroreflex amplification for resistant hypertension: a safety and proof-of-principle clinical study. Lancet 2017;390(10113):2655-61.

22. Bisognano JD, Bakris G, Nadim MK, et al. Baroreflex activation therapy lowers blood pressure in patients with resistant hypertension: results from the double-blind, randomized, placebo-controlled rheos pivotal trial. J Am Coll Cardiol. 2011;58(7):765-73.

23. Inima T, De Leeuw PW, Tan FE, et al. Renal responses to long-term carotid baroreflex activation therapy in patients with drug-resistant hypertension. Hypertension. 2013;61(6):1334-9.

RhoA/Rho—Kinase Signaling Pathway in Vascular Smooth Muscle Contraction: Biochemistry, Physiology, and Pharmacology

R Rajasekar, Packiamary Jerome, Ananthi Mathiyalagan

INTRODUCTION

Hypertension is a systemic disorder, which affects all the systems, especially the cardiovascular system. The increased pressure in the arteries causes alteration in the vascular tone and increased vascular contractility.

VASCULAR SMOOTH MUSCLE CELL

The vascular smooth muscle has a very peculiar character of plasticity. During the adolescent age, the vascular smooth muscle is largely contractile which is helpful for the autoregulation of blood pressure. When the patients age advances, it loses its contractility which is the key factor in the development of atherosclerosis or vessel remodeling. A better knowledge about the regulation of smooth muscle contraction is essential for the management of certain diseases of blood vessels. Several studies are now under process explaining about the role of RhoA Rho kinase (ROCK Rho associated protein kinase) in calcium-independent regulation of smooth muscle contraction.

ROCK Structure

ROCK— Rho associated protein kinase kinase. They belong to serine threonine kinase family. It has a molecular mass of 160 kDa. There are two isoforms of ROCK family. Each isoforms is encoded by two different genes, *ROCK1* and *ROCK2*. *ROCK1* gene is present in chromosome 18 and *ROCK2* gene is present in chromosome 2.[1] ROCK structure comprises of three domains. One is a kinase domain presents at the amino terminus, second containing the Rho binding region and the third is the pleckstrin homology domain with cysteine rich domain. Both isoforms are expressed ubiquitously. Both ROCK1 and ROCK2 are present in visceral smooth muscle and heart, whereas ROCK2 messenger ribonucleic acid (mRNA) is present highly in brain and skeletal muscle.

The upregulation of ROCK proteins is done by angiotensin II, interleukin-1β and also through Pks-nuclear factor-kappa B-dependent pathways.

Distribution

Rho has two forms. One is the guanosine diphosphate (GDP) bound inactive form and the other is the guanosine triphosphate (GTP) bound active form.[2] Rho is usually present in the cytosol of the cells. In the cytosol, it is in the inactive form. Whenever the cell gets stimulated, RhoA moves from the cytosol to the plasma membrane. In the plasma membrane, GDP–GTP exchange takes place. When it is bound to GTP, it interacts with its receptors and targets and initiates the cellular response.[3]

Regulation

The ROCK structure contains two terminal ends. One is the C terminal and the other is the N terminal. The C terminal end contains the pleckstrin homology and Rho binding domains. The N terminal end contains the kinase domains. The normal regulation of ROCK is maintained by these domains. The domains in the C terminal end bind independently to the kinase domain in the N terminus and in turn, it inhibits the enzyme activity. When the ROCK gets activated, the interaction between the C terminal and kinase domain is interrupted. This disruption yields an active kinase (Fig. 1).

The C terminal portions of ROCK in cells act as dominant negatives. Whenever the C terminal portion containing the Rho binding protein and pleckstrin homology domain is cleaved, it becomes an active form. The C terminal portion has an autoinhibitory effect on the kinase domains.

Stimulation

When the active GTP-bound form of RhoA binds to Rho binding domain, the

phosphotransferase activity of ROCK gets stimulated. Arachidonic acid or sphingosine phosphorylcholine increases the ROCK activity effectively.

Inhibition

RhoE is a small G protein. It binds to the N terminal region of ROCK1 which contains the kinase domain. The binding of RhoE to ROCK1 inhibits the activity of ROCK function.

ROCK Substrates

There are more than 15 ROCK substrates identified.

Targets

The targets of ROCK substrates are:
- Myosin phosphatase target subunit 1 (MYPT1)
- CPI-17
- Myosin light chain (MLC)
- Calponin
- Cardiac troponin.

These targets are mainly involved in regularity smooth cell contraction.

One newly diagnosed ROCK substrate is PTEN—phosphatase and tensin homolog. This PTEN substrate is helpful in the dephosphorylation of both proteins and phosphoinositol kinase such as PI-3 kinase/AKT (protein kinase B) pathway which is involved in many of the cellular regulation. When ROCK binds to PTEN, it stimulates its phosphatase activity, such as cell growth, protein synthesis, transcription and cell survival.

The ROCK is also involved in the phosphorylation of IRS-1 (insulin receptor substrate-1) in visceral smooth muscle cells, which leads to inhibition of both insulin induced IRS-1 tyrosine phosphorylation of PI-1 kinase activation.

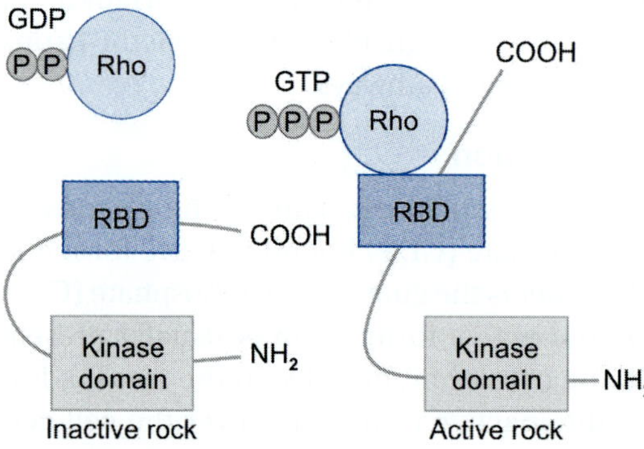

Fig. 1: Rock structure.

ROCK AND VISCERAL SMOOTH MUSCLE CONTRACTION

Myosin light chain is a major molecule involved in the regulation of visceral smooth muscle. The phosphorylation and dephosphorylation of this MLC is essential for regulation of smooth muscle contraction. The rise in calcium activates MLC kinase and consequent phosphorylation of MLC and smooth muscle contraction.

Myosin phosphatase target subunit 1 is the regulatory unit of MLC phosphatase. RhoA-mediated ROCK activation phosphorylates MYPT1 and inhibits its activity. This causes calcium sensitization of the contractile proteins and enhances smooth muscle contraction.

ROCK AND HYPERTENSION

Hypertension occurs as a result of increased peripheral vascular resistance. This increased peripheral vascular resistance is attributed to enhanced contractility of smooth muscles and arterial wall remodeling. In the recent trends, there has several evidence indicating the role of Rho–Rho kinase in the development and maintenance of hypertension, blocking of the ROCK activity with the help of Y27632 has a significant blood pressure lowering effects in rats. Similarly, oral administration of fasudil significantly lowered arterial blood pressure.

The ROCK is also involved in spontaneous tone development under hypertensive conditions. Treatment with Y27632 significantly reduces the arterial vascular tone in rats, but it has no impact on basal tone of normotensive rats.

Not only oral but also direct central administration of ROCK inhibitor has an impact on blood pressure. Alterations in the RhoA or ROCK pathway are most likely the consequence of an upstream event in the hypertensive state. One upstream signaling molecule that seems to be involved is angiotensin II and its receptor type 1 (AT1). Angiotensin II has been the important molecule responsible for hypertension. Y27632 has been shown to be more potent in relaxing arteries from angiotensin II induced hypertension. This highlights the increased sensitivity to ROCK inhibition in animals.

The blockade of AT1 receptors prevents the upregulation of RhoA and ROCK activity.

The other concept which is involved in the regulation of hypertension is the formation of reactive oxygen species (ROS). Oxidative stress plays an important role in the development and maintenance of hypertension. ROS have increased sensitivity toward Y27632 pointing toward an activation of rock pathway. The quantity of membrane bound, active RhoA was increased by ROS.

Air pollution is an important environmental factor involved in the pathogenesis of hypertension. A recent study conducted in rats shows that exposure of rats to air pollution and angiotensin II leads to an increase in blood pressure which is accompanied by a ROS mediated increase in ROCK activity.

Atherosclerosis that often accompanies hypertension might also be in part due to changes in RhoA and ROCK activity.

Several genetic mechanisms are involved in humans in regulation of hypertension. The polymorphisms which occur at amino acid terminal with asparagines have been associated with a greater resting systolic blood pressure. A haplotype block consisting of four single – nucleotide polymorphisms (SNPs) within the ROCKII allele was found to be recessively associated with a lower risk of hypertension.

Increased nitric oxide production will lead to an inhibition of the RhoA ROCK cascade thus protecting against the enhanced contractile and proliferative effects of the pathway.[4]

■ ROCK INHIBITORS[5]

- Y27632 has no specific predilections for ROCK isoforms. It inhibits both isoforms
- *Fasudil/HA-1077:* It also has an inhibitory activity effects on protein kinase A (PKA) and protein kinase C (PKC)
- Hydroxyfasudil, active metabolite of fasudil has a more inhibitory effect on ROCK
- Aminofurazan-based inhibitors— GSK269962A and SB772077B also have inhibitory effects on ROCK-I and II but with a higher potency than Y27632
- H1152P, a potent and specific inhibitor II with weak inhibitory effects on other kinases.

■ CONCLUSION

The emergence of RhoA or ROCK molecule in the future may be a milestone in the treatment of smooth muscle disorders. Further studies are warranted to prove its significance. Targeting the critically involved ROCK isoform under specific cardiovascular pathophysiological conditions might have multiple beneficial effects on vascular function.

■ REFERENCES

1. Amano M, Ito M, Kimura K, et al Phosphorylation and activation of myosin by Rho-associated Kinase. J Biol Chem. 1996;271(34):20246-9.
2. Khalil RA. Chapter 7, Rho Kinase in vascular smooth muscle. Regulation of vascular smooth muscle function. San Rafael (CA), Chapter 7. Morgan & Claypool Life sciences; 2010.
3. Nakagawa O, Fujisawa K, Ishizaki T, et al. Rock–1 & Rock–II, two isoforms of Rho associated coiled–coil forming protein serine/threonine kinase in mice. FEBS Lett. 1996;392(2):189-93.
4. Hahmann C, Schroeter T. Rho-kinase inhibitors as therapeutics: from pan inhibition to isoform selectivity. Cell Mol Life Sci.2010;67:171-7.
5. Jacobs M, Hayakawa K, Swenson L, et al. The structure of dimeric ROCK I reveals the mechanism for ligand selectivity. J Biol C Hem. 2006;281:260-8.

Guidelines and Meta-analysis

Comparison of Various Guidelines in Hypertension—Which is Best for India?

Jagdish C Mohan

■ INTRODUCTION

Arterial hypertension is a major public health issue all over the world. Current data suggest a prevalence of about 25% in Indian adult population with geographic and demographic variations.[1] From these data, it can be estimated that there are at least 200 million adults with hypertension in India of which more than 50% are not even aware of it.[2] Hypertension is the most important risk factor for heart failure, chronic kidney disease and stroke. It plays a significant role in pathogenesis of atherosclerosis and all acute ischemic events. The Department of Health Research, Government of India, estimated in 2018 that hypertension accounts for 10.8% of all deaths in adults.[3] Seminal studies performed half a century back showed a marked reduction in stroke, heart failure, and all-cause mortality with pharmacotherapy.[4] The era of pharmacotherapy soon evolved into an era of clinical guidelines to advise healthcare professionals about optimal management of arterial hypertension. The guidelines documents were a synopsis of detailed analysis of the evidence available till date and then converting that discussed data into summary points. The Americans and the Europeans took the lead in issuing guidelines

periodically followed by a large number of scientific bodies issuing their own guidelines. The American Heart association and American College of Cardiology (AHA/ACC) in conjunction with several other societies published their latest guidelines in November 2017.[5] The European Society of Cardiology (ESC) along with European Society of Hypertension (ESH) issued new guidelines in July 2018.[6] Hypertension Canada and Chinese Hypertension league also released their new guidelines in 2018.[7-8] The National Institute for Health and Care Excellence (NICE), UK is about to bring out their next hypertension guidelines in August 2019.[9] The last Indian guidelines were published in 2013.[10]

As recognition dawned upon physicians that blood pressure (BP) is a dynamic biomarker with significant situational, method-based, circadian, seasonal and frequency variation, nonoffice based measurements gained currency. Thresholds of abnormalcy and desirability of these measurements were also included into guidelines. Over period of time, nonoffice BP measurements have become more important than office BP. The emphasis of guidelines has been on accurate measurement of BP, detection and definition of hypertension based upon arbitrary threshold, staging and classification, recognizing difficult-to-treat hypertension, appropriate investigative data, nonpharmacological measures and their impact, pharmacological therapy, and finally device-related or nonsurgical invasive interventional advice. Over a period of time, threshold for detection has been lowered and more accurate and automatic methods for recording BP have emerged. A major portion of guidelines is based upon opinion of experts since evidence cannot be generated in every aspect of hypertension because of logistic issues. The evidence also needs to be classified as strong with high quality, moderate, and weak with low quality. Typically, concordant undisputed data from multiple adequately powered randomized trials impacting key outcome endpoints is referred to as strong with high quality. Evidence from single randomized trial or small trials with nonmortality benefits is grouped as moderate. Grouping of evidence is not perfect science and these create important differences between guidelines. New guidelines are supposed to resolve unanswered issues and bring uniformity in treatment of hypertension. To suit Indian needs, guidelines have to be simple, pragmatic, and easy to implement without altering the current practice drastically. Let us look at what is new in these guidelines.

■ THE GUIDELINES

Hypertension is a complex condition that covers most of cardiovascular continuum, which makes it impractical to perform outcome clinical trials in all aspects of the hypertension. Thus, some degree of subjectivity will always be there. Most current guidelines include and integrate cardiovascular risk assessment, stages of hypertension and optimizing drug treatment. Health economics dictate that low-risk young patients must be treated with non-pharmacological measures especially if their BP is less than 160/100 mm Hg. Many such

subjects may actually be having white-coat hypertension. However, one size does not fit all. Hence, different thresholds of initiating drug treatment in different situations appear logical. These two cardinal principles have been largely ignored in ACC/AHA 2017 guidelines and hence the controversy.[5]

How Do Guidelines Differ?

Automatically measured office BP has been recommended by most guidelines in preference over nonautomatic methods. The former provide somewhat lower numerical values in a given case and hence lowering of thresholds for definition and initiation of treatment. However, the world would not change over to new automated methods that quickly. Reality in most part of the healthcare horizon needs to be kept in mind. Following are the major areas of differences:

- Definition of hypertension
- Targets in various disease states
- Methods of measuring BP
- Treatment goals and decision-making algorithms for elderly patients
- Defining the first-line antihypertensive drugs
- Role of β-adrenergic receptor blockers
- Role of centrally acting antiadrenergic drugs (frequently used in India but hardly getting any mention in guidelines).

Lowering the Threshold for Definition and Initiating Drug Therapy

The main difference between various recommendations is the definition of arterial hypertension. The ESC/ESH used cut-off of 140 mm Hg and/or 90 mm Hg for systolic and diastolic BP, respectively in their new guidelines which were very similar to their previous guidelines and more in line with NICE guidelines.[6] A few months before, ACC/AHA had reduced these cut-off values to 130 mm Hg and/or 80 mm Hg (Table 1). The ACC/AHA 2017 guidelines target value

TABLE 1: A comparison of ACC/AHA 2017 and ESC/ESH 2018 guidelines with regard to classification and staging.

Reclassification of blood pressure							
AHA/ACC 2017				**ESC/ESC 2018**			
Category	**SBP (mm Hg)**		**DBP (mm Hg)**	**Category**	**SBP (mm Hg)**		**DBP (mm Hg)**
Normal	<120	and	<80	Optimal	<120	and	<80
Elevated	120–129	and	<80	Normal	120–129	or	80–84
				High-normal	130–139		85–89
Hypertension							
Stage 1	130–139	or	80–89	Stage 1	140–159	or	90–99
Stage 2	≥140	or	≥90	Stage 2	≥160	or	≥100
				Stage 3	>180	or	>110

(ACC/AHA: American Heart Association/American College of Cardiology; DBP: Diastolic blood pressure; ESC/ESH: European Society of Cardiology/European Society of Hypertension; SBP: Systolic blood pressure)

of BP less than 130 mm Hg and less than 80 mm Hg for systolic and diastolic BP is for all except for low-risk subjects and those with prior stroke respectively,[5] while in the ESC/ESH guidelines corresponding values are less than 140 mm Hg and less than 90 mm Hg for everyone below the age of 80 years, and for treatment purposes target values of less than 130/80 mm Hg in patients below the age of 65 years only in those who can tolerate drug therapy safely. The target to treat with pharmacotherapy is liberalized to less than 160/90 mm Hg in those above the age of 80 years by the Europeans. Hypertension Canada brought the threshold to 135/85 mm Hg if automatic BP recordings were taken into consideration and 140/90 mm Hg if nonautomatic measurements were done.[7] This appears a pragmatic approach. The draft of NICE Guidelines to be published in August 2019 is in public domain now and their cut-off values are similar to ESC/ESH recommendations.[9] The Indian guidelines are dated in 2013 and hence may not be based upon the latest evidence (Fig. 1).[10]

There is some difference with regard to target of lowering BP in chronic kidney disease in Europe (<140/90 mm Hg) versus America (<130/80 mm Hg). Hypertension Canada has recommended in-between values depending upon the use of equipment and presence or absence of diabetes. New American threshold for detection of hypertension would increase the absolute prevalence of hypertension in the society by about 14%.[11]

Initiating Pharmacotherapy

According to the ACC/AHA 2017 guidelines, therapy should be initiated if BP was more than 130/80 mm Hg systolic and diastolic BP, respectively in patients with prior cardiovascular disease, renal disease, diabetes, and 10-year risk more than 10%. Drug therapy initiation threshold was raised to 140/90 mm Hg only in those with low cardiovascular risk (10-year risk <10%) or prior stroke (Table 2); while, in the ESC/ESH guidelines corresponding values are less than 140 mm Hg and less than 90 mm Hg for

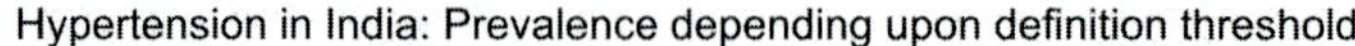

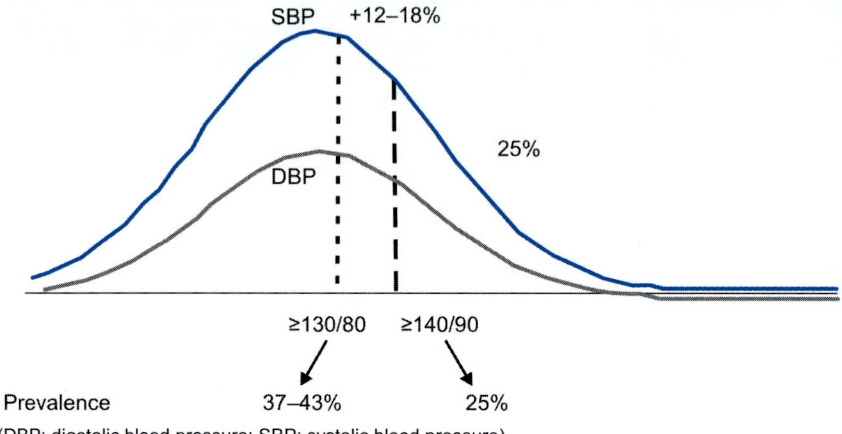

Fig. 1: Actual estimate of hypertension prevalence in India versus projected prevalence with cut-off value of 130/80 mm Hg.[1,11]

every one below the age of 80 years, and less than 130/80 mm Hg in patients below the age of 65 years in those who can safely tolerate drug therapy. The target is liberalized to less than 160/90 mm Hg in those above the age of 80 years. High-normal BP (now rechristened stage I hypertension by the Americans) is associated with left ventricular remodeling that involves cardiac muscle mechanics, diastolic function and hypertrophy.[12] High-normal BP is also related with deterioration of right ventricular function and mechanics, as well as with left atrial function impairment and functional capacity. However, evidence with regard to treating such patients who are now being labeled stage I hypertension by ACC/AHA 2017 guidelines is scant (Table 2).

Changing cut-off values for diagnosis of hypertension, but not for therapy introduction (as suggested by ACC/AHA 2017) might be an important way to make a clarion call to the society and healthcare professionals to follow-up these patients, to persuade them to change their lifestyle and use more non-pharmacological methods to reduce BP, and ultimately to prevent and reduce morbidity and mortality. The other important difference between these guidelines refers to the target values of BP in hypertensive patients who are already on antihypertensive therapy. Hypertension Canada has further queered the pitch by giving different definition of hypertension depending upon presence or absence of diabetes and depending upon the equipment used. It has suggested a cut-off of 140/90 mm Hg if nonautomatic office BP readings are taken into consideration; and for automatic BP recordings, the threshold is 135/85 mm Hg. In diabetes, hypertension has been defined at a cut-off value more than 130/80 mm Hg regardless of the equipment used and risk profile. However, Canadian guidelines recommend initiating drug therapy based upon the risk assessment in other patients like the other guidelines. In low-risk patients (no diabetes or cardiovascular risk factor), the recommendation is to initiate drug therapy only if BP exceeds 160/100 mm Hg. That may be too liberal. The NICE, UK suggest a target of less than 140/90

TABLE 2: One Size Fits All American Guidelines of 2017 for pharmacotherapy initiation.

Clinical condition(s)	BP threshold mm Hg	BP goal mm Hg
General		
Clinical CVD 10-year ASCVD risk ≥10	≥130/80	≥130/80
No clinical CVD and 10 year ASCVD risk <10%	≥140/90	<130/80
Older persons (≥65 years of age; noninstitutionalized, ambulatory, community-living adults)	≥130 (SBP)	<130 (SBP)
Specific comorbidities		
Diabetes mellitus	≥130/80	<130/80
Chronic kidney disease	≥130/80	<130/80
Chronic kidney disease and postrenal transplantation	≥130/80	<130/80
Heart failure	≥130/80	<130/80
Stable ischemic heart disease	≥130/80	<130/80
Secondary stroke prevention	≥140/90	<130/80
Secondary stroke prevention (lacunar)	≥130/80	<130/80
Peripheral arterial disease	≥130/80	<130/80

mm Hg for those below the age of 80 years and less than 150/90 mm Hg for those above the age of 80 years. The NICE recommends classifying in two stages only unlike ESC/ESH which now have three stages. It also suggests initiating drug treatment in young patients (<80 years) with stage I hypertension only if the 10-year cardiovascular risk exceeds 10% (NICE guidelines Draft 2019 to be published in August 2019) or there is established cardiovascular disease or diabetes or renal disease. Chinese guidelines published in 2018 are almost like ESC/ESH 2018 guidelines.[8]

Choice of Drug Therapy

Much has changed since β-receptor anti-adrenergic agents were brought down to level of secondary agents in last guidelines. The NICE guidelines Draft 2019 proposes to bring down β-receptor blocking agents in step 4 and diuretics in step 3. This way, diuretics have been removed as first-line agents in new proposed NICE guidelines. The other guidelines continue to use thiazides and thiazide-like diuretics as first-line antihypertensive agents. Hypertension Canada continues to recommend β-receptor blocking agents as first-line therapy in patients younger than 60 years. The European guidelines have a weak recommendation for β-blocking agents in young hypertensives with sinus tachycardia. Of course, compelling indications are a different story in all situations. The ESC/ESH and Hypertension Canada recommend two-drug combinations as first-line therapy while ACC/AHA 2017 guidelines propose fixed-dose drug combinations in stage II. These guidelines may not be entirely applicable in India where cost and compliance are bigger issues even if the patients are willing to be treated. Pathophysiology of essential hypertension differs in elderly and younger subjects, the latter being related to obesity and increased sympathetic nerve activity and hence β-blockers may have an important role in management of young hypertensive subjects. It may be too early to write their obituary.

Broad Viewpoint

Previous guidelines about categorizing subjects with different BPs had wider acceptability because those were simple and pragmatic. The latest American guidelines are more disruptive. It was easy to label an individual with prehypertension (most did not like it), stage I and stage II hypertension. The Europeans maintained traditional BP categories, with stage I hypertension starting at an office pressure of 140/90 mm Hg but introduced stage III in new guidelines with a cut-off value more than or equal to 180/110 mm Hg. Stage III introduces some kind of urgency in treatment and is a welcome step. The Europeans have not been as aggressive in lowering targets to reflect the SPRINT data,[13] which has been the pivot of ACC/AHA guidelines. The US guidelines recommend lowering BP to less than 130/80 mm Hg for all adults, even those with various comorbidities, who have confirmed hypertension and known cardiovascular disease or a high estimated risk. Evidence for such an approach is limited. The European document establishes target ranges, advising a systolic target of 130 mm Hg, but not lower than 120 mm Hg, for most adults younger than 65 if they can tolerate polypharmacy without adverse effects. For adults 65 years and older, regardless of comorbidities, the treatment target range is the same as the one in younger patients with chronic kidney disease: less than 140 mm Hg, but no lower than 130 mm Hg. This approach would appeal to Indian healthcare professionals.

Relevance in Indian Context

India has sufficient prevalence data on high-normal or elevated BP and hypertension in the general population. We lack indigenously generated multicentric outcome data from randomized trials. Less than 1% of our healthcare professionals use automatic BP methods.

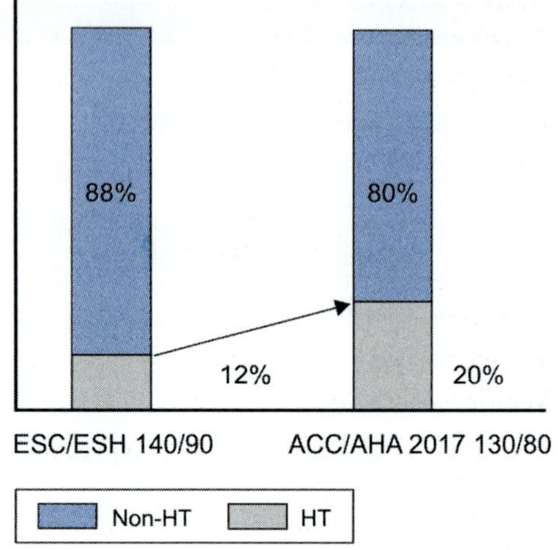

(ACC/AHA: American Heart association/American College of Cardiology; ESC/ESH: European Society of Cardiology/European Society of Hypertension; HT: hypertension)

Fig. 2: Hypertension in age range 18–25 years in India.

Situation is unlikely to change soon. In busy practices, automated equipment which record at least three readings at fixed intervals are time-consuming and hence unwelcome. The BP control data still may reflect casual readings adding to the unreliability. Following additional points are worth considering:

- With implementation of ACC/AHA guidelines, prevalence of hypertension in Indian adults would reach or exceed 40%. This redefinition would have medical, legal, insurance and psychological implications
- Bigger issue would be that every fifth young man or woman in age range 18–25 years would be labeled hypertensive (Fig. 2).[1,11] Would this deprive this population from certain jobs based upon medical ineligibility?
- Based upon a cut-off limit of 130/80 mm Hg and 10-year cardiovascular risk of more than or equal to 10%, a large number of apparently healthy elderly subjects will receive pharmacotherapy. Even American College of Physicians has suggested a

threshold of 150/90 mm Hg for treating individuals with age more than 65 years[14]

- Another aspect is that stage I hypertension becomes a very narrow range now and normal variability of BP may make a person in and out of this stage
- There should be more emphasis on measuring BP in all adults as and when they present to healthcare professionals or other public places where automatic BP equipment can be strategically located. Wider use of automatic BP measurements at offices, public utilities and homes should be encouraged
- For India, a threshold of less than 140/90 mm Hg in adults should be most acceptable. Thus, we may follow ESC/ESH guidelines rather than ACC/AHA guidelines
- Staging hypertension (3 stages) is to be emphasized. This will help people understand the urgency about BP control
- Home BP by cheaper automatic devices which family or families can share should become routine
- Rather than advocating a specific target for all adults, the focus should be on choosing BP targets that allow for a choice based on a patient's risk profile, susceptibility to harm, and treatment preferences. In this aspect, proposed NICE guidelines would be more appropriate for India
- Reinforcement in the new guidelines to utilize single pill or fixed dose combination right from the beginning is a practical step toward improving patient participation and synergy in the healthcare delivery mechanism. Stepped care approach is dead
- In India, the cost for healthcare is mostly and directly borne by individuals and not by a third party. Low-cost rational and effective fixed-drug combinations will go a long way in controlling the menace of hypertension. With first-line recommendations for single-pill combination, physicians should feel encouraged to use these without compunction
- Cardiovascular risk assessment has come to stay. The Joint British Society 3 risk score or WHO-ISH modified risk scores for Southeast Asian region are suited better for Indian population and should be used routinely.[15,16] This will ensure better compliance with nondrug and drug therapy both
- Fragility in elderly needs greater attention. Liberal targets of less than 150 mm Hg systolic BP in those who cannot walk more than 1 m/s regardless of age would be a good idea in author's view.

■ CONCLUSION

Guidelines on management of hypertension attempt to include new information and evidence so that busy clinicians are provided with broad basic advice on how to manage their patients. These are not the Gospel's truth. Sometimes tweaking with evidence is done to stay practical, relevant and free from controversy. However, current guidelines do differ when sheer evidence is contrasted with practicality. In this context, European guidelines are more practical and relevant to India. Auscultatory blood pressure measurement is more common in this country and is usually somewhat over-estimated because of not adhering to usual precautions. A goal of <140/90 mm Hg clinic blood pressure is advisable for most patients and very elderly can be given a latitude of another 10 mm Hg in systolic blood pressure. Individualized therapy based upon global cardiovascular risk is strongly recommended. Long-term adherence and persistence are more important than exact numbers to be achieved.

■ REFERENCES

1. Geldsetzer P, Manne-Goehler J, Theilmann M, et al. Diabetes and hypertension in India: A nationally representative study of 1.3 Million adults. JAMA Intern Med. 2018;178(3):363-72.

2. Sudan P. Ministry of Health & Family Welfare, Govt of India. Release Date November 28, 2017.

3. Dept of Health Research and Indian Council of Medical Research. Release date May 2, 2018.

4. Veterans Administration Cooperative Study Group on Antihypertensive Agents. Effects of treatment on morbidity and hypertension: Results in patients with diastolic pressures averaging 115 through 129 millimeters of mercury. JAMA. 1967;202:1028-34.

5. Whelton PK, Carey RM, Aronow WS, et al. 2017 ACC/AHA/AAPA/ABC/ACPM/AGS/APhA/ASH/ASPC/NMA/PCNA Guideline for the Prevention, Detection, Evaluation, and Management of High Blood Pressure in Adults: Executive Summary: A Report of the American College of Cardiology/American Heart Association Task Force on Clinical Practice Guidelines. Hypertension. 2018;71:1269-324.

6. Williams B, Mancia G, Spiering W, et al. 2018 ESC/ESH Guidelines for the management of arterial hypertension. Eur Heart J. 2018;39:3021-104.

7. Nerenberg KA, Smith EE, Gubitz G. Hypertension Canada's 2018 Guidelines for Diagnosis, Risk Assessment, Prevention, and Treatment of Hypertension in Adults and Children. Canadian J Cardiol. 2018;34(5):506-25.

8. Liu L, Wu Z, Wang J, et al. 2018 Chinese guidelines for the management of hypertension. Chin J Cardiovasc Med. 2019;24:1-46

9. Hypertension in adults: NICE guideline DRAFT. March, 2019.

10. Association of Physicians of India. Indian guidelines on hypertension (IGH)-III-2013. J Assoc Physicians India. 2013;61(2 Suppl):6-36.

11. Gupta R, Deedwania PC, Achari V, et al. Normotension, prehypertension, and hypertension in urban middle-class subjects in India: prevalence, awareness, treatment, and control. Am J Hypertens. 2013;26:83-94.

12. Cuspidi C, Sala C, Tadic M, et al. Pre-hypertension and subclinical cardiac damage: A meta-analysis of echocardiographic studies. Int J Cardiol. 2018;270:302-8.

13. Wright JT Jr, Williamson JD, Whelton PK, et al. A randomized trial of intensive versus standard blood-pressure control. N Engl J Med. 2015;373:2103-16.

14. Qaseem A, Wilt TJ, Rich R, et al. Pharmacologic treatment of hypertension in adults aged 60 years or older to higher versus lower blood pressure targets: A clinical practice guideline from the American College of Physicians and the American Academy of Family Physicians. Ann Intern Med. 2017;166:430-7.

15. World Health Organization Prevention of Cardiovascular Disease Guidelines for Assessment and Management of Cardiovascular Risk. Geneva: WHO; 2007.

16. JBS3 Board. Joint British Societies' consensus recommendations for the prevention of cardiovascular disease (JBS3). Heart. 2014;100(Suppl 2):ii1-ii67.

"Meta-analysis in Hypertension" What We have Learnt and What We have to Learn?

SS Iyengar

INTRODUCTION

We are in an era of "evidence-based medicine (EBM)", and steadily and surely moving into practicing "precision medicine". The evidence has to be derived from clinical studies and guidelines. The hierarchical system of evidence places "meta-analysis" at the top.

Meta-analysis studies in the field of hypertension have dealt with various aspects—epidemiology, diagnosis, treatment thresholds, treatment targets, drugs, and devices. Guidelines from national medical societies have taken the support of the results of these studies in framing their recommendations. Ethnicity, age, gender, drug response, and comorbidities are other factors for consideration in the management of hypertension. Unexplored areas and unmet needs are there and form a fertile field for meta-analysis studies.

META-ANALYSIS

Meta-analysis has received a lot of importance in the practice of EBM. There has been an explosive growth and mass production of meta-analysis in medical literature, accounting for nearly 2,000% increase in number.[1] Obviously, there has been a decline in the quality of meta-analysis.[2] A meta-analysis is a statistical exercise where the results from multiple studies are combined with an objective to increase the power (which would be weak otherwise with individual studies) of the study, and thus try to resolve some uncertainties that remain with individual studies. Meta-analysis is different from systematic review and may be said to be a subset of systematic review.

It should be appreciated that meta-analysis has its own limitations. A meta-analysis is as good as the studies that have been included in the methodological approach. It is associated with certain biases like publication bias, time lag bias, selective reporting bias, and the language bias. Despite this, meta-analysis has contributed a great deal to our understanding and management of hypertension.[3-5]

META-ANALYSES IN HYPERTENSION

Some important meta-analyses that have had an impact on our understanding and practice in the management of hypertension will be discussed briefly in the following sections.

Hypertension and Cardiovascular Disease

A collaborative meta-analysis of 61 prospective observational studies, involving 1 million adults with no atherosclerotic cardiovascular disease (ASCVD) at baseline observed that during 12.7 million person-years at risk, there were about 56,000 vascular deaths and 66,000 other deaths at ages 40–89 years.[6] There were 12,000 strokes and 34,000 ischemic heart diseases (IHD). The study concluded that:

- With every 20/10 mm Hg systolic blood pressure (SBP)/diastolic blood pressure (DBP) increase in blood pressure (BP), the risk of mortality doubles (Fig. 1)
- Age specific associations are similar in men and women
- Throughout the age group of 40–89 years, BP is linearly related to vascular and all-cause mortality, with no evidence of a threshold down to a BP level of 115/75 mm Hg.

This meta-analysis showed that lower BP is better. But, does BP lowering in a patient of hypertension improve cardiovascular (CV) outcome and mortality?

Now let us look at this systematic review and meta-analysis of BP lowering trials, published between 1966 and 2015. 123 studies with 613,815 participants were included in this meta-analysis.[7]

The analysis showed that each 10 mm Hg reduction in SBP significantly reduced the risk of major CVD events, coronary heart disease (CHD), stroke and heart failure. It also resulted in a significant 13% reduction in all-cause mortality. It did not reduce the risk of renal failure significantly. This benefit was similar with higher or lower mean baseline SBP. Patients with underlying diabetes and chronic kidney disease showed smaller, but significant, risk reductions.

This meta-analysis also brought out the effects of different classes of drugs. β-blockers were inferior to other drugs when it comes to preventing major CVD events, stroke and renal failure. Calcium channel blockers (CCBs) were superior in preventing stroke, but inferior in preventing heart failure, where diuretics were found to be superior.

The authors concluded that BP lowering reduces atherosclerotic CV risk across various baseline BP levels and comorbidities. The

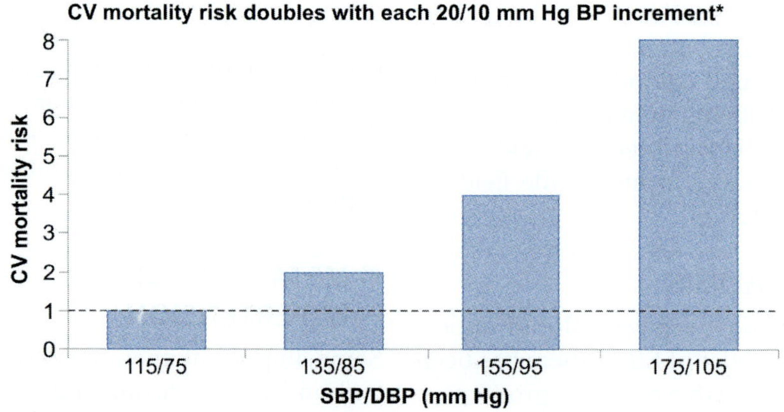

*Individuals aged 40–69 years, starting at BP 115/75 mm Hg.

(CV: cardiovascular; SBP: systolic blood pressure; DBP: diastolic blood pressure)

Fig. 1: Cardiovascular mortality increases with increasing systolic and diastolic blood pressure.

analysis supports lowering SBPs to less than 130 mm Hg and recommends BP lowering in patients with CVD, CHD, stroke, diabetes, heart failure and chronic kidney disease.

Epidemiology—Prevalence, Awareness, and Control of Hypertension in India

A systematic review and meta-analysis of prevalence, awareness, and control of hypertension in Indian rural and urban areas has clearly brought to the attention of the medical community the burden of hypertension and magnitude of the problem in India.[8] The study looked at 142 studies that were published between 1950 and 2013 with definition of hypertension being a BP of 140/90 mm Hg or more, in adults 18 years or older.

Overall, prevalence of hypertension in India was 29.8%; it was 27.6% in rural population and 33.8% in urban population, the difference being statistically significant. Regional estimates are shown in Figure 2. The prevalence of awareness overall was 25.3% for rural population and 42% for urban Indians; for treatment and control it was 25.1% and 10.7% for rural area and 37.5% and 20.2% for urban area.

First-line Drug for Hypertension

There are a number of drugs available that are safe and effective in the management of hypertension. The choice of first-line drug and additional drugs depend on various factors like cost, efficacy and safety of the drugs, comorbidities, and physician's experience.

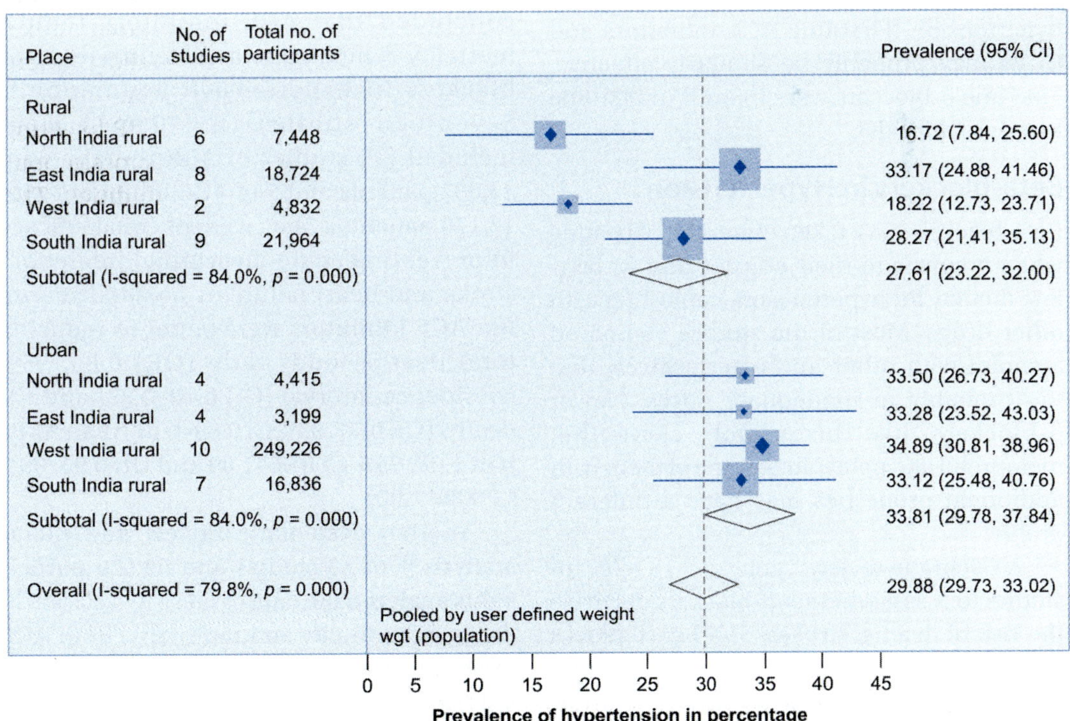

Fig. 2: Prevalence of hypertension in India (rural vs. urban). Overall pooled estimates: region-wise (North, East, West and South) and place-wise (rural and urban).

The results of meta-analysis do guide clinicians in choice of therapy.

A Cochrane database systematic review looked at the studies published till November 2017, and using one of the six major classes of drugs, i.e. thiazides (low-dose and high-dose), β-blockers, CCB, angiotensin-converting enzyme (ACE) inhibitors, angiotensin II receptor blockers (ARBs), and alpha-blockers, in patients with a baseline BP over 140/90 mm Hg.[9] The outcomes assessed were mortality, stroke, CHD, total cardiovascular events (CVS), decrease in systolic and DBP, and withdrawals due to adverse drug effects.

Withdrawals due to adverse effects were seen with thiazide diuretics and β-blockers and this information was not available with ACE inhibitors, ARBs, and CCBs. The authors concluded that first-line therapy with low-dose diuretics reduced morbidity and mortality outcomes in patients with moderate to severe hypertension. First-line ACE inhibitors and CCBs may probably be similarly effective. First-line β-blockers were inferior to first-line low-dose thiazides.

Beta-blockers in Hypertension

Beta-blockers have taken quite a bit of beating when it comes to their efficacy and as first-line therapy for hypertension, contesting with other drugs. Most of the studies compared atenolol with other antihypertensives, that too probably in inadequate doses. Newer β-blockers like bisoprolol, carvedilol, metoprolol and nebivolol—some of them with additional properties may have a different profile.

A Cochrane review[10] analyzed 13 relevant studies to assess whether β-blockers decrease the risk of deaths, strokes, and heart attacks associated with high BP in adults. Atenolol was the β-blocker most used. The analysis found that β-blocker use leads to modest CVD reductions and little or no effects on mortality, and they are inferior to other antihypertensive drugs. However, the reviewers suggest more studies of high quality with newer β-blockers, and in different age groups.

Angiotensin-converting Enzyme Inhibitors or Angiotensin II Receptor Blocker?

Renin–angiotensin–aldosterone system (RAAS) plays a vital role in health and disease of the CV system. It has been the target of therapeutics in hypertension, heart failure, ASCVD, chronic kidney disease and myocardial protection.

Angiotensin-converting enzyme inhibitor entered the therapeutic field about 10 years before ARBs. Ever since, there is an ongoing debate about the superiority of one over the other. This issue has been addressed by some meta-analyses.

One systematic review and meta-analysis concluded that ACE inhibitors reduce mortality compared to angiotensin receptor blockers in hypertensive population.[11] Seventeen studies (n = 73,761) were included (12 studies of ARB therapy with 24,697 patients and 5 of ACE inhibitors with 12,170 patients). They were of equal efficacy in preventing acute myocardial infarction, stroke and heart failure or hospitalization. But ACE inhibitors were better in reducing total deaths [odds ratio (OR) 0.85, 95% confidence interval (CI) 0.78–0.93] and CV deaths (OR 0.77, 95% CI 0.69–0.87) than ARBs (OR 1.02, 95% CI 0.96–1.09 and OR 0.95, 95% CI 0.86–1.06).

Another systematic review and meta-analysis,[12] of 38 studies and 32,528 participants analyzed the data of these two classes of drugs on mortality and morbidity. Both ACE inhibitors and ARBs were equally effective in lowering systolic and DBP, all-cause mortality, CV mortality, fatal and nonfatal myocardial infarction, and stroke. However, ACE inhibitors were more effective in preventing heart failure and hospitalization for heart failure than ARBs (RR: 0.71, 95% CI 0.54–0.93).

Treatment of Hypertension based on Blood Pressure Readings or ASCVD Risk

It is usual clinical practice to treat hypertension based on BP readings, and so did guidelines traditionally recommend treatment based on BP thresholds. Recent guidelines have rightly shown a shift in the strategy. Both—assessment of ASCVD risk and BP readings—should dictate the therapy, and that is the appropriate way and effective method to treat hypertension and reduce its complications and ASCVD risk.

A meta-analysis used individual participant data from the Blood Pressure Lowering Treatment Trialists' Collaboration (BPLTTC) from 1995 to 2013 and compared the two strategies looking at specific SBP thresholds and the spectrum of risk and BP levels.[13]

From 11 trials there were 47,872 participants and during a 4 years of follow-up, 3,566 patients (7.5%) experienced a major CV event. It was seen that a greater number of ASCVD events would be avoided if treated with the ASCVD risk strategy compared with the SBP strategy (area under the curve 0.71 for the CVD risk strategy vs. 0.54 for the SBP strategy).

The study concluded that a BP-lowering treatment strategy based on predicted ASCVD risk is appropriate and more effective than one based on BP levels alone across a range of BP thresholds. It is wise to adopt global risk assessment to guide BP treatment decision-making.

Blood Pressure Targets

Over a period of years, BP targets have changed and the trend is to go for lower targets. Medical societies differ in their recommendations, though based on the same studies in the literature, obviously due to disparate interpretation of the data.

Some information on SBP and DBP targets for drug treatment can be drawn from recent, large meta-analyses of RCTs of BP lowering.

In one of these meta-analyses,[14] the data were collected from randomized-controlled trials (RCTs) of BP lowering treatment between 1966 and 2015. Sixteen trials of 52,235 patients comparing more versus less intense treatment and in 34 trials of 138,127 patients where SBP (active vs. placebo or the more vs. less intense treatment) was below or above three predetermined cutoffs.

Achieved SBP was stratified according to three SBP target ranges (149–140 mm Hg, 139–130 mm Hg and <130 mm Hg). Lowering SBP to less than 140 mm Hg reduced the relative risk of all major CV outcomes (including mortality); similar benefits were seen when SBP was lowered to less than 130 mm Hg (average 126 mm Hg). Importantly, the latter was also true when the achieved SBP in the comparator group was 130–139 mm Hg. An achieved DBP, to either 89–80 mm Hg or less than 80 mm Hg, also showed a reduction in all types of CV outcomes compared with higher DBP values.

Achieving lower SBP levels might result in adverse effects and the patients might discontinue drugs exposing them to a higher ASCVD risk. That is the reason guidelines caution that "advocating more intensive BP-lowering targets for all has to be viewed in the context of an increased risk of treatment discontinuation due to adverse events, which might offset, in part or completely, the limited incremental reduction in CV risk".[15]

■ SUMMARY

Meta-analyses have helped us in understanding the following:
- Hypertension is a risk factor for ASCVD

- Treating hypertension reduces ASCVD risk
- Prevalence of hypertension in India, coupled with a very low level of awareness, treatment, and control is a cause of concern
- Low dose diuretics or ACE inhibitors or ARBs or CCBs may be used as the first-line drug
- Beta-blockers are not as effective as other antihypertensives
- Angiotensin-converting enzyme inhibitors and ARBs are equally effective, with ACE inhibitors having an edge
- Antihypertensive therapy should be based on both BP readings and ASCVD risk
- Lower BP to less than 140/90 mm Hg in all patients. If the treatment is well tolerated, BP values should be targeted to 130/80 mm Hg or lower in most patients.

However, there are many questions that remain unanswered.

Ideal method of measuring BP: Majority of the doctors usually use auscultatory or oscillometric semiautomatic or automatic sphygmomanometers for measuring BP in their clinics. Unattended automated office BP measurement (AOBPM) was used in the SPRINT trial[16] and this generated a lot of debate and discussion about its quantitative relationship to the usual methods of measuring BP in clinics, and the feasibility of using AOBPM in clinical practice has been seriously questioned. We are all aware that conventional office BP measurement has been the basis of all the studies and the data we have on hypertension.

Though there have been advances in home BP monitoring (HBPM) and ambulatory BP monitoring (ABPM), there is uncertainty whether using HBPM or ABPM to guide therapy results in better outcome than conventional office BP-guided treatment. HBPM and ABPM do provide many more indices in understanding hypertension, but continue to remain as research tools and do not yet find a place for routine clinical use.[15]

Role of newer and vasodilator β-blockers: The guidelines available have given their recommendations based on studies that have used atenolol representing β-blockers. It is clear that β-blockers are not a homogenous class. In recent years, there are newer β-blockers with vasodilatory properties and favorable effect on central BP, aortic stiffness, endothelial dysfunction and glycemia. Labetalol, nebivolol, bisoprolol and carvedilol have shown a more favorable clinical profile than old β-blockers. However, there are no large outcome studies with these β-blockers in hypertensive population.[17,18]

Role of antihypertensive treatment in white coat hypertension: White coat hypertension is not entirely benign and persons with white coat hypertension need to be closely followed. Drug treatment for patients with white coat hypertension may have to be considered, particularly in those with a high ASCVD risk. Hypertensive patients on treatment may show higher office BP readings, and whether uptitration of drug dosage in such patients' benefits is debatable.[19]

More understanding of masked hypertension: Registry-based studies have shown that masked hypertension is prevalent in nearly 30% of treated hypertensives and is more common with diabetes and chronic kidney disease. Masked hypertension denotes a higher ASCVD risk. Again, there are no large outcome trials in patients with masked hypertension. It is wise and appropriate to ensure good control of both office BP and out of office BP.[20]

Ethnicities, drugs and response: It is known that ethnicities exhibit differences in prevalence, complications, and response to drugs in hypertension. Socioeconomic status, healthcare access, and facilities also add to the problem. Target organ damage, cardiovascular CV events and renal complications are known to be more common and severe in black patients compared with age-matched white patients at any given BP level.[21] How does Indian ethnicity play its role in a hypertensive patient as compared to others is a subject for studies.

These issues are likely to be addressed by studies and meta-analyses in near future.

■ CONCLUSION

Well-conducted meta-analyses in hypertension have provided robust evidence for guidelines to recommend strategies in the management in most of the situations. Science keeps evolving and studies in future will address the unresolved issues and find answers.

■ REFERENCES

1. Ioannidis JP. The mass production of redundant, misleading, and conflicted systematic reviews and meta-analyses. Milbank Q. 2016;94(3):485-514.

2. Ioannidis JP. Meta-research: the art of getting it wrong. Res Synth Methods. 2010;1(3-4):169-84.

3. Egger M, Davey Smith G, Schneider M, et al. Bias in meta-analysis detected by a simple, graphical test. BMJ. 1997;315(7109):629-34.

4. Egger M, Zellweger-Zähner T, Schneider M, et al. Language bias in randomised controlled trials published in English and German. Lancet. 1997;350(9074):326-9.

5. Dickersin K, Berlin JA. Meta-analysis: State-of-the-science. Epidemiol Rev. 1992;14:154-76.

6. Lewington S, Clarke R, Qizilbash N, et al. Age-specific relevance of usual blood pressure to vascular mortality: a meta-analysis of individual data for one million adults in 61 prospective studies. Lancet. 2002;360(9349):1903-13.

7. Ettehad D, Emdin CA, Kiran A, et al. Blood pressure lowering for prevention of cardiovascular disease and death: a systematic review and meta-analysis. Lancet. 2016;387(10022):957-67.

8. Anchala R, Kannuri NK, Pant H, et al. Hypertension in India: a systematic review and meta-analysis of prevalence, awareness, and control of hypertension. J Hypertens. 2014;32(6):1170-7.

9. Wright JM, Musini VM, Gill R. First-line drugs for hypertension. Cochrane Database Syst Rev. 2018;4:CD001841.

10. Wiysonge CS, Bradley HA, Volmink J, et al. Beta-blockers for hypertension. Cochrane Database Syst Rev. 2017;(8):CD002003.

11. Salvador GL, Marmentini VM, Cosmo WR, et al. Angiotensin-converting enzyme inhibitors reduce mortality compared to angiotensin receptor blockers: Systematic review and meta-analysis. Eur J Prev Cardiol. 2017;24(18):1914-24.

12. Dimou C, Antza C, Akrivos E, et al. A systematic review and network meta-analysis of the comparative efficacy of angiotensin-converting enzyme inhibitors and angiotensin receptor blockers in hypertension. J Hum Hypertens. 2018. [Epub ahead of print].

13. Karmali KN, Lloyd-Jones DM, van der Leeuw J, et al.; Blood Pressure-Lowering Treatment Trialists' Collaboration. Blood pressure-lowering treatment strategies based on cardiovascular risk versus blood pressure: A meta-analysis of individual participant data. PLoS Med. 2018;15(3):e1002538.

14. Thomopoulos C, Parati G, Zanchetti A. Effects of blood pressure lowering on outcome incidence in hypertension: 7. Effects of more vs. less intensive blood pressure lowering and different achieved blood pressure levels - updated overview and meta-analyses of randomized trials. J Hypertens. 2016;34(4):613-22.

15. Williams B, Mancia G, Spiering W, et al. 2018 ESC/ESH Guidelines for the management of arterial hypertension. Eur Heart J. 2018;39(33):3021-104.

16. Wright JT Jr, Williamson JD, Whelton PK, et al.; SPRINT Research Group. A randomized trial of intensive versus standard blood-pressure control. N Engl J Med. 2015;373(22):2103-16.

17. Bakris GL, Fonseca V, Katholi RE, et al. Metabolic effects of carvedilol vs metoprolol in patients with type 2 diabetes mellitus and hypertension: a randomized controlled trial. JAMA. 2004;292(18):2227-36.

18. Ayers K, Byrne LM, DeMatteo A, et al. Differential effects of nebivolol and metoprolol on insulin sensitivity and plasminogen activator inhibitor in the metabolic syndrome. Hypertension. 2012;59(4):893-8.

19. Franklin SS, Thijs L, Asayama K, et al. The cardiovascular risk of white-coat hypertension. J Am Coll Cardiol. 2016;68(19):2033-43.

20. Banegas JR, Ruilope LM, de la Sierra A, et al. High prevalence of masked uncontrolled hypertension in people with treated hypertension. Eur Heart J. 2014;35(46):3304-12.

21. Whelton PK, Einhorn PT, Muntner P, et al. Research needs to improve hypertension treatment and control in African Americans. Hypertension. 2016;68(5):1066-72.

SECTION 14

Miscellaneous

How to Organize and Run a Hypertension Clinic

Sadanand R Shetty

INTRODUCTION

Hypertension still remains a major health problem globally and has affected millions of individuals across continents. It already has a significant impact on mortality and morbidity due to insufficient hypertension prevention and control at community level. A linear relationship of blood pressure (BP) with adverse cardiovascular (CV) outcomes puts hypertensive individuals at increased risk of CV events.[1]

Hypertension is being classified by two major societies—(1) American Heart Association/American College of Cardiology (AHA/ACC) 2017 and (2) European Society of Cardiology/European Society of Hypertension (ESC/ESH) 2018 guidelines. In the ACC/AHA guideline, stage 1 hypertension is defined as office systolic BP (SBP) 130–139 mm Hg or diastolic BP (DBP) 80–89 mm Hg. In contrast, ESC/ESH defines stage 1 hypertension as office SBP values 140–159 mm Hg and/or DBP 90–99 mm Hg, with a similar definition in adults of any age. The European higher threshold is based on evidence from multiple randomized controlled trials (RCTs) that there is a clearer treatment benefit using the higher thresholds.[2]

Indeed, hypertension accounts for more than 5.8% of total deaths, 1.9% of years of life lost and 1.4% disability adjusted life years all over the world. These figures are more dramatic in the formerly socialist economic countries.[3] From India, a recent study done in 1.3 million adults of 18 years and above reported hypertension in 25.3% individuals.[4] With such colossal prevalence of hypertension, screening for hypertension in asymptomatic adults becomes imperative.

Even though hypertension may be simple to treat, it very often remains undiagnosed and inappropriately managed. Despite the availability of useful nondrug therapy and potent medications, treatment is too often ineffective, mainly as a consequence of the lack of patient's compliance with therapeutic regimens. Therefore, hypertension prevention and control in the community is currently a pivotal challenge. This can largely be justified with the implementation of a hypertension clinic serving the needy hypertensive patients.

WHAT IS HYPERTENSION CLINIC?

Hypertension clinic is a specialized center of supremacy for treatment of hypertension with an integrated approach. Hypertension clinic consists of specialists or members working in sync to provide comprehensive hypertensive care. These members may also be working in primary care or institutions or hospitals, but have special interest and expertise in hypertension. Teams working in hypertension clinic are also identified by their high quality expert scientific work in research and clinical management. These teams have potential even to diagnose secondary hypertension with available necessary facilities.

The preparation of a written protocol presenting the purpose, structure, and function of each hypertension clinic is highly recommended. This would certainly help in standardization of hypertension clinics across India.

NEED OF HYPERTENSION CLINIC IN INDIA

As Indian population is rapidly growing, so do hypertensive patients. Hypertensive burden is hampering our healthcare resources, wealth, increasing burden of complications and poor quality of life. A clamp of appropriate and timely treatment needs to be applied to curtail hypertensive complications and improve quality of life.

The main purpose of a hypertension clinic is to provide an expert medical advice and care for patients with hypertension. However, there are clearly quite a number of other objectives of a BP service delivered through a clinic, which are important to the healthcare system. The final shape and organization or structure of a hypertension clinic may depend on the objectives which may differ among clinics, different local health care systems, and change with time. Other clinics may not necessarily address all the possible purposes described below.

Hypertension clinics should:
- Provide high level of expertise and facilities for BP measurement
- Round the clock hypertension emergency services for the patients
- Have the ability to estimate total CV risk by assessing established indices of organ damage
- Well-equipped ambulance offering basic and advanced life support systems
- Be involved in clinical research
- Patient education
- Rehabilitation programs
- Be affiliated with other local diagnosing centers of excellence.

OBJECTIVES OF THE HYPERTENSIVE CLINIC

The objective of any hypertension clinic needs to be specific by providing qualitative and holistic hypertensive care. Other objective includes:
- *Medical service:* To deliver optimal integrated and coordinated clinic care, including assessment, investigation, treatment, ongoing monitoring, and auditing of therapeutic response and outcomes
- *Education:* To provide structured training facilities for doctors, nurses and other health professionals. Patients' education aiming to improve understanding of relevant health issues to aid long-term compliance with treatment is an additional important objective
- *Referral center:* To act as a center of excellence that receives patients with difficult, secondary, complicated hypertension referred by primary care physicians
- *Research:* To recruit patients into clinical trials and facilitate follow-up of patients in long-term trials, in collaboration with other centers of excellence and regulatory authorities.

■ WHO CAN RUN A HYPERTENSION CLINIC?

As discussed earlier, doctors working in hypertension clinic need to be an expert in managing hypertension. Long years of experience in managing hypertension can make a person expert. Doctors can be assisted by various medical and paramedical staff to carry out various other activities related to diagnosis and management of hypertension. Various societies like ACC/AHA and ESC are providing short expertized courses on overall management of hypertension, which can help you in set up of a hypertension clinic.

Organizing or Building a Set Up

Creation of a hypertension clinic providing aggregated hypertensive care is very important. It needs to be unique apart from other clinics providing hypertension care. Various aspects which can be looked upon are (Fig. 1):

- Blood pressure assessment:
  - o Standardized BP in clinic measurements with help of qualified expert physician and nurses
  - o Standardized office measurements with help of electronic devices, hybrid devices, self-measurements, or Bluetooth
  - o *Standardized out-of-office BP measurement methods*: Controlled and unbiased ambulatory and home BP monitoring need to be done
  - o *Mercury sphygmomanometers*: Still an option in some countries; which needs to be replaced by aneroid or digital instrument followed by timely calibration
  - o *Professional automated oscillometric arm devices*: It is also preferred in countries where mercury devices are banned and/or large numbers of staff measuring BP
  - o Device validation can be done by using established protocols (ESH International protocol, British Hypertension Society protocol, American Association for the Advancement of Medical Instrumentation)
  - o New technology provides automated repeated measurements and averaging, Bluetooth communication, simultaneous both arms measurements, etc.
  - o *Nurse taken BP measurements*: Preferred to physicians, if available

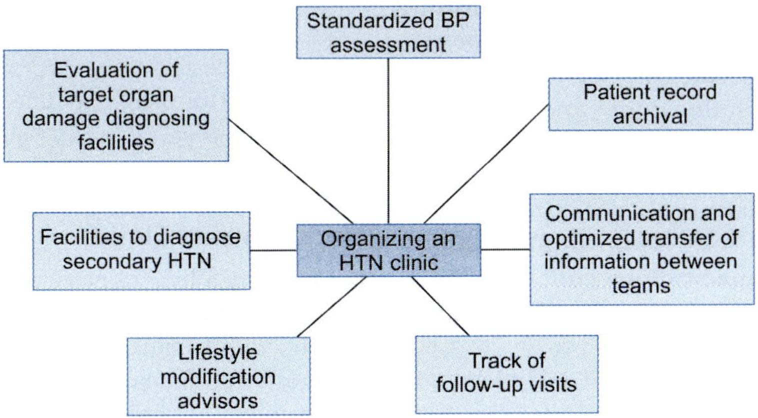

(HTN: hypertension)

Fig. 1: Schematic diagram highlighting various components involved in organizing a hypertensive clinic.

- o *Automated office BP measurements*: Office measurements taken by automated devices while patients are alone in the office examination room can be done
- o *Ambulatory BP monitoring*: Device validation required using established protocols (ESH International protocol, British Hypertension Society protocol, American Association for the Advancement of Medical Instrumentation).
- *Evaluation of target organ damage:* It can be done with the help of following tests which play a pioneer role in managing hypertension and its complications
  - o Electrocardiography
  - o Echocardiography
  - o Fundoscopy
  - o Urine dipstick
  - o Microalbuminuria (spot urine for albumin: creatinine ratio)
  - o Ankle brachial index (ABI)
  - o Carotid wall thickening (where available)
  - o Pulse wave velocity (PWV) (where available).
- *Investigation for secondary hypertension:* Direct access is required to tertiary hospitals or laboratories performing appropriate tests excluding endocrine, renal or renovascular hypertension
- *Lifestyle modification and other risk factors:* Integrated treatment plan to include consultation and follow-up of nonpharmacological intervention (diet and exercise); lipid lowering or other medication; and need for a multidisciplinary team to deliver these treatments
- *Follow-up monitoring:* It includes audit and review of individual cases and the overall BP control in the patients attending the clinic. Ideally, it plays a major role in

linking treatment impact on CV events in the population
- Communication and optimized transfer of information between the clinic and the patient and primary care and other specialist medical teams
  - o Telemedicine to improve compliance, e.g. home BP monitoring; patients' memo and appointments; and communication for unattended appointments
  - o Development of other models of continuing care such as "shared care" with general practice or "intermediate care" with specialist nurse teams for BP, diabetes, lipids, etc.
- *Patient record archival:* Establishment of database management system and computer software designed to collect, store and retrieve patients' data to be done in a structured way. The system should be designed to:
  - o Facilitate prompt monitoring of all CV risk factors and target organ damage
  - o Implement and interpret office and out-of-office BP measurements
  - o Calculate total CV risk annually
  - o Highlight major problems of individual patients
  - o Aid communication with patients, primary care and other relevant services
  - o Audit of drug use, effectiveness and outcomes.

Effective Running of a Hypertensive Clinic

For running a hypertensive clinic effectively, it needs to create a network of hypertensive patients with an aim to improve the accuracy of diagnosis and management of hypertension. Involvement of clinic in multicenter clinical research activities needs to be done further enhancing hypertensive research.

Training your staff on timely basis and guiding them in conductance of various diagnostic procedures is of paramount importance. Certified and well-qualified staff creates an edge over other clinics treating hypertension.

Dietary and Exercise Advice

To be an expert clinic, it needs to touch every aspect involved in management of hypertension. Changes in diet can lower BP, prevent the development of hypertension and reduce the risk of hypertension-related complications. Dietary strategies for the prevention of hypertension include reducing sodium intake (<5 g/day), limiting alcohol consumption, increasing potassium intake and adopting an overall dietary pattern such as the DASH (dietary approaches to stop hypertension) diet or a Mediterranean diet.[5] Moderate physical activity in form of brisk walking is also recommended by various cardiology societies.[6,7] A trained physiotherapist at the clinic would help the patient to make understand the concept of brisk walking further providing effective therapeutic care.

Hypertension Clinic as a Center of Excellence

To become a center of excellence, hypertension clinic needs to play a pivotal role in management of hypertensive patients along with improvement in quality of life. This can be done by implementation of a set of interventions mainly focused on:

- Development and management of standardized hypertension diagnostic and management systems
- Development of integrated hypertension management interventions based on interdisciplinary and intersectoral collaboration with other clinics

- Intensified public health education about disease and its complications
- Continued education programs and supply of material for public, hypertensive patients, internal staff, and doctors
- Building partners in community will help to pool many hypertensive patients to clinic and reduce burden of hypertension complications
- Advertisement about a specialized hypertension clinic creates noise and further enlarges the pool of patients to clinic.

■ CHALLENGES IN SETTING UP A HYPERTENSION CLINIC

The challenge is basically to make understand people that hypertension is a silent killer. Delay in diagnosis and lack of medication with inappropriate dosage will lead to higher morbidity and mortality. While setting a hypertension clinic, it is critical that all your staff is well trained with necessary certifications. Accredited laboratories, specialized machines, timely calibration of instruments and standardized procedures need to be followed on regular bases at all hypertensive clinics (Flowchart 1).

■ CONCLUSION

Management of hypertension with holistic care is need of day. Treatment needs to be revolutionized as per emerging standards and to match the international standards of care. This can only be achieved with the help of experts working in a hypertension clinic by providing highest level of consultative care thereby improving hypertensive care and quality of life. Additionally, hypertensive clinic can disseminate knowledge through clinical research and educational programs.

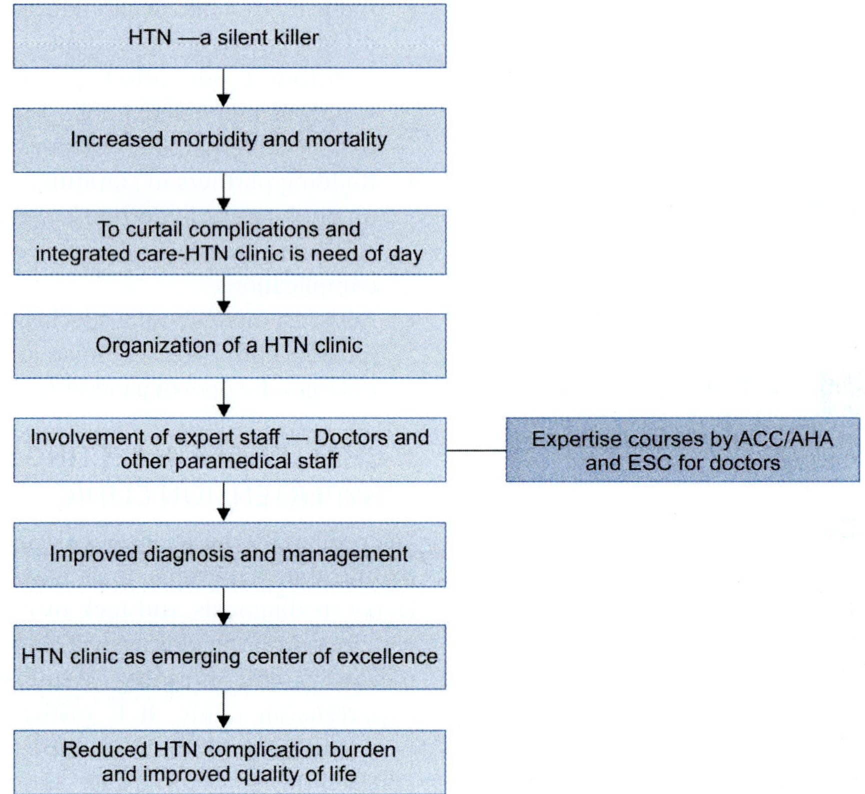

(ACC: American College of Cardiology; AHA: American Heart Association; ESC: European Society of Cardiology; HTN: hypertension)

Flowchart 1: Flowchart indicating importance of a hypertension clinic in society.

■ REFERENCES

1. Lewington S, Clarke R, Qizilbash N, et al. Age-specific relevance of usual blood pressure to vascular mortality: a meta-analysis of individual data for one million adults in 61 prospective studies. Lancet. 2002;360:1903-13.

2. American College of Cardiology. (2018). 2018 ESC/ESH Guidelines for Management of Arterial Hypertension. [online] Available from: https://www.acc.org/latest-in-cardiology/ten-points-to-remember/2018/09/04/14/41/2018-esc-esh-guidelines-for-the-management-of-arterial [Last Accessed March, 2019].

3. Murray CJL, López AD. The global burden of disease. Cambridge, Mass.: Harvard University Press; 1996.

4. Geldsetzer P, Manne-Goehler J, Theilmann M, et al. Diabetes and hypertension in India a nationally representative study of 1.3 million adults. JAMA Intern Med. 2018;178:363-72.

5. Bazzano LA, Green T, Harrison TN, et al. Dietary approaches to prevent hypertension. Curr Hypertens Rep. 2013;15(6): 694-702.

6. Williams B, Mancia G, Spiering W, et al. 2018 ESC/ESH Guidelines for the management of arterial hypertension. Eur Heart J. 2018;39(33)3021-104.

7. American College of Cardiology. (2018). 2017 High Blood Pressure Clinical Practice Guideline. [online] Available from: https://www.acc.org/latest-in-cardiology/ten-points-to-remember/2017/11/09/11/41/2017-guideline-for-high-blood-pressure-in-adults [Last Accessed March, 2019].

Dilemmas in Hypertension Management

YP Munjal, Niharika Aggarwal, Ghan Shyam Pangtey

■ INTRODUCTION

Hypertension is a leading cause of global disease burden and is independent risk factor for coronary heart disease, congestive heart failure, cerebrovascular accident, renal failure and peripheral vascular diseases. The morbidity and mortality associated with hypertension is considerable. World Health Organization (WHO) defined hypertension as "a humanitarian tragedy on a planetary scale." It is estimated that due to hypertension up to 7 million people die prematurely and around 64 million disability adjusted life years (DALY) are lost. Prevalence of hypertension in India is around 29.8%[1] (with definition of cut-off values 140/90 mm Hg) with urban prevalence around 33% and rural prevalence around 25%. The prevalence in western countries is even higher, up to 40% of western population are living with high blood pressure (BP).

First comprehensive guidelines for detection and management of high BP was published in 1977 by National Heart, Lung and Blood Institute (NHLBI) of National Institute Health (NIH) of United States of America and in subsequent years a series of Joint National Committee (JNC) on detection, evaluation and treatment of high BP guidelines were published to improve management and awareness about hypertension.

Hypertension is a leading noncommunicable public health problem and the morbidity and mortality associated with it is considerable worldwide. In recent times, noncommunicable diseases (NCD) have overtaken communicable diseases as the leading cause of death, it is estimated that 50% of global disease burden is due to NCD.

There has been rapid advancement in knowledge, evaluation, diagnosis and management of hypertension, but we are still unable to control hypertension epidemic. We are still not able to manage various dilemmas of hypertension; from availability of proper calibrated BP equipment, release of multiple guidelines with different targets and different recommendations by different scientific societies creating more confusion, refractory hypertension and complex evaluation algorithms for secondary hypertensions which are difficult to interpret and follow by general practitioners, and white coat hypertension and masked hypertension, etc.

The important issues and dilemmas in hypertension management are shown in box 1. We will need to solve these dilemmas for

---

Box 1: Dilemmas in hypertension management.

- **Sphygmomanometer:** Aneroid/oscillometric digital blood pressure device
- Calibration of sphygmomanometer
- Ambulatory blood pressure measurement
- Central aortic pressure versus peripheral blood pressure
- White coat or masked hypertension
- **Multiplicity of guidelines:** Joint National Committee-8/AHA 2017

---

better control of BP and achieving reduction in target organ damage and reduced mortality and morbidity.

MEASUREMENT OF BLOOD PRESSURE

Mercury sphygmomanometer was considered ideal since and "gold standard" since immemorial, however with knowledge of neurotoxin hazard of mercury, it has to be withdrawn and banned. Aneroid sphygmomanometer is considered error prone and requires frequent calibrations. In present time, majority of the physicians use either aneroid sphygmomanometer or oscillometric battery operated BP equipment. The battery-operated oscilloscope has become very popular for home based self-monitoring of BP. There are few advantages in use of these oscillometric devices. These battery-operated BP devices are very popular with general physicians as well as patients. The various advantages of oscillometric/digital devices include ease of use, cheap, easy to use, read and interpret compared to aneroid sphygmomanometers. Some of these digital instruments may also have memory function with it for remembering and recording previous BP records. WHO also recommends its use in resource limited countries due to its cost-effectiveness and minimal need for trained manpower. These digital

BP instrument remove the terminal digit preference seen with aneroid and mercury instrument and also help in diagnosing and correcting white coat hypertension. However, in present time, the majority of oscillometric devices are sold in the market without any rigorous validation or check.[2] Since the algorithms to calculate the diastolic pressure and systolic pressure from the measured mean are proprietary in nature, each model must be authorized separately before being promoted. The digital oscilloscope BP instruments are still not validated for use in elderly population, diabetic patient, pregnant females and in patient with arrhythmias. Therefore, its use should be with caution in patient with these conditions and there is urgent need for further trials in these group of patients to show their consistency in BP recording.

CALIBRATION OF SPHYGMOMANOMETER

The sphygmomanometer should be of standardized quality and specification. The various standardization recognized in the world includes—United States Food and Drug administration (USFDA), European CE, British Standard Institute (BSI) and in India, Bureau of Indian Standards (BIS) or ISO. Every sphygmomanometer should be calibrated regularly from every 6 months or every year as per WHO recommendation, depending upon manufacturer's instructions. In case the BP instrument is not calibrated regularly then it may faulty provide readings and lead to mismanagement. The calibration technique involves testing pressure readings between a standard pressure meter, which could either be a digital pressure gauge or a mercury sphygmomanometer, and a test device, using a Y-connector to the cuff, which is wrapped around a rigid cylinder. As to possible replacement of aneroid for mercury devices, recent articles stated that when aneroid devices were calibrated and maintained suitably, they performed equally or even better than the mercury counterparts.[2]

A study was conducted on aneroid sphygmomanometer readings against mercury manometer in Brazil's capital São Paulo between 2009 and 2010, in both private and public hospitals.[3] The aneroid BP device was considered out of calibration when the differences in reading between test and control instrument were 4 mm Hg or more. The study found that 56.2% of manometers were not calibrated. It was also observed that in 70.2% cases, no periodic evaluation was done. There were significant number of equipment with aged/damaged rubber extension, leaking valve and manometer not pointing to zero during rest.

AMBULATORY BLOOD PRESSURE MONITORING

Ambulatory BP monitoring (ABPM) has been given much importance in recent American College of Cardiology/American Heart Association (ACC/AHA) 2017 guidelines as office recordings are 15–20/5–10 mm Hg higher compared from home BP monitoring (HBPM) and average 24 hour ABPM, thus preventing inappropriate diagnosis and ruling out white collar hypertension.[4] It is also useful in optimization of therapy and thus prevents postural hypotension and poor compliance. Other indication for ABPM are resistant hypertension, autonomic dysfunction and episodic hypertension.

CENTRAL AORTIC PRESSURE

There are recent evidences of central aortic systolic pressure (CASP) being better predictor of cardiovascular events compared to brachial pressures.[5] Using pulse wave in conjunction with systolic blood pressure (SBP) and diastolic blood pressure (DBP) readings from traditional inflatable cuff, CASP values are computed with 99% correlation with actual surgically measured CASP readings particularly more important in young people as peripheral arteries are compliant so central and peripheral BP may differ.

WHITE COAT OR MASKED HYPERTENSION

When BP recordings are relatively higher in office as compared to home recording, the condition of raised BP is called "masked hypertension". The diagnosis of white coat hypertension is challenging to make. Although it can occur at any age, it is more common in older men and women. White coat hypertension is the result of an exaggerated white coat effect of physician, which may be a conditioned anxiety response. Masked and situational hypertension known as "white coat hypertension" must be considered in this situation. Home and office BP measurements as well as 24-hour ambulatory BP monitoring may be helpful in diagnosing this condition and help in avoiding unnecessary drug treatment which may be harmful too.

MULTIPLICITY OF GUIDELINES

In recent years there has been sudden increase in number of guidelines by various professional bodies for hypertension evaluation, diagnose and management. There is no doubt that development of guidelines will lead to improvement in disease knowledge and better management and ultimately to reduced cardiovascular deaths. The NHLBI and NIH have been historically involved in development of hypertension guidelines since 1977. The last hypertension guideline by NHLBI was published in 2014 as JNC-8 guideline. The controversies started to erupt since year 2017 when up to 9 hypertension guidelines were published in USA from different societies. The controversy reached next level when the ACC/AHA 2017 reduced the BP threshold to 130/80 for diagnosis of hypertension. The controversy aggravated to maximum peak with publication of 2018 European Society of Cardiology/European Society for Hypertension (ESC/EHS) guideline which did not agree to reduction in BP threshold sighting inadequate evidence. Although critical assessment of current science may expose ambiguities and uncertainties, conflicting references may create dilemmas into physician's mind and confuse the physicians and possibly undermine the credibility of all recommendations. Therefore, the guidelines should be based on strong evidence only and to be made with consensus. These recent guidelines have created more confusion, than solving the issue.

Joint National Committee Classification of Hypertension

Joint National Committee-7 was published in year 2003. It defined and classified BP into four categories given in Table 1.[6] They introduced the term prehypertension (systolic BP: 120–139 mm Hg and diastolic BP: 80–89 mm Hg).

TABLE 1: Classification of blood pressure for adults according to Joint National Committee-7.

BP Classification	SBP mm Hg		DBP mm Hg
Normal	<120	AND	<80
Prehypertension	120–139	AND	80–89
Stage 1 hypertension	140–159	OR	90–99
Stage 2 hypertension	≥160	OR	≥100

BP: Blood pressure; SBP: Systolic blood pressure; DBP: Diastolic blood pressure

JNC-8 classification was published in 2014. It kept same classification of hypertension as Joint National Committee-7 but gave treatment goals in general population, diabetic and chronic kidney disease cohort and antihypertensive agent of choice in these cohorts (Tables 2 and 3).[6]

American College of Cardiology/ American Heart Association 2017

American College of Cardiology/American Heart Association released their combined hypertension guidelines in 2017.[4] ACC/AHA 2017 definition left out prehypertension and isolated systolic hypertension. The major change was lowering of the cut-off values for hypertension definition in order to increase awareness in population at large and timely initiation of lifestyle modification (Table 4). This reduction of threshold for diagnosis of hypertension (SBP/DBP: >120/>80 mm Hg) has major implications. Firstly, it increased the prevalence of hypertension in society manifold and secondly, it labeled millions of people diseased with high BP, who were previously known to have only borderline high normal blood pressure. This increased burden of hypertension after ACC/AHA guideline has created major challenges for resource limited developing countries. First-line agents are advised that include angiotensin converting enzyme (ACE) inhibitor/aldosterone receptor blocker (ARB)/calcium channel blocker (CCB)/ thiazide diuretic (TD). Nonpharmacological treatment of hypertension includes weight loss in overweight and obese patients, heart healthy diet in form of omega three fatty acids,

TABLE 2: Treatment goals in management of hypertension.

	General population	General population	Diabetic patients	Chronic kidney disease
Age (years)	18–59	≥60	≥18	≥18
Blood pressure (mm Hg)	<140/90	<150/90	<140/90	<140/90

TABLE 3: Antihypertensive agents of choice in various cohorts.

General population	General population	Diabetic patient	Diabetic patient	Chronic kidney disease	Chronic kidney disease
Black	Non-black	Black	Non-black	Black	Non-black
• CCB • TD	• ACE • ARB • CCB • TD	• CCB • TD	• ACE • ARB • CCB • TD	• ACE • ARB	• ACE • ARB

(ACE: angiotensin converting enzyme; ARB: aldosterone receptor blocker; CCB: calcium channel blocker; TD: thiazide diuretic)

TABLE 4: Blood pressure categories as per ACC/AHA 2017 in adults.*

BP category	SBP		DBP
Normal	<120 mm Hg	AND	<80 mm Hg
Elevated	120–129 mm Hg	AND	<80 mm Hg
Stage 1 hypertension	130–139 mm Hg	OR	80–89 mm Hg
Stage 2 hypertension	≥140 mm Hg	OR	≥90 mm Hg

*Individuals with SBP and DBP in two categories should be designated to higher BP category.
BP: Blood pressure; SBP: Systolic blood pressure; DBP: Diastolic blood pressure

TABLE 5: European Society for Hypertension 2018 guidelines for diagnosis of hypertension.

Category	Systolic (mm Hg)		Diastolic (mm Hg)
Optimal	<120	AND	<80
Normal	120–129	AND	80–84
High normal	130–139	OR	85–89
Grade 1 hypertension	140–159	OR	90–99
Grade 2 hypertension	160–179	OR	100–109
Grade 3 hypertension	≥180	OR	≥110
Isolated systolic hypertension	≥140	AND	<90

low sodium and potassium rich diet and limitation of alcohol intake to two standard drinks per day in men and one standard drink per day in women, smoking cessation and finally physical activity and exercise schedule.

European Society of Cardiology/ European Society for Hypertension Guidelines 2018

European Society for Hypertension published their latest guidelines in 2018 (Table 5).[7]

In 2018 ESC-ESH guidelines kept the old definition for diagnosis of hypertension (>140/80 mm Hg) instead of ACC/AHA 2017 guideline which reduce the diagnosis threshold for hypertension to 130/80 mm Hg. According to ESC/ESH experts, there is not much evidence that BP >130/80 can lead to excessive morbidity and mortality. Although the ESC/EHS guideline agreed to keep BP target of 130/80 mm Hg for known hypertensives similar to 2017 ACC/AHA guideline.

CHANGING CONCEPTS IN DEFINITION AND MANAGEMENT

- Thresholds for hypertension has been decreased from ≥140/90 mm Hg to ≥130/80 mm Hg (ACC/AHA 2017) with impact of increasing prevalence of hypertension in general population however leading to increase awareness and timely initiation of lifestyle changes but with increased prevalence and burden to society and health care
- Isolated systolic hypertension and pre-hypertension terms has been removed from latest hypertension guidelines (2017–2018) and has been clubbed in stage 1/2 hypertension categories thus making classification easier and less cumbersome
- Importance of HBPM and ABPM has increased in diagnosis and management of hypertension compared to office readings
- Incorporation of risk assessment scores has been recommended in deciding therapeutic plan for the patient as in form of ACC/AHA pooled risk equation estimator and Framingham's risk scoring
- Treatment thresholds have been reduced in all cohorts of patients including diabetes, chronic kidney disease with or without transplant, heart failure, stable ischemic heart disease and peripheral vascular disease from ≥140/90 to ≥130/80
- Revision of BP treatment goals. BP treatment goals have been revised and targets have been reduced from what JNC-8 recommended
- Although first-line antihypertensive agents remain similar to JNC-8 guidelines in the form of ACE/ARB/CCB/TD, however, when to initiate monotherapy versus combination therapy is defined. Stage 1 hypertensive patients with clinical atherosclerotic cardiovascular disease or 10-year cardiovascular disease risk >10% should be initiated with monotherapy with gradual up titration of doses and those in stage 2 hypertension or with BP more than 20/10 mm Hg above treatment goals should be started on 2 first-line agents of different class either separately or as fixed dose combination with monthly follow-ups till targets are met.

REFERENCES

1. Anchala R, Kannuri N, Pant H, et al. Hypertension in India. J Hypertens. 2014;32(6):1170-7.
2. Ogedegbe G, Pickering D. Principles and techniques of blood pressure measurement. Cardiol Clin. 2010;28(4):571-86.
3. De-Souza ST, de-Andrade TG, Lima de GJ, et al. Evaluation of the conditions of use of sphygmomanometers in hospital services. Acta paul Enferm. 2012;25(6):940-6.
4. Whelton P, Carey R, Aronow W, et al. 2017 ACC/AHA/AAPA/ABC/ACPM/AGS/APhA/ASH/ASPC/NMA/PCNA Guideline for the Prevention, Detection, Evaluation, and Management of High Blood Pressure in Adults. J Am Coll Cardiol. 2018;71(19):e127-e248.
5. McEniery CM, Cockcroft JR, Roman MJ, et al. Central blood pressure: current evidence and clinical importance. Eur Heart J. 2014;35(26):1719-25.
6. Chobanian AV, Bakris GL, Black HR, et al. Seventh report of the Joint National Committee on Prevention, Detection, Evaluation, and Treatment of High Blood Pressure. Hypertension. 2003;42:1206-52.
7. Williams B, Mancia G, Spiering W, et al. 2018 ESC/ESH Guidelines for the management of arterial hypertension. Eur Heart J. 2018;39(33):3021-104.

Natural History of Hypertension

BC Kalmath

INTRODUCTION

High blood pressure (BP) is considered to be one of the most relevant and prevalent risk factors for disability and death in the world. Over 1 billion people suffer from hypertension, causing approximately 9.4 million fatalities each year. Overall, the prevalence of hypertension is around 40% of the world population, and it shows a steep rise with increase in age with 7% in people in the age of 18–39 years and as high as 65% in people greater than 59 years. BP is directly and strongly associated with cardiovascular and overall mortality in the middle and older age people.

A continuous log-linear connection is found between BP and vascular events across a broad spectrum by prospective cohort studies, seemingly starting at 115 mm Hg systolic BP and 75 mm Hg for diastolic with no apparent threshold. Considering this, most cardiovascular complications associated with BP happen in people with prehypertension.

Approximately, half of patients with hypertension develop associated end-organ damage if BP remains untreated for 7–10 years. The rest of the patients show a less impactful course with slowly occurring hypertensive complications. Less than 5% of individuals with high BP enter a very expeditious, sometimes malignant course with rapid cardiovascular, kidney and neurological function deterioration.

SUBTYPES OF HYPERTENSION

According to National Health and Nutrition Examination Survey (NHANES), different subtypes of hypertension are:

- Isolated systolic hypertension (ISH) is defined as a systolic BP >140 mm Hg and diastolic BP <90 mm Hg
- Isolated diastolic hypertension (IDH) is defined as a diastolic BP >90 mm Hg and a systolic BP <140 mm Hg
- Systolic diastolic hypertension (SDH) is defined as a diastolic BP >90 mm Hg and a systolic BP >140 mm Hg.

PHYSIOLOGY OF VARIOUS SUBTYPES

- An increase in the stiffness of the aorta and large elastic arteries not accompanied by a rise in arteriolar resistance may lead to ISH
- A predominant rise in arteriolar resistance with increase in arterial stiffness may lead to combined SDH
- An increase in arteriolar resistance without increase in arterial stiffness leads to IDH.

EFFECT OF AGE ON VARIOUS SUBTYPES

Isolated diastolic rise could be considered a marker of good elasticity of big arteries and aorta, which may be due to a lack of atherosclerotic lesions.

On the contrary, because the rigidity of aorta and large arteries tends to enhance with age, systolic BP also tends to rise with age, leading to an increased ISH frequency in the elderly people. The decrease in diastolic BP with increasing age was correlated with the advancement of aortic atherosclerosis, reported by one study by the emergence of new calcifications or the expansion of old calcified fields.

One of the confounding factors in the evaluation of subtypes of hypertension is the progressive amplification of the pressure wave during transmission from the aorta to the peripheral arteries, which is a phenomenon that predominates in young people and reduces with aging. Brachial diastolic BP can therefore overestimate aortic BP, especially in young people.

EFFECT OF VARIOUS SUBTYPES ON PROGRESSION OF HYPERTENSION

According to Framingham Heart Study and HARVEST (Hypertension and Ambulatory Recording Venetia Study) report, the risk of developing hypertension over the years may vary according to hypertension subtype in the screening phase. Young-to-middle-age subjects with ISH at baseline screening had an increased likelihood of developing hypertension during subsequent years compared to subjects with BP <140/90 mm Hg. The risk was smaller than in persons with SDH. Patients with IDH entry also have an increased likelihood of developing hypertension with a

significant adjusted odds ratio, only slightly greater than those with ISH.

Major intervention trials (ALLHAT, CONVINCE, HARVEST) have shown that drug treatment usually generates a higher degree of diastolic than systolic BP control; therefore, it is now reported that high systolic BP is more hard to manage, particularly among the elderly people. More than 90% of participants accomplished diastolic BP normalization in the Hypertension Optimal Treatment (HOT) study; whereas, less than 50% attained systolic BP normalization.[1] Approximately, 90% of subjects had their diastolic BP normalized after 2 years of therapy in the Antihypertensive and Lipid-Lowering Trial to Prevent Heart Attack (ALLHAT) and the Controlled Onset Verapamil Investigation of Cardiovascular Events (CONVINCE) trials, while about 50% attained systolic BP normalization.[2,3]

Among the hypertensive patients who received treatment, those having uncontrolled systolic BP were having higher risk of cardiovascular disease as compared to those with uncontrolled diastolic BP after confounding variables had been adjusted. Therefore, the true challenge and the main focus of treatment is effective systolic BP control.

TARGET ORGAN DAMAGE

Only a small proportion of the hypertensive population has an elevation of BP alone, while additional cardiovascular risk factors are present in most of the patients. When elevated BP is related with other cardiovascular risk factors, the total cardiovascular risk exceeds the sum of its individual components.

Pathophysiology of Target Organ Damage

Structural modifications in arteries, arterioles, and target organs is produced by hypertension in many patterns, which is a result of mechanical effects of BP and shear stress, and the action of neurohormonal systems, comprising the endothelins, catecholamines, renin–angiotensin-aldosterone system, and agents produced in perivascular fat and inflammatory mediators. A significant role may be played by resistance arteries in development of hypertension. Resistance arteries can also contribute in the pathogenesis of complications related to cardiovascular system. Chronic high BP generates vascular stretching, which induces complex cascades of signal transduction that leads to vascular remodeling. One of the renin–angiotensin-aldosterone system's final products, i.e. angiotensin II may initiate vascular remodeling and injury through many processes comprising cell growth, production of reactive oxygen species (ROS), vasoconstriction, and inflammation. Also, the endothelium is also an important vascular tone regulator. Function of endothelium is impaired in patients of hypertension, with decreased nitric oxide-mediated vasodilation and enhanced vascular tone related with proinflammatory and prothrombotic state and vascular remodeling.

The prehypertension phase can be defined as the combination of normal plus high-normal BP categories (for systolic BP, values range from 120 mm Hg to 139 mm Hg and for diastolic 80–89 mm Hg). During this phase, recurrent perturbations of cardiovascular homeostasis happen, which reflect an array of environmental and hereditary factors. Over the time, these small modifications accumulate and produce larger changes in pathophysiology that can be recognized as early hypertension. Early functional perturbations can be minor and reversible, while subsequent major chronic changes tend to be slower, larger, and irreversible.

Difference of Pathophysiological Mechanism of Target Organ Damage with Age

Vascular remodeling occurs in small arteries and arterioles in younger people with high BP. Usually, it is eutrophic with decreased lumen diameter and normal cross section of the media, decreased or increased stiffness, and enhanced deposition of the extracellular matrix and connected with endothelial dysfunction.

Systolic BP tends to enhance with age, which results in an increased frequency of ISH related with high pulse pressure in the elder people. This form of hypertension may represent diffuse atherosclerotic procedures. It is therefore regarded a significant cardiovascular risk determinant. When BP stays elevated for an extended period of time, especially in patients over 55 years of age, vascular changes happen mainly in large and conduit arteries (i.e. aorta). These arteries become stiffer as arteriosclerosis develops, which lead to enhanced pulse pressure.

■ REFERENCES

1. Hansson L. The Hypertension Optimal Treatment study and the importance of lowering blood pressure.J Hypertens Suppl. 1999;17(1):S9-13.
2. ALLHAT Officers and Coordinators for the ALLHAT Collaborative Research Group. Major outcomes in high-risk hypertensive patients randomized to angiotensin-converting enzyme inhibitor or calcium channel blocker vs diuretic: The Antihypertensive and Lipid-Lowering Treatment to Prevent Heart Attack Trial (ALLHAT).JAMA. 2002;288(23):2981-97.
3. ack HR, Elliott WJ, Grandits G, et al. Principal Results of the Controlled Onset Verapamil Investigation of Cardiovascular End Points (CONVINCE) Trial. JAMA. 2003;289(16):2073-82.

Lipid and Hypertension

Raman Puri

INTRODUCTION

Dietary cholesterol intake is also among one of factors known to have major impact on blood pressure (BP).[1]

A well-established causal risk has been associated for coronary heart disease (CHD) between low-density lipoprotein (LDL), cholesterol, and BP. Risk of CHD is persistent irrespective of threshold LDL levels described in guidelines. So, patients with moderately elevated LDL-cholesterol (LDL-C) level or BP level are at higher risk of developing a CHD compared to those with lower levels. CHD risk is known to increase with prolonged exposure to higher LDL-C.[2,3]

Both American and European guidelines recommend dietary and statin therapy intervention for a patient having dietary cholesterol 190 mg/dL or higher as an indication statement.[4,5] Treating hypertension only reduces CHD risk by approximately 25%. Treating hypercholesterolemia in hypertensive patients reduces residual CHD risk by more than 35%.[6]

Patients with elevated BP and normal lipid levels may be benefitted with intensive cholesterol reduction. This also helps in reduction of large arterial stiffness. A study done by Ferrier found a greater reduction in systolic arterial pressure (SAP), mean arterial pressure (MAP), and diastolic arterial pressure (DAP).[7]

Few more studies have demonstrated benefit of additional statin therapy producing a greater reduction in systolic blood pressure (SBP), MAP, and diastolic blood pressure (DBP) in both controlled hypertensive and hypercholesterolemic patients.[8,9]

Combination of hypertension and dyslipidemia is deadly and contributes to increased risk of cardiovascular disease (CVD) and coronary artery disease (CAD) than individual contribution. It is known that controlling BP alone would prevent 37% of CHD events, whereas optimal control of BP prevents 62% and a combination of BP and cholesterol leads to reduction in 76% of CHD events.[10]

CORRELATION BETWEEN HYPERTENSION AND HYPERLIPIDEMIA

Several studies have shown that most of the hypertensive patients undergo inconsistent treatment, and there was significant instability of serum total cholesterol (TC), triglycerides (TG), high-density lipoprotein (HDL), and LDL in hypertensive patients.[11-13]

It has been found that elevated BP is strongly associated with increased risk of CVD and CHD events regardless of presence or extent of dyslipidemia. This highlights that when BP is elevated, risk is elevated, regardless of the presence of dyslipidemia.[14]

The "co-existence and interplay of dyslipidemia and hypertension" produces a marked increase in CVD risk; this is term as "LIPITENSION" by Dalal et al. (2012) which may help clinicians in management and easy identification of the two conditions together, ultimately arrest cardiovascular event, and can significantly improve the outcomes.[15] HDL levels were slightly lower among Asians compared with non-Asians, a population who require further study and targeted intervention.[16]

Statins are known speculated via improvement in endothelial function, which may produce reduction in large artery stiffness. Also it was found that more the reduction in LDL-C, better the reduction in arterial stiffness.[17] As per recent study, cardiologists prescribe combination antihypertensive therapies more likely than endocrinologists.[18]

COMPLICATIONS OF BOTH HYPERTENSION AND HYPERLIPIDEMIA

Some studies concluded saying patients having a combination of both hypertension and hyperlipidemia may impair cognition in later life and treatment with respective drugs may help overcome this problem.[19-23]

It is well documented that high LDL-C and low HDL-C are related to future risk of cardiovascular events.[24] As the person gets old, there is a strong possibility of older people having both dyslipidemia and hypertension. But, only 10% of populations having both are under control.[25]

Prevention of around 80% CHD events could be possible as quoted by the Framingham heart study.[26] Dyslipidemia and high BP in diabetic patients increase the risk of microvascular and macrovascular complications.[27] Hypertension and dyslipidemia are often associated with insulin resistance and aggravation of diabetic kidney disease.[28,29]

Hypertension and dyslipidemia both are aggravating factors of diabetic nephropathy, thus more attention to dyslipidemia and appropriate treatment of hypertension could attenuate progression of diabetic kidney disease.[30]

MANAGEMENT OF DYSLIPIDEMIA AND HYPERTENSION EVIDENCES

The evidence from clinical trial data suggests a mutualism between blood pressure control and lipid lowering. The first interaction between simvastatin and antihypertensives was published by Sposito et al. (1999).[9]

In a study of a small population of patients with hypertension and high serum TC, the results of the antihypertensive effect of enalapril or lisinopril was significantly enhanced by pravastatin or lovastatin concomitantly administered. It was verified from a trial that a "small" mean reductions in BP (2–4 mm Hg) correlate to a significant difference in CHD risk.[31]

Goode et al. evidenced from eight controlled, lipid-lowering trials with populations totaling 18,000 individuals showed reductions in SBP ranging from 1.3 mm Hg to 6 mm Hg among those receiving lipid-lowering therapy.[32]

In clinical trials, Glorioso et al. and Bandinelli et al. reported non–placebo controlled trials, which showed reductions in SBP and in DBP of 8 mm Hg and 5 mm Hg, respectively with pravastatin and atorvastatin.[33,34]

In a study showed apparent synergy between atorvastatin and the amlodipine +/- perindopril regimen were less likely to suffer any of the major CV end points evaluated in the trial when the results of Anglo-Scandinavian Cardiac Outcomes Trial—Blood Pressure Lowering Arm (ASCOT-BPLA) and Anglo-Scandinavian Cardiac Outcomes Trial-Lipid-Lowering Arm (ASCOT-LLA) were viewed together.[35]

In a comparative study of combined therapy of lipanthyl (fenofibrate) 200 mg with rosuvastatin 10 mg and monotherapy by rosuvastatin 20 mg in diabetic type 2 patients with hypertension, 40 patients (40–65 years old) with high level of TGs and LDL-C blood with pressure between 140/90 mm Hg and 180/110 mm Hg were studied. In group a significantly reduction of BP was found after 12 weeks, systolic—26.6% (p <0.001) and diastolic—18.0%; and improved lipid range.[36]

■ STUDIES

Both developed and developing countries are facing challenge of increased incidence of diabetes. This will ultimately increase number of cardiovascular events, cerebral vascular events, and peripheral vascular, and other cardiovascular illness.[37]

A study was done to quantify impact of long-term exposure of moderately elevated LDL-C and BP on risk of developing a CHD from a 16-year follow-up in the Framingham heart study. The Western Electric Study analyzed relation of nutrient intake to change in BP for a period of 9 years and postulated a positive result about annual increase in BP with intake of dietary cholesterol.[38]

A study was done to assess effect of dietary cholesterol on BP (International Study of Macro-/Micronutrients on Blood Pressure—INTERMAP study) in both men and women was studied in four countries. In total, 83 nutrients were studied on 4,680 participants from United States of America, United Kingdom, China, and Japan. Dietary cholesterol was directly related to SBP

in all multivariate models studied with a difference of around 0.6–1.4 mm Hg in high dietary cholesterol intake group. As serum cholesterol is strongly correlated with endothelial dysfunction and reduced nitric oxide production, improvement in dietary cholesterol may improve BP in body.[39]

Another dietary intervention study showed lowering of SBP with consumption of vegetarian diet, dietary fiber, vegetable protein, potassium, magnesium, high PUFA diet along with reduced intake of dietary cholesterol, and total and saturated fat.[40]

A study also highlighted lowering of BP in hyperlipidemic patients by cutting down fats (25% of energy), and restricting cholesterol to less than 150 mg/day with or without addition of dietary fiber intake.[41]

Reduction in dietary cholesterol was also a part of two DASH (Dietary Approaches to Stop Hypertension) feeding trials which produced a reduction in both pre-hypertensive and hypertensive adults. Trial results are concordant with concept of reduction in dietary cholesterol contributes to reduction in BP.[42,43]

The large Fenofibrate Intervention and Event Lowering in Diabetes (FIELD) study and the Brisighella Heart Study have already shown that effective reduction in BP with usage of statin and fibrates.[44,45]

Pathogenic role of LDL-C on hypertensive was evaluated on 84 patients suffering from Cushing's disease. Study noted patients having high LDL-C also had significant high levels of body mass index (BMI), SBP, cholesterol, TG, and apolipoprotein B (apoB). LDL-C remained positively associated with SBP even after adjusting the covariates. Irrespective of statin intake, patients with LDL-C more than or equal to 3.37 mmol/L had higher SBP than patients with LDL-C less than 3.37 mmol/L. So, an independent association was found between LDL-C and SBP in Cushing's disease patients. Study speculated that LDL-C may be a pathogenic factor for producing hypertension in patients.[46]

Patients suffering with diabetes, chronic kidney disease (CKD), and CHD or those having heavy pill burden should be encouraged for combination antihypertensive therapies instead of heavy pill burden to improve treatment compliance and target BP rates. A study was done on 17,096 Chinese hypertensive dyslipidemia patients receiving lipid-lowering treatment for more than 3 months. Aim was to assess BP and LDL-C goal attainment. Also, factors interfering with BP, or BP and LDL-C goal attainment rates and antihypertensive treatment patterns were analyzed. Overall, goal attainment rates for combined BP and LDL-C as well BP or LDL-C targets were 22.9%, 31.9%, and 60.1%, respectively. Here, combination therapies failed to show benefit for BP goal achievement particularly.[47]

Another big 16-year follow-up outcome study called Anglo-Scandinavian Cardiac Outcomes Trial (ASCOT) showed beneficial effects of antihypertensive treatment on top of lipid-lowering therapy. ASCOT was a multicenter randomized control trial with UK-based patients with hypertension. Patients were followed up for all-cause and cardiovascular mortality for a median of 15.7 years. Patients were randomized to either beta-blocker or calcium channel blocker treatment for control of hypertension. It was found significantly 29% lower stroke rate deaths in calcium channel blocker group. Significant cardiovascular death reduction occurred by 15% among patients on statin treatment. Trial concluded showing mortality benefits with long-term antihypertensive and lipid-lowering treatments.[48]

Antihypertensive and Lipid-Lowering to prevent Heart Attacks Trial (ALLHAT) is the other trial to study CV outcome on patients taking both antihypertensive and lipid-lowering drugs and compared different monotherapy. In ALLHAT, pravastatin was compared with usual care, but the results were not much satisfactory. Both ASCOT and ALLHAT assessed the potential benefits of statins in patients with hypertension. In ASCOT, atorvastatin was compared with placebo. Unfortunately, in ALLHAT, many patients in the usual care group received statins and only a small difference in cholesterol was detected between the treatment groups, which resulted in the trial being underpowered to compare effects on major cardiovascular endpoints.[49]

A trial called Heart Outcomes Prevention Evaluation-3 (HOPE-3) compared effects of BP and lipid-lowering drug on cognition. Patients without known CVD were randomized to candesartan plus hydrochlorothiazide and also to rosuvastatin. Both drugs were compared against placebo to assess if combination of these drugs can slow down cognitive decline in older people. After a median follow-up for 5.7 years, BP drug duo reduced SBP by 6 mm Hg and lipid-lowering reduced LDL-C by 24.8 mg/dL. Though there was reduction in both BP and LDL-C, but study found that results were not significant.[50]

One major study called the Cardiovascular Health Study was done to assess combined association of lipids and BP and their relation to incident CVD in elderly. Study was done in 4,311 participants aging more than 65 years with no prior history of CVD. Relationship of LDL, HDL, or non-HDL cholesterol combined with BP categories to know risk of incident CVD including CHD [angina, myocardial infarction (MI), angioplasty, coronary bypass surgery, or CHD death], stroke, claudication, and CVD death over 15 years was evaluated. CVD rates were lower around 38.4 when BP recording was <120/80 mm Hg and LDL-C <100 mg/dL. Rates were higher around 94.8 when BP was ≥160/100 mm Hg and LDL-C ≥160 mg/dL, and were around 28.9 when BP <120/80 mm Hg and HDL >60–87.1 mg/dL for a BP ≥160/100 mm Hg and HDL-C

<40 mg/dL. Hazard ratios for CVD event rates were high around 2.1 times when BP was ≥160/100 mm Hg and LDL-C ≥160 mg/dL and 2.1 times when BP ≥160/100 mm Hg and HDL-C <40 mg/dL (all p <0.01). The authors conclude that increased BP is associated with increased CVD risk in elderly person across all lipid levels. Low HDL-C can add risk in hypertensive and LDL-C added risk even if BP <140/90 mm Hg.[14]

Continued evaluation of both BP and lipid levels in elderly persons is necessary. In the Multiple Risk Factor Intervention Trial (MRFIT), CHD event rates were 10 times higher in lowest quintile of TC and SBP to highest quintile for both. It also meant both SBP and TC increased CHD risk regardless of baseline levels. Lower treatment rates for both diseases increases CHD event risk.[51]

Another study was done to investigate the association between serum lipid and BP level in type 2 diabetics (mellitus T2DM. 60 patients having T2DM were enrolled in the study. A significant correlation between serum cholesterol and SBP/DBP was found.[30] It is noteworthy to understand hypertension is linked to development of CKD and may also aggravate dyslipidemia.[52,53]

A study was done to found association between serum lipid profiles in both hypertensive and normotensive control subjects in Bangladesh. In this study, 159 hypertensive patients and 75 normotensive controls were enrolled. Mean SBP and DBP of participants was 137.94 ± 9.58 mm Hg and 94.42 ± 8.81 mm Hg, respectively, which was found higher in hypertensive patients (p = 0.001). The serum levels of TC, TG, and LDL were higher while HDL levels were lower in hypertensive subjects compared to normotensives, which was statistically significant (p = 0.001). The logistic regression analysis showed that hypertensive patients had 1.1 times higher TC and TG, 1.2 times higher LDL, and 1.1 times lower HDL than normotensives, which was

statistically significant (p = 0.05). Study concluded by saying hypertensive patients have close association with dyslipidemia and need measurement of BP and lipid profile at regular intervals to prevent CVD, stroke, and other comorbidities.[54]

It was also found as hypertension increases risk of CVD, even dyslipidemia is known to increase risk of kidney disease in diabetes patients. A survey was done to assess progress in concurrent hypertension in hyper-cholesterolemia patients called the National Health and Nutritional Examination Surveys (NHANES) from 1988 to 2010. Hypertension was defined by BP ≥140/≥90 mm Hg, current medication treatment, and two-fold hypertension status; BP <140/<90 mm Hg defined control. Hypercholesterolemia was defined by Adult Treatment Panel III (ATP III) criteria based on 10-year CHD risk, LDL-C, and non-HDL cholesterol; values below diagnostic thresholds defined control. Across surveys, 60.7–64.3% of hypertensives were hypercholesterolemic. Even though patients had combination of hypertension and hypercholesteromia, control of both diseases also increased during the survey. In conclusion, authors said that prescribing antihypertensive and antihyperlipidemic medications to achieve treatment goals, especially for older, minority, diabetic, and CVD patients, and accessing healthcare at least biannually could improve concurrent risk factor control and CHD prevention.[6]

The Systolic Hypertension in Elderly Patients (SHEP) study documented non-HDL cholesterol is known to predict atherosclerotic cardiovascular disease (ASCVD) risk equally well irrespective of TG levels. But, in the study it was found that LDL-C lost its predictive value once TG levels exceeded 400 mg/dL.[55]

Treatment and Guidelines

As per American College of Cardiology/ American Heart Association (ACC/AHA) guidelines, maximally tolerated statin therapy needs to be started in patients with clinical ASCVD to lower their LDL-C levels by at least 50%. When a patient's 10-year risk of ASCVD is 20% or more, an effort needs to be taken to reduce LDL-C levels by at least 50%. Also, the same goal can be kept even for people with clinical ASCVD. When a patient has coronary artery calcium (CAC) score of zero, statin treatment can be delayed but not in patients having diabetes, current smoker, and family history of premature ASCVD.[56]

As per AHA 2018 Cholesterol Guidelines, focus is to reduce risk of ASCVD through cholesterol management. Top 10 key home messages are been delivered to reduce ASCVD risk.[57]

1. Every individual must follow heart healthy lifestyle.
2. In established ASCVD patient, reduction in LDL-C by ≥50% needs to be done with high intensity statin therapy or maximally tolerated statin therapy.
3. In very high risk ASCVD patients, LDL-C to be brought under threshold of <70 mg/day. If failed to achieve threshold, nonstatin drugs like ezetimibe or PSCK-9 inhibitors to be added.
4. In patients with LDL-C ≥190 mg/dL, high intensity statin therapy needs to be started even without calculation of 10-year ASCVD risk. If LDL-C >100 mg/dL still remains high even after statin treatment, addition of ezetimibe to be done. If still not under control, add proprotein convertase subtilisin/kexin type 9 (PCSK-9) inhibitor.
5. Diabetes mellitus patients with age between 40 years and 75 years, and LDL-C ≥70 mg/dL, moderate intensity statin therapy needs to be started (reducing LDL-C level by 50%) without calculation of 10-year ASCVD risk.
6. For primary ASCVD prevention in patients aged 40–75 years, clinician patient discussion needs to be done for shared decision making. Calculation of ASCVD risk and benefits/adverse effects of statin therapies need to be discussed.
7. In adults aging 40–75 years without diabetes mellitus and LDL-C ≥70 mg/dL and a 10-year risk ≥7.5%, moderate-intensity statin needs to be started if found favorable.
8. In adults aging 40–75 years without diabetes mellitus and 10-year risk of 7.5–19.9% (intermediate risk), initiation of statin therapy needs to be done based on risk factors.
9. In adults aging 40–75 years without diabetes mellitus and with LDL-C levels ≥70 mg/dL to 189 mg/dL, having a 10-year ASCVD risk of ≥7.5–19.9%, if decision to begin about statin therapy is uncertain, consider measuring CAC.
10. Regular assessment of adherence and percentage response to LDL-C lowering drugs and life style changes. Lipid measurement needs to be repeated 4–12 weeks after statin initiation or dose adjustment. Later repeat measurements to be done every 3–12 months.

The ACC/AHA 2017 guidelines did not specify treatment when a patient has both diseases. It did mention usage of high-dose angiotensin-receptor blocker (ARB) therapy in hypertensive patients having comorbidity of metabolic syndrome. Traditional beta-blocker use may predispose patient to dyslipidemia, dysglycemia, and hamper ability to lose weight. But the new vasodilating beta-blockers (like labetalol, carvedilol, nebivolol) have shown neutral or favorable effects on metabolic profiles compared with the traditional beta-blockers.[58]

Even the European Society of Cardiology (ESC) 2018 guidelines support beneficial administration of statin to patients without history of CV event and analysis been supported by findings from the Justification for the Use of Statins in Prevention: an

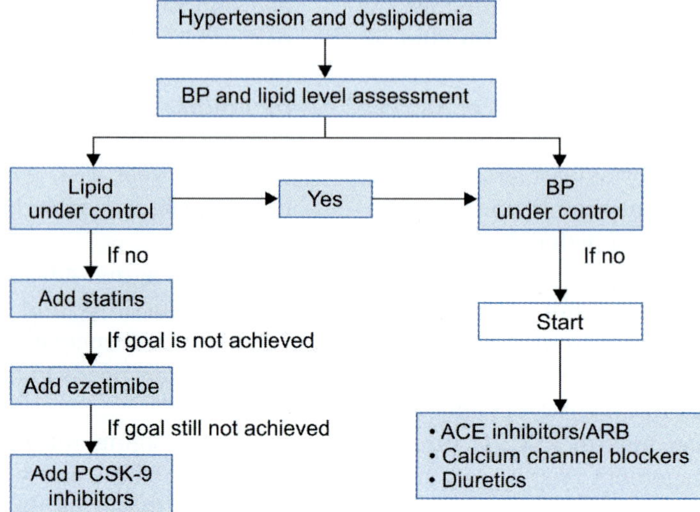

(ACE: angiotensin-converting enzyme; ARB: angiotensin-receptor blocker; BP: blood pressure; PCSK-9: proprotein convertase subtilisin/kexin type 9)

Flowchart 1: A combined approach to lipid and hypertension management.

Intervention Trial Evaluating Rosuvastatin (JUPITER) and HOPE-3 studies highlighting lowering in LDL-C can lead to reduction in CV events between 44% and 24%. To achieve LDL-C <70 mg/dL or reduction of ≥50% from baseline, statin therapy needs to be considered. In patients having high CV risk, an LDL-C goal of <100 mg/dL or a reduction of ≥50% from baseline is recommended (Flowchart 1).[59]

CONCLUSION

Hypertension and dyslipidemia are independent risk factors for CVD. Combination of both is deadly and predisposes patient to high risk of CV event. Assessment of lipid and BP levels at regular intervals needs to be done in all patients. Keeping the BP and lipid levels under control are key success factors in prevention of a cardiovascular event. Appropriate management with beneficial drugs will help the patient in living a healthy life.

REFERENCES

1. Stamler J, Stamler J, Brown IJ, et al. Relation of raw and cooked vegetable consumption to blood pressure: the INTERMAP Study. J Hum Hypertens. 2014;28(6):353-9.
2. Lewington S, Clarke R, Qizilbash N, et al. Age-specific relevance of usual blood pressure to vascular mortality: a meta-analysis of individual data for one million adults in 61 prospective studies. Lancet. 2002;360:1903-13.
3. Lewington S, Whitlock G, Clarke R, et al. Blood cholesterol and vascular mortality by age, sex, and blood pressure: a meta-analysis of individual data from 61 prospective studies with 55,000 vascular deaths. Lancet. 2007;370:1829-39.
4. Stone NJ, Robinson JG, Lichtenstein AH, et al. 2013 ACC/AHA guideline on the treatment of blood cholesterol to reduce atherosclerotic cardiovascular risk in adults: a report of the American College of Cardiology/American Heart Association Task Force on Practice Guidelines. J Am Coll Cardiol. 2014;63:2889-934.
5. Piepoli MF, Hoes AW, Agewal S, et al. 2016 European Guidelines on cardiovascular disease prevention in clinical practice: The Sixth Joint Task Force of the European Society of Cardiology and Other Societies on Cardiovascular Disease Prevention in Clinical Practice (constituted by representatives of 10 societies and by invited experts) Developed with the special contribution of the European Association for Cardiovascular Prevention & Rehabilitation (EACPR). Eur Heart J. 2016;129:557-67.

6. Egan BM, Li J, Qanungo S, et al. Blood pressure and cholesterol control in hypertensive hypercholesterolemic patients: national health and nutrition examination surveys 1988-2010. Circulation. 2013;128:29-41.

7. Ferrier KE, Muhlmann MH, Baguet JP, et al. Enoxaparin after high-risk coronary stenting. JACC. 2002;39:1020-5.

8. Borghi C, Prandin MG, Costa FV, et al. Use of statins and blood pressure control in treated hypertensive patients with hypercholesterolemia. J Cardiovas Pharmacol. 2000; 35:549-55.

9. Sposito AC, Mansur AP, Coelho OR, et al. Emerging insights into hypertension and dyslipidaemia synergies. Am J Cardiol. 1999;83:1497-9.

10. Lopez VA, Franklin SS, Tang S, et al. Hypertension in older people: part 1. J Clin Hypertens (Greenwich). 2007;9:436-43.

11. Bambara R, Mittal Y, Mathur, A. Evaluation of lipid profile of North Indian hypertensive subjects. Asian J Biomed Pharm Sci. 2013;3:38-41.

12. Il Ijeh, CECC Ejike, U Okorie. Serum lipid profile and lipid pro-atherogenic indices of a cohort of Nigerian adults with varying glycemic and blood pressure phenotypes Int J Biol Chem Sci. 2010;4(6):2102-12.

13. Isezuo S, Badung SL, Omotoso AB. Comparative analysis of lipid profiles among patients with type 2 diabetes mellitus, hypertension and concurrent type 2 diabetes, and hypertension: a view of metabolic syndrome. J Natl Med Assoc. 2003;95:328.

14. Wong ND, Lopez V, Tang S, et al. Prevalence, treatment and control of combined hypertension and hypercholestemia in the United States. Am J Hypertens. 2010;23:161-7.

15. Dalal JJ, Padmanabhan TN, Jain P, et al. LIPITENSION: Interplay between dyslipidemia and hypertension. Indian J Endocrinol Metab. 2012;16(2):240-5.

16. Karthikeyan G, Teo KK, Islam S, et al. Lipid profile, plasma apolipoproteins, and risk of a first myocardial infarction among Asians: an analysis from the INTERHEART Study. J Am Coll Cardiol. 2009;53(3):244-53.

17. Orr JS, Dengo AL, Rivero JM, et al. Arterial destiffening with atorvastatin in overweight and obese middle-aged and older adults. Hypertension. 2009;54:763-8.

18. Wang J, Song J, Huang, QF, et al. Sacubitril/valsartan. J Hypertens. 2015;33(1):e124.

19. Verghese J, Lipton RB, Hall CB, et al. Low blood pressure and the risk of dementia in very old individuals. Neurology. 2003;61:1667-2.

20. Qiu C, Winblad B, Viitanen M, et al. Hypertension, cognitive decline and dementia. Arch Neurol. 2003;60:223-8.

21. Gifford KA, Badaracco M, Liu D, et al. Verbal fluency in elderly with and without hypertension and diabetes from the FIBRA study. Arch Clin Neuropsychol. 2013;28:649-64.

22. Gottesman RF, Sharrett AR. Associations between midlife vascular risk factors and 25-year incident dementia in the Atherosclerosis Risk in Communities (ARIC) Cohort. JAMA Neurol. 2014;71:1218-27.

23. Macedo AF, Taylor FC, Casas JP, et al. Unintended effects of statins from observational studies in the general population: systematic review and meta-analysis. BMC Med. 2014;12:13.

24. Wong ND, Black HR, Gardin JM. Preventive Cardiology: A Practical Approach.: New York: McGraw-Hill; 2005. pp. 183-211.

25. Wong ND, Lopez V, Tang S. LIPITENSION: Interplay between dyslipidemia and hypertension. Am J Cardiol. 2006;98:204-8.

26. Lopez VA, Franklin SS, Tang S, et al. Antihypertensive combination therapy: optimizing blood pressure control and cardiovascular risk. J Clin Hypertens. 2007;9:436-43.

27. Baradaran A. Lipoprotein(a), type 2 diabetes and nephropathy; the mystery continues. J Nephro Pathol. 2012;1: 126-9.

28. Nasri H, Yazdani M. Oxford-MEST classification in IgA nephropathy patients: A report from Iran. Kardiol Pol. 2006;64:1364-8.

29. Danquah I, Bedu-Addo G, Terpe K, et al. Diabetes mellitus type 2 in urban Ghana: characteristics and and associated factors. BMC Public Health. 2012;12:210.

30. Nasri H, Rehradmanesh S, Ahmadi A, et al. Association of serum lipids with level of blood pressure in type 2 diabetic patients. J Renal Inj Prev. 2014;3(2):43-6.

31. ALLHAT. Major outcomes in high-risk hypertensive patients randomized to angiotensin-converting enzyme inhibitor or calcium channel blocker vs diuretic: The Antihypertensive and Lipid-Lowering Treatment to Prevent Heart Attack Trial (ALLHAT). J Am Med Assoc. 2002;288(23):2981-97.

32. Goode GK, Miller JP, Heagerty AM. Hyperlipidaemia, hypertension, and coronary heart disease. Lancet. 1995;345: 362-4.

33. Glorioso N. Effect of the HMG-CoA reductase inhibitors on blood pressure in patients with essential hypertension. Hypertension. 1999;34:1281-6.

34. Bandinelli S, Bertolotto L, Pucci L, et al. Hypotensive effects of statins: preliminary data with atorvastatin. J Hypertens. 1999;17(3):59-60.

35. Poulter N. Treating both hypertension and dyslipidemia: a synergistic approach. Medicographia. 2013;35:411-7

36. Maglapheridze Z. Treatment of dyslipidemia in diabetic type 2 patients with hypertension. Atherosclerosis. 2017; 263:e217.

37. Rydén L, Grant PJ, Anker SD, et al. ESC Guidelines on diabetes, pre-diabetes, and cardiovascular diseases developed in collaboration with the EASD: the Task Force on diabetes, pre-diabetes, and cardiovascular diseases of the European Society of Cardiology (ESC) and developed in

collaboration with the European Association for the Study of Diabetes (EASD). Eur Heart J. 2013;34(39):3035-87.

38. Stamler J, Elliott P, Dennis B. Eight-year blood pressure change in middle-aged men. Hypertension. 2002;39: 1000-6.

39. Sakuraia M, Stamler J, Miura K, et al. Relationship of dietary cholesterol to blood pressure: the INTERMAP study. J Hypertens. 2011;29(2):222-8.

40. Rouse IL, Beilin LJ, Armstrong BK, et al. Blood-pressure-lowering effect of a vegetarian diet: controlled trial in normotensive subjects. Lancet. 1983;1:5-10.

41. Jenkins DJ, Kendall CW, Vuksan V, et al. Soluble fiber intake at a dose approved by the US Food and Drug Administration for a claim of health benefits: serum lipid risk factors for cardiovascular disease assessed in a randomized controlled crossover trial. Am J Clin Nutr. 2002;75:834-9.

42. Appel LJ, Moore TJ, Obarzanek E, et al. A clinical trial of the effects of dietary patterns on blood pressure. N Engl J Med. 1997;336:1117-24.

43. Sacks FM, Svetkey LP, Vollmer WM, et al. Effects on blood pressure of reduced dietary sodium and the Dietary Approaches to Stop Hypertension (DASH) diet. DASH-Sodium Collaborative Research Group. New Engl J Med. 2001;344:3-10.

44. Keech A, Simes RJ, Barter P, et al. Effects of long-term fenofibrate therapy on cardiovascular events in 9795 people with type 2 diabetes mellitus (the FIELD study): randomised controlled trial. Lancet. 2005;366:1849-61.

45. Borghi C, Dormi A, Veronesi M, et al. Association between different lipid-lowering treatment strategies and blood pressure control in the Brisighella Heart Study. Am Heart J. 2004;148:285-92.

46. Lang Qi, Xiaoxia Liu, Xiaoming Zh, et al. Evaluation of lipid profile and its relationship with blood pressure in patients with Cushing's disease. Endocr Connect. 2018;7:637-44.

47. Yan X, Li Y, Dong Y, et al. Blood pressure and low-density lipoprotein cholesterol control status in Chinese hypertensive dyslipidemia patients during lipid-lowering therapy. Lipid Health Dis. 2019;18:32.

48. Gupta A, Mackeey J, Whitehouse A, et al. Long-term mortality after blood pressure-lowering and lipid-lowering treatment in patients with hypertension in the Anglo-Scandinavian Cardiac Outcomes Trial (ASCOT) Legacy study: 16-year follow-up results of a randomised factorial trial. Lancet. 2018;e 92(10153):P1127-37.

49. Han BH, Sutin D, Williamson JD, et al. Effect of statin treatment vs usual care on primary cardiovascular prevention among older adults: The ALLHAT-LLT Randomized Clinical Trial. JAMA Intern Med. 2017;177(7): 955-65.

50. Jackie B, O'Donnell M, Swaminathan B, et al. Effects of blood pressure and lipid lowering on cognition: Results from the HOPE-3 study. Neurology. 2019;92:e1435-e1446.

51. Neaton JD, Wentworth D. Serum cholesterol, blood pressure, cigarette smoking, and death from coronary heart disease. Overall findings and differences by age for 316,099 white men. Multiple Risk Factor Intervention Trial Research Group. Arch Intern Med. 1992;152:56-64.

52. Petitti DB, Imperatore G, Palla SL, et al. Serum lipids and glucose control: the SEARCH for Diabetes in Youth study. Arch Pediatr Adolesc Med. 2007;161:159-65.

53. Kamara NT, Asiimwe S. Dyslipidaemia and hypertension among adults with diabetes in rural Uganda. Trop Doct. 2010;40:41-2.

54. Chowdhury KN, Mainuddin AKM, Wahiduzzaman M, et al. Serum lipid profile and its association with hypertension in Bangladesh. Vascular Health and Risk Management. Vascu Health Risk Manag. 2014;10:327-32.

55. Frost PH, Burlando AJ, Curb JD, et al. Serum lipids and incidence of coronary heart disease. Findings from the Systolic Hypertension in the Elderly Program (SHEP). Circulation. 1996;94:2381-8.

56. Abbasi J. Medical News & Perspectives, New Cholesterol Guidelines Personalize Risk and Add Treatments, JAMA. 2019.

57. Grundy SM, Stone NJ, Bailey AL, et al. 2018 Guideline on the Management of Blood Cholesterol. [online] Available from https://www.acc.org/~/media/Non-Clinical/Files-PDFs-Excel-MS-Word etc/Guidelines/2018/Guidelines-Made-Simple-Tool-2018-Cholesterol.pdf. [Last Accessed April 2019].

58. Whelton PK, Carey RM, Aronow WS, et al. 2017 ACC/AHA/AAPA/ABC/ACPM/AGS/APhA/ASH/ASPC/NMA/PCNA Guideline for the Prevention, Detection, Evaluation, and Management of High Blood Pressure in Adults: A Report of the American College of Cardiology/American Heart Association Task Force on Clinical Practice Guidelines. J Am Coll Cardiol. 2018;71:e127-e248.

59. Willaims B, Mancia G, Spiering W, et al. 2018 ESC/ESH Guidelines for the management of arterial hypertension. Eur Heart J. 2018;39(33):1-98.

Role of Vitamin D3 and Hypertension

RK Jha, Ashish Mishra, Kamlesh Patidar, Akash Singh

INTRODUCTION

Following the exposure of ultraviolet rays over the skin, a steroid prohormone called vitamin D is synthesized. Vitamin D can be supplemented by dietary intake.

Hypertension is a leading noncommunicable disease and is one of the essential modifiable risk factors for cardiovascular disease (CVD) and hence prevention of which is a vital public health measure.

In conjunction with obesity, sedentary lifestyle, high salt intake, lately vitamin D deficiency has also been considered as a modifiable factors associated with hypertension.

There is a growing body of evidence from animal and clinical studies that vitamin D-mediated reduction of hypertension involves increased activation of the renin–angiotensin-aldosterone system, which is the main regulator of electrolyte and volume homeostasis that contributes to the development of arterial hypertension.

PHYSIOLOGY OF VITAMIN D

Irradiation of ultraviolet B rays on 7-Dehydrocholesterol in the skin leads to synthesis of vitamin D in humans. Vitamin D is further metabolized to the primary circulating vitamin D compound [25-hydroxyvitamin D [25(OH)D]] and then to the hormonal form [1,25-dihydroxyvitamin D (1,25D)] (Table 1).

The primary function of vitamin D is to augment the active absorption of consumed calcium and phosphate ions. Most nucleated cells, including vascular smooth muscle cells, macula densa and juxtaglomerular cells bear the vitamin D receptors.

Vitamin D has direct effects to enhance bone and muscle function. It helps in building

TABLE 1: Nomenclature of vitamin D precursors and metabolites.

Common name	Clinical name	Comments
7-Dehydrocholesterol	Provitamin D3	Lipid in cell membranes
Cholecalciferol	Previtamin D3	Synthesis in skin
Ergocalciferol	Previtamin D2	Precursor for active vitamin D
Calcidiol	25-hydroxyvitamin D	Best reflects vitamin D status
Calcitriol	1,25-hydroxyvitamin D	Active form of vitamin D, highly regulated

TABLE 2: Vitamin D—deficiency and sufficiency.

25(OH)D level (ng/mL)	Laboratory diagnosis
<20	Deficiency
20–32	Insufficiency
54–90	Normal in sunny countries
>100	Excess
>150	Intoxication

in younger age groups. It also helps in making sure that the bone does not get resorbed in order to maintain calcium concentration in the blood (Table 2).

Based on calcium control and musculoskeletal function, target levels of 25(OH)D in blood are at least 50–60 nmol/L.

■ VITAMIN D AND RENIN–ANGIOTENSIN SYSTEM

Vitamin D and the renin–angiotensin system (RAS) dietary sodium and increased activity of the RAS are known to contribute to hypertension; salt restriction and inhibition of RAS activity reduce blood pressure.

Vitamin D inhibits the RAS by reducing renin gene expression. This mechanistic link between vitamin D and the RAS has been translated to cross-sectional studies in humans.

More recently, Tomaschitz et al. showed that both 25(OH)D and 1,25(OH)D were inversely associated with plasma renin and angiotensin II concentrations in a cohort referred for coronary angiography.[1]

■ HOMEOSTASIS OF VITAMIN D, RENIN–ANGIOTENSIN SYSTEM, AND CALCIUM

Calcium homeostasis is associated with regulation of the blood pressure. 1,25-dihydroxyvitamin D aids in influx of calcium ions into vascular smooth muscle cells and these calcium ions plays a crucial role in regulating the vascular tone and hence, the intracellular calcium ion concentrations were positively associated with blood pressure.[2]

Because the accumulation of intracellular calcium ions in juxtaglomerular cells results in inhibition of renin secretion, it was hypothesized that sodium-regulating hormones (the RAS) and calcium-regulating hormones (vitamin D) may be collective factors in the progress of hypertension (Table 3).

TABLE 3: Various causes of vitamin D deficiency.

Causes	Example
Reduced skin synthesis	Sunscreen, skin pigment, season/time of day, aging, cystic fibrosis, celiac disease, Crohn's disease
Decreased absorption	Gastric bypass, medications that reduce cholesterol absorption
Increased sequestration	Obesity (body mass index >30)
Increased catabolism	Anticonvulsant, glucocorticoid
Breastfeeding	Exclusively without vitamin D supplementation
Decreased synthesis of 25(OH) vitamin D	Hepatic failure
Increased urinary loss of 25(OH) vitamin D	Nephrotic proteinuria
Decreased synthesis of 1, 25(OH) vitamin D	Chronic renal failure
Inherited disorders	Vitamin D resistance

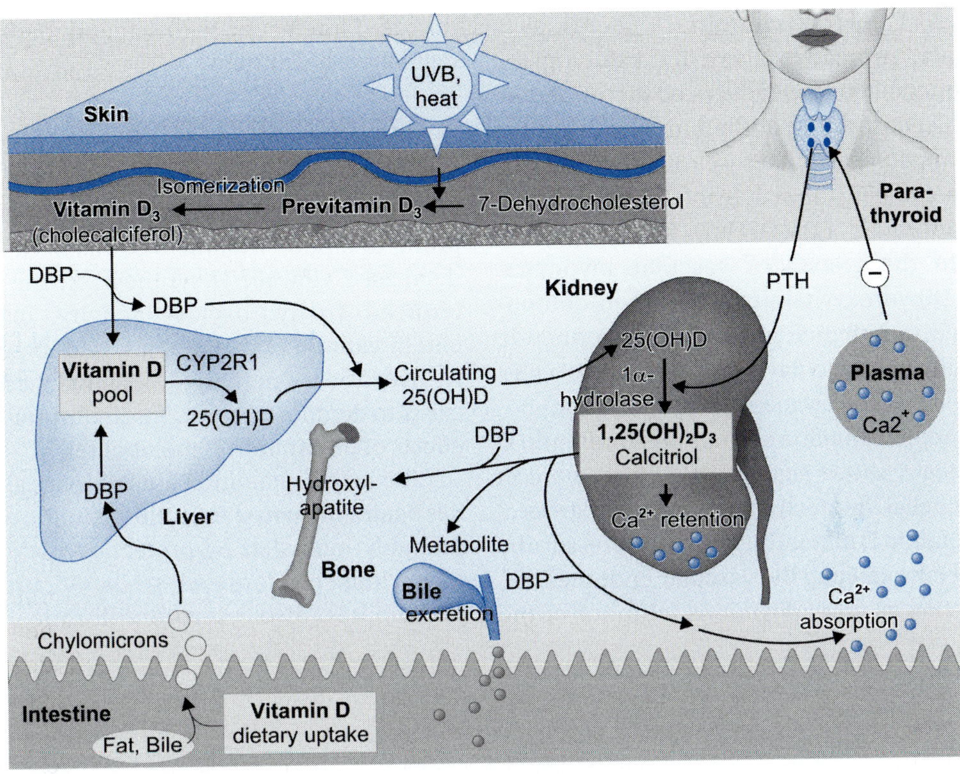

(DBP: vitamin D-binding protein; PTH: parathyroid hormone; UVB: ultraviolet B)

Fig. 1: Molecular mechanisms of vitamin D3 action.

TABLE 4: Vitamin D tolerance dosages for children and young people.

Age group	Tolerable upper limit
Neonates	Up to 1,000 IU/day (25 mg/day)
Infants and children aged 1 month to 10 years	Up to 2,000 IU/day (50 mg/day)
Children and adolescents aged 11–18 years	Up to 4,000 IU/day (100 mg/day)
Adults and the elderly	Up to 10,000 IU/day (250 mg/day)

Earlier studies revealed that dietary salt loading in humans lead to elevated concentrations of 1,25(OH)2D. Moreover, subjects with the considerable salt-induced elevations in 1,25(OH)2D presented with the greatest salt-induced elevations in blood pressure, supposedly because of elevated concentrations of intracellular calcium ions (Table 4). Neither the mechanism of the salt-induced elevation of 1,25(OH)2D concentrations nor the role of salt and RAS components in 1,25(OH)2D-mediated calcium influx has yet been elucidated (Fig. 1).

VITAMIN D EFFECT ON OTHER VASCULAR MECHANISMS

In addition to potential effects of vitamin D on the RAS and regulation of vascular tone, many other direct effects of vitamin D on vascular endothelium and smooth muscle cells has been hypothesized, regarding the association between vitamin D and hypertension.

1,25-Dihydroxyvitamin D serves as a vascular protective agent by reducing the detrimental effect of advanced glycation end products on the endothelium, lowering the inflammatory and atherosclerotic parameters, and enhancing the activity of the NO system.

Moreover, 1,25(OH)2D has been related to the growth of vascular myocytes. 1,25-Dihydroxyvitamin D has been demonstrated to enhance prostacyclin production in cultured vascular smooth muscle cells, possibly via the cyclooxygenase pathway.

Supplementation of vitamin D in vitamin D deficiency shows significant improvement in endothelial dysfunction and oxidative stress.

Vitamin D may influence blood pressure by indirectly affecting the vascular endothelium, by acting as an endogenous inhibitor of the RAS, and interacting with salt and the RAS to regulate vascular tone.

■ NEPHROPROTECTIVE EFFECT OF VITAMIN D

Patients with chronic kidney diseases are prone to a poor vitamin D status because of decreased vitamin D synthesis in the skin, reduced 1α-hydroxylase activity, urinary loss of vitamin D metabolites, and increased 24-hydroxylase activity. Collective evidence exists to demonstrate various neuroprotective effects of the vitamin D metabolites.[3]

The active vitamin D analog (paricalcitol) has been shown to exert antiproteinuric effects probably mediated by protecting podocytes in various randomized trials. Vitamin D metabolites also exert antifibrotic, anti-

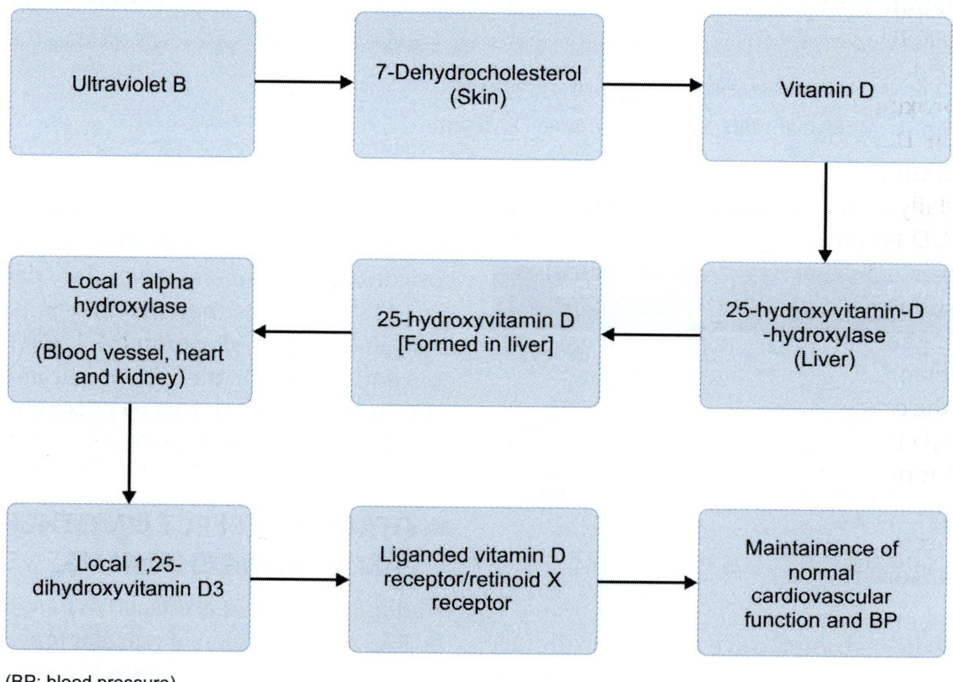

(BP: blood pressure)

Fig. 2: Association of vitamin D and hypertension.

inflammatory (e.g. reduced highly sensitive C-reactive protein), and immunomodulating actions and that may diminish renal damage. Vitamin D has a nephroprotective role due to its antifibrotic properties as well as suppression of renin due to vitamin D metabolites (Fig. 2).

Among the different effects of vitamin D on immune system, it should be emphasized that vitamin D supplementation decreases tumor necrosis factor-alpha (TNF-alpha) and increases T regulatory cells.

T regulatory cells are considered to protect against autoimmune processes. Furthermore, vitamin D deficiency is a significant risk factor for CVD events and mortality in patients with chronic kidney disease.

TREATMENT

Target 25(OH)D levels of at least 30 ng/mL is recommended.

Vitamin D supplementation in doses up to 10,000 IU per day over longer time periods is considered safe. About 10,000 IU per day is approximately equal to the increases in vitamin D status that can be achieved by natural sunlight exposure.

A daily intake of 1,000 IU vitamin D raises 25(OH)D levels by approximately 10 ng/mL. However, significant interindividual variability should be considered. Obese individuals need higher vitamin D doses compared with lean persons to increase their 25(OH)D levels.

In the case of an ongoing vitamin D therapy, 25(OH)D levels should not be checked earlier than 3 months after initiation of treatment to allow for a plateau to be reached.

Moreover, it should be noted that in comparison with (natural) vitamin D supple-

mentation, supplementation of the active vitamin D aims to correct low serum levels of 1,25(OH)2D and not of 25(OH)D. Moreover, active vitamin D is more expensive and has a relatively narrow therapeutic window. Active vitamin D supplementation/therapy is mainly confined to patients with advanced chronic kidney disease.

CONCLUSION

High blood pressure is one of the leading causes of early mortality worldwide and the problem is progressing. Low 25-hydroxyvitamin D levels are correlated to higher prevalence of blood pressure.

Evidence from meta-analysis of cohort studies revealed that enhanced risk of all-cause mortality, CVD and hypertension occurs in relation with vitamin D deficiency.

Certain mechanisms proposed that vitamin D decreases blood pressure. However, further studies are necessary to find the role of vitamin D on blood pressure in normal individuals as well as in patients with chronic hypertension.

REFERENCES

1. Tomaschitz A, Pilz S, Ritz E, et al. Independent association between 1,25-dihydroxyvitamin D, 25-hydroxyvitamin D and the renin-angiotensin system: the Ludwigshafen Risk and Cardiovascular Health (LURIC) Study. Clin Chim Acta. 2010;411:1354-60.
2. Cui C, Xu P, Li G, et al. Vitamin D receptor activation regulates microglia polarization and oxidative stress in spontaneously hypertensive rats and angiotensin II-exposed microglial cells: Role of renin-angiotensin system. Redox Biol. 20198;26:101295.
3. Milovanov IuS, Kozlovskaia LV, Milovanova LI. The role of D2 vitamin metabolite paricalcitol in nephroprotective strategy. Ter Arkh. 2011;83(6):70-3.

Creating Effective Delivery Systems for Hypertension Control

Marc G Jaffe, Norm RC Campbell, Pedro Ordunez, Sonia Y Angell, Donald J DiPette

■ INTRODUCTION

Even though effective treatment for hypertension has been available for decades, hypertension control rates (<140/90 mm Hg) remain low in most parts of the world. There are many barriers to effective blood pressure control, including lack of awareness (undiagnosed hypertension), awareness without treatment, and inadequate treatment. This situation is even more dire in low- and middle-income countries where a large proportion of communities do not have access to more than one blood pressure-lowering medicine and, even when available, they are often not affordable.[1] To identify and effectively treat individuals with hypertension, these issues must be addressed, and a systematic approach to addressing each of these issues must be designed and implemented.[2]

■ LEADERSHIP

Systemization of care for large populations requires effective health sector leadership, preferably in the context of a functional health system with good quality, access and coverage. Key stakeholders, administrators, thought leaders, and advocates are often necessary to identify hypertension as a priority issue, particularly in an environment with many other competing initiatives and priorities. Active and visible support from health sector leadership can facilitate allocation of financial resources, intellectual capital, media attention, and most importantly, empower other parties to focus energy on addressing hypertension in an organized way. Securing the support of key leaders often allows groups to spend the time and effort needed to thoughtfully organize, develop, implement, measure, and refine a hypertension care improvement program. To increase the likelihood of sustainability, programs should integrate interventions that progressively transform the existing model of chronic care rather than expand in parallel to the existing care model.

■ DIAGNOSIS

Hypertension Screening

Screening the at-risk population is important to identify individuals who have hypertension yet are unaware of their condition and remain undiagnosed.[3] This is particularly challenging for populations with low access and low coverage of care, such as vulnerable groups including those living in rural or remote communities. Though an important part of a population-focused hypertension treatment program, screening programs alone are not sufficient to achieve high control rates for people with hypertension. In environments where the majority of adults visit a medical center at least annually, universal blood pressure measurement of all adult patients may be effective. Alternatively, screening can be performed using outreach, where members of a community are systematically identified and targeted, often by community health workers using lists of individuals living in the community.

Population Outreach

Other systematic screening methods, such as mandatory annual workplace screening, have been implemented in some locations (e.g. Mongolia) and can reach very large numbers of individuals.[4] Screening fairs or booths set up in the community, such as in community centers, places of worship or popular shopping destinations, are likely to capture only a small fraction of affected individuals. Although screening tables may help promote greater awareness in the community, their impact is limited unless established as part of a more comprehensive program. Both opportunistic and outreach screening strategies can be used in the same community, simultaneously or sequentially, to complement other efforts and provide some redundancy that increases screening rates.

Patient Follow-up

Once outreach has been performed, it is necessary to have a mechanism for transfer of information and to support patient navigation to a clinical location to confirm the hypertension diagnosis and initiate treatment. Without such a system, patients who screen positive for hypertension (or potential hypertension) often fail to follow-up with appropriate providers, leading to large numbers of people who may be aware of their elevated blood pressure but do not receive proper monitoring or treatment. A follow-up system can take many forms, such as a direct referral to the care center or a list of people with suspected hypertension. A staff member can be tasked with reviewing the list to check for people who failed to appear after having been directed to the referral site.

■ TREATMENT PROTOCOLS

Protocols versus Guidelines

Simple protocols or clinical pathways for pharmacologic treatment of hypertension are also necessary to achieve high rates of blood pressure control. A protocol is distinct from a guideline, as most guidelines are quite long (often several hundred pages), very detailed, serve as a framework, and describe many possible options. Many guidelines contain detailed instructions for the diagnosis of hypertension, however, these may be too complicated to effectively implement in primary healthcare settings.

Guidelines may recommend that blood pressure be taken many times, in different arms, with results mathematically averaged, and that people make repeated visits for re-evaluation. Ideally, validated automated blood pressure monitors and specifically trained personnel should be utilized to avoid both false-positive and false-negative hypertension diagnoses. Some guidelines suggest using equipment that may not be readily available in many (or most) primary healthcare sites, such as ambulatory blood pressure monitoring (ABPM), automated office blood pressure (AOBP), or home blood pressure measurement. Because satisfying all these criteria may represent a barrier to diagnosis, developing and adopting streamlined and practical approaches that acknowledge the challenges in primary care settings is essential.

Characteristics of Protocols

A practical protocol is short (often one page), contains basic information suitable for most patients, and provides limited treatment options. Characteristics of an effective treatment protocol include recommending a single specific drug and dose at each step, reduction or elimination of different drug and dose options, and selection of drugs based on value (low cost and high efficacy), ready availability, low risks of adverse events, reduced need for laboratory monitoring, and ability to be taken once daily, with consideration for single-pill combination therapy.[5] Simple standard protocols and validated blood pressure devices are necessary for consistent and accurate diagnosis and to facilitate proper treatment and follow-up. In addition, training activities can be simplified and errors reduced as treatment becomes more standardized using a shared protocol.

The process of creating a drug treatment protocol can serve as a focal point for starting the systematic treatment of hypertension in a population. A protocol consensus conference is often held with a clinical leader and a multidisciplinary team, consisting of individuals representing academic leaders, administrators, pharmacy and procurements specialists, clinical specialists (such as family physicians, cardiologists, internal medicine physicians, and nephrologists), ministries of health and other key stakeholders.

▪ MEDICATIONS

Access

Access to medications is another critical element of a successful hypertension program. Though many appropriate hypertension drugs may be in the system formulary, identifying and promoting use of a core set of high-quality recommended medications is optimal. This allows for better drug forecasting and procurement and can lead to more economical purchasing of large quantities of medications, as well as improve other logistical issues such as distribution and storage. Drugs that are low-cost or free to patients are preferable to more expensive alternatives. Although existing prescription practices may favor the use of higher-cost branded medications, the use of quality assured inexpensive generic drugs benefits both patients and health systems. To improve medication adherence, once-daily medications are preferred over those taken two or more times daily.

Single-pill Combinations

Single pills that combine two or more medications (single-pill combination) are becoming increasingly more common and have many advantages over tablets containing a single medication.[6] Single-pill combination tablets are available that cost the same as the constituent drugs purchased separately, increase adherence, simplify logistics, reduce pill burden for patients, and can accelerate treatment because the majority of people with hypertension require two or more drugs for appropriate blood pressure control.[7] Most single-pill combination medications consist of drugs that treat blood pressure through different physiologic pathways with complementary mechanisms of action, resulting in a greater magnitude of blood pressure reduction at lower doses and with reduced side effects.

▪ TASK SHARING

Task sharing using nonphysician health workers can help improve hypertension care delivery.[8] In environments with limited resources and insufficient numbers of physicians, this may the only way to provide hypertension care to large numbers of individuals. In systems with adequate resources, the use of a mix of providers with difference skill sets is used to increase the efficiency of the delivery system. In many situations, the current scope of permissible care as defined by licensure may allow many nonphysicians to participate in a variety of care activities, although they often are not practicing at the highest level allowable by their position. Training, supervision and support can increase the actual scope of clinical practice so that team members can function to the fullest of their allowable functions.

Encouraging the team to identify all steps necessary to systematically treat hypertension, then assigning tasks based on maximal allowable scope of practice, can be more effective than relying on physicians to provide most services. For example, nurses operating under protocol may be able to initiate and/or adjust medications for patients without complications. Medical assistants may be trained to accurately and reliably measure blood pressure as well as contact individuals overdue for services.

■ MONITORING AND REPORTING

Standardized and regular reporting of hypertension quality performance metrics allows health care leadership, administrators, implementors, and care teams to understand their performance over time, in relation to others, and to understand where care gaps exist.[9] The exact definition of the hypertension quality metric is less important than having metrics that can be measured easily, shared widely, and distributed regularly. For example, continuous measurement of the total number of individuals diagnosed with hypertension every quarter, the number of people who had controlled blood pressure documented at their last clinic encounter in the past 12 months, or the percentage of people who started treatment 6 months ago who have blood pressure controlled in the past quarter are all useful to help understand

which sites are performing well and which may need improvement. Other metrics can be designed to identify a specific intervention. For example, a monthly list of patients who failed to follow-up 3 months after an elevated blood pressure reading may lead to changes such as reminder contacts prior to a scheduled visit or a system to have community health workers visit individuals in their homes.

■ PROGRAM DESIGN

The approach to designing a system of hypertension care for large populations, using many of the previously mentioned elements, is similar in populations of differing sizes. Small clinic settings may choose to have a simple metric and focus on team-based care with task sharing, while larger settings such as health systems may focus on standardization of metrics and training. Larger systems, such as counties and states, may focus on consensus building and protocol development. All of these elements can play important roles in increasing the quality of care for people with hypertension.

■ PROGRAM SUCCESSES

California

In Kaiser Permanente Northern California, a United States-based integrated care delivery system with more than 4 million members, hypertension control improved from 42% to nearly 90% from 2001 to 2014 using an evidence-based protocol, a hypertension patient registry, regular performance feedback, task sharing with medical assistants performing blood pressure follow-up visits, and promoting use of a single-pill combination medication for initial treatment of most people with hypertension.[10] The simple treatment protocol was evaluated every 2 years with slight modifications to reflect emerging evidence, and strong support from key stakeholders was continuously present for the program's duration. Though drug choices were always at the discretion of treating clinicians, the medications on the protocol were promoted widely, with training and supporting materials easily available, to reduce barriers to using the recommended drugs. The system of continuous quality metric reporting was initially available quarterly, later modified to monthly to allow more rapid cycles of quality improvement.

South Carolina

South Carolina, a US state with a population of 5 million, ranked 51st out of 52 states and territories for cardiovascular disease (CVD)-related mortality in 1995 and had been recognized as the center of the "Stroke Belt", an area in the southern US with very high rates of cerebrovascular disease. In 1999, community and academic stakeholders in South Carolina collaborated and began a hypertension initiative. This was a population-based, community-wide approach not specifically associated with a health system or integrated practices that targeted primary care with subspecialists serving as local leaders and trainers. In 2000, the program began promotion of healthy lifestyles, access to effective medical care and medications, public education, and continuing education to healthcare providers, particularly physicians. Medical practices of all sizes and locations were recruited into a community-based practice network. Practice data was acquired on a regular basis, initially on data cards mailed in to a central data site and subsequently by electronic medical records, with prompt and timely feedback given to providers as a quality improvement tool. The network grew to 197 practices with approximately 1.6 million patients, of which about 700,000 had hypertension. From 2000 to 2005, the hypertension control rate (defined by systolic blood pressure <140 mm Hg and diastolic blood pressure <90 mm Hg) rose from 49% to 66%. Over this same period, South Carolina's ranking in CVD mortality improved from 51st to 35th. From 1995 to 2006, coronary heart disease deaths declined by 43% and stroke deaths by 42%, with cardiovascular deaths declining to a greater extent in South Carolina compared to all other "Stroke Belt" states.[11]

New York

New York City launched a citywide hypertension initiative that extends beyond a single delivery system. Utilizing multisector engagement that bridges clinical and community systems with an emphasis on shared goals and agreed metrics, "Take the Pressure Off, NYC!" is supported by a coalition of more than 100 member organizations. In Upstate New York, Common Ground Health and the Greater Rochester Chamber of Commerce organized more than 200 volunteers from 70 organizations. Community participants range from barbers and hair stylists trained to take blood pressure in their workplaces, to faith-based congregations forming an Interdenominational Health Ministry Coalition, to chief executive officers of the area's largest employers. A hypertension registry was created that included more than 200,000 patients from 198 practices in nine counties across the area.[12] Quality improvement work leveraged this data by sharing both population and practice-level comparative data to providers, coupled with practice-level quality improvement assistance. Across the nine counties, hypertension control rates improved from 61.9% in 2011 to 69.5% in 2016. Those at highest risk, with blood pressures ≥160/100 mm Hg, were observed to experience the greatest reductions. A lesson reported by this group was to continuously seek best practices and assess barriers to continued success.

Canada

In Canada, a program to improve hypertension control was initiated in 2000. The program was based on annually updated scientific recommendations, a formal implementation (education) process with surveillance, monitoring and evaluation. Implementation was based on transforming the scientific recommendations into simplified, standardized public and primary healthcare education with extensive sustained dissemination. Over the next 6–7 years, there were marked increases in the antihypertensive drug prescription rate, with the national hypertension control rate improving from 13% to 66% and a reduction in the national death and hospitalization rates for stroke, myocardial infarction, and heart failure.[13] This illustrates the potential to increase hypertension control through an extensive simplified sustained hypertension education program.

WHO Region of the Americas

Hypertension control is also a priority for the WHO Region of the Americas. The Pan American Health Organization (PAHO), with support from the US Centers for Disease Control and Prevention (CDC), launched the Standardized Hypertension Treatment and Prevention (SHTP) Project in 2013, which later evolved to Global HEARTS,[14] a global initiative led by WHO. The HEARTS in the Americas program emphasizes using available resources, continuous performance improvement, active support from leadership, and enhanced technical capabilities. By using a health system strengthening approach, improved quality of care as well as high hypertension control rates are expected to be achieved, although program sustainability will require institutionalization of the model into routine health system practice. The HEARTS intervention to improve hypertension control has been implemented using a standardized package to improve primary care services in more than 30 health centers in eight PAHO countries, with commitments by the Ministries of Health and local stakeholders in Argentina, Barbados, Chile, Colombia, Cuba, Ecuador, Panama, and Trinidad and Tobago.[15] The intervention includes introducing a simplified hypertension treatment algorithm with a core set of medications, establishing a registry and monitoring control of hypertensive patients, and training primary health care providers. This innovative model of service delivery has resulted in improvements in system coverage and increased hypertension control rates in a short period of time, and the countries are working on expanding the intervention and scaling up programs nationally.

■ DISCLOSURE

PO is staff member of the Pan American Health Organization. He alone is responsible for the views expressed in this publication, and do not necessarily represent the decisions or policies of the Pan American Health Organization.

■ CONCLUSION

Addressing hypertension care in large populations can be successfully accomplished using several strategies, including engaging leadership, screening with linkage to follow-up, protocols for diagnosis and treatment, access to medications including single-pill combination therapy, task sharing, quality metric reporting, and connecting to the broader community of stakeholders. There are many examples of successful systems which have used many of these core elements to effectively increase hypertension control in many communities, and the lessons learned from these programs should serve as examples to other communities across the world committed to improving hypertension care.

■ REFERENCES

1. Attaei MW, Khatib R, McKee M, et al. Availability and affordability of blood pressure-lowering medicines and the effect on blood pressure control in high-income, middle-income, and low-income countries: an analysis of the PURE study data. Lancet Public Health. 2017;2:e411-9.

2. Angell SY, De Cock KM, Frieden TR. A public health approach to global management of hypertension. Lancet. 2015;385:825-7.

3. Mangat BK, Campbell N, Mohan S, et al. Resources for blood pressure screening programs in low resource settings: A guide from the World Hypertension League. J Clin Hypertension. 2015;17:418-20.

4. Mattke S, Liu H, Caloyeras J, et al. Workplace wellness programs study: final report. RAND Health Quarterly. 2013;3:7.

5. Patel P, Ordunez P, DiPette D, et al. Improved blood pressure control to reduce cardiovascular disease morbidity and mortality: The Standardized Hypertension Treatment and Prevention Project. J Clin Hypertension. 2016;18:1284-94.

6. DiPette DJ, Skeete J, Ridley E, et al. Fixed-dose combination pharmacologic therapy to improve hypertension control worldwide: Clinical perspective and policy implications. J Clin Hypertension. 2019;21:4-15.

7. Mensah GA, Bakris G. Treatment and control of high blood pressure in adults. Cardiol Clin. 2010;28:609-22.

8. He J, Irazola V, Mills KT, et al. Effect of a community health worker-led multicomponent intervention on blood pressure control in low-income patients in Argentina: a randomized clinical trial. JAMA. 2017;318:1016-25.

9. Campbell NRC, Ordunez P, DiPette DJ, et al. Monitoring and evaluation framework for hypertension programs. A collaboration between the Pan American Health Organization and World Hypertension League. J Clin Hypertension. 2018;20:984-90.

10. Jaffe MG, Young JD. The Kaiser Permanente Northern California story: improving hypertension control from 44% to 90% in 13 years (2000 to 2013). J Clin Hypertension. 2016;18:260-1.

11. Egan BM, Laken MA, Shaun Wagner C, et al. Impacting population cardiovascular health through a community-based practice network: Update on an ASH-supported collaborative. J Clin Hypertension. 2011;13:1751-76.

12. Fortuna RJ, Rocco TA, Freeman J, et al. A community-wide quality improvement initiative to improve hypertension control and reduce disparities. J Clin Hypertension. 2019;21:196-203.

13. Campbell NR, Sheldon T. The Canadian effort to prevent and control hypertension: can other countries adopt Canadian strategies? Current Opinion in Cardiology. 2010;25:366-72.

14. World Health Organization. HEARTS: technical package for cardiovascular disease management in primary health care. Geneva: World Health Organization; 2016. Also available from https://www.who.int/cardiovascular_diseases/hearts/en. [Last accessed September, 2019].

15. Pan American Health Organization. Hypertension control project in the Americas. Washington: Regional Office for the Americas of the World Health Organization; 2017. Also available from https://www.paho.org/hq/index.php?option=com_content&view=article&id=13755. [Last accessed September, 2019].